TO RALPH & KARLEEN

VERY BEST WISHES

Rich

2013

ASK THE PHARMACIST

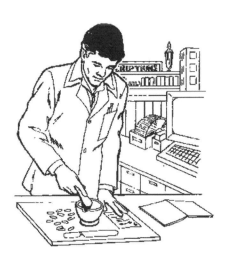

ASK THE PHARMACIST

Drug & Health Information
For The Consumer
Last Edition

Richard P. Hoffmann, RPh, PharmD

iUniverse, Inc.
Bloomington

Ask The Pharmacist
Drug & Health Information For The Consumer

iUniverse books may be ordered through booksellers or by contacting:

iUniverse
1663 Liberty Drive
Bloomington, IN 47403
www.iuniverse.com
1-800-Authors (1-800-288-4677)

ISBN: 978-1-4759-4838-7 (sc)
ISBN: 978-1-4759-4839-4 (hc)
ISBN: 978-1-4759-4840-0 (ebk)

Printed in the United States of America
iUniverse rev. date: 09/13/2012

To Mom and Dad,
who were proud that I became a pharmacist.

Contents

Preface

This book is a collection of previously published "Ask The Pharmacist" newspaper columns. It contains useful and easy to understand answers to questions about medications and is written by one of America's most trusted healthcare professionals, the pharmacist. Dr. Hoffmann provides answers to commonly asked questions about a variety of medication and health topics. This information is needed more than ever before due to rapidly growing advances in drug research and medical technology, along with the explosion of direct-to-consumer advertising. Add to this the faster approval of new drugs by the Food and Drug Administration and switches from prescription to over-the-counter medication availability, and the complexity of drug use increases. Approximately 70% of consumers say that currently available healthcare information is overwhelming and confusing. This confusion is only part of the overall problem of medication use in America, where adverse effects from drugs are now a leading cause of death. "Ask The Pharmacist" provides information to assist consumers in making informed decisions about their medication needs.

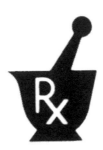

Acknowledgments

This book and my weekly "Ask The Pharmacist" newspaper column would not have been possible without the loving support, encouragement, and assistance of my wife, Meg. She truly complements my life in every way possible.

I would also like to thank the Citrus County Chronicle for giving me the opportunity to create a column and share my ideas and information as part of their newspaper and Chronicle Online web site for the past 16 years. Also, many thanks to all the readers who provided me with unending topics and questions to write about.

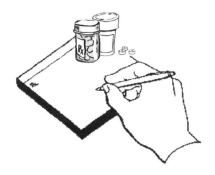

CHAPTER 1
PROPER MEDICATION USE

PRESCRIPTION ABBREVIATIONS

QUESTION: What do all the abbreviations on my prescriptions mean?

ANSWER: Most of the abbreviations or shorthand used in writing prescriptions come from Latin phrases. I have listed below and on the following pages some of the more commonly used abbreviations, the Latin phrase or word the abbreviation represents on the line below it, followed by its meaning.

Abbreviation
Latin Phrase or Word; Meaning

- **ac**
  Ante cibum; Before meals
- **ad**
  Aurio dextra; Right ear
- **am**
  Ante meridiem; Morning
- **as**
  Aurio sinister; Left ear

- **au**
  Aures ultrae; Each ear
- **bid**
  Bis in dies; Twice daily
- **c**
  Cum; With
- **d**
  Dies; Day
- **disp**
  Dispensa; Dispense
- **gtt**
  Gutta; A drop
- **h**
  Hora; Hour
- **hs**
  Hora somni; At bedtime
- **od**
  Oculus dexter; Right eye
- **os**
  Oculus sinister; Left eye
- **ou**
  Oculo uterque; Each eye
- **pc**
  Post cibos; After meals
- **pm**
  Post meridiem; Afternoon or evening
- **po**
  Per os; By mouth
- **prn**
  Pro re nata; As needed
- **qh**
  Quiaque hora; Every hour
- **qid**
  Quater in die; Four times daily
- **qs**
  Quantum sufficiat; A sufficient quantity
- **RX**
  Recipe; Take, a recipe

- **s**
  Sine; Without
- **sig**
  Signa; Label
- **ss**
  Semis; One-half
- **stat**
  Statim; Immediately
- **supp**
  Suppositorium; Suppository
- **syr**
  Syrupus; Syrup
- **tab**
  Tabella; Tablet
- **tid**
  Ter in die; Three times daily
- **ung**
  Unguentum; Ointment
- **ud or ut dict**
  Ut dictum; As directed

INFORMATION YOU NEED

QUESTION: What information should I have about the medications that I take?

ANSWER: Every patient or their caretaker should have some basic information about any medication (prescription or nonprescription) that they take. Your doctor or pharmacist should provide you with this information and if they don't, you should make sure that you ask them to. In general, you should know the following facts about your medications:

1. The name of the medication (trade name and/or generic name) and what it is supposed to do. If you see more than one doctor, you should always inform each doctor of all the medications that you take—prescription or not.

2. When and how to take it. For instance, should you take it before meals, with meals, or on an empty stomach? What times of the day or night should you take it? Does three times a day mean every 8 hours? What does "as needed" or "as directed" mean? Do you need to shake it prior to use, etc.?
3. How long you can expect to take the medication. Is it short-term or long-term therapy?
4. Can anything in the medicine cause an allergic reaction? Some medicines contain multiple ingredients that can produce an allergic reaction. Keep your doctor and pharmacist informed about any medication allergies that you may have.
5. Should you avoid alcohol, certain foods, or any other medications while on this medicine? Many drugs can interact with foods, other drugs, and alcohol causing a harmful effect.
6. Side effects that can be expected. All medications can cause side effects, but many are not serious or common. Your pharmacist and doctor can help you anticipate and understand these side effects and help you deal with them. You should report any suspected side effects to your doctor or pharmacist.
7. Is a generic version of the drug available? If there is an appropriate generic drug available, it can save you a lot of money.
8. What to do if you miss a dose. Don't panic and take a double dose. Ask your pharmacist or doctor what to do ahead of time.
9. Pregnant women and women of child bearing age should also know whether it is safe to take the medication while pregnant or when breast feeding. Some drugs can cause birth defects and some pass into breast milk affecting the baby.
10. How the medicine should be stored. Many drugs lose their effectiveness if stored incorrectly. The medicine cabinet in the bathroom is not a good place for storage because of the moisture and heat. Remember, when in doubt about any of this information, ask your pharmacist or doctor.

GENERAL GUIDELINES FOR MEDICATION USE

QUESTION: I often have questions about or problems with taking my medication. What general guidelines can you give me about taking medicine?

ANSWER: Here are some general recommendations to consider when taking medication:

General Principles

- Learn the names of all medications you are taking and the dosage strengths. Know why you are taking them, i.e., high blood pressure, heart, water, etc. Carry a list of your medications in your wallet for quick reference.
- If you are allergic to any medications, learn their names and carry a medic-alert card.
- Take only the medications that have been prescribed for you. Take medications only at the times ordered and in the amount ordered. Two pills are not necessarily better than one and, in fact, can be dangerous. Only stop taking your medication on your doctor's advice or if you think you are having an allergic reaction.
- Any medication may produce an allergic or unexpected reaction, even if you have no known allergies. Contact your doctor or pharmacist to explain unusual signs or symptoms such as rash, fever, bruising, vomiting, and diarrhea.
- Keep all medications in a secure place out of reach of children.
- Do not take medication that is more than several months old without checking with your pharmacist to see if it is still safe and effective to take. Outdated medication may be ineffective and/or even harmful.

Instructions For Taking

- Always take medication exactly as ordered by your doctor. The directions are usually based on how long the drug stays in the body and the special effects of the drug.

- Be sure you understand fully the directions on the label (four times daily may mean every 6 hours around the clock or four times during the waking hours). Ask your doctor or pharmacist to clarify any questions.
- If the label reads "Take with meals," this is usually done to lessen the chance of any stomach upset the medication may cause. "Before or after meals" directions are ordered because food may decrease the action of some drugs. The drug should be taken about one half hour before or 1-2 hours after meals. Milk may alter some medications, but water is almost always okay. Take your medication with water unless otherwise advised by your doctor.
- If an extended-release tablet is prescribed, do not break, crush, or chew it before swallowing.

Side Effects
- All drugs can cause unwanted side effects. This may include dizziness, drowsiness, dry mouth, diarrhea, constipation, headache, blurred vision, rashes, etc. In some cases, the side effect is short term and will not require medical attention. If any side effect appears, it is a good idea to ask your physician or pharmacist about it. They will be able to tell you if it is serious or will pass as your body adjusts to the drug. Some drugs are known to cause drowsiness and you should avoid driving a car or operating machinery while taking them.

Drug Interactions
- Before drinking any alcoholic beverages, it's a good idea to check with your pharmacist. Present him/her with a list of medications you are on and he will tell you if there will be any problems. Alcohol and certain drugs can have very dangerous reactions.
- When adding a new drug to your regimen, check with the pharmacist to see if there may be side effects with your current medication.

Storage
- All medications should be stored in a cool, dry place away from direct sunlight. Care should be taken to be sure there is no easy access of medications by children. Open medication bottles should not be within reach of children.

DRUG USE IN THE ELDERLY

QUESTION: How does aging affect medication use and are there drugs that should be used with caution in the elderly?

ANSWER: The normal aging process is associated with many changes in the body, which can affect how drugs work. To begin with, body fat increases while total body water and proteins in the blood decrease with age. This change can affect how drugs are distributed in the body. Fat-soluble drugs will have increased effects, but water-soluble will have reduced effects. Age-related changes in liver and kidney function can affect the activity of drugs taken by the elderly. Although there are many differences in individuals, both liver and kidney function decrease as we age. Because of this there is a reduced ability to metabolize (detoxify) and get rid of (excrete) medications that are taken. This can lead to an increase in drug activity and side effects. Gastrointestinal changes that occur with aging may also affect how drugs are absorbed into the body and cardiovascular changes can alter the response to some drugs. Furthermore, the elderly have an increased sensitivity to drugs that affect the central nervous system and therefore dosage reductions are needed for these medications. In addition, age-related hormonal changes and immune function can affect the action of drugs. Finally, the control of bowel and bladder function decreases with age and numerous drugs can affect these physiologic activities.

Because of these age-related changes in body functions, many drugs must be used with caution or in decreased doses to prevent side effects and other problems. In general, the use of sedative-hypnotic drugs, antibiotics, cardiac drugs, antidepressants and antipsychotics, and anticoagulants are of special concern for older individuals.

I have listed some specific oral drugs that can cause problems in the elderly population. Please note that this is not a complete listing and you need to check with your doctor and pharmacist if you have any questions regarding the medication that is prescribed for you or your loved one.

Some Drugs Of Concern In The Elderly
Drug (Some Trade Names) or Drug Class
What Drug Is Used For
Notes

- Amitriptyline (Elavil)
  Depression
  Many side effects including sedation
- Antihistamines
  Colds, etc.
  Non-sedating OK, others cause many side effects
- Barbiturates
  Sedative
  Many side effects
- Chlordiazepoxide (Librium, Libritabs)
  Sedative
  Oversedation
- Chlorpropamide (Diabenese)
  Diabetes
  Long-action can cause side effects
- Diazepam (Valium)
  Sedative, muscle relaxant
  Oversedation
- Digoxin (Lanoxin)
  Heart problems
  May need to reduce dose
- Dipyridamole (Persantine)
  Antiplatelet agent
  Can reduce blood pressure in elderly
- Disopyramide (Norpace)
  Abnormal heart rhythm
  Many side effects
- Doxepin (Sinequan)
  Anxiety, depression
  Many side effects including sedation
- Flurazepam (Dalmane)
  Sleep aide
  Oversedation

- Indomethacin (Indocin)
  Pain, inflammation
  Central nervous system side effects
- Iron supplements (over 325 mg/day
  Anemia
  Constipation
- Meperidine (Demerol)
  Pain
  Other drugs more effective, neurotoxicity
- Meprobamate (Equanil, Meprospan, Miltown)
  Sedative
  Oversedation, addicting
- Methydopa (Aldomet)
  High blood pressure
  Can slow heart rate and cause depression
- Metoclopramide (Reglan)
  Gastrointestinal disorders
  May cause movement disorders
- Muscle relaxants & antispasmotics
  Many side effects in elderly
- Pentazocine (Talwin NX, Talacen)
  Pain
  Central nervous system side effects
- Propoxyphene (Darvon, Darvon N, Darvocet)
  Pain
  Use acetaminophen (Tylenol) instead
- Reserpine
  High blood pressure
  Many side effects
- Ticlopidine (Ticlid)
  Antiplatelet agent
  More side effects than aspirin
- Trimethobenzamide (Tigan, T-Gen, Trimazide)
  Nausea & Vomiting
  Many side effects

QUESTION: What prescription medications can be inappropriate for people over 65?

<u>ANSWER</u>: Numerous prescription medications are more dangerous in people over 65 because they have side effects like memory impairment, dizziness, blurred vision, or other effects. Many of these medications should be avoided unless no other options exist. A recent Johns Hopkins Health Alert (**www.johnshopkinshealthalert.com**, 2009) reviewed this topic and provided the following list of potentially dangerous medications in people over the age of 65. If you are over 65 and are taking a medication on this list, please discuss this issue with your doctor to see if any other alternative medication can be used.

<u>Inappropriate Medications</u>
Barbiturates (amobarbital, butabarbital, pentobarbital, phenobarbital, secobarbital)

Flurazepam (Dalmane, Somnol, Novo-Flupam, Apo-Flurazepam)

Meprobamate (Equanil, Meprospan 200, Meprospan 400, Probate, ApoMeprobamate)

Chlorpropamide (Diabinese, Novo-Propamide, Apo-Chlorpropamide)

Meperidine (Demerol)

Pentazocine (Talwin, Talwin Nx)

Trimethobenzamide (Benzacot, Stemetic, Tebamide, Tigan, Tribenzagan, Trimazide)

Dicyclomine (Bentyl, Bentylol, Spas—moban, Formulex)

Hyoscyamine (Anaspaz, A-Spas-S/L, Cystospaz, Levbid, Levsin, Levsinex Timecaps, Symax SL)

Propantheline (Pro-Banthine)

Belladonna alkaloids/phenobarbital (Barbidonna, Donnatal)

<u>Rarely Appropriate Medications</u>
Chlordiazepoxide (Librium)

Diazepam (Valium)

Propoxyphene (Darvon, Darvon-N)

Carisoprodol (Soma)

Chlorzoxazone (Remular-S, Paraflex, Parafon Forte DSC)

Cyclobenzaprine (Flexeril)

Metaxalone (Skelaxin)

Methocarbamol (Robaxin)

Sometimes Appropriate Medications

Amitriptyline (Elavil)
Doxepin (Sinequan)
Indomethacin (Indocin)
Dipyridamole (Persantine)
Ticlopidine (Ticlid)
Methyldopa (Aldomet)
Reserpine (Serpasil, Serpalan, Novoreserpine)
Disopyramide (Norpace, Norpace CR)
Oxybutynin (Ditropan, Ditropan XL)
Chlorpheniramine (Aller-Chlor, Chlorate, ChloAmine, ChlorTrimeton)
Cyproheptadine (Periactin)
Diphenhydramine (Benadryl)
Hydroxyzine (Atarax, Rezine, Vistaril)
Promethazine (Phenergan)

QUESTION: I have poor vision and memory. What can I do to avoid mistakes with my medications?

ANSWER: Medication errors are a big problem with some 1.5 million preventable adverse drug events occurring in the United States every year. A recent Johns Hopkins Health Alert (**www.johnshopkinshealthalerts. com**, 2009) provides some useful information for people with poor vision or memory that can help prevent medication mistakes. I have outlined these tips for you:

If You Have Vision Loss

- Use a medication organizer or "dosette" to keep track of your pills, and put larger-type labels on each compartment so that you can read the days of the week and the times of day. Ask a family member or friend to fill the medication organizer for you each week.
- Keep a magnifier handy with your pills.
- Ask your pharmacist to use different-size bottles when dispensing similarly shaped pills. Or ask about talking pill bottles. They play a recorded message telling you the name of the medication and your prescription information.

If You Have Memory Loss

- Try wrapping rubber bands around each pill bottle equaling the number of daily doses. Remove one band each time you take the medication, and then replace all of the bands for the following day.
- Keep a medication chart in order to record whether you have taken your pills. This can be a simple dry-erase board on the refrigerator door; put a check next to each medication after you take it.
- Use an alarm on your watch or cell phone to remind you when it's time to take your medication. Some fancier versions of dosettes come with built-in alarms. There are even automated medication dispensers that announce when it's time to take your medication, and then dole out the appropriate pill.

QUESTION: Can some medications increase your risk of falls?

ANSWER: Yes, in fact researchers at the University of North Carolina at Chapel Hill have recently put together a list of prescription drugs that may increase the risk of falling for people aged 65 and older. Falls are the leading cause of both fatal and non-fatal injuries for adults 65 and older. The prescription drugs on this list represent many different categories (i.e., antidepressants, seizure medications, pain relievers, sedatives, sleep medication, etc.) but they all work by depressing the central nervous system, which can make patients less alert and slower to react. It is recommended that if patients see a drug that they are taking on the list, they should not stop taking it, but the next time they see their doctor they should talk about the risk of falling and possible alternative medications. In addition, some nonprescription allergy medications, sleep aids, and cough/cold remedies that can cause drowsiness can put you at increased risk of falling, so be sure to read the labeling carefully.

Prescription Medications That Can Increase
The Risk Of Falls In People Age 65 & Older
Generic Name (Brand Name)

Alprazolam (Xanax)
Amitriptyline (Elavil)
Amobarbital (Amytal)
Amoxapine (Asendin)

Aripiprazole (Abilify)
Baclofen (Lioresal)
Bupropion (Wellbutrin, Wellbutrin SR)
Buspirone (Buspar)
Butabarbital
Carbamazepine (Tegretol, Tegretol XR, Carbatrol)
Chloral hydrate
Chlorazepate (Tranxene)
Chlordiazepoxide (Librium, Limbitrol, Librax)
Chlorpromazine (Thorazine)
Citalopram (Celexa)
Clidinium-chlordiazepoxide (Librax)
Clomipramine (Anafranil)
Clonazepam (Klonopin)
Clozapine (Clozaril)
Codeine (Tylenol with Codeine)
Desipramine (Norpramin)
Diazepam (Valium)
Digoxin (Lanoxin)
Disopyramide (Norpace)
Divalproex sodium (Depakote, Depakote ER)
Doxepin (Sinequan, Zonalon, Prudoxin)
Duloxetine (Cymbalta)
Escitalopram (Lexapro)
Estazolam (Prosom)
Ethosuximide (Zarontin)
Felbamate (Felbatol)
Fentanyl (Duragesic)
Fluoxetine (Prozac)
Fluphenazine (Permitil, Prolixin)
Flurazepam (Dalmane)
Fluvoxamine (Luvox)
Gabapentin (Neurontin)
Halazepam (Paxipam)
Haloperidol (Haldol)
Hydrocodone (Vicodin)
Hydromorphone (Dilaudid)
Imipramine (Tofranil)

Isocarboxazid (Marplan)
Levetiracetam (Keppra)
Levorphanol (Levo-Dromoran)
Lorazepam (Ativan)
Loxapine (Loxitane, Loxitane C)
Maprotiline (Ludiomil)
Mephobarbital
Meprobamate (Miltown, Equanil)
Mesoridazine (Serentil)
Methadone (Dolophine)
Methsuximide (Celontin)
Mirtazapine (Remeron)
Molindone (Moban)
Morphine (MS Contin)
Nefazodone (Serzone)
Olanzapine (Zyprexa, Zyprexa Zydis)
Oxazepam (Serax)
Oxcarbazepine (Trileptal)
Oxycodone (Percocet)
Oxymorphone (Numorphan)
Paraldehyde (Paral)
Paroxetine (Paxil)
Pentobarbital (Nembutal)
Perphenazine (Trilafon)
Phenelzine (Nardil)
Phenobarbital
Phenytoin (Dilantin)
Pimozide (Orap)
Pregabalin (Lyrica)
Primidone (Mysoline)
Propoxyphene (Darvon, Darvocet)
Protriptyline (Vivactil)
Quazepam (Doral)
Quetiapine (Seroquel)
Risperidone (Risperdal)
Secobarbital (Seconal)
Sertraline (Zoloft)
Temazepam (Restoril)

Thioridazine (Mellaril)
Thiothixene (Navane)
Tiagabine (Gabatril)
Topiramate (Topamax)
Tranylcypromine (Parnate)
Trazodone (Desyrel)
Triazolam (Halcion)
Trifluoroperazine (Stelazine)
Trimipramine (Surmontil)
Venlafaxine (Effexor, Effexor XR)
Ziprasidone (Geodon)
Zolpidem (Ambien)
Zonisamide (Zonegran)

USE CAUTION WITH GRAPEFRUIT

QUESTION: I am a Floridian and love grapefruit and grapefruit juice. Is it true that grapefruit can interact with some medications?

ANSWER: Yes. Although much more study and research is needed, we now know that grapefruit juice (or whole grapefruits) can interfere with a number of medications. This may be of even greater concern for people who take many of their medications at breakfast time, while enjoying grapefruit. It appears that some of the substances found in grapefruits (maybe bioflavonoids) interfere with an important enzyme in the intestinal tract, which allows more of certain medications to be absorbed. Because of this, it is like taking a much higher dose of the drug, which can cause toxic side effects. For example, antihypertensive drugs may lower blood pressure too much, which can lead to an increased heart rate, flushing, and headache. Some studies indicate that this grapefruit effect can last for up to as long as 24 hours. A solution to this problem would be to avoid grapefruit or grapefruit juice while taking medications. Orange juice does not appear to cause the same problem and is a good alternative juice. Allowing at least 6 to 8 hours separation between taking medication and grapefruit may also lessen the possibility of a significant interaction. Changing medication may be another solution for diehard grapefruit fans. I have listed many of the drugs that can potentially interact with grapefruits or grapefruit juice. **Please note**, however, that not all drugs have been studied for this potential problem and much more information is needed.

<u>**Potential Drug Interactions With Grapefruit**</u>
Type of Drug or Use
Generic Name (Example Trade Names(s))

- AIDS treatment
    Indinavir (Crixivan)
    Saquinavir (Fortovase, Invirase)
- Anticoagulant
    Warfarin (Coumadin)
- Anticonvulsant
    Carbamazepine (Tegretol)
- Antihistamines
    Fexofenodine (Allegra)
    Loratadine (Claritin)
- Anxiety
    Buspirone (BuSpar)
- Blood pressure or heart medication
    Felodipine (Plendil)
    Nifedipine (Adalat, Procardia)
    Nisoldipine (Sular)
    Verapamil (Calan, Isopin, Verelan)
    Amlodipine (Norvasc)
    Nimodipine (Nimotop)
    Propafenone (Rythmol)
    Nitrendipine (Baypress)
- Caffeine
    Many products
- Cholesterol-lowering agents
    Lovastatin (Mevacor, Altoprev)
    Simvastatin (Zocor)
    Atorvastatin (Lipitor)
- Estrogens
    Estradiol (Estinyl, Estrace)

- Heartburn
    Cisapride (Propulsid)
- Impotence
    Sildenafil (Viagra)
- Leg cramping
    Cilostazol (Pletal)
- Organ transplant drug
    Cyclosporine (Sandimmune, Neoral)
    Sirolimus (Rapamune)
    Tacrolimus (Prograf)
- Sedative/hypnotic
    Triazolam (Halcion)
    Alprazolam (Xanax)
    Midazolam oral (Versed)

QUESTION: Where can I find information about what prescription drugs can interact with grapefruit juice?

ANSWER: I often get questions about drug interactions with grapefruit juice, especially from Florida residents. Grapefruit juice contains a natural substance that can affect the way certain prescription medications are broken down (metabolized) by the body. This substance blocks an enzyme known as CYP3A4 in the intestinal tract that helps the body get rid of certain drugs. By blocking this enzyme, grapefruit juice allows more of the drug to enter the bloodstream, which can lead to adverse effects in some situations. However, most prescription drugs do not interact with grapefruit juice and most studies suggest that it is safe to consume grapefruit juice while taking nonprescription medication. To help consumers and healthcare professionals find information about drug interactions with grapefruit juice, a new Internet web site was recently established by the University of Florida and Tufts University. This site lists drugs by category, compound name, and brand name that may interact with grapefruit juice. The web site **is www.druginteractioncenter.org**. For those of you who do not have Internet access, I have listed below drugs by trade name and generic name that may have a strong or moderate interaction capability with grapefruit juice. **Please note** that not all trade names or combination products may be listed and that you should always consult with your doctor and pharmacist if you have any questions or concerns about your medication and its use with grapefruit juice.

Strong Interaction

Altocor (Lovastatin)
Altoprev (Lovastatin)
BuSpar (Buspirone)
Diastat (Diazepam)
Dizac (Diazepam)
Halfan (Halofantrine)
Mevacor (Lovastatin)
Valium (Diazepam)
Zocor (Simvastatin)

Moderate Interaction

44 Magnum (Caffeine)
357 HR Magnum (Caffeine)
Activella Tablets (17 Beta-Estradiol)
Adalat (Nifedipine)
Adalat CC (Nifedipine)
Afeditab CR (Nifedipine)
Agenerase (Amprenavir)
Alertness Al (Caffeine)
Allegra (Fexofenadine)
Alprazolam Intensol (Alprazolam)
AmVaz (Amlodipine)
Babee Cof (Dextromethorphan)
Benylin Adult Formula (Dextromethorphan)
Benylin Pediatric (Dextromethorphan)
Biaxin (Clarithromycin)
Biaxin XL (Clarithromycin)
Biltricide (Praziquantel)
Cafcit (Caffeine)
Caffedrine (Caffeine)
Calan (Verapamil)
Calan SR (Verapamil)
Cardizem (Diltiazem)
Cardizem CD (Diltiazem)

Cardizem IV (Diltiazem)
Cardizem LA (Diltiazem)
Cardizem SR (Diltiazem)
Cartia XT (Diltiazem)
Children's ElixSure Cough (Dextromethorphan)
Clarinex (Desloratadine)
Clarinex RediTabs (Desloratadine)
Clozaril (Clozapine)
Coumadin (Warfarin)
Covera-HS (Verapamil)
Cozaar (Losartan)
Creo-Terpin (Dextromethorphan)
Crestor (Rosuvastatin)
Crixivan (Indinavir)
Delsym (Dextromethorphan)
DexAlone (Dextromethorphan)
Di-Phen (Phenytoin)
iabetuss (Dextromethorphan)
Digitek (Digoxin)
Digoxin Elixir (Digoxin)
Dilacor XR (Diltiazem)
Dilantin (Phenytoin)
Dilt-CD (Diltiazem)
Dilt-CD Extended Release Capsules (Diltiazem)
Diltia XT (Diltiazem)
E-Mycin (Erythromycin)
EES (Erythromycin)
Elixophyllin (Theophylline)
Enerjets (Caffeine)
Ery-Tab (Erythromycin)
ERYC (Erythromycin)
EryPed (Erythromycin)
Erythrocin (Erythromycin)
Estinyl (Ethinylestradiol)
Estrace (17 Beta-Estradiol)
Estradiol Tablets (17 Beta-Estradiol)
Etopophos (Etoposide)
Fastlene (Caffeine)

Fazaclo (Clozapine)
Fortovase (Saquinavir)
Gengraf (Cyclosporine)
Gynodiol (17 Beta-Estradiol)
Halcion (Triazolam)
Haloperidol Tablets (Haloperidol)
Hold DM (Dextromethorphan)
Honey Tussin Cough (Dextromethorphan)
Ilosone (Erythromycin)
Innofem (17 Beta-Estradiol)
Invirase (Saquinavir)
Isoptin (Verapamil)
Isoptin SR (Verapamil)
Jantoven (Warfarin)
Keep Alert (Caffeine)
Keep Going (Caffeine)
Ketek Pak (Telithromycin)
Ketek (Telithromycin)
Lanoxicaps (Digoxin)
Lanoxin (Digoxin)
Lescol (Fluvastatin)
Lescol XL (Fluvastatin)
Little Colds Cough Formula (Dextromethorphan)
Lucidex (Caffeine)
Luvox (Fluvoxamine)
Maximum Strength Stay Awake (Caffeine)
Medrol (Methylprednisolone)
Menostar (Ethinylestradiol)
Methylprednisolone Tablets (Methylprednisolone)
Methylpred (Methylprednisolone)
Midazolam Syrup (Midazolam)
Molie (Caffeine)
My-E (Erythromycin)
Neoral (Cyclosporine)
Nifediac CC (Nifedipine)
Nifedical XL (Nifedipine)
Nimotop (Nimodipine)
NoDoz (Caffeine)

NoDoz Maximum Strength (Caffeine)
Norvasc (Amlodipine)
Overtime (Caffeine)
PCE Dispertab (Erythromycin)
Phenytek (Phenytoin)
Pletal (Cilostazol)
Pravachol (Pravastatin)
Prefest Tablets (17 Beta-Estradiol)
Prilosec OTC (Omeprazole)
Prilosec (Omeprazole)
Procardia XL (Nifedipine)
Procardia (Nifedipine)
Quibron T (Theophylline)
Quibron T/SR (Theophylline)
Quick Pep (Caffeine)
Quin-Tab (Quinine)
Quinadure (Quinine)
Quinaglute (Quinine)
Quinidex (Quinine)
Quinine Capsules (Quinidine)
Quinine Tablets (Quinidine)
Quinora (Quinine)
Respbid (Theophylline)
Revatio (Sildenafil Citrate)
Revive (Caffeine)
Robitussin Cough Calmers (Dextromethorphan)
Robitussin Honey Cough (Dextromethorphan)
Robitussin Maximum Strength Cough (Dextromethorphan)
Robitussin Pediatric Cough (Dextromethorphan)
Sandimmune (Cyclosporine)
SangCya (Cyclosporine)
Scopace (Scopolamine)
Scopolamine Tablets (Scopolamine)
Scot-Tussin Diabetic (Dextromethorphan)
Scot-Tussin DM Cough Chasers (Dextromethorphan)
Silphen DM (Dextromethorphan)
Simply Cough (Dextromethorphan)
Slo-bid (Theophylline)

Slo-Phyllin (Theophylline)
Snap Back (Caffeine)
Sporanox (Itraconazole)
Stay Alert (Caffeine)
Sucrets Cough Control Formula (Dextromethorphan)
T-Phyl (Theophylline)
Taztia XT (Diltiazem)
Theo-24 (Theophylline)
Theo-Bid Duracap (Theophylline)
Theo-Dur (Theophylline)
Theo-Dur Sprinkle (Theophylline)
Theo-X (Theophylline)
TheoCap (Theophylline)
Theochron (Theophylline)
Theolair (Theophylline)
Theolair SR (Theophylline)
Theovent LA (Theophylline)
Tiamate (Diltiazem)
Tiazac (Diltiazem)
Toposar (Etoposide)
Truxophyllin (Theophylline)
Tussin Honey Cough Syrup (Dextromethorphan)
Ultra Pep-Back (Caffeine)
Uni-Dur (Theophylline)
Uniphyl (Theophylline)
Valentine (Caffeine)
VePesid (Etoposide)
Verelan (Verapamil)
Verelan PM (Verapamil)
Versed (Midazolam)
Verv (Caffeine)
Viagra (Sildenafil citrate)
Vicks 44 Cough Medicine (Dextromethorphan)
Vicks 44 Cough Relief (Dextromethorphan)
Vivarin (Caffeine)
Wakespan (Caffeine)
Waykup (Caffeine)
Xanax XR (Alprazolam)

Xanax (Alprazolam)
Zegerid (Omeprazole)
Zoloft (Sertraline)

ASPIRIN INTERACTIONS

QUESTION: What drugs can interact with aspirin?

ANSWER: A number of potential drug interactions can occur when aspirin is used in combination with other medications. Acetaminophen (Tylenol) is usually recommended instead of aspirin in these situations. I have summarized some of these interactions for you:

Drug or Drug Class
Some Example Products
Potential Problem

- ACE inhibitors
     Capoten (Captopril), Altace, Monopril, Prinivil or Zestril (lisinopril), Vasotec (enalapril), Accupril, Aceon
     Worsening of high blood pressure or congestive heart failure.
- Anticoagulants
     Coumadin (warfarin)
     Risk of bleeding.
- Ginkgo
     Various herbal products
     Increased bleeding tendency.
- Ibuprofen
     Motrin, Advil
     Interference with anticoagulant effect of aspirin.
- Methotrexate in high doses
     Methotrexate
     Risk of methotrexate toxicity.
- Sulfonylureas for diabetes
     Diabenese (chlorpropamide), Tolinase (tolazamide), Orinase (tolbutamide), Glucotrol (glipizide), Amaryl, Diabeta, Micronase, Glynase, Glyburide

    Low blood sugar.
- Uricosurics for gout
    Probenecid, Anturane (sulfinpyrazone)
    Worsening of gout.
- Valproic acid for seizures
    Depakote (valproic acid)
    Increased side effects such as drowsiness or behavioral problems.

USING NASAL PRODUCTS

QUESTION: What is the best way to use nasal sprays or nasal inhalers?

ANSWER: If your nasal spray or inhaler is not used correctly, not only will you decrease its effectiveness, but you will also waste a lot of money. The proper way to use both of these products is as follows:

- Blow your nose gently to clear your nostrils.
- Clean the outer portion of your nose with a damp tissue.
- Wash your hands with soap and warm water and dry them.
- Shake the medication container. If you think a nasal inhaler might be empty, test it by removing the metal canister and placing it in a container of water. If the canister floats, it is empty. Call your pharmacist to get a refill. Reassemble the inhaler if the canister sinks; it is not empty.
- Keep your head upright. Press a finger against the side of your nose to close one nostril. With your mouth closed, insert the tip of the pump, spray, or inhaler into the open nostril. Sniff in through the nostril while quickly and firmly squeezing the spray container or activating the pump or inhaler.
- Hold your breath for a few seconds and then breathe out through your mouth.
- Repeat this procedure for the other nostril only if directed to do so.
- Rinse the spray, pump, or inhaler tip with hot water and replace the cap on the container.
- Wash your hands.

QUESTION: What is the best way to use nose drops?

ANSWER: It can be difficult giving yourself nose drops. If possible, have someone else administer the drops as follows:

- Have the patient blow his or her nose gently to clear the nostrils. Use a bulb syringe to gently clear the nostrils of an infant.
- Clean the outer portion of the nose with a damp tissue.
- Wash your hands with soap and warm water and dry them.
- Lie down (or have the patient lie on his or her back) on a bed with the head tilted back and the neck supported (allow the head to hang over the edge of the bed or place a small pillow under the neck and shoulders). Cradle an infant in your arms with the head tilted back.
- Shake the nose drops container.
- Insert the dropper tip into the nostril about 1/3 inch, and place the prescribed dose or number of drops in the nostril. Try not to touch the nose with the dropper tip.
- Stay (or have the patient stay) in the same position for at least five minutes.
- Unless otherwise directed, repeat these steps for the other nostril.
- Rinse the dropper tip with hot water and replace the cap on the container.
- Wash your hands.

USING EYE DROPS

QUESTION: What is the proper way to use eye drops?

ANSWER: Almost everyone uses eye drops at one time or another. Eye drops are used to treat eye infections, to soothe dry or irritated eyes, to treat allergies, or to treat other conditions such as glaucoma. When eye drops are not used properly the full benefit of the medication may not be realized and there may be spillage and waste if the drop does not fall directly onto the eye. In order to use eye drops correctly you should follow these steps:

- Always wash your hands first before administering eye drops.
- Shake the bottle if indicated on the label. If the bottle has been refrigerated, warm it between your hands to room temperature.
- Gently clean the eyelids if they are crusty with discharge by wiping the lid from the inner corner to the outer corner with the eye closed, using a cotton ball dampened with warm water.
- Tilt back the head, or lie down, and look upward. Using the thumb and index finger, gently pinch and pull the lower eyelid downward to form a pocket.
- Place the eye drop or drops into the pouch formed in the lower lid, not directly into the eye. If an eye ointment is used, place a ¼ inch line of ointment into the lower lid pouch. Be careful that the dropper or ointment tube does not touch the eye.
- Close your eye gently for 1 to 3 minutes or as instructed by the doctor to allow the medication to be absorbed. Some doctors recommend pressing the finger against the inner corner of the eye to keep the medication from going into the tear duct.
- If another drop of eye medication is needed, wait at least 5 to 10 minutes before administering the second eye drop so the first drop will not be washed out of the eye. The small pouch formed by the lower lid will only hold one drop at a time, and extra drops will either flow into the tear duct (and out of the eye) or down the face.
- Always recap the bottle or tube immediately after use. Never wipe or rinse the tip of the dropper to avoid contamination.
- Never wear contact lenses while using eye drops or ointments unless instructed to do so by your doctor.
- If you are told to use an eye drop and an eye ointment at the same time, use the eye drop first, wait a few minutes, and then use the ointment.
- Most eye drops should not be used longer than one month after the bottle is opened, unless otherwise stated on the label.

USING METERED DOSE INHALERS

QUESTION: I currently use both Proventil and Vanceril inhalers to treat my asthma. What is the best way to use these medications?

ANSWER: Proventil or albuterol (al-byoo-ter-ole) is a drug that expands the breathing tubes and is known as a bronchodilator. Vanceril or beclomethasone (beck-loe-meth-a-sone) on the other hand is an anti-inflammatory drug and is known as a corticosteroids. They are commonly used together to treat symptoms of difficult breathing in patients with chronic asthma. Asthma is considered to be an inflammatory disease that involves the airways and proper treatment will prevent asthma attacks and possible death. Inhalers (also called metered dose inhalers) provide an effective way to deliver medications directly to the airways where they can work.

The best way to use your inhaler is to use the bronchodilator (Proventil) first, wait a minute, and then use your anti-inflammatory medication (Vanceril). This will allow your bronchodilator to dilate or expand your airways so that the anti-inflammatory drug can be transported deeper into the lungs. This will result in greater effectiveness of the medications and better control of symptoms. Some general guidelines for using a metered dose inhaler (MDI) are as follows:

- Shake the inhaler first. If you think the inhaler may be empty, place the canister in a bowl of water. If the canister floats, it's empty. If the canister sinks to the bottom of the bowl, it's full. If the canister floats at an angle, it's partially full and you should consider refilling the prescription as it starts to float closer to the surface of the water.
- After shaking, remove the mouthpiece cover, invert the canister so that the mouthpiece is in front of the mouth or between the lips above the tongue.
- Choose one of the following three acceptable methods for administering inhaler medication (choose the method that is easiest for you):
  - ❖ The preferred way is to place the MDI two finger widths in front of your open mouth.

- ❖ A spacer can be attached to the inhaler and the mouthpiece of the spacer placed between the teeth.
- ❖ The mouthpiece of the inhaler can be placed between the teeth, above the tongue, with the lips closed around the mouthpiece.
- Tip the head back slightly. Breathe out fully. Expel as much air as possible.
- Begin to breathe in. As you begin to take in a breath, press down on the canister and continue to breathe in the spray released by the metered dose inhaler. Close your mouth after the spray has been inhaled and count to ten.
- Exhale through your nose.
- If you are using an inhaler with a medication to dilate or open your airways when you are short of breath, use that medication first. Wait one minute and then use the inhaler with the steroid medication, using the same procedure. If you are using a spacer, the procedure is different and these instructions do not apply. The directions on the spacer device must be followed. At the end of your treatment, rinse your mouth and throat with water. Do not swallow the rinse water, spit it out. Also, rinse the mouthpiece of the MDI. Shake out the water and reassemble the inhalers.
- Check the quantity of medication remaining in your canisters before returning them to their storage place. Refill prescriptions as necessary so that you never run out of them.
- If you do not experience improved breathing after your inhaler treatment, contact your physician and your pharmacist.

STORAGE OF MEDICATIONS

QUESTION: What is the best way to store medications? How long are drugs good for?

ANSWER: Storing medications correctly is very important because many drugs will become ineffective if they are not stored properly. The bathroom medicine cabinet is <u>not</u> a good place to keep medicine because the room's moisture and heat speed up the chemical breakdown of drugs. In addition, drugs should never be stored in a car's glove compartment, as it can reach a very high temperature. Storing medication in the refrigerator is also not a good idea because of the moisture inside the unit. Some easily spoiled drugs do require refrigeration, but these should be labeled as needing to be kept in the refrigerator. Light and air can also affect drugs, but dark-tinted bottles and air-tight caps can keep these effects to a minimum. A closet is probably your best bet for storage of your medications. Pick a high shelf out of the reach of children, and be sure to use child-resistant safety caps if you have children, grandchildren or pets around.

Medications should not be used beyond their expiration date. Many medications become ineffective over time, but some drugs like tetracycline can actually become dangerous if used past their expiration date. Expiration dates, however, only apply to medicine that has been stored under good conditions. All medications should be stored in the original container and it is a good idea to throw away any medicine that has not been used in six months. Be especially sure to get rid of any solid medications that have a foul odor, have cracked coatings, or have changed color. All medications should be labeled with expiration dates, but if there is any doubt, ask your pharmacist.

DRUG DISPOSAL

QUESTION: Local authorities have advised me not to dispose of outdated or unused medications in the trash or down the toilet. The pharmacies I checked with won't take them either. What should I do?

ANSWER: The proper disposal of outdated or unused prescription and nonprescription drugs is a concern all over the United States. When I did an Internet search on this topic, over 6 million web sites were identified. Flushing medications down the toilet may be associated with environmental damage. When medicines are flushed down a toilet, they usually go to one of two places—a septic tank or through a series of sanitary sewers into a wastewater treatment plant. In both of these situations, medicines can harm the beneficial bacteria that are responsible for breaking down waste. In addition, sewage treatment plants are not designed to remove medications and many drugs have been identified in lakes, rivers, and groundwater. In fact, in some cities researchers have reported lethargic fish swimming in water containing drugs that affect the nervous system and fish with both male and female sex organs in waterways that contain human hormones. Antibiotics are of particular concern and an increase in bacterial resistance to multiple antibiotics has been attributed to their increased release into the environment. In addition, some medications contain mercury compounds, which can pose a potential risk to humans and wildlife that consume fish from polluted waters. Issues regarding the disposal of medications in the trash include potential access of the drugs to children, pets, wildlife, and drug abusers. Furthermore, privacy may be a problem if prescription vials are thrown away with patient names on them. So what should the consumer do? There are no specific government guidelines for the disposal of drugs by consumers. Probably one of the most appropriate methods of medication disposal is via incineration, but this process is not readily available in many communities and a collection program could be difficult to set up. State and Federal rules may also interfere with drug disposal efforts. For example, the State Boards of Pharmacy, the Drug Enforcement Agency (DEA), the Department of Transportation (DOT), the Food and Drug Administration (FDA), and the Environmental Protection Agency (EPA), all have rules and regulations that may impact any disposal program. We need a national effort to develop an appropriate and practical drug disposal program in our country. In order to do this, all pertinent governmental agencies should be involved in the process along with pharmaceutical manufacturers, drug wholesalers, drug return companies, large pharmacy corporations, and national pharmaceutical organizations. Until this happens, there is no good answer to your question.

QUESTION: I got a flyer with my prescription for OxyContin about how to dispose of any unused medication. What is this all about?

ANSWER: About 6,300 pharmacies around the country have signed up for a 26—week pilot project with the Substance Abuse and Mental Health Services Administration (SAMHSA). The purpose of this pilot program is to provide practical advice to consumers on how to properly store and dispose of unused medications that have a high potential for abuse (e.g., oxycodone (OxyContin, etc.), hydrocodone (Vicodin, etc.), certain sleep aids, etc. When these drugs are dispensed at any of the participating pharmacies, consumers will receive an information sheet about how to dispose of any unused medication. This new program is important because prescription drug abuse is on the rise, and research suggests that more than half of people who misuse these drugs get them from a friend or relative. Hopefully, with this information consumers can play a major role in helping to eliminate prescription drug abuse, particularly among teens and young adults. Advice on disposing of unused medications with abuse potential includes the following:

- Don't flush unused drugs down the toilet, unless they're one that expressly advises that on the prescription label.
- Crush or dissolve leftover medicine in a little water. Then mix with a yucky substance—cat litter, coffee grounds, even dog waste—in a sealed plastic bag or other unmarked container, and put in the trash. That renders the drug unpalatable if a child, animal or drug abuser rummages through the trash.
- Remove and destroy the prescription label and any other personal identifying information from the original drug container before throwing it away.
- An alternative is to call pharmacies or local environmental or hazardous waste collection sites, to see if they run drug "take-back" programs.

QUESTION: What medications should be flushed down the toilet?

ANSWER: I've written about the disposal of unused medicines in past columns and most of these medications should not be flushed down the sink or toilet due to potential environmental problems. Unused or expired medicines that do not have flushing directions in the label can be disposed of safely in the household trash by:

- Mixing them with something that will hide the medicine or make it unappealing, such as kitty litter or used coffee grounds.
- Placing the mixture in a container such as a sealed plastic bag.
- Throwing the container in your household trash.

Drug take-back programs for disposal can be another good way to remove unwanted or expired medicines from the home and reduce the chance that someone may accidentally take the medicine.

On the other hand, certain medicines may be especially harmful and, in some cases, fatal in a single dose if they are used by someone other than the person the medicine was prescribed for. For this reason, these medicines have special disposal directions that indicate they should be flushed down the sink or toilet after the medicine is no longer needed. If you dispose of these medicines down the sink or toilet, they cannot be accidentally used by children, pets, or anybody else. Recently the FDA has identified numerous prescription medications that should be flushed to get rid of them right away and help keep your family and pets safe. I have listed these medicines below. More information on this subject can be obtained at **www.fda.gov** or by calling the FDA at 1-888-463-6332.

Medicine/Active Ingredient

Actiq, oral transmucosal lozenge/Fentanyl Citrate
Avinza, capsules (extended release)/Morphine Sulfate
Daytrana, transdermal patch system/Methylphenidate
Demerol, oral solution */Meperidine Hydrochloride
Demerol, tablets */Meperidine Hydrochloride
Diastat/Diastat AcuDial, rectal gel/Diazepam
Dilaudid, oral liquid */Hydromorphone Hydrochloride
Dilaudid, tablets */Hydromorphone Hydrochloride
Dolophine Hydrochloride, tablets */Methadone Hydrochloride
Duragesic, patch (extended release) */Fentanyl
Embeda, capsules (extended release)/Morphine Sulfate; Naltrexone
Fentora, tablets (buccal)/Fentanyl Citrate
Kadian, capsules (extended release)/Morphine Sulfate
Methadone Hydrochloride, oral solution */Methadone
Methadose, tablets */Methadone Hydrochloride
Morphine Sulfate, oral solution */Morphine Sulfate
Morphine Sulfate, tablets (immediate release) */Morphine Sulfate
MS Contin, tablets (extended release) */Morphine Sulfate
Onsolis, soluble film (buccal)/Fentanyl Citrate
Opana ER, tablets (extended release)/Oxymorphone
Opana, tablets (immediate release)/Oxymorphone

Oramorph SR, tablets (sustained release)/Morphine Sulfate
Oxycontin, tablets (extended release) */Oxycodone
Percocet, tablets */Acetaminophen; Oxycodone
Percodan, tablets */Aspirin; Oxycodone
Xyrem, oral solution/Sodium Oxybate

*These medicines have generic versions available or are only available in generic formulations.

ACCESSORY LABELS

QUESTION: Would you please explain some of the sticker labels that are put on prescription containers?

ANSWER: Pharmacists frequently put stickers or "accessory labels" on vials or bottles that contain prescription drugs to provide reminders or additional information to patients. Use of these labels can help to prevent side effects or drug interactions and can assist patients in using their medications correctly. An explanation of some of the most common accessory labels is provided below, but if you ever have any questions about using or storing your medicine, be sure to ask your pharmacist:

"Take On An Empty Stomach"
Foods and beverages in your stomach may interfere with the absorption of certain medications, or slow the time it takes them to begin working. To avoid these problems, take the medication either one hour before, or two hours after eating or drinking. You should take all medication with a full glass of water.

"Take With Food"
On the other hand, many medications can irritate or upset the stomach. They should be taken with food or right after a meal.

"Avoid Prolonged Exposure To Sunlight"
This means you, not the medication. Certain medications, such as sulfa drugs and tetracyclines (as well as others), may make you more sensitive

to sunlight or tanning lamps, causing you to burn more easily. You should limit exposure to the sun when you are taking these medications. If your skin does become more sensitive, use a sunscreen (SPF 15 or more), avoid spending a long time in the sun, and wear protective clothing.

"Keep In The Refrigerator"
Medications requiring storage in the refrigerator should generally be kept at a temperature of 36 to 46 degrees Fahrenheit to maintain their potency. Refrigerate only those medications that have this instruction. Refrigerating other medications could cause them to lose their effectiveness because of low temperatures and high humidity. Medication should not be kept in the freezer unless specifically instructed to do so.

"May Cause Discoloration Of Urine Or Feces"
Some medications may change the color of your urine or stools. This effect is not harmful and will stop when the medication is discontinued. If you wear soft contact lenses you may not want to wear them while using this type of drug, as the medication may also discolor your tears and permanently stain the contact lenses.

"Shake Well"
The active ingredient in many liquid medications is in the form of a fine powder, which can settle to the bottom of the bottle. To be sure that you get the right dose, shake the bottle for 15 to 30 seconds every time you take or give the medication.

NON-STEROIDAL ANTI-INFLAMMATORY DRUGS (NSAIDS)

QUESTION: You've written several columns about non-steroidal anti-inflammatory drugs (NSAIDs) and their possible gastrointestinal problems. What is the best way to take these medications to prevent these side effects?

ANSWER: Numerous prescription and non-prescription medications known as NSAIDs are available to treat pain and inflammation. Older drugs like aspirin, ibuprofen (Motrin, Advil), diclofenac (Voltaren, Cataflam), naproxen (Anaprox, Aleve), ketoprofen (Orudis, Actron), and many others are probably more likely to cause GI side effects like ulcers and or bleeding compared to the new types of NSAIDs called COX-2 inhibitors (Celebrex) but the jury is still out on this question. These side effects can be a big problem for heavy users of NSAIDs like patients with arthritis. It has been estimated that there are about 20,000 hospitalizations and 2,600 deaths each year in the U.S. alone due to side effects from these types of drugs amongst rheumatoid arthritis patients. Your question is timely because recent study results from the UK have shown that if you take NSAIDs with meals, the risk of ulcer bleeding is reduced by about 50%. On the other hand, if you take these medications one hour or more before a meal you have twice the risk of GI bleeding. Lying down after taking NSAIDs and smoking also appear to significantly increase the risk of GI side effects. It was no surprise in this study that patients with GI bleeding were more likely to take high doses of these drugs and to take them more often than twice a day. However it was a surprise that alcohol had no effect of the risk of ulcer bleeding with NSAID use in the study. The bottom line is that you should always take these medications with food. In addition, you should avoid lying down after taking them and avoid smoking if possible. Never use these medications in a higher dose or more frequently than recommended on the product package or as prescribed by your doctor.

PLEASE NOTE: Celebrex now has a black-box warning in its labeling about an increased risk of serious and potentially life-threatening gastrointestinal and cardiovascular events associated with use of this drug.

QUESTION: I take nonprescription naproxen for arthritis. How can I reduce the risk of upset stomach and stomach bleeding from this drug?

ANSWER: Naproxen is known as a non-steroidal anti-inflammatory drug or NSAID for short. Numerous NSAIDs are available as prescription drugs or over-the-counter (OTC) products. Other nonprescription

NSAIDs include ibuprofen, aspirin, and ketoprofen. Commonly used OTC brand-name products containing one of these NSAIDs include Motrin, Advil, Orudis, Excedrin, and Aleve. They are also contained in many common OTC cold and flu products such as Advil Cold and Sinus, Dimetapp Sinus, Motrin IB Sinus, and Aleve Cold and Sinus. It is estimated that every day more than 30 million people take OTC and prescription NSAIDs for relief from pain, headaches, and arthritis. These drugs have been available for a long time, but like all drugs they can produce side effects. NSAIDs can cause serious gastrointestinal problems ranging from upset stomach to stomach bleeding, stomach pain, ulcers (a hole in the lining of the stomach), and even death. These side effects lead to more than 100,000 hospitalizations and 16,000 deaths each year in the U.S. alone. Some people are at a greater risk of these side effects, including people:

- Over the age of 60.
- Have had previous ulcers.
- Taking steroid medications such as prednisone.
- Taking blood thinners such as warfarin (Coumadin).
- Consuming alcohol on a regular basis.
- Taking high doses of NSAIDs.
- Taking several different medications that contain NSAIDs.
- Taking NSAIDs for a long period of time.

While about 80% of people who have serious stomach problems from NSAIDs have no warning symptoms, you should see your doctor immediately if you have stomach pain; have dark black, tarry, or bloody stools; or are vomiting blood or materials that look like coffee grounds.

There are several measures that you can take to reduce your risk of developing a serious stomach problem from taking NSAIDs. These include the following steps:

- Read the product label and follow instructions carefully. Do not take more than the recommended dose or for a longer time than recommended. Know all of the ingredients in the medications that you take. If unsure, ask your doctor or pharmacist.

- Make sure your doctor and pharmacist know all the medications that you take.
- Avoid or limit the use of alcohol when taking NSAIDs.
- Take NSAIDs with food, milk, or antacids.
- Consider taking acetaminophen (Tylenol) or one of the newer NSAIDs that may cause fewer stomach problems. Ask your doctor and pharmacist about possible alternative NSAID medications, or other drugs that can help reduce your risk of stomach problems if taking NSAIDs.
- Do not take aspirin without talking to your doctor or pharmacist.
- Report all side effects to your doctor and pharmacist.
- Review the risk factors noted above.

ALCOHOL AND MEDICATION USE

QUESTION: I drink alcohol occasionally. What medicines can cause problems when taken with alcohol?

ANSWER: Alcohol use can be dangerous when combined with many types of prescription or non-prescription medication, including some herbal preparations. Alcohol produces depressant effects on the central nervous system and when combined with other drugs that affect the nervous system numerous side effects can occur. Because of this, the use of alcohol can be dangerous when it is combined with sedatives, sleeping medication, antidepressants, tranquilizers, and some prescription pain relievers. Alcohol can also affect blood sugar levels and therefore caution needs to be observed when using alcohol with anti-diabetic medications. In addition, the use of alcohol can lead to gastrointestinal irritation and liver damage, which can be magnified when other drugs are used in combination with it. In the table below I have listed some of the more common drug interactions with alcohol. Please note that this list is not complete and if you have any questions about the use of alcohol with medications that you are taking please be sure to "Ask The Pharmacist" or your physician for advice.

Some Types of Drug Interactions With Alcohol
Drug Type
Some Examples
Problem

Non-Prescription Medications

* Antihistamines
  Diphenhydramine (Benadryl), chlorpheniramine
  (Chlor-Trimeton), clemastine (Tavist)
  Increased sedative effects, drowsiness, confusion
* Herbals
  Kava kava, St. Johns Wort
  Increased sedative effects, drowsiness
* Pain Relievers—Non-Steroidal Antiinflammatory Drugs (NSAIDs)
  Ibuprofen (Motrin, Advil), aspirin, ketoprofen (Actron,
  Orudis), naproxen (Aleve)
  Possible stomach and intestinal ulceration or bleeding
* Pain Relievers—Other
  Acetaminophen (Tylenol)
  Increased risk of liver problems

Prescription Medications

* Antidepressants
  Amitriptyline (Elavil), clomipramine (Anafranil),
  desipramine (Norpramin), doxepin (Sinequan), imipramine
  (Tofranil), protriptyline (Vivactil), maprotiline (Ludiomil),
  mirtazapine (Remeron), trazodone (Desyrel), bupropion
  (Wellbutrin), venlafaxine (Effexor), nefazodone (Serzone)
  Increased sedative effects, confusion
* Anti-diabetic
  Chlorpropamide (Diabenese), tolazamide (Tolinase), glipizide
  (Glucotrol), glyburide (Micronase), metformin (Glucophage)
  May cause dangerous drops in blood glucose and other side
  effects
* Anti-infective
  Metronidazole (Flagyl)
  Reaction causing facial flushing, headache, nausea, stomach pain
* Heart medication
  Nitroglycerin

     May produce a dangerous drop in blood pressure
- Pain relievers
  NSAIDs (See some examples above); Narcotics and narcotic-like drugs (codeine, morphine, propoxyphene (Darvon, Darvocet), fentanyl (Actiq, Duragesic), methadone (Dolophine), oxycodone (Oxycontin, Tylox), hydrocodone (Vicodin, Lortab), pentazocine (Talwin, Tramadol (Ultram)) Possible stomach and intestinal ulceration or bleeding; Excessive depressant effects (drowsiness, sedation, confusion), difficult breathing
- Sedatives, Tranquilizers
  Alprazolam (Xanax), chlorazepate (Tranxene), chlordiazepoxide (Librium), diazepam (Valium), lorazepam (Ativan), oxazepam (Serax), hydroxyzine (Vistaril), meprobamate (Equanil)
  Increased sedative effects, drowsiness

DRUG INFORMATION SOURCES

QUESTION: Where can I get good information about the medications that I take?

ANSWER: Besides the "Ask The Pharmacist" column there are many other useful sources of drug information available. Everyone should become better informed about their illnesses and medications that they take, both prescription and non-prescription. Patients need to know why they are taking each medication and what benefits can be expected from them. They should also know exactly how to take medications, if drugs, foods, or alcohol should be avoided, and what side effects are possible. Most pharmacies now provide printed drug information with new prescriptions so that patients can be better informed. If they don't, or if you have additional questions, be sure to ask the pharmacist or your doctor. The local library is another good place to find medical and drug information. Most libraries have a special section with health-related books. The reference section of the library will also usually carry an up to date copy of the Physician's Desk

Reference (PDR) or similar references. If you have access to the Internet (and most libraries provide this service), you can find many good medical and drug information resources available on the World Wide Web. You should note, however, that there is a great deal of misleading or inaccurate information on the Internet. A few useful and accurate sites include: **www.drugs.com**; **www.consumermedsafety.org** has a search feature where patients can enter the name of a prescription drug they are taking and the site searches for safety information and features of that drug; Medlineplus (**www.medlineplus.gov**) which has a wealth of information about drugs and diseases; Food and Drug Administration information for consumers (**www.fda.gov/opacom/morecons. html**) which provides information regarding newly approved drugs, proper use of prescription drugs, and herbal products; **www.fda.gov/ Drugs/GuidanceComplianceRegulatoryInformation/Surveillance/ ucm090385.htm** which provides risk summaries of approved drugs based upon health reports from companies, consumers, and physicians after drugs are approved; MayoClinic.com (**www.mayohealth.org/ home**) and Johns Hopkins Medicine (**www.johnshopkinshealthalerts. com**) which cover illnesses, drugs, and wellness; The Merck Manual Home Edition (**www.merckhomeedition.com**) with a variety of health and drug information for consumers; The Natural Pharmacist (**www.tnp.com**) with information on herbs and dietary supplements including drug interactions; **www.my.webmd.com** with extensive medical information including diseases, drugs and herbals, health and wellness; Pharmacy and You (**www.pharmacyandyou.org/**) covering medications, self-care, and pharmacist's services; and the National Council on Patient Information and Education (NCPIE) provides a wide variety of consumer-oriented medication information (**www. talkaboutrx.org**).

QUESTION: I heard that the FDA has a new web site to obtain drug information. What is it?

ANSWER: The FDA recently launched a new Internet web site to help consumers and health professionals find information they need about drug products. I've tried it. It is easy to use and provides a wide variety of information about prescription and over-the-counter drugs. To get to the site, you need to have access to a computer connected to the Internet (all local library branches have these computers available for public use). The FDA's Home Web site is **www.fda.gov**. At this site click on "Drugs" in the left hand column on the screen. Then click on Drugs@ FDA. Once you are at the Drugs@FDA screen you can search for drug information by entering at least 3 characters of the drug name (generic or trade name). At this site you can obtain a wealth of information about most FDA approved drug products, including Consumer Information Sheets, Medication Guides, and product labeling. You can also find information about generic drug products that are available for brand name drugs. In addition, information can be obtained to help identify therapeutically equivalent drugs for prescription medicines, and alternative nonprescription drug products with the same active ingredient. It should be noted, however, that the Drugs@FDA site does not include information about dietary supplements (because they do not require FDA approval), drugs for animals, or prescription drugs sold in countries other than the U.S. This drug information site is updated daily. More information about this new information source can be obtained by calling 1-888-INFO-FDA (1-888-463-6332) or via e-mail at druginfo@cder.fda.gov.

QUESTION: I heard about a new FDA web site for drug safety information. What can you tell me about it?

ANSWER: The FDA recently created a new web page with drug safety information for patients and health care professionals. You can now go to a single page on the U.S. Food and Drug Administration's web site to find a wide variety of safety information about prescription drugs. This web page, **http://www.fda.gov/cder/drugSafety.htm**, provides links to information in the following categories:

- Drug labeling, including patient labeling, professional labeling, and patient package inserts;
- Drugs that have a Risk Evaluation and Mitigation Strategy (REMS) to ensure that their benefits outweigh their risks;
- A searchable database of postmarket studies that are required from, or agreed to by, drug companies to provide the FDA with additional information about a drug's safety, efficacy, or optimal use;

- **Clinicaltrials.gov**, a searchable database of clinical trials, including information about each trial's purpose, who may participate, locations, and useful phone numbers;
- Drug-specific safety information, including safety sheets with the latest information about the drug as well as related FDA press announcements, fact sheets, and drug safety podcasts;
- Quarterly reports that list certain drugs that are being evaluated for potential safety issues, based on a review of information in the FDA's Adverse Event Reporting System (AERS);
- Warning Letters, Import Alerts, Recalls, Market Withdrawals, and Safety Alerts;
- Regulations and guidance documents;
- Consumer information about using medications safely and disposing of unused medicines;
- Instructions how to report problems to the FDA through its MedWatch program;
- Consumer articles on drug safety; and
- The FDA's response to the Institute of Medicine's 2006 report on the future of drug safety.

By providing these up-to-date resources on a single page, the FDA hopes to help consumers and healthcare professionals find drug safety information faster and easier.

HEALTH INFORMATION ONLINE

QUESTION: What online health information sites do you recommend?

ANSWER: The number of online health-related information web sites is overwhelming to say the least. Much of the information posted online is unreliable, outdated, or misleading. The web site address can provide some help in determining the accuracy of the information it contains. For example, web site addresses that end in ".gov" (government agencies), ".edu" (educational institutions), or ".org" (professional organizations) may be more reliable than those that end in ".com", which are often trying to sell a product or service. You can also try to check how current the information is by looking at the last revision date, usually located at the bottom of the web site page. Other useful clues to determine the validity of the information provided on a web site include: is the name of the person/group who sponsors the web site listed, is contact information (e-mail, phone number, address, etc.) given, is your privacy protected, and does the web site make claims that seem too good to be true? Some online health information web sites that can be recommended include:

- American Cancer Society (**www.cancer.org**)
- American Diabetes Association (**www.diabetes.org**)
- American Heart Association (**www.heart.org**)
- National Heart, Lung, and Blood Institute (**www.nhlbi.nih.gov**)
- CDC (**www.cdc.gov**)
- FDA (**www.fda.gov**)
- American Academy of Family Physicians' FamilyDoctor.org (**www. familydoctor.org**)
- U.S. Department of Health & Human Services' healthfinder.gov (**www.healthfinder.gov**)
- KidsHealth (**www.kidshealth.org**)
- Mayo Clinic (**www.mayoclinic.com**)
- National Library of Medicine's MedlinePlus (**www.medlineplus.gov**)

If you have any questions regarding the information that you receive on a web site, please discuss it with a healthcare professional before making any health-related decisions.

<u>DRUGS AND FOOD</u>

<u>QUESTION</u>: How do I know if I should take my medication with food or not?

<u>ANSWER</u>: Always check with your pharmacist if you are not sure if you should take your medication with food or on an empty stomach. Pharmacists will usually label your prescription if it is important to take certain drugs with or without food, but sometimes these instructions

can be overlooked. Drugs taken by mouth must be absorbed through the lining of either the stomach or the small intestine and sometimes foods can affect this process. Some drugs are absorbed better when given with certain foods, but the absorption of drugs can be blocked by certain foods and prevent the medication from getting into the bloodstream. In addition, some drugs need to be taken with food to help reduce gastrointestinal irritation and other side effects. In general "Take On An Empty Stomach" usually means one hour before or two hours after a meal, while "Take With Food" means that the medication should be taken with food or right after a meal. In the table below I have listed some examples of drugs that should be taken with food and some drugs that are usually taken on an empty stomach. However, in some situations this decision is not clearcut, so be sure to ask your pharmacist or doctor what is best for you. For example, some drugs are better absorbed on an empty stomach, but may need to be taken with food to reduce stomach upset. Some examples of drugs that should or should not be taken with food are found below.

With Food

Aldactone, Ceftin, Corgard, Dilantin, Dyazide, Dynabac, Fortovase, Griseofulvin, Inderal, Lithium, Macrodantin, Mevacor, NSAIDs (ibuprofen-Motrin, naproxen-Naprosyn, Aleve, many others), Potassium, Tegretol, Tenormin

Without Food

Accolate, Adalat/Procardia, Capoten, Carafate, Cardizem, Cipro, Erythromycin (some formulations), Ferrous salts, Isoniazid, Lopid, Penicillins, Persantine, Reglan, Synthroid, Tetracycline

DRUGS AND DRIVING

QUESTION: What medications can affect the driving ability of an elderly person?

ANSWER: Numerous medications can affect your driving ability by causing drowsiness, dizziness, or by affecting your vision, hearing, or judgment. In addition, the normal aging process is associated with many changes in the body, which can affect how drugs work. For example, body fat increases while total body water and proteins in the blood decrease with age. These changes can affect how drugs are distributed in the body and how they act. Fat-soluble drugs will have increased effects, but water-soluble drugs will have reduced effects. Age-related changes in liver and kidney function can also affect the activity of drugs taken by the elderly. In general, both liver and kidney functions decrease with age and there is a reduced ability to metabolize (detoxify) and get rid of (excrete) medications that are taken. This can lead to an increase in drug activity and side effects that can affect your ability to drive. Gastrointestinal changes that occur with aging may also affect how drugs are absorbed into the body, making some drugs more or less effective. Furthermore, the elderly have an increased sensitivity to drugs that affect the central nervous system, making them more potent.

Drugs that should be used with caution when driving would include those that can produce drowsiness, dizziness, blurred vision, ringing in the ears, confusion, mental alertness, or alter reaction time. It is beyond the scope of this column to list all the medications that can produce these effects so I will only provide a few examples here. Many different types of drugs can cause drowsiness, dizziness, or confusion, including sedatives, sleep medication, pain relievers, muscle relaxants, antidepressants, anti-psychotics, blood pressure medications, and antihistamines. Even some herbal products like St. Johns Wort or Kava can cause these effects. Several of these drugs can also slow down a person's reaction time. In addition, blurred vision is a common side effect of numerous drugs. Stimulant-like medications used for weight control or congestion can potentially affect a person's driving ability by producing a false sense of alertness or by causing nervousness. Diabetic patients taking insulin or oral agents to control their blood sugar should also have the potential for developing low blood sugar (hypoglycemia), which can affect their mentation and driving ability. Finally, some drugs like salicylates can affect one's hearing ability or produce ringing in the ears, which may affect driving ability. It should be noted that the use of alcohol can enhance many of these potentially dangerous drug side effects. All drivers need to carefully read all package labeling and prescription labeling to determine if their medication can produce side effects and impair their driving ability. If you are not sure, make sure that you ask your doctor and pharmacist about the side effects of all medications (prescription and non-prescription) that you take.

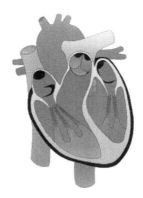

CHAPTER 2
CARDIOVASCULAR PROBLEMS

HEART FAILURE
AND ITS TREATMENT

<u>QUESTION</u>: What types of drugs are used to treat heart failure?

<u>ANSWER</u>: Heart failure or congestive heart failure (CHF) affects nearly 5 million people in the U.S., with more than 400,000 new cases diagnosed every year. For people over age 65, heart failure is one of the most frequent causes of hospitalization. Furthermore, as the population ages CHF will become an even more common medical problem.

CHF is caused by an inefficient heart that cannot pump blood effectively out to the various body parts. This leads to a backup of blood flow and causes swelling of the arms, legs, or abdomen, decreased urination, fatigue, and shortness of breath. Some causes of heart failure include coronary heart disease, high blood pressure, heart muscle diseases, heart defects, severe anemia, and alcohol abuse.

If the cause of CHF is known and can be treated, then this is the first step in treating someone with heart failure. However, for most patients a combination of 3 or 4 different types of medications are used for the treatment of CHF. These include: a water tablet (diuretic) to remove excess fluid from the body; digoxin to increase the heart's pumping ability; an ACE inhibitor which improves blood flow by expanding blood vessels; and a beta-blocker to prevent damage to heart cells caused by hormones. Sometimes other drugs can be used if a person cannot tolerate these medications or if other medical problems are present. The use of these drugs can result in decreased mortality, fewer hospitalizations, and a general improvement in symptoms allowing for a better quality of life. Your doctor can determine which medication or combination of medications is best for you. I have listed below some examples of drugs used to treat congestive heart failure.

Drug Type
Generic Name (Trade Name)

- **Diuretic (water tablets)(used to decrease excess fluid)**
  Furosemide (Lasix); Bumetanide (Bumex); Ethacrynic acid (Edecrin); Torsemide (Dermadex); Amiloride (Midamor); Spironolactone (Aldactone); Triameterene (Dyrenium)
- **ACE Inhibitor (used to increase blood flow)**
  Quinapril (Accupril); Ramipril (Altace); Captopril (Capoten); Fosinopril (Monopril); Lisinopril (Prinivil, Zestril); Enalapril (Vasotec)
- **Digoxin (used to increase pumping ability of heart)**
  Digoxin (Lanoxin)
- **Beta Blocker (used to block hormone damage to the heart)**
  Carvedilol (Coreg); Metoprolol (Lopressor)

PLEASE NOTE: Other types of drugs used to treat CHF in some patients are not included in this listing.

QUESTION: I get short of breath and my ankles swell up now and then. I'm taking Celebrex for back pain and I wonder if this is OK?

ANSWER: Shortness of breath and swollen ankles are signs of congestive heart failure and you should see a physician for an evaluation.

The drug Celebrex is a medication that falls into the class of drugs known as nonsteroidal anti-inflammatory drugs or NSAIDs. NSAIDs are useful agents to treat pain and inflammation but one of their side effects is fluid retention and edema. Because of this, caution must be used when using this medication in patients with heart failure, high blood pressure, or other conditions that can cause fluid retention. In fact, a recent study showed that the use of NSAIDs by elderly patients doubles the risk of being hospitalized for CHF, and for those with a history of heart disease it increases the risk by more than 10 times. The newer NSAIDs like Celebrex were not included in this study, but until they can be proven to be safer, they should be used with caution in the elderly. Patients taking NSAIDs should immediately contact their physician if they get short of breath. Other commonly used NSAIDs include Voltaren (diclofenac), Lodine (etodolac), Nalfon (fenoprofen), Ansaid (flurbiprofen), Motrin or Advil (ibuprofen), Indocin (indomethacin), Orudis, Actron, or Oruvail (ketoprofen), Toradol (ketorolac), meclofenamate, Relafen, Naprosyn or Anaprox (naproxen), Daypro (oxaprozin), Feldene (piroxicam), Clinoril (sulindac), and Tolectin (tolmetin).

PLEASE NOTE: Celebrex now has a black-box warning in its labeling about an increased risk of serious and potentially life-threatening gastrointestinal and cardiovascular events associated with use of this drug.

QUESTION: I heard about a new drug on TV that is supposed to help people with heart failure. What can you tell me about it?

ANSWER: The news you heard is really about an old drug called spironolactone or Aldactone. As I discussed in an earlier column, heart failure or congestive heart failure (CHF) is a very common disorder, especially in the elderly. It is caused by an inefficient heart that cannot pump blood effectively out to various parts of the body. This leads to a backup of blood flow and causes swelling of the arms, legs, or abdomen; decreased urination; fatigue; and shortness of breath. Treatment of this medical problem usually includes a water tablet (diuretic) to remove excess fluid from the body; digoxin to increase the heart's pumping ability; an ACE inhibitor to improve blood flow; and a beta-blocker to prevent damage to the heart caused by hormones. Recently a very important study showed that if a low dose of spironolactone was added to the therapy in patients with severe CHF, the risk of death or hospitalization was reduced by approximately 30%. In fact, this study was stopped before it was finished because of the excellent results. How spironolactone works in CHF is not exactly known, but it probably prevents progressive heart failure by blocking a hormone known as aldosterone. This appears to have a protective effect on the heart and also prevents sodium retention and potassium loss by the body. Spironolactone, a diuretic that increases potassium levels, has been used for decades to treat a variety of medical conditions. Some of its potential side effects include gastrointestinal problems (cramping, diarrhea, gastritis, etc.), drowsiness, headache, confusion, skin rash, erectile dysfunction, irregular menses, abnormal hair growth, and breast pain or enlargement in males. In the recent CHF study, the drug was fairly well tolerated according to the researchers. Because of these study results, many more physicians will probably be using spironolactone in combination with other drugs to treat patients with heart failure.

QUESTION: I've read that a drug used for heart failure has caused many deaths from side effects. What can you tell me about it?

ANSWER: In 1999 a major study found that by adding the drug spironolactone or Aldactone to other standard treatments for congestive heart failure could reduce the risk of death by approximately 30%. Since that time its use has increased dramatically and the number of prescriptions for spironolactone has gone up 5 times. Unfortunately, hospitalizations and deaths due to high potassium levels caused by the drug have also tripled in this time period. Spironolactone is a diuretic (water pill) that helps to relieve the excess water and congestion of heart failure. It also appears to have a protective effect on the heart. Spironolactone, however, can cause potassium levels to build up in the blood, leading to irregular heart rates or sudden death. This can especially be a problem for heart failure patients with diabetes and kidney problems, or those eating potassium-rich foods. Patients taking nonprescription medications or herbal products containing large amounts of potassium could also be at greater risk when receiving spironolactone. This problem has created a dilemma for doctors who want to prescribe spironolactone for its beneficial effects, but also wants to avoid the potential complications of high potassium levels. In view of this, researchers have recommended that doctors closely monitor their patients potassium levels when spironolactone is prescribed and take into account other medical conditions or medications (prescription and nonprescription), and foods that can also increase potassium levels in the blood.

QUESTION: I heard on the news about a new drug for heart failure. What can you tell me about it?

ANSWER: Many different types of oral drugs are used to treat CHF. These include diuretics to remove excess fluid from the body, digoxin to increase the heart's pumping ability, ACE inhibitors to improve blood flow by expanding blood vessels, and beta-blockers to prevent damage to heart cells caused by hormones. The new drug you heard about is Natrecor (generic name nesiritide), which is only given intravenously. It is the first injectable drug approved for heart failure in over a decade. It will be used in hospitals for patients with acute congestive heart failure who have difficult breathing when they are at rest or with minimal activity so that they can breathe more easily. Natrecor is a new biotechnology drug that is similar to a naturally occurring hormone in the body that aids healthy functioning of the heart. Natrecor works to correct CHF by helping to expand (dilate) blood vessels and it also has diuretic activity. Clinical studies have shown that Natrecor can significantly improve patient breathing and it provides physicians with another tool for acute heart failure. The major side effect of Natrecor is low blood pressure (hypotension) so patients need to be closely monitored when the drug is given intravenously. Approximately one million people are hospitalized each year in the U.S. due to acute CHF.

QUESTION: I heard that a new drug was approved to treat heart failure in black patients only. What can you tell me about it?

ANSWER: The FDA recently approved BiDil to treat heart failure (HF) in black patients only, which makes it the first medicine to be targeted for a specific racial group. HF is an epidemic in the U.S., affecting an estimated 5 million people. Among black individuals, the estimated prevalence of HF is 3.1% for men and 3.5% for women compared to 2.5% and 1.9% for white men and white women. African

Americans have a higher incidence of cardiovascular disease, and death rates are also higher for black males and females with HF compared to the white population. It is estimated that 750,000 African Americans have been diagnosed with HF and this number is expected to grow to approximately 900,000 people in 2010. While the exact cause(s) of heart failure are complex, it has been shown that a chemical known as nitric oxide (NO) may be involved. Several studies have reported that there are reduced levels of NO in black patients, which may make them more likely to develop heart failure. BiDil contains two different drugs that have been used for a long time to treat high blood pressure and angina. It contains isosorbide dinitrate and hydralazine, which help to expand blood vessels, reducing blood pressure and improving blood flow. Isosorbide dinitrate is converted to NO in blood vessels and leads to blood vessel expansion (vasodilation). Meanwhile, hydralazine has been shown to prolong these vasodilating effects by protecting the NO formed by isosorbide dinitrate from breaking down (deactivating). Hydralazine is a vasodilator agent and is also an antioxidant. The FDA approved the use of BiDil based upon a large study in black patients with HF. In this study, the use of BiDil resulted in a 43% reduction in deaths and a 39% decrease in hospitalizations for HF compared to those who did not receive BiDil. In addition, the quality of life was much better for patients taking BiDil. BiDil is usually taken 3 times a day in conjunction with other drugs used to treat heart failure.

PLAVIX AND ASPIRIN

QUESTION: Why are Plavix and aspirin sometimes given together to prevent blood from clotting?

ANSWER: Both Plavix (clopidogrel) and aspirin are known as anti-platelet drugs. The means by which blood coagulation (clotting) takes place is a very complex process. The first step in this process occurs when blood platelets adhere (stick) to each other when a blood vessel wall is damaged. Platelets are small, oval disks found in the blood. This initial activity of platelets then initiates a complicated pathway of events that leads to the formation of fibrin that reinforces the platelets that are stuck together, forming a clot. Both Plavix and aspirin prevent blood from clotting by inhibiting the platelets to aggregate (stick together). However, they each do this in a different way. Basically, aspirin prevents platelets from clumping together by inhibiting an enzyme (cyclooxygenase) that is needed to produce a substance that promotes platelet stickiness. It should be noted that an estimated 5% to 45% of patients might be resistant to the anti-platelet effects of aspirin. Plavix on the other hand, inhibits a chemical (ADP) that is also needed for platelets to clump together and form a linkage between them. Thus, by giving both Plavix and aspirin together you provide a two-pronged approach to prevent blood from clotting. Plavix and aspirin have been used together to prevent clotting in patients with acute coronary syndromes (e.g., unstable angina, acute myocardial infarction) and for interventions used to reverses coronary artery blockage such as angioplasty or stent placement. However, the use of Plavix and aspirin in combination can also increase the risk of bleeding.

PLEASE NOTE: On March 12, 2010 the FDA announced that the manufacturers of clopidogrel (Plavix) will place a new Black Box Warning into the drug's prescribing information. This Black Box Warning will caution healthcare providers of the reduced effectiveness of clopidogrel in patients who are "poor metabolizers" of the drug, and suggest that they consider the use of other antiplatelet medications or alternative dosing strategies for clopidogrel in these patients. Patients can determine if they are "poor metabolizers" by taking a genetic test.

PLAVIX AND PRILOSEC

QUESTION: Can Prilosec interfere with Plavix?

ANSWER: We don't know yet, but there is some concern that certain drugs known as proton pump inhibitors (PPIs) may make Plavix (clopidogrel) less effective. Plavix, an anti-clotting drug, is commonly used to prevent blood clots that could lead to heart attacks or strokes in cardiac patients. However, many people receiving Plavix may also take a proton-pump inhibitor to prevent internal bleeding and ulcers associated with Plavix. Proton-pump inhibitors include Prilosec (omeprazole), Zegerid (omeprazole), Nexium (esomeprazole), Prevacid (lansoprazole), Protonix (pantoprazole), and Aciphex (rabeprazole). In order to better understand how drugs like PPIs may affect the effectiveness of Plavix, the FDA has asked the makers of Plavix to work with them in conducting studies to obtain more information about combining these drugs. It appears that the reduced effectiveness of Plavix in some patients may be due to genetic differences in the way the body breaks down (metabolizes) Plavix or that other drugs (like PPIs) can interfere with the metabolism of Plavix. However, it could take several months to complete the studies and analyze the results. Until further information is available the FDA recommends the following:

- Healthcare providers should continue to prescribe and patients should continue to take Plavix as directed, because Plavix has demonstrated benefits in preventing blood clots that could lead to a heart attack or stroke.
- Healthcare providers should re-evaluate the need for starting or continuing treatment with a PPI, including Prilosec OTC, in patients taking Plavix.
- Patients taking Plavix should consult with their healthcare provider if they are currently taking or considering taking a PPI, including Prilosec OTC.

PLEASE NOTE: On March 12, 2010 the FDA announced that the manufacturers of clopidogrel (Plavix) will place a new Black Box Warning into the drug's prescribing information. This Black Box Warning will caution healthcare providers of the reduced effectiveness of clopidogrel in patients who are "poor metabolizers" of the drug, and suggest that they consider the use of other antiplatelet medications or alternative dosing strategies for clopidogrel in these patients. Patients can determine if they are "poor metabolizers" by taking a genetic test.

PLAVIX AND DRUG INTERACTIONS

QUESTION: I heard that some drugs can make Plavix less effective. What can you tell me about this?

ANSWER: Plavix is a blood thinner that is used by millions of Americans to reduce the risk of heart attacks and strokes. However, when taken together with other medications its anti-blood clotting effects can be reduced significantly, because these other drugs can block the conversion of Plavix into its active form. In view of this potential drug interaction, the FDA is warning patients to avoid certain drugs, if possible, when taking Plavix. Medications that may be a problem when combined with Plavix include:

* Diflucan (generic name: fluconazole)
* Felbatol (generic name: felbamate)
* Intelence (generic name: etravirine)
* Luvox (generic name: fluvoxamine)
* Nexium (generic name: esomeprazole) *
* Nizoral (generic name: ketoconazole)
* Prilosec (generic name: omeprazole) *
* Prozac, Serafem, and Symbyax (generic name: fluoxetine)
* Tagamet (generic name: cimetidine)
* Ticlid (generic name: ticlopidine)
* VFEND (generic name: voriconazole)

In addition, there are ongoing studies looking at other drugs that may interact with Plavix. Patients taking Plavix should not stop taking any of these drugs until they have discussed this with their doctor. It's dangerous to stop taking any medication without medical advice. Patients taking Plavix should call their doctor to discuss all the other drugs and supplements they are taking, including over-the-counter medications.

* May reduce the risk of gastrointestinal bleeding in patients taking Plavix plus aspirin.

PLEASE NOTE: On March 12, 2010 the FDA announced that the manufacturers of clopidogrel (Plavix) will place a new Black Box Warning into the drug's prescribing information. This Black Box Warning will caution healthcare providers of the reduced effectiveness of clopidogrel in patients who are "poor metabolizers" of the drug, and suggest that they consider the use of other antiplatelet medications or alternative dosing strategies for clopidogrel in these patients. Patients can determine if they are "poor metabolizers" by taking a genetic test.

GENERIC PLAVIX NOW AVAILABLE

QUESTION: I heard that Plavix is now available as a generic drug. What can you tell me about this?

ANSWER: On May 17, 2012 the U.S. Food and Drug Administration approved generic versions of the blood thinning drug Plavix (clopidogrel bisulfate), which helps reduce the risk of heart attack and stroke by making it less likely that platelets in the blood will clump and form clots in the arteries. Clopidogrel is FDA-approved to treat patients who have had a recent heart attack or a recent stroke, or have partial or total blockage of an artery (peripheral artery disease). Clopidogrel has a boxed warning to alert health care professionals and patients that the drug may not work well for those with certain genetic factors that affect how the body metabolizes the drug. Patients can be tested for these genetic factors to ensure that clopidogrel is the right choice for them. Also, certain medicines, such as proton pump inhibitors Prilosec (omeprazole) and Nexium (esomeprazole), reduce the effect of clopidogrel, leaving a person at greater risk for heart attack and stroke. Clopidogrel may cause bleeding, which can be serious and sometimes lead to death. While taking the drug, people may bruise and bleed more easily, be more likely to have nose bleeds, and it may take longer for all bleeding to stop. Clopidogrel is dispensed with a patient Medication Guide that provides important instructions on its use and drug safety information. Dr. Reddy's Laboratories, Gate Pharmaceuticals, Mylan Pharmaceuticals, and Teva Pharmaceuticals have gained FDA approval for 300 milligram (mg) clopidogrel. Apotex Corporation, Aurobindo

Pharma, Mylan Pharmaceuticals, Roxane Laboratories, Sun Pharma, Teva Pharmaceuticals, and Torrent Pharmaceuticals have received approval for 75 mg clopidogrel. Generic drugs approved by the FDA are of the same high quality and strength as brand-name drugs. The generic manufacturing and packaging sites must pass the same quality standards as those for brand-name drugs. This new approval of generic Plavix should make the drug much more affordable for many patients.

RISK FACTORS FOR
<u>HEART DISEASE</u>

<u>QUESTION</u>: It seems like everyone I know is taking a statin drug to lower his or her cholesterol. Is this a good idea?

<u>ANSWER</u>: There are currently six statin drugs available to treat high levels of LDL (bad) cholesterol-Mevacor or Altocor (also available as a generic, lovastatin), Zocor (also available as a generic, simvastatin), Pravachol (also available as a generic, pravastatin), Lescol, Lipitor and Crestor. All of these drugs block an enzyme in the liver that is involved in producing LDL cholesterol, high levels of which have been associated with heart disease. They are very effective in lowering LDL cholesterol levels and it has been suggested half-jokingly that statins should be put in the drinking water. They are one of the most profitable and widely promoted types of drugs. The LDL cholesterol "bar" is also being lowered and many more people are having these drugs prescribed for them. Because of the emphasis that has been placed on the use of statin drugs, we sometimes lose sight of the fact that there are many other controllable risk factors for heart disease that are just as important or even more important than bad cholesterol levels. Additional important risk factors that we can control include:

- High blood pressure
- High blood sugar
- High levels of homocysteine
- Cigarette smoking

- Obesity
- Lack of regular exercise
- Inflammation in blood vessels (high C-reactive protein levels)
- Low HDL (good cholesterol) levels

We may also overlook the fact that statin drugs, while very effective in lowering cholesterol, may also cause side effects such as muscle or liver problems. Other long-term use concerns such as their effect on mental function or other disease links are unknown at this time. In summary, statin drugs are very useful agents for many people with high cholesterol levels to reduce their risk of heart disease, but side effects are possible and there are numerous other important controllable risk factors that should not be ignored.

QUESTION: Is it true that statin drugs may help some people with normal cholesterol levels reduce heart disease?

ANSWER: Yes, a large new study, known as the JUPITER study, suggests that many people could have cardiovascular benefits from taking statin drugs, even if they have low cholesterol levels. This is very important because it is known that almost half of all heart attacks and strokes occur in people with normal or low cholesterol levels. The JUPITER study involved almost 18,000 people who did not have high cholesterol or a history of heart disease, but they did have high levels of a protein in the blood known as C-reactive protein or CRP. High levels of CRP are associated with inflammation in the body. It is thought that inflammation may play a crucial role in heart attacks and strokes by causing fatty deposits inside arteries to rupture, triggering blood clots that block blood flow. In addition to lowering "bad" cholesterol (LDL) and raising "good" cholesterol (HDL), statin drugs also reduce inflammation. In the JUPITER study, men and women were given either the statin drug Crestor (rosuvastatin) or a "dummy" pill (placebo) and were to be followed for 3 to 4 years to see who had the most cardiovascular problems, such as a heart attack or stroke. However, the study was stopped after only 2 years because people receiving the statin drug were over 40% less likely to have a heart attack or stroke or need angioplasty or bypass surgery than people getting the "dummy" pill. They were also 20% less likely to die. While these study results are dramatic, it is not known whether lowering cholesterol, reducing inflammation, or a combination of both is responsible for these effects. In addition, many other risk factors for heart disease such as obesity, smoking, high blood pressure, or diabetes are still very important considerations in preventing cardiovascular problems. Crestor (rosuvastatin) is the most potent statin drug currently available, but numerous others are on the market, including Lipitor (atorvastatin), Lescol (fluvastatin), Mevacor, Altoprev (lovastatin), Pravachol (pravastatin), and Zocor (simvastatin). Lovastatin, pravastatin, and simvastatin are also available as generic drugs. Your physician can determine if statin therapy is appropriate for you.

PLEASE NOTE: There are currently seven statin drugs available: atorvastatin (Lipitor), fluvastatin (Lescol), lovastatin (Mevacor, Altoprev), pitavastatin (Livalo), pravastatin (Pravachol), rosuvastatin (Crestor), and simvastatin (Zocor). Atorvastatin, lovastatin, pravastatin, and simvastatin are also available as generic drugs.

HIGH BLOOD PRESSURE (HYPERTENSION)

QUESTION: I take medication for high blood pressure and use a home monitor to measure my blood pressure. Why is my blood pressure higher in the morning?

ANSWER: A few years ago a group of expert doctors and researchers developed new guidelines for classifying blood pressure. This new classification is based upon current scientific information that has been reviewed by the National Institutes of Health. Normal blood pressure is now less than 120/80. A blood pressure of 120-139 over 80-89 is now called "prehypertension". The higher number refers to your systolic blood pressure, which is the pressure in your blood vessels when the heart contracts to force blood out into the circulation. The lower number is the diastolic blood pressure, which is the pressure in your blood vessels between heartbeats when the heart relaxes. High blood pressure or hypertension causes our heart to work harder and can lead to an enlarged heart, heart attack, or stroke. High blood pressure is called the "silent killer" because there are usually no symptoms unless the pressure is very high.

Blood pressure can vary throughout the day depending upon foods eaten, physical activity, and emotional stress. Unfortunately, for some people, their blood pressure may be too high in the morning, which is referred to as "morning hypertension". Blood pressure can increase in the morning because the body releases hormones such as adrenaline and noradrenaline into the bloodstream. These hormones give you a boost of energy, but can also raise your blood pressure. The morning increase in blood pressure is usually seen between 6:00 am and noon. People with morning hypertension may have a higher risk of a heart attack or stroke due to this increase in blood pressure. In fact, the risk of sudden death, heart attack, and stroke is 30% to 50% higher in the early morning hours. People at risk for morning hypertension include those with high blood pressure, diabetes, or over the age of 65. You may also be at risk if you use tobacco or alcohol, are overweight, or have high cholesterol levels.

The use of a home monitor is a good idea for people to check their blood pressure. Your blood pressure should be checked in the morning, about an hour after you wake-up, and in the evening, about an hour before you go to sleep, using the same arm each time. Taking 3 consecutive measurements (about 1 minute apart) will provide a more accurate understanding of your "true" blood pressure. Avoid food, caffeine, or tobacco at least 30 minutes before the measurement. Sit in a chair with your legs and ankles uncrossed and your back supported. Your arm should be at the same level as your heart and rested on a table or counter. You should also keep a log of your blood pressure readings and bring it to your doctor every appointment. Your doctor may make changes in your medications based on your home blood pressure readings, which may include changing the type of medication or the time you take it.

QUESTION: I've heard that plain old "water pills" are just as good as newer, more expensive drugs for treating high blood pressure. Is this true?

ANSWER: Recent results from a very large study have shown that thiazide diuretics ("water pills") may work as well as or even better at lowering high blood pressure than more costly newer drugs known as ACE inhibitors and calcium channel blockers. Some widely available thiazide diuretics include chlorothiazide (Diuril), hydrochlorothiazide (Hydrodiuril, Esidrix), methyclothiazide (Enduron, trichlormethiazide (Metahydrin, Naqua) and chlorthalidone (Hygroton). In this study over 33,000 people over the age of 55 who had high blood pressure (hypertension) and at least one other coronary heart disease risk factor (e.g., high cholesterol, family history of heart disease at an early age, diabetes, obesity, lack of exercise, smoking) were followed from 1994 to 2002. Some of the study patients received chlorthalidone (Hygroton) while others received either amlodipine (Norvasc)-a calcium channel blocker, or lisinopril (Prinivil, Zestril)-an ACE inhibitor. Results from this study (known as ALLHAT) showed that all 3 of these medications were equally effective at preventing fatal coronary heart disease and nonfatal heart attacks. The thiazide diuretic (chlorthalidone) also proved to be more effective than the other two drugs for preventing heart failure. In view of these study results, many physicians now feel that thiazide diuretics should be the first drug prescribed for patients with hypertension. They may not only be better, but far less expensive with many generic products available. The treatment of high blood pressure, however, can be complicated. Your physician can best determine which anti-hypertensive medication is most appropriate for your individual situation. More information about this landmark study can be found on the Internet at **www.nhlbi.nih.gov/health/allhat/ index.htm**. It should also be noted that the National Heart, Lung, and Blood Institute (NHLBI) recently revised its blood pressure guidelines and people with blood pressure between 120/80 and 139/89 are now placed in a category called "pre-hypertension", which raises a person's risk of stroke, heart failure, and kidney disease. The new guidelines recommend that pre-hypertension is best treated with exercise, weight loss, and a more balanced diet. Medications such as a diuretic are usually recommended when the blood pressure exceeds 140/90, and more than one drug may be necessary in some situations.

QUESTION: Are water pills useful for high blood pressure?

ANSWER: Yes, they are and this subject has been recently reviewed in a Johns Hopkins Health Alert (**www.johnshopkinshealthalerts.**

com, 2011). Very few medicines have been studied as intently or used as successfully for as many years as diuretics. Whether they are taken alone or in combination with other hypertension drugs, diuretics have consistently been shown to be safe, effective, and relatively inexpensive. Often referred to as fluid or water pills, diuretics help reduce blood pressure by increasing the removal of sodium and fluid from the blood into the urine by the kidneys. Probably more important, some diuretics also lower blood pressure by promoting dilation of small blood vessels. There are three types of diuretics and each one acts on a different site in the kidney.

- **Thiazide diuretics**—These are the most commonly used diuretics. Examples include hydrochlorothiazide and chlorthalidone.
- **Loop diuretics**—These diuretics, such as furosemide (Lasix), are more powerful for salt and water excretion than thiazides and are often used in people with heart failure or kidney disease.
- **Potassium-sparing diuretics**—These medications may be used in combination with a thiazide diuretic to counteract potassium loss. Some examples are triamterene (Dyrenium), spironolactone (Aldactone) and eplerenone (Inspra).

Despite their declining popularity over the years, diuretics have been vindicated by recent studies showing that this class of drugs is not only as effective as other hypertension drugs but may in fact provide better protection from cardiovascular disease, heart failure, stroke and other complications. The seminal study to reassert the effectiveness of diuretics was the Antihypertensive and Lipid-Lowering Treatment to Prevent Heart Attack Trial (ALLHAT), which followed about 33,000 people with hypertension who had at least one other risk factor for heart disease (for example, type 2 diabetes or smoking). The participants were randomly assigned to receive the thiazide diuretic chlorthalidone or one of two newer drugs—the ACE inhibitor lisinopril (Prinivil, Zestril) or the calcium channel blocker amlodipine (Norvasc). Chlorthalidone was found to be superior to the ACE inhibitor in terms of lowering risk of stroke, heart failure and angina (chest pain) and more effective at preventing heart failure than the calcium channel blocker. Several studies in the past few years have re-examined the ALLHAT data and come to similarly positive conclusions. Nevertheless, thiazide diuretics are not always the choice drugs for everyone. A beta-blocker may be the preferred option for someone with coronary artery disease and an ACE inhibitor may be the first choice for a person with kidney disease.

High blood pressure or hypertension is a very common problem that affects about 50 million people in the U.S. and nearly one-third of them don't know they have it. While high blood pressure produces few symptoms, if it is not corrected it can lead to a stroke, heart attack, or heart disease. It is often referred to as the "silent killer". Many people are concerned about high cholesterol levels, but high blood pressure is even more important to be concerned about. In most cases, the cause of high blood pressure is unknown. The regulation of blood pressure is very complex and a number of body systems are involved including the nervous system, the kidneys, blood vessels, the heart, and various enzymes or hormones.

QUESTION: I've heard that the numbers for high blood pressure have changed. What are they now and what can be done to treat this problem?

ANSWER: A few years ago, a group of expert doctors and researchers developed new guidelines for classifying blood pressure. This new classification is based upon current scientific information that has been reviewed by the National Institutes of Health. Normal blood pressure is now less than 120/80. The higher number refers to your systolic blood pressure, which is the pressure in your blood vessels when the heart contracts to force blood out into the circulation. The lower number is the diastolic blood pressure, which is the pressure in your blood vessels between heartbeats when the heart relaxes. High blood pressure or hypertension causes our heart to work harder and can lead to an enlarged heart, heart attack, or stroke. High blood pressure is called the "silent killer" because there are usually no symptoms unless the pressure is very high. In order to classify your blood pressure, an average of two or more blood pressure measurements is made after you have been seated quietly for at least 5 minutes. A blood pressure of 120-139 over 80-89 is now called "prehypertension". If you are in this "prehypertensive" range, lifestyle changes such as weight reduction, dietary changes, regular exercise 30-45 minutes per day several days a week, stopping smoking, lowering alcohol consumption, and limiting your sodium intake can be helpful. People with a blood pressure of 140-159 over 90-99 are classified as having stage 1 hypertension, and people with a blood pressure of 160 or higher over 100 or higher are classified as having stage 2 hypertension. If one of the numbers is high, but the other number is within the range, you fall into the higher category. In most people over 50, the upper number is more important. If you have a blood pressure greater than 140/90 you may need medication to lower your blood pressure. Usually a diuretic (water pill) is used initially. Other medications or combinations of medications may also be used if you have another medical problem such as diabetes, kidney disease, or heart disease. Your doctor can determine if medication is necessary and which ones are best for you.

QUESTION: I heard about a new combination drug for high blood pressure. What can you tell me about it?

ANSWER: The regulation of blood pressure is very complex and a number of body systems are involved including the nervous system, the kidneys, blood vessels, the heart and various enzymes or hormones. In view of this complexity, a number of different drugs are utilized to help lower high blood pressure. Some drugs act on the kidneys, such as water tablets or diuretics. Others work on the nervous system or heart. Still others work to expand blood vessels, which help lower blood pressure. Sometimes a combination of drugs is used to treat hypertension because they work together on different body systems and produce an "additive" effect.

The new combination drug recently approved for hypertension is Tekturna HCT. It is a once daily medication that contains two drugs that work together to produce additive effects for lowering blood pressure. It contains aliskiren, which works by blocking an enzyme in the kidneys known as renin, which is associated with the regulation of blood pressure. By blocking this enzyme, it prevents a chemical from being produced that constricts (narrows) blood vessels and raises blood pressure. It also contains a diuretic that works to lower blood pressure by riding the body of unneeded water and salt. The most common side effects of Tekturna HCT include dizziness, flu-like symptoms, diarrhea, cough, and tiredness. However, it can also cause injury and death to a developing fetus and must not be used by someone who is pregnant.

QUESTION: I heard that a new triple-drug combination tablet was approved for high blood pressure. What can you tell me about it?

ANSWER: The FDA recently approved Tribenzor, a new three-in-one combination product for the treatment of high blood pressure (hypertension). Tribenzor is not indicated for the initial therapy of hypertension, but instead may be useful for people with high blood pressure that cannot be controlled by a combination of other types of anti-hypertensive medications. The active ingredients in Tribenzor target 3 separate mechanisms involved in blood pressure regulation. The 3 ingredients in Tribenzor are: amlodipine, a calcium channel blocker that blocks blood vessels from narrowing/constricting; olmesartan, which blocks an enzyme in the body preventing both the narrowing/constricting of blood vessels as well as the retention of sodium in the body; and hydrochlorothiazide, a diuretic. Together these drugs allow blood vessels to relax so that blood can flow more easily. All of these individual medications have been available for quite some time to treat hypertension, but Tribenzor is the first product to contain all three. High blood pressure affects approximately 74 million adults in the United States and if left untreated can lead to heart attacks and stroke. It is estimated that up to 85% of people with hypertension may need multiple medications and many need 3 or more to control their blood pressure. Tribenzor is taken once daily and its most common side effects include dizziness, edema, headache, fatigue, inflammation of the nose and throat, muscle spasms, nausea, upper respiratory tract infection, diarrhea, urinary tract infections, and joint swelling.

QUESTION: I heard about a new combination drug for high blood pressure. What can you tell me about it?

ANSWER: The FDA recently approved Tekamlo, a new two-in-one combination product for the treatment of high blood pressure (hypertension). Tekamlo is indicated for initial therapy in patients likely to need multiple drugs to lower their blood pressure to an appropriate level. The two active ingredients in this product include amlodipine, a widely used calcium channel blocker that lowers blood pressure by relaxing blood vessel walls and aliskiren (Tekturna) that blocks an enzyme made by the kidneys that leads to blood vessel narrowing and high blood pressure. Both of these medications allow the blood to flow more easily and lower blood pressure. Tekamlo is taken once daily and its blood pressure lowering effects are attained within one to two weeks. The most common side effect of Tekamlo is peripheral edema, which can occur in more than 2% of patients.

QUESTION: I heard that a new triple-drug combination tablet was approved for high blood pressure. What can you tell me about it?

ANSWER: The FDA recently approved Amturnide, a new three-in-one combination product for the treatment of high blood pressure (hypertension). Amturnide is not indicated for the initial therapy of hypertension, but instead may be useful for people with high blood pressure that cannot be controlled by a combination of other types of anti-hypertensive medications. The active ingredients in Amturnide target 3 separate mechanisms involved in blood pressure regulation. The 3 ingredients in Amturnide are: amlodipine, a calcium channel blocker that blocks blood vessels from narrowing/constricting; aliskiren, which blocks an enzyme in the body preventing both the narrowing/constricting of blood vessels as well as the retention of sodium in the body; and hydrochlorothiazide, a diuretic. Together these drugs allow blood vessels to relax so that blood can flow more easily. All of these individual medications have been available for some time to treat hypertension, but Amturnide is the first product to contain all three. Amturnide is taken once daily and its most common side effects include dizziness, edema, headache, fatigue, and inflammation of the nose and throat.

QUESTION: What generic drugs are available to treat high blood pressure?

ANSWER: Since there are so many different drugs available to treat hypertension, I have only listed below and on the next page some common examples of generic antihypertensive medications that are available.

Generic Medications Used To Lower Blood Pressure
Type of Drug (Class)
Generic Name (Trade Name)

- **Diuretics (water pills)**

    Hydrochlorothiazide(Hydrodiuril);Chlorthalidone(Hygroton); Methyclothiazide (Enduron); Hydroflumethiazide (Diucardin); Trichlormethiazide (Naqua); Furosemide (Lasix)

- **Beta-Blockers**

    Propranolol (Inderal); Atenolol (Tenormin); Timolol (Blocarden); Sotalol (Betapace); Acebutolol (Sectral); Nadolol (Corgard); Labetolol (Normodyne)

- **Calcium Channel Blockers**

    Nifedipine extended-release (Adalat CC, Procardia XL); Nicardipine (Cardene); Diltiazem extended-release (Cardizem CD, Dilacor XR, Diltia XT, Tiazac, Cartia XT); Verapamil (Calan)

- **ACE Inhibitors**

    Captopril (Capoten); Lisinopril (Prinivil, Zestril); Enalapril (Vasotec)

- **Alpha-Blockers**

    Prazosin (Minipress); Doxazosin (Cardura)

QUESTION: My doctor switched me from an ACE inhibitor to Cozaar for my high blood pressure. I also take hydrochlorothiazide and triamterene. What can you tell me about these drugs?

ANSWER: Cozaar is known as an angiotensin II receptor blocker or ARB for short. It lowers blood pressure by blocking the action of angiotensin II, which causes blood vessels to narrow or constrict. This helps to expand blood vessels and lower blood pressure. ACE inhibitors (e.g., Capoten, Captopril, Monopril, Lotensin, Prinivil, Zestril, Lisinopril, Vasotec, Enalapril, Accupril, Aceon, etc.) block an enzyme known as ACE (angiotensin-converting enzyme), which helps to produce angiotensin II and also prevents blood vessels from narrowing to lower blood pressure. So in simple terms these two types of drugs work in a similar way to lower blood pressure, but are different. Sometimes a doctor will switch from one type of drug to another because the patient has side effects, or the first drug may not be working well to lower blood pressure. For example, many people cannot take ACE inhibitors because they can cause a chronic cough as a side effect. On the other hand, ACE inhibitors may be more useful in patients with diabetes. Hydrochlorothiazide is a diuretic (water pill) that lowers blood pressure. When used in combination with an ACE inhibitor or ARB, diuretics help to lower blood pressure to a greater extent. Triamterene is also a diuretic, but it helps the body to retain potassium, which is lost when using other diuretics like hydrochlorothiazide. Treatment of high blood pressure is very important and the drug or drugs used depend upon your individual situation. Various health problems such as diabetes, kidney disease, or heart disease help to determine what drugs should be used. You should discuss your specific drug therapy with your doctor. I will be reviewing new high blood pressure guidelines in a future column.

QUESTION: I take propranolol (Inderal) for high blood pressure. Can it cause me to have bad dreams or nightmares?

ANSWER: Yes, propranolol (Inderal) and other similar medications known as beta-blockers can cause frequent or bizarre dreams, and nightmares. Other common beta-blockers include atenolol (Tenormin), metoprolol (Lopressor), timolol (Blocadren), sotalol (Betapace), nadolol (Corgard), labetalol (Normadyne, Trandate), carvediol (Coreg), and others. These drugs can influence dreaming by altering the amounts of certain chemicals in the brain during sleep. It is not known why dreaming occurs during sleep, but everyone dreams. Usually people dream for about 2 hours each night but only about 5% of dreams are recalled when awaken. A nightmare is nothing more than a dream about engulfment, persecution, trauma, or terror. The most vivid and active dreams always occur during sleep when there are rapid eye movements under the sleeper's eyelids. This is known as REM (rapid eye movement) sleep. Some researchers have suggested that REM sleep is a time when the mind processes the day's experiences similar to a computer uploading files and updating its programs. In general, other medications that may affect dreaming or cause nightmares include some drugs used to treat depression, insomnia, high blood pressure, malaria, Parkinson's disease (PD), HIV, and Alzheimer's disease (AD). Barbiturates and opiod drugs can also alter dream patterns. Please note that I have not listed all the drugs that can affect dreaming and if you want to know about the medication that you take, make sure to "Ask The Pharmacist" or your doctor for advice.

QUESTION: What medications or supplements should I avoid that can make my high blood pressure worse?

ANSWER: A number of medications and dietary supplements can worsen blood pressure and this topic was recently discussed in a Johns Hopkins Health Alert (**www.johnshopkinshealthalerts.com**, 2010). Medications that can worsen hypertension include ibuprofen (Motrin, Advil); corticosteroids like prednisone; cyclosporine (Gengraf, Neoral, Sandimmune; used to suppress the immune system); epoetin alfa (Epogen, Procrit; used to treat anemia in cancer patients); estrogens such as those in hormone replacement therapy; migraine drugs such as sumatriptan (Imitrex); the weight loss drug sibutramine (Meridia); and nasal decongestants. Over-the-counter cough, cold, and asthma medications also may raise blood pressure, so always check with your doctor before using one. It's also important to get your doctor's approval before using any dietary or herbal supplements. These products are not regulated by the FDA, but in some cases, they can be just as powerful as any drug. For example, the herbal supplement ephedra has caused numerous deaths due to its deleterious effects on blood pressure and the heart. Appetite suppressants can also raise blood pressure to dangerous levels. Make sure all of your doctors know that you have high blood pressure and be sure to ask whether any new medication or supplement will have a negative effect on your blood pressure control.

QUESTION: You've recently written about medications to treat high blood pressure. What can someone do to reduce his or her blood pressure without drugs?

ANSWER: New recommendations from the Joint National Committee on the Prevention, Detection, Evaluation, and Treatment of High Blood Pressure (JNC7) now emphasizes that the risk of cardiovascular disease begins to increase at lower blood pressure levels than previously thought. A new classification of blood pressure now includes a category known as "prehypertension", which includes people with an upper blood pressure (systolic) reading of 120-139 and a lower (diastolic) reading of 80-89. For people in this new "prehypertension" category, the importance of "lifestyle" changes are recommended to stop the blood pressure from getting higher and causing actual hypertension. I have listed below and on the next page some lifestyle changes and how they can help to lower your blood pressure.

Lifestyle Change #1: Reduce Weight

Recommendation: Maintain normal weight
Average Reduction In Systolic Pressure (mm Hg)*: 5-20 per 22 pounds of weight lost

Lifestyle Change #2: Watch What You Eat

Recommendation: Adopt a diet rich in fruits, vegetables, and low-fat dairy products with reduced intake of saturated and total fat
Average Reduction In Systolic Pressure (mm Hg) *: 8-14

Lifestyle Change #3: Reduce Salt Intake

Recommendation: Reduce dietary sodium intake
Average Reduction In Systolic Pressure (mm Hg)*: 2-8

Lifestyle Change #4: Increase Exercise

Recommendation: Regular aerobic physical activity such as brisk walking at least 30 minutes per day, most days of the week
Average Reduction In Systolic Pressure (mm Hg) *: 4-9

Lifestyle Change #5: Reduce Alcohol Consumption

Recommendation: Men: Limit of 2 drinks/day; Women: Limit of 1 drink/day
Average Reduction In Systolic Pressure (mm Hg)*: 2-4

*(Upper Number)

QUESTION: I heard about a new combination drug for high blood pressure. What can you tell me about it?

ANSWER: The new combination drug recently approved for hypertension is Twynsta. It is a once daily medication that contains two drugs that work together to lower blood pressure. It contains telmesartan, which works by blocking an enzyme in the kidney that leads to constriction (narrowing) of the blood vessels. It also contains amlodipine, which produces relaxation of blood vessels by blocking calcium from going into blood vessel cells. Together, telmisartan and amlodipine have additive effects in lowering blood pressure. Telmisartan is also available by itself in the product Micardis, while amlodipine is available by itself as a generic product.

QUESTION: I heard about a new combination drug for high blood pressure. What can you tell me about it?

ANSWER: The new combination drug recently approved for hypertension is Valturna. It is a once daily medication that contains two drugs that work together to lower blood pressure. It contains aliskiren, which works by blocking an enzyme in the kidneys known as renin, which is associated with the regulation of blood pressure. By blocking this enzyme, it prevents a chemical from being produced that constricts (narrows) blood vessels and raises blood pressure. It also contains valsartan, which also works on the renin system in the kidneys, but at a different point. Together, aliskiren and valsartan have additive effects in lowering blood pressure. Aliskiren is also available by itself in the product Tekturna, while valsartan is available by itself in the product Diovan.

The most common side effects of Valturna include fatigue, inflammation in the nose and throat, diarrhea, flu-like symptoms, and dizziness. It can also cause injury and death to a developing fetus and must not be used by someone who is pregnant.

HIGH BLOOD PRESSURE
AND CHOLESTEROL

QUESTION: I heard about a new pill to treat both high blood pressure and high cholesterol. What can you tell me about it?

ANSWER: Both high blood pressure (hypertension) and high cholesterol levels are risk factors for developing coronary heart disease.

Approximately 30 million Americans have both of these risks and are at much greater risk of suffering a heart attack or stroke than those who have only one of these conditions. Other risk factors for coronary heart disease include: being over the age of 45 for men or 55 for women; a family history of premature heart disease; cigarette smoking; obesity; lack of exercise; diabetes; and a low level of "good" cholesterol (HDL).

Because many people have both high blood pressure and high cholesterol, a new prescription combination drug product was developed to treat both of these conditions at once. The product is named Caduet and it contains a "statin" drug to lower cholesterol (atorvastatin or Lipitor) along with a "calcium channel blocker" to lower the blood pressure (amlodipine or Norvasc). "Statin" drugs like Lipitor lower cholesterol levels by blocking its production in the liver. "Calcium channel blockers" like Norvasc lower blood pressure by helping to expand blood vessels (vasodilation) and lower resistance to blood flow. While neither of these medications are new, combining them into a single tablet may make it more convenient for patients to take and help people with complicated drug therapy regimens. People with both high blood pressure and high cholesterol should discuss this therapy with their physician to determine if Caduet is appropriate for them.

QUESTION: What can you tell me about the "polypill"?

ANSWER: The so-called "polypill" or "polycap" is a combination of six medications in one pill or capsule taken once a day to prevent heart attacks and strokes. The polypill (Polycap) is a combination of three blood pressure-lowering drugs in low doses (thiazide diuretic, atenolol, and ramipril), a statin drug (simvastatin), low dose aspirin, and folic acid-all in one capsule. All of these medications are available as generics so it should not be very expensive if the polypill ever comes to market, which could be several years from now. A recent study tested the polypill (Polycap) in about 2,000 people at 50 centers across India. The study participants were aged 45 to 80 years old without cardiovascular disease, but had at least one risk factor for heart disease—high blood pressure, high cholesterol, obesity, diabetes, or smoking. Some of the participants received the polypill (Polycap) once a day while others received aspirin alone, simvastatin alone, thiazide diuretic alone, combinations of blood pressure-lowering drugs alone, or combinations of blood pressure-lowering drugs plus aspirin. Results from this preliminary study showed that people taking the polypill (Polycap) lowered their blood pressure by about 7 units compared to those given no blood pressure-lowering medication. The polypill (Polycap) also reduced LDL (bad) cholesterol by about 23% and triglycerides by about 10%. Anti-clotting effects of the polypill (Polycap) were about the same as aspirin alone and reductions in heart rates were also about the same as other people taking atenolol. Side effects of the polypill (Polycap) were about the same as the other treatment groups. While these results are only preliminary and much more study is needed, the study researchers concluded that the polypill (Polycap) formulation could be conveniently used to reduce multiple risk factors and cardiovascular risk. A much larger study is now needed to see whether the polypill (Polycap) actually does cut heart attacks and strokes.

MEMORY TIPS FOR TAKING YOUR BLOOD PRESSURE MEDICATION

QUESTION: How can I help myself remember to take my blood pressure medication?

ANSWER: A recent Johns Hopkins Health Alert (**www. johnshopkinshealthalerts.com**, 2009) provided the following tips and information to help people remember to take their blood pressure medications:

- Buy an inexpensive plastic pillbox (available at pharmacies). Look for one with seven compartments that correspond to the days of the week (Sunday through Saturday), as well as times of day (morning, noon, evening), and keep your medication there.
- Leave a Post-It note on the refrigerator or bathroom mirror, or anywhere else you're likely to see it, as a reminder to take your pills.
- Take your blood pressure pills at the same time each day, and at the same time as an everyday activity (for example, eating breakfast or

brushing your teeth). This will make taking your medication a part of your daily routine.

- Medical pagers and electronic pillboxes are also available. These products make a beeping noise when it's time for your blood pressure medication.

- Each time you take your blood pressure medication, write it down in a log or on a calendar, including the date and time that you took it.

Additional Advice

- If you forget to take your blood pressure medicine, don't "double up" with an extra dose to make up for the lapse. Instead, just take your next scheduled dose.

- When you travel, make sure to pack an adequate supply of blood pressure pills in your carry-on luggage, purse, or briefcase. Also, bring some extra pills with you in case your return home is delayed.

- Never stop taking your blood pressure medication (or adjust its dose) on your own without first discussing it with your physician. Doing so can cause a dangerous spike in your blood pressure. Nor should you take a smaller dose (or skip a dose) in order to make your medicine last longer.

- Let your doctor know if you're having difficulty sticking with or paying for your pill regimen, and he or she may have some suggestions. In addition, don't forget to refill your prescription with plenty of time to spare so you don't run out of pills.

QUESTIONS TO ASK ABOUT YOUR BLOOD PRESSURE MEDICATION

QUESTION: What questions should I ask my doctor about my blood pressure medications?

ANSWER: Many people take one or more medications for high blood pressure to reduce their risk of heart attacks and strokes. A Johns Hopkins Health Alert (**www.johnshopkinshealthalerts.com**, 2009) reviewed 6 questions that patients should ask their doctor about blood pressure medications in order to get the most benefit from them:

1. What is the name of my blood pressure medicine? Is that the brand or generic name? How much will it cost? It's always a good idea to know both the generic and brand names of the medications you take, particularly in a medical emergency or when you visit a new doctor. If medication costs are an issue, let your doctor know. Many blood pressure drugs are available in less expensive, generic formulations that work just as well as the brands.

2. Should I be on a diuretic? Experts now say that most people with high blood pressure should take a diuretic, either alone or in combination with other blood pressure drugs. That's because diuretics of the thiazide type effectively lower blood pressure, reduce the risk of heart attacks and strokes, and cause few if any side effects.

3. What are the possible side effects of my medicine? Blood pressure drugs can cause side effects. Knowing in advance what side effects might occur can help you and your doctor decide which drug is best for you. Also find out what to do if you experience a side effect: Should you call your doctor right away or wait and see if it goes away on its own? Is it safe to drive if you're experiencing a side effect?

4. What time of day should I take my blood pressure drugs? Blood pressure varies over 24 hours. For example, it is typically low during the night and high when you wake up in the morning. Some blood pressure medications work better when taken at one time of day than at another, so ask your doctor about dose timing.

5. What foods and dietary supplements should I avoid while taking this medicine? Some drugs are made less effective or more powerful when taken with certain foods or beverages. For example, grapefruit juice can increase blood levels of calcium channel blockers.

6. What should I do if I forget to take my blood pressure medicine at the recommended time? Everyone occasionally forgets to take a dose of medication. Be prepared for this situation by asking for advice before it happens. Whether your physician recommends that you take your medication as soon as you remember or that you wait until the next dose will depend on how long it has been since your last dose.

Richard P. Hoffmann, RPh, PharmD

ASPIRIN TO
PREVENT HEART ATTACKS

QUESTION: What's the latest information about daily aspirin use?

ANSWER: I've written several columns in the past about the use of daily aspirin to prevent cardiovascular problems and/or cancer. Aspirin has numerous effects in the body including the prevention of blood clotting and anti-inflammatory properties. The anti-clotting effect of aspirin is a two-edged sword—it may help prevent heart attacks and strokes, but can also lead to serious gastrointestinal bleeding. Therefore, any potential benefits of regular daily aspirin use must be weighed against its potential risks. Recently (2012), researchers reviewed and analyzed 9 studies of aspirin use in the United States, Europe, and Japan that included over 100,000 participants who had never had a heart attack or stroke. Results from this retrospective analysis reported in the journal Archives of Internal Medicine showed that regular aspirin users were 10% less likely to have any type of heart attack and 20% less likely to have a nonfatal heart attack compared to non-aspirin users. However, aspirin users were also about 30% more likely to have a serious gastrointestinal bleeding event. The overall risk of dying during the study was the same for aspirin users and non-aspirin users as was the risk of dying from cancer. The study researchers concluded that the regular use of aspirin in people without prior cardiovascular disease might be more harmful than it is beneficial, but that treatment decisions need to be considered on a case-by-case basis depending on the individual's risk factors and family history. Risk factors for heart disease include high blood pressure, obesity, lack of exercise, smoking, diabetes, or high cholesterol levels. Risk factors for gastrointestinal bleeding can include a history of gastrointestinal bleeding, alcohol use, smoking, or the use of medications such as NSAIDs, corticosteroids, or blood thinners in addition to aspirin. Anyone regularly using aspirin or planning to start regular aspirin use should discuss this therapy with their physician.

QUESTION: I am 50 years old. Is it a good idea to take aspirin to prevent a heart attack?

ANSWER: According to a report from the U.S. Preventive Services Task Force, the benefits of aspirin therapy seem to outweigh the risks for men over age 40 and for postmenopausal women. Besides being useful to treat pain, inflammation, and fever, aspirin also helps to keep the blood from clotting. It does this by preventing the platelets in your blood from sticking together and forming clots. Platelets are small, oval discs found in the blood. However, aspirin therapy can also cause side effects such as upset stomach and constipation, as well as internal bleeding and ulcers. Therefore, people with active peptic ulcer or with bleeding disorders should not take aspirin. In addition, aspirin can interact with other medications and you should talk to your doctor and pharmacist about possible drug interactions. Although the optimum dose of aspirin for preventing heart attacks is not known, doses of 75-150 mg per day appear to be cardioprotective. Low-dose aspirin tablets contain 81 mg of aspirin and regular dose aspirin tablets contain 325 mg of aspirin. The daily use of aspirin may also be beneficial in younger adults who have other risk factors for heart disease such as high blood pressure, smoking, diabetes, or high cholesterol levels. People with these risk factors should talk to their physician about using aspirin for protection against heart attacks. For people who use the Internet, an interesting and easy to use "Coronary Heart Disease Risk Calculator" can be found at **www.intmed.mcw.edu/clincalc/heartrisk.html**. At this site you plug in your age, sex, smoking status, diabetic status, blood pressure, along with cholesterol levels and your risk of developing heart disease within 10 years is quickly estimated for you.

QUESTION: I've heard that taking aspirin can help if you are having a heart attack. What kind of aspirin should I take if this happens?

ANSWER: A heart attack occurs when a blood clot forms in a narrowed artery, blocking the flow of blood to the part of the heart muscle supplied by that artery. Other medical terms for this condition include coronary thrombosis, coronary occlusion, or myocardial infarction (MI). In order to survive a heart attack it is important to promptly recognize the warning signs and get immediate medical attention. If you feel an uncomfortable pressure, fullness, squeezing, or pain in the center of your chest that may spread to your shoulders, neck, or arms, and it lasts for 2 minutes or more, you may be having a heart attack.

Sweating, dizziness, fainting, nausea, indigestion, or shortness of breath may also occur, but not in all cases. More than 300,000 heart attack victims died in 1999 before reaching the hospital, many because they did not take their symptoms seriously and waited too long for help.

Studies have now shown that taking an aspirin tablet as soon as possible when having the symptoms described above can reduce the risk of dying by approximately 23%. Aspirin works by blocking the formation of a substance called thromboxane. Thromboxane causes blood vessels to narrow (constrict) and also promotes the formation of clots by helping blood platelets to stick to each other. Aspirin, therefore, help to prevent this vasoconstriction and blood clotting. Since time is so important when having a heart attack, you want to take aspirin that gets into the bloodstream as quickly as possible so that it can do its work. Research has demonstrated that the best way to do this is by chewing a regular uncoated aspirin tablet (325 mg) and swallowing with water if possible. Aspirin will usually get into the bloodstream within 3-5 minutes when taken this way. If the aspirin tablet is swallowed whole, it may take 20 minutes or longer for it to get into the blood. Do not use coated aspirin tablets, especially enteric coated tablets (e.g., Ecotrin, Halfrin, Easprin, etc.) or extended release aspirin (e.g., Zorprin, Bayer 8 hour caplets, etc.) since the coatings will delay the absorption of aspirin. It's probably a good idea to keep a small supply of uncoated aspirin tablets handy because you never know when you will need them. However, aspirin tablets can breakdown (smell like vinegar) and lose their potency over time or if stored improperly, so make sure your supply is fresh.

STATINS AND STROKE

QUESTION: Can statin drugs help to prevent strokes?

ANSWER: Yes, there is evidence that statin drugs may be helpful in stroke prevention, especially in patients at high risk for cardiovascular disease. In addition, a recent study has also shown that statins may be useful in the prevention of strokes in people who have had an ischemic stroke (not a hemorrhagic stroke) or a transient ischemic attack (TIA or mini stroke) within the previous six months. It is not known exactly how statin drugs may help to prevent strokes, but it may not be entirely related to their cholesterol-lowering effects. In addition to blocking the production of cholesterol in the liver, statins also have a number of other effects that may help to prevent strokes. Statins have anti-inflammatory activity, anti-clotting effects, plaque stabilizing actions, and can improve blood flow in vessels. All of these effects may aid in the prevention of a blocked artery in the brain causing a stroke. Over 600,000 people have a stroke each year in the U.S. Over two-thirds of all strokes occur in people over the age of 65. About 80% of strokes are due to a blocked artery to the brain (ischemic stroke) and the other 20% are due to a blood vessel rupture resulting in bleeding in or around the brain (hemorrhagic stroke). There are currently seven statin drugs available: atorvastatin (Lipitor), fluvastatin (Lescol), lovastatin (Mevacor, Altoprev), pitavastatin (Livalo), pravastatin (Pravachol), rosuvastatin (Crestor), and simvastatin (Zocor). Atorvastatin, lovastatin, pravastatin, and simvastatin are also available as generic drugs. Your physician can determine if statin therapy is appropriate for you.

STATIN USE

QUESTION: You have written several columns about the potential benefits of using a statin drug. What about statin side effects?

ANSWER: Statin drugs are very effective in reducing "bad" cholesterol (LDL) levels and are recommended for use in conjunction with diet and exercise to reduce the risk of heart attacks and strokes in patients with coronary heart disease, or those who are at high risk of coronary heart disease. In the past I have written columns about studies suggesting that statin use may be associated with a lower risk of fatal prostate cancer and that it possibly lowers the risk of death in elderly patients hospitalized due to the flu, but more study is needed. Besides lowering cholesterol levels, statin drugs have also been shown to have multiple effects including anti-inflammatory and anti-blood clotting properties. However, like all drugs, statins can also cause a number of side effects. Two serious side effects of statins include muscle problems which can lead to kidney failure, and liver problems. Fortunately, these side effects are not common and can be monitored by the patient and physician. In addition, all statins are contraindicated during pregnancy due to the possibility of birth defects. Other more common side effects of statins include diarrhea, upset stomach, muscle and joint pain, and alterations in some laboratory tests. Many additional side effects and drug interactions can occur with statin use, so patients should get as much information as possible from their physician, pharmacist, and other drug information sources. As more study data becomes available, new side effects of statins may be identified. For example, recent study data associates statin use with lung problems in smokers and former smokers, while other data suggests the risk of diabetes may be greater in statin users. As new information is discovered, the risk to benefit ratio of statins may change, but for now the potential benefits of statin therapy to reduce heart attacks and strokes in high-risk patients appear to outweigh the potential risks.

There are currently seven statin drugs available: atorvastatin (Lipitor), fluvastatin (Lescol), lovastatin (Mevacor, Altoprev), pitavastatin (Livalo), pravastatin (Pravachol), rosuvastatin (Crestor), and simvastatin (Zocor). Atorvastatin, lovastatin, pravastatin, and simvastatin are also available as generic drugs.

STATINS AND
RHEUMATOID ARTHRITIS

QUESTION: I have rheumatoid arthritis and high cholesterol. You recently wrote about new safety changes in the labeling for statin drugs. Should I stop taking my statin?

ANSWER: You should not stop taking your statin medication without consulting with your doctor. Rheumatoid arthritis (RA) is a chronic inflammatory disease that is associated with an increased risk of death from cardiovascular disease. In addition to lowering high cholesterol levels, statin drugs also have anti-inflammatory effects, which may be beneficial in people with RA. In fact, a recent population-based Canadian study (2011) involving more than 4,000 statin users who had RA revealed that patients who discontinued their statin medications had a 60% increased risk of death due to cardiovascular disease than those who did not discontinue their statin medication. The researchers emphasized the importance of patient compliance with statin therapy in people with RA. In addition, another recent study (2011) from Finland involving over 60,000 statin users with diabetes also showed that good adherence to statin therapy was associated with a significantly reduced incidence of a major coronary event like a heart attack compared to patients with poor adherence to statin therapy. Statin products include: Lipitor (atorvastatin), Lescol (fluvastatin), Mevacor (lovastatin), Altoprev (lovastatin extended-release), Livalo (pitavastatin), Pravachol (pravastatin), Crestor (rosuvastatin), and Zocor (simvastatin). Combination products include: Advicor (lovastatin/niacin extended-release), Simcor (simvastatin/niacin extended-release), and Vytorin (simvastatin/ezetimibe).

ANTIBIOTICS AND BLOOD PRESSURE MEDICATIONS

QUESTION: Can some antibiotics interfere with my blood pressure medication amlodipine?

ANSWER: A recent report published in the Canadian Medical Association Journal (January 17, 2011) warns that older people who are taking common blood pressure medications called calcium channel blockers face an increased risk of developing dangerously low blood pressure and possibly going into shock if they also take the commonly used antibiotic erythromycin (Ery-Tab, PCE) or clarithromycin (Biaxin). Oral calcium channel blockers include amlodipine (Norvasc), diltiazem (Cardizem, others), felodipine, isradipine (DynaCirc), nicardipine (Cardene), nifedipine (Adalat, Procardia), nisoldipine (Sular), and verapamil (Verelin). The researchers in this study collected data on people 66 and older who were taking a calcium channel blocker between 1994 and 2009. Results from the study found that 7,100 of these patients had been hospitalized for low pressure or shock, and that taking either erythromycin or clarithromycin was associated with an increased risk of trouble. The researchers reasoned that these antibiotics interfere with an enzyme in the liver that is needed to break down (metabolize) the calcium channel blocker causing it to accumulate in the blood stream and cause the blood pressure to drop too much. Study researchers also point out that grapefruit juice can also interfere with calcium channel blockers in the same way. However, a limitation of this study is not knowing how many of these patients had low blood pressure or shock from the infection for which they were receiving the antibiotic. In addition, it was not known how many of these patients consumed grapefruit juice. Nevertheless, the researchers point out that it is important for practitioners, pharmacists, and patients to be aware of this potential problem

CANCER AND AVAPRO

QUESTION: Is there an increased risk of getting cancer from taking Avapro for my high blood pressure?

ANSWER: No, not that I am aware of, but the FDA recently announced that drugs like Avapro do not increase the risk of cancer. The U.S. Food and Drug Administration announced on June 2, 2011 that a group of medications used to control high blood pressure, called angiotensin receptor blockers (ARBs), do not increase the risk of developing cancer in patients using the medications. In July 2010, the FDA reported that a safety review of ARBs would be performed after a published study found a small increased risk of cancer in patients taking an ARB compared to those patients not taking an ARB. For this safety review, the FDA evaluated 31 randomized clinical trials, comparing patients taking an ARB to patients not taking an ARB, looking for the incidence of cancer. The FDA has completed its review of controlled trial data on more than 155,000 patients randomized to ARBs or other treatments and found no evidence of an increased risk of cancer in patients who take an ARB.

ARBs are medications used alone or in combination with other medications to treat high blood pressure and other heart-related conditions. A list of ARBs is listed below.

Brand Names (Generic Names) Include:

- Atacand (candesartan)
- Avapro (irbesartan)
- Benicar (olmesartan)
- Cozaar (losartan)
- Diovan (valsartan)
- Micardis (telmisartan)
- Teveten (eprosartan)
- Several combination drug products

Sustained elevated blood pressure (hypertension) increases the risk of death, heart attacks, stroke, heart failure and kidney failure. That is why it is important to keep blood pressure at normal levels. There are many treatments available to control elevated blood pressure and ARBs are an important group of such treatments. The FDA has determined that any concern about a relationship between ARB use and development of cancer has been resolved by this analysis. People currently taking any antihypertensive medication should not stop taking it without talking to their health care professional first. Adverse events associated with ARB medications should be reported to the FDA MedWatch program at **www.fda.gov/medwatch**.

LASIX AND POTASSIUM LEVELS

QUESTION: My doctor increased my Lasix dose and added a prescription for potassium, which I can't get filled right away. How can I make sure that my potassium is OK until I get the prescription filled?

ANSWER: As you know, Lasix (generic name furosemide) is a diuretic (water tablet) that helps you get rid of excess fluids from the body. In doing this, it also removes potassium, which can lead to low potassium levels in the blood known as hypokalemia. Potassium is a very important element, essential for muscle contraction and nerve conduction. Low potassium levels can cause muscle weakness, dizziness, excessive urination, intestinal problems, and heart problems.

Severe hypokalemia can even lead to total paralysis and cardiac arrest. Therefore, it is extremely important to maintain proper potassium levels in the blood—not too high and not too low. Your doctor prescribed potassium chloride to take in conjunction with Lasix in order to prevent a possible potassium deficiency. Since you cannot get the potassium chloride prescription filled right away, food sources of potassium may be a good alternative. Excellent sources of potassium include cereals, dried peas and beans, fresh vegetables, fresh or dried fruits like bananas, fruit juices such as orange or prune, sunflower seeds, watermelon, nuts, molasses, cocoa, fresh fish, beef, ham, and poultry. People with adequate dietary potassium intake usually do not develop severe hypokalemia and may not need potassium supplements. There are also some non-prescription potassium products available, but be sure to check with your doctor before using them. Your doctor will also perform periodic blood tests to determine if your potassium levels are OK.

DRUG COMBINATIONS

QUESTION: I am a 75-year-old lady who takes Lanoxin and gemfibrozil each day. Is it OK to take these two drugs together?

ANSWER: Yes. Lanoxin or digoxin is a commonly used medication that has been available for a long time to help the heart pump blood more effectively and to slow down a heart that beats too fast. It should, however, be used with special care in the elderly because kidney function is reduced as you get older. If your kidneys are not working properly, the amount of Lanoxin can increase in the blood and produce toxic effects. Low levels of potassium in the blood can also increase the chances of toxicity. Numerous drugs can interact with Lanoxin to cause problems but gemfibrozil, which lowers fat levels in the blood, is not one of them. Because there are many drugs, both non-prescription and prescription, which can cause problems when taken with Lanoxin, always ask your pharmacist or doctor if it is OK before taking them. You should also notify your doctor if you develop a loss of appetite, lower stomach pain, nausea, vomiting, diarrhea, unusual tiredness or weakness, drowsiness, headache, blurred or yellow vision, skin rash or hives, or mental depression. These symptoms may indicate Lanoxin toxicity and a blood test may be necessary to see if you are having a problem from the Lanoxin.

LOWERING CHOLESTEROL

QUESTION: My doctor said that my cholesterol level is too high. How can I lower it?

ANSWER: High blood cholesterol can increase your risk of developing coronary heart disease, which is the main cause of death in the United States. Coronary heart disease may lead to a heart attack, or the need for bypass surgery or other procedures to increase the amount of blood going to your heart from your coronary blood vessels. In addition to high cholesterol levels, other "risk factors" for coronary heart disease include a family history of heart disease at an early age, high blood pressure, diabetes, smoking, a high-fat or high-cholesterol diet, obesity, lack of exercise and being over 45 years old for men or 55 for women.

A diet that is low in saturated fat and cholesterol may help to lower your blood cholesterol level. Saturated fat is found in meats and dairy products, "creamy" salad dressings and many other foods. Vegetables, fruits, and grains are low fat foods and many other low fat packaged foods are now available. Exercise may also help lower blood cholesterol levels. With your doctor's approval you may want to start an exercise program such as daily walking or other activities.

If your cholesterol level is not lowered enough after several months on your new eating and exercise program, a cholesterol lowering medication may be needed in addition to diet and exercise. On the next page I have put together a list which provides some information about cholesterol lowering medications.

<u>**Cholesterol Lowering Medications**</u>
Drug Name
How It Works
Possible Side Effects

- **Questran or Colestid**

   Traps cholesterol in your intestinal tract so that it will pass through your body

   Indigestion, gas, bloating, constipation

- **Niacin**

   Decreases the amount of cholesterol coming from your liver into the blood

   Flushing, itching, fatigue, stomach upset

- **Mevacor, Lescol, Crestor, Pravachol, Zocor, Lipitor & others**

   Blocks the manufacture of cholesterol in the body

   Headache, nausea, muscle aches

- **Lopid, gemfibrozil**

   Lowers fats (triglycerides) in the blood

   Indigestion, nausea, stomach pain, diarrhea, gas

<u>QUESTION :</u> Can niacin lower cholesterol levels?

<u>ANSWER:</u> Niacin (nicotinic acid or vitamin B3) helps to convert food into energy and is needed to keep your skin, blood cells, brain, and nervous system healthy. People who don't get enough niacin can develop pellagra, which causes scaly skin sores, inflamed mucous membranes, diarrhea, and mental confusion and delusions. Pellegra is a very rare condition in the U.S. today, because many of the foods we eat have niacin added to them. Niacin is also used to treat high cholesterol and it can lower LDL (bad) cholesterol and triglycerides in the blood. It also raises the levels of HDL (good) cholesterol. However, niacin products approved for treating high cholesterol are available only by prescription. Niacin is available in three different kinds of dosage forms and this can be confusing and potentially harmful if they are not used correctly. Prescription niacin products include an "immediate-release" formulation (Niacor) and an "extended-release" formulation (Niaspan). Niacor is given two to three times per day while Niaspan is taken once daily at bedtime. The extended-release niacin (Niaspan) reduces the skin flushing and itching seen with immediate-release niacin (Niacor).

Nonprescription or dietary supplement products containing niacin can be either an "immediate-release" formulation or a "sustained-release" formulation (also marketed as "long-acting", "controlled-release", or "timed-release" niacin) and this can lead to confusion and safety concerns. These "sustained-release" products were developed to reduce skin flushing and itching, but unfortunately, they can also cause liver problems in some people. Serious liver problems have occurred in people who stopped using immediate-release niacin products and began using the same dose of sustained-release niacin. In view of this potential for confusion and safety issues, if you have high cholesterol it may not be a good idea to treat it on your own with nonprescription niacin containing products. It should also be noted that nonprescription niacin supplements have not been approved for treating high cholesterol and may not contain the proper amount or type of niacin. Your physician can decide if a cholesterol lowering medication is necessary and what product is best for you

QUESTION: Is Vytorin any better than Zocor for high cholesterol?

ANSWER: Vytorin is a cholesterol-lowering prescription medication that contains ezetimibe (the active ingredient in Zetia) and the statin drug simvastatin (the active ingredient in Zocor). Each of these drugs works in different ways to lower cholesterol and when used in combination have additive effects on cholesterol lowering. Ezemtimibe reduces blood cholesterol by blocking the absorption of cholesterol in the small intestine. Simvastatin, on the other hand, lowers cholesterol by blocking the manufacture of cholesterol in the liver. When these drugs are combined they can lower cholesterol significantly more than when either one is used by itself. Recently, the results of a 2-year clinical study showed that Vytorin might not be more effective than Zocor alone in reducing the buildup of fatty plaque in arteries, which can lead to a heart attack or stroke. This study involved 720 patients with a genetic condition that causes very high cholesterol levels (over 300). About half of the patients received Vytorin and the other half Zocor alone for their high cholesterol levels. After 2 years of drug therapy, patients receiving Vytorin had a 58% reduction in their "bad" cholesterol (LDL) and those receiving Zocor alone had a 41% reduction. However, in spite of the greater reduction in "bad" cholesterol in patients taking Vytorin, there was no significant difference in fatty plaque buildup in the neck arteries using ultrasound measurements compared to patients taking Zocor alone. In fact, patients receiving Vytorin may have experienced slightly more fatty plaque buildup in the arteries. Both medicines in this study were generally well tolerated and side effects were similar in each treatment group. Additional larger studies are also currently underway to determine if Vytorin and Zetia are effective for preventing heart attacks, strokes, and deaths, but study results are not expected until 2011. Patients taking Vytorin or Zetia should consult with their doctors for advice regarding their cholesterol-lowering therapy.

QUESTION: I am a diabetic heart patient taking Lopid for high triglycerides and Pravachol for high cholesterol. Is there any problem in taking these medications together?

ANSWER: This is a very good question, but the answer is difficult. As you mentioned, Pravachol (pravastatin) is used along with dietary changes to help lower high cholesterol levels in the blood. It lowers both total cholesterol and LDL (bad) cholesterol levels by preventing their production in the liver. Pravachol along with Mevacor, Zocor, and Lescol are scientifically known as HMG-CoA Reductase inhibitors. Lopid (gemfibrozil) on the other hand prevents the production of triglycerides (a fatty substance) by the liver and is used along with dietary changes to lower high blood levels of triglycerides. High triglyceride levels commonly occur in patients with diabetes. Lopid works differently than Pravachol and is called a fibrate drug. When these drugs are used together both abnormally high cholesterol and triglyceride levels are lowered, which decreases the risk of heart disease. There is, however, a potential problem when using these drugs together. A drug very similar to Pravachol named Mevacor (lovastatin) has been shown to cause a serious side effect in some patients, particularly when it is used along with Lopid. This side effect is known as myositis (my-o-si-tis) or rhabdomyolysis (rab-do-my-ol-i-sis), which is an inflammation or actual destruction of muscle tissue possibly leading to kidney failure. During a few studies of patients who received both Lopid and Pravachol together, this serious side effect did not occur but these studies were done in only a relatively small number of people, which may not be enough to identify a serious side effect that only occurs infrequently.

For example, to have a good chance of identifying a side effect that only occurs in 1 person out of 1,000 who takes the drug, over 3,000 patients would have to be studied. Therefore, we really don't know if this serious side effect will occur when Pravachol is used with Lopid. Because of this, the FDA has required the manufacturers of Pravachol and Lopid to put a warning or precaution in their labeling that goes with the product. This warning says that the use of these drugs together should be avoided unless the benefit in lowering the cholesterol and triglyceride blood levels is more important than the risk of serious side effects. Certainly, anyone who takes these drugs together must be monitored very closely. If a patient develops muscle pain, tenderness or weakness, they should contact their physician immediately. A blood test can be done (CK or creatine kinase) to determine if there is myositis and if so, the drugs must be discontinued. I hope that this discussion is helpful to you.

QUESTION: I heard about a new combination drug product to lower your cholesterol levels. What can you tell me about it?

ANSWER: The FDA recently approved a cholesterol-lowering prescription medication named Vytorin that contains ezetimibe—the active ingredient in Zetia, and simvastatin—the active ingredient in Zocor. Each of these ingredients works in different ways to lower cholesterol and when used in combination have additive effects on cholesterol lowering. Ezemtimibe reduces blood cholesterol by blocking the absorption of cholesterol in the small intestine. Simvastatin, on the other hand, lowers cholesterol by blocking the manufacture of cholesterol in the liver. When these drugs are combined they can lower cholesterol significantly more than when either one is used by itself. By putting both of these drugs in a single tablet it will make it more convenient for patients to take. The approval of Vytorin coincides with the release of new scientific treatment guidelines that call for people who have had heart attacks or who are at risk for heart disease to lower their LDL cholesterol (bad cholesterol) much more than previously recommended. Like other cholesterol-lowering medications, Vytorin should be used in addition to dietary changes aimed at reducing cholesterol levels. Because Vytorin contains a "statin" drug, it may increase the risk of severe muscle problems known as myopathy or rhabdomyolysis. Because of this, patients taking Vytorin that develop any unexplained muscle pain, tenderness, or weakness should report this to their doctor immediately. Liver problems can also occur and liver function tests should be performed when indicated. In addition, numerous drug interactions are possible with Vytorin and these need to be monitored by the doctor and pharmacist. Vytorin is taken once a day as a single dose in the evening, with or without food.

QUESTION: Are there differences between the "statin" drugs used to lower cholesterol?

ANSWER: Since the first cholesterol-lowering statin drug, lovastatin (Mevacor), was introduced 16 years ago, there are now a total of 7 statin drugs available. All statin drugs work in the same way to lower cholesterol. They block a key enzyme that controls how much cholesterol is made in the liver. This results in lower levels of "bad" cholesterol (LDL), lower triglyceride levels, and an increase in "good" cholesterol (HDL). The main differences between all of these statins are their potency, cost, their interactions with other drugs, and when they are taken during the day. Side effects are about the same for all seven of these products. In the following list, I have outlined some of the major differences between these statin drugs.

Statin Drug: Atorvastatin (Lipitor)
Beginning Daily Dose: 10 mg
Usual Decrease In LDL Cholesterol: 35-40%
When To Take: Anytime

Statin Drug: Fluvastatin (Lescol)
Beginning Daily Dose: 20 mg
Usual Decrease In LDL Cholesterol: 20-25%
When To Take: Evening

Statin Drug: Lovastatin (Mevacor); (Generic); (Altoprev)
Beginning Daily Dose: 20 mg; 20 mg; 20 mg
Usual Decrease In LDL Cholesterol: 25-30%; 25-30%; 20-25%
When To Take: Evening (with food); Evening (with food); Evening (with food)
Statin Drug: Pitavastatin (Livalo)

Beginning Daily Dose: 2 mg
Usual Decrease In LDL Cholesterol: 35-40%
When To Take: Anytime

Statin Drug: Pravastatin (Pravachol)
Beginning Daily Dose: 40 mg
Usual Decrease In LDL Cholesterol: 30-35%
When To Take: Evening

Statin Drug: Rosuvastatin (Crestor)
Beginning Daily Dose: 10 mg
Usual Decrease In LDL Cholesterol: 40-50%
When To Take: Anytime

Statin Drug: Simvastatin (Zocor)
Beginning Daily Dose: 20 mg
Usual Decrease In LDL Cholesterol: 35-40%
When To Take: Evening

QUESTION: Are statin drugs safe to take for a long time?

ANSWER: Apparently so, according to the results of a large long-term study recently published online in The Lancet journal. This study was a follow-up of patients who were enrolled the Heart Protection Study (HPS). In the HPS, over 20,000 patients at increased risk of vascular disease such as a heart attack or stroke were given simvastatin (Zocor) 40 mg daily or a placebo ("dummy pill") for about 5 years. Results from this study showed that patients treated with simvastatin lowered their LDL (bad) cholesterol and experienced a 23% decrease in major vascular events such as a heart attack or stroke compared to those getting a placebo. In order to determine if a statin drug was safe and effective in the long run, these patients were followed for an additional 6 years and the results are now in. In this follow-up study, simvastatin was found to provide lasting reductions in serious vascular events such as a heart attack or stroke. In addition, the researchers found no differences in cancer deaths or cancer incidence in patients receiving the statin medication. Furthermore, there were not any differences in non-vascular mortality nor were there any identifiable adverse effects that would not support the long-term treatment with statins. The authors of this study concluded that their research findings provide support for the prompt initiation of statin therapy in patients at risk of vascular disease and that the extended use of a statin drug is safe with respect to possible risk of cancer and non-vascular mortality.

QUESTION: I am taking Zocor 20 mg at bedtime for high cholesterol. Now all my cholesterol levels are within the normal range. Will I need to take Zocor for the rest of my life?

ANSWER: You should discuss this question with your doctor. High blood cholesterol can increase your risk of developing coronary heart disease, which is the main cause of death in the United States. Coronary heart disease may lead to a heart attack, or the need for bypass surgery or other procedures to increase the amount of blood going to your heart from your coronary blood vessels. In addition to high cholesterol levels, other "risk factors" for coronary heart disease include a family history of heart disease at an early age, high blood pressure, diabetes, smoking, a high-fat diet or high-cholesterol diet, obesity, lack of exercise and being over 45 years old for men or 55 for women. Furthermore, since people with normal cholesterol levels also develop coronary heart disease and have heart attacks, additional factors besides cholesterol are probably involved in this disease process.

A diet that is low in saturated fat and cholesterol may help to lower your blood cholesterol. Saturated fat is found in meats and dairy products, "creamy" salad dressings and many other foods. Vegetables, fruits, and grains are low fat foods and many other low fat packaged foods are now available. Exercise may also help lower bad blood cholesterol levels.

If your cholesterol is not lowered enough after several months on a good diet and exercise program, cholesterol-lowering medication may be needed. Zocor is a "statin" drug, which blocks the manufacture of cholesterol in the body. If someone cannot tolerate a "statin" drug due to side effects, there are several other medication options available. A lower dose of Zocor may also be an option if your cholesterol levels are well controlled. You should discuss the various treatment choices with your doctor, who can decide what is best for your particular situation.

QUESTION: I heard that the FDA is warning about using high-dose simvastatin (Zocor) to lower cholesterol levels. What can you tell me about this?

ANSWER: On June 8, 2011 the U.S. Food and Drug Administration (FDA) announced safety label changes for the cholesterol-lowering medication simvastatin. The highest approved dose of 80 milligram (mg) has been associated with an elevated risk of muscle injury (myopathy), particularly during the first 12 months of use. The FDA recommends that simvastatin 80 mg be used only in patients who have been taking this dose for 12 months or more and have not experienced any muscle injury. It should not be prescribed to new patients. There are also new contraindications and dose limitations for when simvastatin is taken with certain other medications.

Simvastatin is used together with diet and exercise to reduce the amount of "bad cholesterol" (low-density lipoprotein cholesterol or LDL-C) in the blood. High levels of LDL-C are linked to a higher risk of heart attack, stroke and cardiovascular death. In 2010, about 2.1 million patients in the United States were prescribed a product containing simvastatin 80 mg. The changes to the label for simvastatin-containing medications are based on the FDA's review of the results of the 7-year Study of the Effectiveness of Additional Reductions in Cholesterol and Homocysteine clinical trial, other clinical trial data, and analyses of adverse events submitted to the FDA's Adverse Event Reporting System. All showed that patients taking simvastatin 80 mg daily had an increased risk of muscle injury compared to patients taking lower doses of simvastatin or other statin drugs. The risk of muscle injury is highest during the first year of treatment with the 80 mg dose of simvastatin, is often the result of interactions with certain other medicines, and is frequently associated with a genetic predisposition for simvastatin-related muscle injury.

Simvastatin is sold under the brand-name Zocor and as a single-ingredient generic product. It is also sold in combination with ezetimibe as Vytorin and in combination with niacin as Simcor. The FDA has revised the drug labels for simvastatin and Vytorin to include the new 80 mg dosing restrictions. The agency also revised the labels for simvastatin, Vytorin and Simcor to include new dosing recommendations when these drugs are used with certain medications that interact to increase the level of simvastatin in the body, which can increase the risk for myopathy. Patients who are unable to adequately lower their level of LDL-C on simvastatin 40 mg should not be given the higher 80 mg dose of simvastatin. Instead, they should be placed on an alternative LDL-C-lowering treatment(s). It should also be noted that patients should consult with their physician before discontinuing any of their medications.

QUESTION: I was switched from Zocor to Welchol for cholesterol control because I developed severe muscle pain. What can you tell me about Welchol?

ANSWER: I have heard similar stories from several other people taking Zocor or other drugs that lower cholesterol levels. Zocor is a "statin" drug that lowers cholesterol by blocking the production of cholesterol in the liver. "Statins" are very effective in lowering cholesterol levels but they can cause serious side effects including liver problems and muscle damage. "Statin" products include Mevacor (lovastatin), Zocor (simvastatin), Pravachol (pravastatin), Lescol (fluvastatin), and atorvastatin (Lipitor). Welchol (colesevelam) is known as a bile acid sequestrant and was approved by the FDA in May 2000. Welchol works differently than the "statins" drugs to lower cholesterol levels. During normal digestion, bile acids produced from cholesterol are secreted into the intestinal tract from the liver to help with the digestion of fats in the diet. Bile acids are reabsorbed in the intestine and returned to the liver. Welchol binds with these bile acids, preventing their reabsorption. Because of this, more bile acids are made from cholesterol to replenish them, thus lowering cholesterol levels. Welchol appears to be fairly well tolerated. The most common side effects of Welchol involve the gastrointestinal tract and include constipation and indigestion. The recommended dose of Welchol is 3 tablets twice a day with meals or 6 tablets once a day with a meal. Welchol is not absorbed and is passed through the body in the stool.

QUESTION: I heard about a new type of drug to lower cholesterol. What can you tell me about it?

ANSWER: The FDA recently approved Zetia (generic name ezetimibe) for lowering high levels of cholesterol when used in conjunction with a diet low in cholesterol and saturated fat. Zetia can be used alone or in combination with "statin" drugs (e.g., Mevacor, Zocor, Pravachol, Lescol, or Lipitor) to lower cholesterol levels in the blood. "Statin" drugs are more effective in lowering cholesterol, but Zetia will probably be used by itself in people who have less severe high cholesterol or in patients who cannot tolerate "statins" due to side effects or drug interactions. When Zetia is prescribed in combination with a "statin" drug, additive effects are obtained and cholesterol levels are reduced by more than the "statin" drug used alone. The combination may also allow a smaller dose of "statin" medication to be prescribed, which could lower the potential for serious "statin" side effects. Although both Zetia and "statin" drugs lower cholesterol levels, they do it in different ways. "Statins" lower cholesterol by blocking its production in the body. Zetia, on the other hand, lowers cholesterol levels by blocking the absorption of cholesterol in the small intestine. Because they work in different ways they have "additive" effects on lowering blood cholesterol. Zetia seems to be well tolerated with mild side effects such as back pain, joint pain, or diarrhea. Zetia is given as a 10 mg tablet once daily.

QUESTION: I take Metamucil daily and sprinkle grapefruit fiber on my cereal for breakfast. Can this help lower my cholesterol?

ANSWER: It may help some if used in conjunction with a low fat diet and exercise. Both grapefruit fiber and Metamucil are dietary fiber supplement products. Simply put, fiber is the undigested residue from plant food sources and has been referred to as roughage or bulk. Not much information is available concerning grapefruit fiber and its effect on cholesterol levels. Grapefruit fiber contains a carbohydrate known as pectin, which is an absorbent and bulk-forming agent. It has been used for the management of diarrhea and constipation for a long time. It can also interact with certain medications including lovastatin (Mevcor) interfering with this drug's cholesterol-lowering effects. Much more information is available for psyllium, which is the active ingredient in Metamucil. Psyllium is a soluble fiber product that is used as a bulk-forming laxative. Psyllium fiber has also been used for the treatment of irritable bowel syndrome, diverticular disease, and hemorrhoids. In addition, studies have shown that psyllium may be useful in helping to lower cholesterol levels in some people when used in conjunction with a low fat diet and exercise. It may do this by binding to bile acids in the intestinal tract, preventing them from being absorbed. Since the liver makes bile acids from cholesterol, serum cholesterol levels can be lowered as cholesterol is used to make more bile acids. Psyllium may also interfere with fat and cholesterol absorption from food intake. To help control cholesterol levels, psyllium is usually taken at a dose of 3.4 grams three times a day in a full 8 ounce glass of water. Psyllium can also interfere with certain medications, so make sure that you talk to your doctor and pharmacist before using these dietary fiber supplements and remember to carefully read all product labeling.

QUESTION: I heard about a new drug for high cholesterol. What can you tell me about it?

ANSWER: The FDA recently approved Crestor (generic name rosuvastatin) for the treatment of high cholesterol and high triglyceride levels. This new prescription medication is used in combination with diet and exercise to help lower cholesterol and triglyceride levels in the blood that can increase your risk of heart disease. Crestor works by blocking the production of cholesterol and is known as a "statin" drug. Other "statin" drugs include Mevacor (lovastatin), Zocor (simvastatin), Pravachol (pravastatin), Lescol (fluvastatin), and Lipitor (atorvastatin). All the "statin" drugs work in the same way, but some are more potent than others. They may also have different types of drug interactions. Crestor appears to be the most potent "statin" drug currently available and has been referred to as a "superstatin". In clinical studies it has been shown to lower "bad" cholesterol (LDL-C) to a greater extent than the other "statin" drugs. It also lowers triglyceride levels and increases "good" cholesterol (HDL-C). In addition, Crestor may interact with fewer drugs compared to some of the other "statins". The most commonly reported side effects of Crestor include muscle pain, stomach pain, nausea, constipation, and weakness. It should not be used by women who are pregnant or who are nursing, or anyone with liver problems. Because all "statin" drugs can cause serious muscle-related problems, patients receiving Crestor should promptly report any unexplained muscle pain, tenderness, or weakness to their doctor. Crestor is taken in a single dose at any time of day, with or without food.

QUESTION: Was another statin drug approved for high cholesterol?

ANSWER: Yes, the FDA recently approved the seventh statin drug to lower high cholesterol levels in conjunction with diet and exercise. The new statin drug is named Livalo (pitavastatin) and was approved to reduce total cholesterol, lower LDL (bad) cholesterol, reduce triglycerides, and to increase HDL (good) cholesterol. Since the first cholesterol-lowering statin drug, lovastatin (Mevacor), was approved in 1987, there are now a total of 7 statin drugs available. All statin drugs work in the same way to lower cholesterol. They block a key enzyme that controls how much cholesterol is made in the liver. The main differences between all of these statins are their potency, cost, their interactions with other drugs, and when they are taken during the day. Side effects are about the same for all 7 of these drugs. The most common side effects of Livalo during clinical studies were muscle pain, back pain, joint pain, and constipation. Other available statin drugs include Lipitor (atorvastatin), Lescol or Lescol XL (fluvastatin), Mevacor or Altoprev (lovastatin), Pravachol (pravastatin), Crestor (rosuvastatin), and Zocor (simvastatin). Lovastatin, pravastatin, and simvastatin are also available as generic products.

QUESTION: I heard that the FDA recently announced important safety changes in the labeling for statins. What can you tell me about this?

ANSWER: On February 28, 2012 the FDA announced important safety changes for some widely used cholesterol-lowering drugs known as statins. These products, when used with diet and exercise, help to lower a person's "bad" cholesterol (low-density lipoprotein cholesterol). The products include: Lipitor (atorvastatin), Lescol (fluvastatin), Mevacor (lovastatin), Altoprev (lovastatin extended-release), Livalo (pitavastatin), Pravachol (pravastatin), Crestor (rosuvastatin), and Zocor (simvastatin). Combination products include: Advicor (lovastatin/niacin extended-release), Simcor (simvastatin/niacin extended-release), and Vytorin (simvastatin/ezetimibe).

The changes to the statin labels are:
- The drug labels have been revised to remove the need for routine periodic monitoring of liver enzymes in patients taking statins. FDA

now recommends that liver enzyme tests should be performed before starting statin therapy, and as clinically indicated thereafter. FDA has concluded that serious liver injury with statins is rare and unpredictable in individual patients, and that routine periodic monitoring of liver enzymes does not appear to be effective in detecting or preventing this rare side effect. Patients should notify their health care professional immediately if they have the following symptoms of liver problems: unusual fatigue or weakness; loss of appetite; upper belly pain; dark-colored urine; yellowing of the skin or the whites of the eyes.

- Certain cognitive (brain-related) effects have been reported with statin use. Statin labels will now include information about some patients experiencing memory loss and confusion. These reports generally have not been serious and the patients' symptoms were reversed by stopping the statin. However, patients should still alert their health care professional if these symptoms occur.

- Increases in blood sugar levels (hyperglycemia) have been reported with statin use. The FDA is also aware of studies showing that patients being treated with statins may have a small increased risk of increased blood sugar levels and of being diagnosed with type 2 diabetes mellitus. The labels will now warn healthcare professionals and patients of this potential risk.

- Health care professionals should take note of the new recommendations in the lovastatin label. Some medicines may interact with lovastatin, increasing the risk for muscle injury (myopathy/rhabdomyolysis). For example, certain medicines should never be taken (are contraindicated) with Mevacor (lovastatin) including drugs used to treat HIV (protease inhibitors) and drugs used to treat certain bacterial and fungal infections.

Healthcare professionals and patients are encouraged to report adverse events or side effects related to the use of these products to the FDA's MedWatch Safety Information and Adverse Event Reporting Program:

- Complete and submit the report online: **www.fda.gov/MedWatch/ report.htm**
- Download form or call 1—800-332-1088 to request a reporting form, then complete and return to the address on the pre-addressed form, or submit by fax to 1-800-FDA-0178

NEW CHOLESTEROL GUIDELINES

QUESTION: My doctor recently put me on a "statin" drug because of new cholesterol treatment guidelines. What's that all about?

ANSWER: In 2001 the National Cholesterol Education Program (NCEP) within the National Institutes of Health (NIH) issued guidelines for physicians to consider using when prescribing drugs for patients with high cholesterol levels. Since that time, several major clinical studies of "statin" drugs have shown that lower "bad" cholesterol (LDL) levels are much better for people with a high risk for heart attacks. People at high-risk are those with cardiovascular disease, or diabetes, or with 2 or more risk factors like smoking or high blood pressure. People at very high-risk are those with cardiovascular disease together with either multiple risk factors (especially diabetes), or who have severe and poorly controlled risk factors (such as continued smoking), or who are overweight and have high triglyceride levels and low "good" cholesterol (HDL). The updated guidelines issued in 2004, call for an LDL cholesterol goal of less than 100 for high-risk patients and an option of less than 70 for very high-risk patients. In addition, lower LDL goals are recommended for some people who are at moderately high-risk for coronary heart disease. The updated guidelines also stress the importance of nutrition, physical activity, and weight control for managing cholesterol. In the future these guidelines will probably be changed again as more information becomes available.

COREG

QUESTION: I take Coreg for my heart. Is there a generic available?

ANSWER: The FDA recently approved the first generic versions of Coreg (generic name carvedilol). Coreg is a widely used medication that is approved to treat high blood pressure (hypertension), mild to severe chronic heart failure, and to improve heart function in people who have had a heart attack. Carvedilol is classified as a beta-blocker, which works by blocking a hormone (norepinephrine) in your body that can raise blood pressure and heart rate. By reducing the effects of this hormone, beta-blockers can lower blood pressure and heart rate, which reduces the workload of the heart and enables it to not pump as hard. In people with weakened hearts and reduced function, carvedilol also helps to lower the heart rate and increase the heart's ability to pump blood better and supply the body with oxygen. In addition, for people who have had a heart attack that reduced how well the heart works, carvedilol can take the strain off the heart, helping to reduce the risk of another heart attack. Coreg was the 30th top selling brand name drug in 2006. As I've noted many times before, the FDA approves all generic drugs using strict guidelines, including checking for the generic drug's chemistry by evaluating its formulation, potency, stability, and purity. The generic drug must also pass bio-equivalency testing that compares the delivery into the bloodstream of the generic drug's active ingredient to that of the brand name drug. Generic drugs are less expensive than brand-name products, and account for about 56% of prescriptions dispensed.

BENECOL AND TAKE CONTROL

QUESTION: My cholesterol is high, but I don't want to try drug treatment yet. Can the newly marketed cholesterol lowering margarines help me?

ANSWER: Yes, they may. Over 98 million adults in the U.S. (myself included) have total blood cholesterol levels of 200 or higher, which can be a significant risk factor for heart disease. The risk is even greater if levels of "bad" cholesterol (LDL) are too high and/or levels of "good" cholesterol (HDL) are too low. Usually a low fat, low cholesterol diet in conjunction with exercise is the first step in managing cholesterol levels. If these measures fail, then the addition of drug therapy may be necessary.

The recent introduction of two new "functional food" products in the U.S. may help to reduce the need for drug therapy in some people. The available margarine-like products are named Benecol (marketed by McNeil Consumer Healthcare) and Take Control (marketed by

Unilever/Lipton). "Functional foods" are foods that contain a particular ingredient added solely to provide the consumer with a specific healthy benefit. Because they are considered to be foods and not drugs, only their safety had to be proven to the FDA and not their actual effectiveness in lowering cholesterol. This allowed the companies to bring theses products to the market more quickly and cheaply. Both of these products contain ingredients from natural plant sources known as "sterols" or "stanols" that have cholesterol-lowering properties. The active ingredients in Benecol are derived from wood pulp, while those in Take Control come from soybeans. These margarines lower cholesterol by blocking the absorption of cholesterol in the intestinal tract, thus preventing it from getting into the bloodstream. Even though these products are not considered to be drugs, several studies have shown that they can begin to lower blood cholesterol levels within about two weeks of use. One study showed a 23% reduction in total cholesterol and a 20% reduction in "bad" (LDL) cholesterol after seven weeks of use (3 grams per day). In another study lasting 12 months, total cholesterol levels were reduced by 10% and "bad" (LDL) cholesterol decreased by 14%. These products do not appear to affect "good" (HDL) cholesterol levels. During clinical studies, product side effects appeared to be the same as those who received placebo products (without active ingredients). The recommended "dose" of Benecol is one serving (1 gram) with breakfast, lunch, and dinner while the Take Control product recommends one or two servings per day. Additional types of similar products are also being introduced, including a line of salad dressing.

BENECOL SMART CHEWS

QUESTION: I recently received a sample of Benecol Smart Chews for lowering cholesterol. How do they work?

ANSWER: Benecol Smart Chews, which come in chocolate or caramel flavors, have recently been marketed by the makers of Benecol Spread (McNeil). Both of these products contain plant stanol esters as the cholesterol-lowering ingredient. Plant stanol esters are derived from natural plant components known as sterols found in vegetable oils, corn, beans, and wood. Plants do not make cholesterol like animals, but instead make waxy sterol compounds that are similar to cholesterol. Like cholesterol in animals, plant sterols are essential for life where they are a part of plant cell membranes and hormonal systems. Plant sterols are effective in lowering cholesterol, but because they are not very soluble, large quantities are needed (10 to 20 grams per day), and they cannot be easily made into food products. Because of this, plant sterols have been modified chemically to form plant stanol esters. These ester compounds are much more effective in lowering cholesterol and can easily be made into fat-based "functional food" products like Benecol. "Functional foods" are foods that contain a particular ingredient added solely to provide the consumer with a specific healthy benefit. Plant stanol esters found in Benecol spread and the tasty Smart Chews lower cholesterol by blocking the absorption of cholesterol in the intestinal tract, thus preventing it from getting into the bloodstream. Studies have shown that the daily intake of 2 to 3 grams of plant stanol esters can decrease LDL (bad) cholesterol levels by about 10% to 15%. However, HDL (good) cholesterol levels do not appear to be affected. Benecol Smart Chews contain 0.85 grams of plant stanol esters and the recommended dose is 1-2 Chews twice daily with meals or snacks. Benecol products should be used as part of a healthy diet and exercise program to help manage cholesterol.

LOWERING TRIGLYCERIDES

QUESTION: I'm taking Tricor to lower my triglycerides and have muscle pain and weakness. Is this a "statin" drug like Baycol and can it cause this?

ANSWER: Tricor (generic name fenofibrate) is used along with dietary changes for the treatment of adults with very high levels of triglycerides in the blood. Triglycerides are fats or lipids like cholesterol and very high levels can lead to inflamation of the pancreas (pancreatitis), which can be a serious medical problem. Tricor is not a "statin" drug like Baycol, which was recently removed from the market. However, Tricor can also cause inflamation of muscle tissues (myositis) and muscle disease (myopathy). Tricor is a "fibrate" drug and the use of fibrates alone or in combination with "statins" have been associated with the destruction of muscle tissue known as rhabomyolysis (rab-do-my-ol-i-sis), which can lead to kidney failure. That is why the FDA recommended that Baycol be removed from the market in 2001. Other "fibrates" include Lopid (generic name gemfibrozil) and Atromid-s (generic name clofibrate). "Statin" products still on the market include Zocor (generic name simvastatin), Pravacol (generic name pravastatin), Lescol (generic name fluvastatin), Lipitor (generic name atorvastatin) and Mevacor (generic name lovastatin). People who take "fibrates" or "statins" (alone or in combination) and who develop muscle pain, tenderness, or weakness should have prompt medical evaluation for muscle tissue problems. A blood test known as creatine kinase or CK can be performed to help diagnose this side effect. Creatine kinase is an enzyme present in muscle tissue and levels in the blood increase when muscle tissue is damaged. If muscle problems are suspected you should see your doctor as soon as possible.

QUESTION: I have high levels of triglycerides in my blood. What drugs are used for this?

ANSWER: Triglycerides are a type of fat found in the body that serves as an energy source. When triglycerides attach themselves to certain proteins they can travel throughout the bloodstream and are called lipoproteins. Blood levels of triglycerides below 250 are desirable and are usually measured after an overnight fast. Higher levels are known as "hypertriglyceridemia". The significance of high levels of triglycerides is uncertain, but there is mounting evidence that they may increase the risk of heart disease. Extremely high levels of triglycerides can also lead to problems with the pancreas. Causes of hypertriglyceridemia include obesity, lack of exercise, alcohol abuse, diabetes, kidney disease, stress, certain drugs, liver problems, and heredity. In general, the best treatment for people with high triglyceride levels is to lose weight if they are overweight, reduce the amount of fat and cholesterol in their diet, decrease alcohol use, control diabetes if present, and increase exercise. If these lifestyle changes are not effective in lowering triglyceride levels, several drug treatments are available. These include fibric acid derivatives like clofibrate (Atromid-S), gemfibrozil (Lopid), or fenofibrate (Tricor).

Niacin (Niaspan, Niacor) and statin drugs like simvastatin (Zocor), pravastatin (Pravachol), rosuvastatin (Crestor), fluvastatin (Lescol) or atorvastatin (Lipitor) may be useful. Fish oil (omega-3-fatty acids) also helps to reduce triglyceride levels. Your physician can determine which treatment would be best for you.

QUESTION: I take Tricor for high triglycerides and it's expensive. Is there a generic available?

ANSWER: Yes, the Food and Drug Administration (FDA) recently approved a generic form of Tricor capsules (generic name fenofibrate) and it should soon be available at your pharmacy. As I've noted before, the FDA approves all generic drugs using strict guidelines, including checking for the generic drug's chemistry by evaluating its formulation, potency, stability, and purity. The generic drug must also pass bio-equivalency testing that compares the delivery into the bloodstream of the generic drug's active ingredient to that of the brand name drug. Generic drugs are less expensive than brand name drugs and account for about 40 percent of all prescriptions dispensed.

Fenofibrate is used to lower high levels of triglycerides in the blood. Triglycerides are a type of fat found in the body that serves as an energy source. When triglycerides attach themselves to certain proteins they can travel throughout the bloodstream and are called lipoproteins. Blood levels of triglycerides below 250 are desirable and are usually measured after an overnight fast. Higher levels are known as "hypertriglyceridemia". The significance of high levels of triglycerides is uncertain, but there is mounting evidence that they may increase the risk of heart disease. Extremely high levels of triglycerides can also lead to problems with the pancreas. Causes of hypertriglyceridemia include obesity, lack of exercise, alcohol abuse, diabetes, kidney disease, stress, certain drugs, liver problems, and heredity. In general, the best treatment for people with high triglyceride levels is to lose weight if they are overweight, reduce the amount of fat and cholesterol in their diet, decrease alcohol use, control diabetes if present, and increase exercise. If these lifestyle changes are not effective in lowering triglyceride levels, several drug treatments are available, including fenofibrate. Your physician can determine which treatment would be best for you.

BLOOD THINNERS

QUESTION: My doctor put me on Coumadin because I have an irregular heartbeat. What should I know about this medicine?

ANSWER: Coumadin (generic name warfarin sodium) is known as a blood thinner because it works to prevent your blood from forming clots that can block your blood vessels. It is widely used for a common heartbeat problem called atrial fibrillation where the upper chambers of your heart beat too fast. When this irregular heartbeat occurs, blood flow is impaired which can cause clots to form and lead to strokes or other problems. Coumadin prevents blood clots because it interferes with the liver's ability to make chemicals that help to form clots. These chemicals also need vitamin K to work. Coumadin or warfarin was first used around 1948 as a product to kill rodents by causing internal bleeding and death. Later it was found to have beneficial effects in humans.

While you are taking Coumadin you must have regular blood tests taken to check how quickly your blood clots, to insure that the right dose is used. You should take this medication at the same time each day and you should keep your diet steady. By keeping your diet steady, your intake of vitamin K remains consistent which is important, as vitamin K affects the way Coumadin works as I noted earlier. Vitamin K helps your blood make clots. If you forget to take a dose, tell your doctor. The missed dose should be taken as soon as possible on the same day. Do not take a double dose the next day or it will change the clot prevention action.

Many other things can affect blood clotting while taking Coumadin, such as sickness, other medicines (prescription and non-prescription, including herbal remedies), and physical activities. Keep your doctor informed about changes in your health or lifestyle so that your Coumadin dose can be adjusted if necessary. Numerous medicines can interact with Coumadin to make it stronger or weaker. I can't go over all these interactions in this column but it is very important that you tell your doctor and pharmacist about all other medicines that you take while on Coumadin—including non-prescription and herbal remedies. Alcohol can also affect blood-clotting times and should be avoided while taking this drug.

The most common side effect of Coumadin is bleeding. Let your doctor know immediately if you experience any of the following: A serious fall or other injury; fever or developing illness, including vomiting, diarrhea, infection, pain, swelling discomfort, or other unusual symptoms; prolonged bleeding from cuts or nosebleeds, unusual bleeding from your gums, increased menstrual flow or vaginal bleeding; red or dark brown urine; red or tarry stools; unusual bruising; pregnancy or planned pregnancy. Coumadin is a very safe and effective medicine, but you must be careful while using it.

QUESTION: How do aspirin and Coumadin thin the blood?

ANSWER: Both aspirin and Coumadin (generic name warfarin) prevent the blood from clotting but do so in different ways. Blood coagulation occurs when blood cells clump together to form a clot. This clotting can occur within a blood vessel or when an injury occurs, allowing blood to escape from a blood vessel. The means by which blood coagulation takes place is a very complex process. The first step in this process occurs when blood platelets adhere to each other and to the edges of the injured blood vessel and form a plug that covers the area. Platelets are small, oval discs found in the blood. This initial activity of the platelets then initiates a complicated pathway of events that leads to the formation of fibrin that reinforces the platelets that are stuck together, forming a clot. Fibrin is a protein substance that forms a threadlike network within the clot—almost like a glue. Many different substances and clotting factors are involved in this complex process. The body also produces a number of "natural anticoagulants" to prevent the blood from clotting so that blood can remain liquid and flow through the vessels.

In simple terms, aspirin prevents the blood from clotting by interfering with the platelets sticking together (platelet aggregation). The way it does this is also very complicated, but involves aspirin interfering with the making of hormone-like chemicals called prostaglandins or eicosanoids. Low doses of aspirin (160 mg daily) are effective in producing this antiplatelet effect. Coumadin (warfarin) on the other hand prevents the blood from clotting in another way, after the platelets stick together. Coumadin interferes with the production of a number of blood coagulation factors in the liver. The making of these factors also requires vitamin K and that is why people taking Coumadin must be careful about eating foods with a lot of this vitamin. Vitamin K can actually help the blood to make clots. Although this explanation is a simplification of the differences between aspirin and Coumadin, I hope it is helpful to you.

ANGINA

QUESTION: How does aspirin and nitroglycerin help someone with angina?

ANSWER: Angina is caused by a lack of oxygen in the heart muscle due to a blockage in the coronary arteries, which bring oxygen-rich blood to the heart. The symptoms of angina include pain or discomfort in the chest, arms, back, neck or jaw. Sometimes the pain may feel like a tightness or crushing sensation, or it may be a stabbing pain or seem like numbness. Some people even mistake anginal pain as indigestion or gas pain. This anginal discomfort may occur in some people when they over-exert themselves or when they get upset or excited. Usually they can tell what activities cause this discomfort, which goes away in a few minutes. This type of angina is called "stable" angina. However, other people have anginal discomfort when they are resting, or suddenly develop moderate or severe discomfort or have a marked increase in the frequency of discomfort. These people have "unstable" angina and are at a greater risk of having a heart attack. Both aspirin and nitrates are commonly used to treat patients with "unstable" angina.

About 25 years ago, doctors discovered that aspirin keeps the body from forming blood clots. Aspirin blocks your body's production of substances called prostaglandins (pros-ta-glan-dins) which make the platelets in your blood stick together and form clots to stop bleeding. These clots can prevent your heart from receiving enough blood and lead to an anginal attack or a heart attack. Research has shown that people with "unstable" angina taking one aspirin tablet daily can reduce the risk of a heart attack or death. Aspirin therapy can also cause side effects such as stomach upset and constipation, as well as internal bleeding and ulcers. Therefore, people with an active peptic ulcer or with bleeding disorders should not take aspirin. In addition, aspirin can interact with other medications and you should talk to your doctor and pharmacist about possible drug interactions.

Nitrates (usually nitroglycerin or isosorbide) are also used to treat people with "unstable" angina. Nitrates have the ability to open (dilate) blood vessels and increase the blood flow to the heart, making it easier for the heart to work. Nitrates come in tablets that you put under your tongue (sublingual), oral tablets, sustained release capsules, a topical cream, and patches that you can apply to your skin. You may feel dizzy, lightheaded, or experience headaches after taking nitrates. These effects are due to the blood vessels expanding (dilating). Several other medications such as beta-blockers are also used to treat "unstable" angina.

In addition to medication, the following lifestyle changes will also help to prevent blockages in the coronary arteries:

- Stop smoking
- Eat foods that are lower in fat
- Keep your weight down
- Increase your physical activity
- Control your blood pressure if it is high
- Lower stress in your life

LEG CRAMPING

QUESTION: I get terrible pain and cramping in my legs when I walk. I heard there is a new medicine for this problem and would like some information about it.

ANSWER: You're probably talking about a new prescription drug named Pletal (generic name cilostazol, pronounced sil-os-tah-zol) for the treatment of intermittent claudication, also called "angina of the legs". Approximately four million people in the U.S. have this problem. Blocked arteries in the legs cause this condition, which produces an aching, cramping, crippling sensation felt in the legs when walking. The way the drug works is not exactly known, but it is believed that Pletal improves the symptoms by blocking an enzyme in the body that results in better blood flow in the legs. The drug causes the blood vessels to expand (dilate) and helps to prevent the blood from forming clots. This allows people with this condition to walk farther and with less pain in their legs. Pletal is the first drug in 15 years to be approved for this problem. Studies have shown that people taking this medication were able to walk an average 1.3 city blocks further than those who did not take the drug. The most common side effects of Pletal are headache, diarrhea, abnormal stools, dizziness, palpitations, and increased heart rate. It is also important to know that Pletal should not be taken by anyone with congestive heart failure. The usual recommended dose of Pletal is a 100-mg tablet twice a day, taken at least half an hour before or two hours after breakfast and dinner. The beneficial effects of Pletal usually take two to four weeks of treatment, but some people may need up to 12 weeks of treatment before the drug produces any relief. Also, be sure to let your pharmacist know about any other medications that you take, because a number of drug interactions are possible with Pletal. Grapefruit juice also interferes with Pletal, so it should be avoided when using this new medication.

NEW USES FOR ASPIRIN

QUESTION: I keep hearing about new uses for aspirin. What is it good for?

ANSWER: If aspirin were a new drug today, it would be considered a real medical wonder drug and probably would be available by prescription only. Besides treating pain, inflammation, and fever, this 100-year-old drug has now been shown to be beneficial for a number of other medical problems. The FDA now believes that aspirin may be useful in reducing the possibility of:

• Stroke in people who have had a previous stroke or who have had a warning sign (transient ischemic attack—TIA or ministroke).
• Heart attack in people who had a previous heart attack or those who experience angina (chest pain).

- Death or complications from a heart attack if aspirin is taken at the first signs of a heart attack.
- Blockage of the blood vessels for people who have had heart bypass surgery or other procedures to clear blocked arteries, such as balloon angioplasty or carotid endarterectomy.

The dose of aspirin recommended for these cardiovascular uses are lower than what is recommended for pain, inflammation, or fever (325 mg-650 mg every 4-6 hours). Only 50 mg to 325 mg once a day appears to be an effective dose for the prevention of strokes, heart attacks, or artery blockage. These lower doses also reduce the risk of side effects from aspirin.

Side effects of aspirin can include irritation of the stomach, ringing in the ears in high doses, allergic reactions (especially in people with asthma), and bleeding. Chronic alcohol users may be at greater risk of stomach bleeding from aspirin use. Because of the risk of Reye's syndrome (a rare but serious disease) aspirin should not be used in children or teenagers for flu-like symptoms or chicken pox. Pregnant women and people with peptic ulcer disease, uncontrolled high blood pressure, or bleeding disorders should also avoid aspirin. In addition, patients with severe kidney or liver problems should not take aspirin.

Because of the potential for side effects, the long-term use of aspirin should always be discussed with your physician. Numerous drug interactions are also possible with aspirin and other drugs, so be sure to let your pharmacist and doctor know that you are taking aspirin when other medications are prescribed.

ASPIRIN-IBUPROFEN INTERACTIONS

QUESTION: I heard that ibuprofen could interfere with the aspirin that I take for my heart. Is this true?

ANSWER: Yes, there is some evidence that the pain reliever ibuprofen (Motrin, Advil, etc.) can counteract the benefits of taking aspirin to prevent heart attacks and strokes. Results from a recent study that was published in the New England Journal of Medicine show that ibuprofen may block the effects of aspirin in reducing the risk for cardiovascular disease. The study also found that three other drugs (rofecoxib (Vioxx), diclofenac (Voltaren), and acetaminophen or Tylenol) did not interfere with aspirin's effects. Aspirin protects against heart attacks by helping to prevent the blood from forming clots. It does this by binding to an enzyme in the blood that helps blood to clot. It appears, however, that ibuprofen also binds with this enzyme and does not allow aspirin to work. It's like having a room with only one chair in it. If ibuprofen gets to the chair first, aspirin cannot sit in the chair and prevent blood clots from forming. Because of this, it might be better to take aspirin early in the day and ibuprofen later in the day if needed. If the ibuprofen is taken several times a day, aspirin may never get a chance to "sit in the chair". If a patient needs to take aspirin and a pain reliever, perhaps a different agent such as acetaminophen may be a better choice. Much more research is needed on this topic, and patients should consult with their doctor and pharmacist to try and prevent any unwanted drug interactions.

ATRIAL FIBRILLATION

QUESTION: I heard that a new blood thinner was approved that might replace Coumadin (warfarin). What can you tell me about this?

ANSWER: The FDA recently approved the oral anticoagulant Pradaxa (dabigatran) for preventing strokes and blood clots in patients with abnormal heart rhythm (atrial fibrillation). Atrial fibrillation, which affects more than 2 million Americans, involves very fast and uncoordinated contractions of the heart' s two upper chambers (atria) and is one of the most common types of abnormal heart rhythm. Because the heart is not pumping blood properly in people with this condition, they are at a higher risk of developing blood clots, which can cause a disabling stroke if the clots travel to the brain. During a large clinical study involving more than 18,000 people with atrial fibrillation, Pradaxa was shown to reduce the risk of blood clots and strokes compared to warfarin. A major advantage of Pradaxa over warfarin is that periodic monitoring with blood tests is not necessary. In addition, Pradaxa does not have as many drug and food interactions as warfarin. The most common side effects of Pradaxa are gastritis-like symptoms and bleeding. Pradaxa is taken orally, twice a day.

QUESTION: Can my heart medication, Multaq, cause liver problems?

ANSWER: On January 14, 2011 the FDA alerted healthcare professionals and patients about cases of rare, but severe liver injury, including two cases of acute liver failure leading to a liver transplant in patients taking the heart medication Multaq (dronedarone). Multaq is an antiarrhythmic drug used to treat an abnormal heart rhythm known as atrial fibrillation or atrial flutter. However, it should not be used in patients with severe heart failure or who have recently been in the hospital for heart failure. According to the FDA, about 492,000 prescriptions for Multaq were dispensed and about 117,000 patients filled prescriptions at U.S. pharmacies for Multaq from the time of drug approval in July 2009 through October 2010. The two cases of acute liver failure that required transplantation occurred in female patients approximately 70 years of age at 4 ½ and 6 months after starting Multaq. Prescribing information for Multaq will now be updated to include this information about the risk of liver injury with Multaq. The FDA advises patients taking Multaq to:

- Contact your healthcare professional if you develop itching, yellow eyes or skin, dark urine, loss of appetite, nausea, vomiting, fever, malaise, right upper quadrant pain, or light-colored stools. These may be signs of liver injury.
- Talk to your healthcare professional about any concerns you have with this medication.
- Do not stop taking dronedarone unless told to do so by your healthcare professional.
- Report any side effects you experience to the FDA MedWatch program at 1-800-332-1088.

Read the Medication Guide when picking up a prescription for dronedarone. It will help you understand the potential risks and benefits of this medication.

PLEASE NOTE: On December 19, 2011 the U.S. Food and Drug Administration (FDA) completed a safety review of the heart drug Multaq (dronedarone). This review showed that Multaq increased the risk of serious cardiovascular events, including death, when used by patients in permanent atrial fibrillation (AF). The Multaq drug label has been revised with the following changes and recommendations (see the revised Multaq label for all changes):

- Healthcare professionals should not prescribe Multaq to patients with AF who cannot or will not be converted into normal sinus rhythm (permanent AF), because Multaq doubles the rate of cardiovascular death, stroke, and heart failure in such patients.
- Healthcare professionals should monitor heart (cardiac) rhythm by electrocardiogram (ECG) at least once every 3 months. If the patient is in AF, Multaq should be stopped or, if clinically indicated, the patient should be cardioverted.
- Multaq is indicated to reduce hospitalization for AF in patients in sinus rhythm with a history of non-permanent AF (known as paroxysmal or persistent AF)
- Patients prescribed Multaq should receive appropriate antithrombotic therapy.

Patients should contact their healthcare professional if they have any questions or concerns about Multaq. Patients should not stop taking Multaq without talking to their healthcare professional.

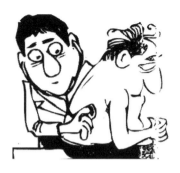

CHAPTER 3
MEN'S CONCERNS

PROSTATE PROBLEMS

QUESTION: What drugs are used to treat an enlarged prostate?

ANSWER: An enlarged prostate gland (also called "benign prostatic hyperplasia" or BPH) is one of the most common problems affecting elderly men. Approximately 80% of men aged 80 years or older have BPH, and 30% of men will need treatment for it at some point in their lives. It is rare in men under 40 and its cause is unknown.

The prostate gland makes some of the milky fluid (semen) that carries sperm. It is about the size of a walnut and is located just under the bladder, which stores urine. The prostate gland wraps around a tube (the urethra) that carries urine from the bladder out through the penis. During a man's orgasm, muscles squeeze the semen into the urethra where it meets up with sperm from the testicles. The prostate gland is normally soft and pliable, but when it becomes enlarged it can become rigid and constrict or totally close off the urethra. This makes urination difficult and causes a "backup" of urine. Symptoms of BPH related to a blockage in urine flow include a decreased force of urine stream, hesitancy in urinating, abdominal straining to urinate, dribbling of urine, and incomplete emptying of the bladder. Other irritating symptoms can include the need to urinate at night, increased frequency of urination, urgency to urinate, and painful urination.

The treatment of BPH includes both medical and surgical options to decrease the obstruction in urine flow, reduce symptoms, and improve quality of life. It should be noted that many medications can aggravate BPH and should be avoided if possible. Avoidance of coffee, alcohol, or large quantities of fluids after dinner can also be helpful. Most of the drugs used to treat BPH are known as "alpha-adrenergic blocking agents". They work by relaxing the smooth muscle in the neck of the bladder and in the prostate to improve urine flow. However, they also relax blood vessels and can cause hypotension, dizziness, or headache. Examples of these drugs include Minipress, Hytrin, Cardura, and Flomax. Another type of drug used to treat BPH is Proscar or finasteride. It works to slow the growth of the prostate gland by blocking hormones that stimulate its growth. It appears to be most effective in patients with significantly enlarged prostates. Proscar may take up to 6 months of treatment to see effects and it can cause a decreased libido, ejaculatory disorders, and erectile dysfunction. Finally, the herbal supplement saw palmetto has also been shown to be effective in treating BPH. I have also reviewed this product in a previous column.

QUESTION: I heard that combining two different drugs to treat an enlarged prostate might be more effective. What are these drugs?

ANSWER: A recent study that was published in the New England Journal of Medicine has shown that combining two different drug therapies may be more effective than either drug alone for the treatment of benign prostatic hyperplasia (BPH) or an enlarged prostate gland. In this 5-year study the drug doxazosin (Cardura) was combined with the drug finasteride (Proscar) to treat men with BPH. Each of these drugs work in a different way to help control the symptoms of BPH such as a decreased force of urine stream, hesitancy in urinating, incomplete emptying of the bladder, the need to urinate at night, urgency to urinate, or painful urination. Doxazosin is known as an "alpha-adrenergic blocking agent" and works by relaxing the smooth muscle in the neck of the bladder and in the prostate to improve urine flow. Other similar drugs include terazosin (Hytrin), and tamsulosin

(Flomax). On the other hand, finasteride works to slow the growth of the prostate gland by blocking hormones that stimulate its growth. When these drugs are used together you have a two-pronged treatment approach. This combination treatment is similar to that used to treat high blood pressure or diabetes where just one drug is not adequate for some people. Approximately 50% of men between 50 and 60 have an enlarged prostate while as many as 90% of those over 80 have that condition. It is rare in men under 40 and its cause is unknown. It has been estimated that about 40% of men with BPH may be considered for this combination therapy.

QUESTION: I heard that combining two different drugs might be better for treating an enlarged prostate. What can you tell me about this?

ANSWER: I reported in an earlier column that a combination of the drugs Cardura (doxazosin) and Proscar (finasteride) might be more effective than either drug alone for the treatment of benign prostatic hyperplasia (BPH) or an enlarged prostate gland. More recently, results from a study in the journal European Urology showed that a combination of two other drugs might also be more effective in treating this common urologic condition in men. In the 4-year study, which involved more than 4,800 men with PBH, the combination of Flomax (tamsulosin) and Avodart (dutasteride) was compared to using either drug alone. Results from the study showed that patients taking the combination were 67% less likely to have acute urinary retention and 70% less likely to require BPH-related surgery than those taking Flomax (tamsulosin) alone. They were 19% less likely to suffer from either of these complications than those taking Avodart (dutasteride) alone. Each of these drugs work in a different way to help control symptoms of BPH, such as decreased force of urine stream, hesitancy in urinating, incomplete emptying of the bladder, the need to urinate at night, urgency to urinate, or painful urination. Flomax (tamsulosin) is known as an "alpha-adrenergic blocking agent", which works by relaxing the smooth muscle in the neck of the bladder and in the prostate to improve urine flow. On the other hand, Avodart (dutasteride) works by blocking an enzyme that changes testosterone into a chemical that promotes prostate growth. When these drugs are used together you have a two-pronged treatment approach.

QUESTION: I heard that a new combination drug was approved for an enlarged prostate. What can you tell me about it?

ANSWER: The FDA recently approved Jalyn to treat the urinary symptoms of men with benign prostatic hyperplasia or BPH. Actually this new drug is a combination of two drugs that have been used as individual agents for many years to treat the symptoms of BPH. The two drugs in Jalyn are dutasteride (Flomax) and tamsulosin (Avodart or generic). Recently, results from a study in the journal European Urology showed that a combination of these two drugs might be more effective in treating this common urologic condition in men. In the 4-year study, which involved more than 4,800 men with PBH, the combination of Flomax (tamsulosin) and Avodart (dutasteride) was compared to using either drug alone. Results from the study showed that patients taking the combination were 67% less likely to have acute urinary retention and 70% less likely to require BPH-related surgery than those taking Flomax (tamsulosin) alone. They were 19% less likely to suffer from either of these complications than those taking Avodart (dutasteride) alone.

Each of these drugs work in a different way to help control symptoms of BPH, such as decreased force of urine stream, hesitancy in urinating, incomplete emptying of the bladder, the need to urinate at night, urgency to urinate, or painful urination. Flomax (tamsulosin) is known as an "alpha-adrenergic blocking agent", which works by relaxing the smooth muscle in the neck of the bladder and in the prostate to improve urine flow. On the other hand, Avodart (dutasteride) works by blocking an enzyme that changes testosterone into a chemical that promotes prostate growth. When these drugs are used together you have a two-pronged treatment approach.

QUESTION: I take Proscar for an enlarged prostate. Is there a generic drug available?

ANSWER: Yes, the FDA recently approved a generic version of Proscar (generic name finasteride). It will be available from TEVA Pharmaceuticals and is indicated for the treatment of men with an enlarged prostate to improve symptoms and to reduce the risk of the need for prostate surgery.

Finasteride works to slow the growth of the prostate gland by blocking hormones that stimulate its growth. It appears to be most effective in patients with significantly enlarged prostates. Finasteride may take up to 6 months of treatment to see effects and it can cause a decreased libido, ejaculatory disorders, and erectile dysfunction.

As I've noted many times before, the FDA approves all generic drugs using strict guidelines, including checking for the generic drug's chemistry by evaluating its formulation, potency, stability, and purity. The generic drug must also pass bio-equivalency testing that compares the delivery into the bloodstream of the generic drug's active ingredient to that of the brand name drug. Generic drugs are less expensive than brand-name products, and account for about 50 percent of prescriptions dispensed.

QUESTION: I take Flomax for an enlarged prostate. Is a generic product available?

ANSWER: The FDA recently approved the first generic versions of Flomax capsules (tamsulosin) to treat the signs and symptoms of benign prostatic hyperplasia (BPH) or enlarged prostate. IMPAX Laboratories and Sun Pharmaceutical will manufacture the generic products with the same prescribing information and safety warnings as those for Flomax capsules. Under FDA regulations, the generic version of tamsulosin must meet the same standards as the brand drug. Flomax (tamsulosin) is classified as an "alpha-adrenergic blocking agent" that works by relaxing the smooth muscle in the neck of the bladder and the prostate to improve urine flow.

QUESTION: What's the difference between using generic Flomax or doxazosin for an enlarged prostate?

ANSWER: As I noted in a previous column, Flomax is now available as the generic drug tamsulosin. Doxazosin (Cardura) and tamsulosin (Flomax) are known as "alpha-adrenergic blocking agents" or "alpha-blockers" for short. In general, alpha-blockers work by relaxing smooth muscle, which is found in blood vessels and in the neck of the bladder, among other places. Doxazosin is approved to treat both high blood pressure (hypertension) and enlargement of the prostate gland (benign prostatic hypertrophy or BPH). Tamsulosin, however, is only approved to treat BPH. The reason that tamsulosin is not approved to treat hypertension is that it is a "uroselective" alpha-blocker which primarily relaxes smooth muscle in the neck of the bladder and prostate, but not in blood vessels. For the treatment of BPH, there do not appear to be major differences in overall effectiveness among the alpha-blockers used to treat this condition. However, since tamsulosin is more selective for smooth muscle in the urinary tract it may be a better choice for men who cannot tolerate doxazosin and its blood pressure lowering effects. On the other hand, doxazosin may be a better choice for the treatment of BPH in men who also have hypertension.

QUESTION: I heard about a new long-acting medication for treatment of an enlarged prostate. What can you tell me about it?

ANSWER: The newly approved medication for BPH is UroXatral (generic name alfuzosin). It is called an "alpha-blocker" and is used to treat symptoms of an enlarged prostate. It works by helping to relax the muscles in the prostate and the bladder, which may decrease urinary tract symptoms of BPH and improve urine flow. Alpha-blockers improve symptoms in about 30-40% of patients. Other similar drugs include Hytrin (terazosin), Cardura (doxazosin), and Flomax (tamsulosin). UroXatral utilizes an oral controlled drug-release system that allows it to be taken only once a day. The most common side effects of UroXatral include dizziness, headache, and fatigue. This new agent may interact with some other drugs, so make sure that your doctor and pharmacist know all our other medications. UroXatral has been available in Europe for about 10 years.

QUESTION: What drugs should be used with caution by someone with an enlarged prostate gland?

ANSWER: When you have this condition, numerous drugs should be avoided or used with caution because they can aggravate the problem and make it worse. They usually do this by preventing muscle contractions in the bladder, which decreases urine outflow even more, or they can actually promote further growth of the prostate gland. I have outlined many of these drugs in the list that follows. Please note that this list is not all-inclusive, so be sure to read all labeling precautions on non-prescription medication packaging and ask your doctor and pharmacist about any potential problems with prescription drugs.

Examples Of Drugs That Should Be Used With Caution
In Patients With An Enlarged Prostate
Drug Type (Class)
Generic Name (Product Names)

Analgesics
Codeine
Hydrocodone
Hydromorphone (Dilaudid)
Meperidine (Demerol)
Methadone (Dolophine)
Morphine (Duramorph, MS Contin, Roxanol)
Oxycodone (OxyContin, Roxicodone)
Propoxyphene (Darvon)

Androgens
Methyltestosterone
Testosterone (Android, Testred, Andro, Depo-Testosterone, Testoderm)
DHEA (?)
Androstendione (?)

Antiarrthymic
Disopyramide (Norpace)

Anticholinergics
Benztropine (Cogentin)
Selegiline (Eldepryl)
Trihexyphenidyl (Artane)
Meclizine (Antivert, Bonine)
Propantheline (Pro-Banthine)
Glycopyrrolate (Robinul)
Hyoscyamine (Anaspaz, Levsin)

Ipratropium (Atrovent)
Oxybutynin (Ditropan)

Anti-Depressants
Amitriptyline (Elavil)
Amoxapine (Asendin)
Clomipramine (Anafranil)
Desipramine (Norpramin)
Doxepin (Sinequan)
Nortriptyline (Aventyl, Pamelor)
Imipramine (Tofranil)
Protriptyline (Vivactil)
Maprotiline (Ludiomil)

Anti-Emetics
Prochlorperazine (Compazine)
Promethazine (Phenergan)
Thiethylperazine (Torecan)

Antihistamines
Chlorpheniramine (Chlor-Trimeton)
Clemastine (Tavist-1)
Diphenhydramine (Benadryl)
Hydroxyzine (Atarax, Vistaril)
Cyproheptadine (Periactin)

Antipsychotics
Clozapine (Clozaril)
Olanzapine (Zyprexa)
Chlorpromazine (Thorazine)
Haloperidol (Haldol)
Loxapine (Loxitane)
Fluphenazine (Prolixin)
Perphenazine (Trilafon)

Trifluoperazine (Stelazine)
Thioridazine (Mellaril)
Thiothixene (Navane)

Decongestants
Pseudoephedrine (Dexatrim, Sudafed, Novafed)

Muscle Relaxant
Orphenadrine (Norflex, Myophen)

QUESTION: I heard about a new drug for an enlarged prostate. What can you tell me about it?

ANSWER: The FDA recently approved Avodart (generic name dutasteride), a new drug for treating men with BPH. Avodart works by blocking an enzyme that changes testosterone into a chemical that promotes prostate growth. It actually blocks two types of this enzyme and is called a dual-acting inhibitor. It is similar to the drug Proscar, which has been available for a number of years. In clinical studies, Avodart was shown to significantly lower the incidence of urinary retention and the need for surgery to correct the problem. Improvement in urine flow usually occurs after about one month of treatment but it may take up to 3 months of treatment for symptoms to improve. The most common side effects of Avodart include impotence, decreased libido, and ejaculation disorders, which may diminish with continued treatment. The drug can also cause enlarged breasts and breast tenderness. In addition, a number of interactions with other drugs are possible. Avodart is taken as a capsule (0.5 mg) once a day.

QUESTION: I heard about a new long-acting medication for treatment of an enlarged prostate. What can you tell me about it?

ANSWER: The newly approved medication for BPH is Rapaflo (generic name silodosin). It is called an "alpha-blocker" and is used to treat symptoms of an enlarged prostate. It works by helping to relax the muscles in the prostate and the bladder, which may decrease urinary tract symptoms of BPH and improve urine flow. Alpha-blockers improve symptoms in about 30-40% of patients. Other similar drugs include Hytrin (terazosin), Cardura (doxazosin), UroXatral (alfuzosin), and Flomax (tamsulosin). Rapaflo is taken once a day to relieve the signs and symptoms of BPH. The most common side effect seen with Rapaflo is reduced or no semen during orgasm. This side effect does not pose a safety concern and is reversible with discontinuation of the product. Other side effects included dizziness, light-headedness, diarrhea, orthostatic hypotension (drop in blood pressure upon standing), headache, nasopharyngitis (a contagious viral infection of the nose and upper portion of the throat), and nasal congestion. Patients planning cataract surgery must notify their ophthalmologist that they are taking Rapaflo because of the possibility of a condition called Intraoperative Floppy Iris Syndrome (IFIS), a complication associated with cataract surgery in patients on alpha-blocker medications. In IFIS the iris of the eye becomes limp and moves in waves as a result of increases in fluid levels within the eye. This can result in a painful and extended recovery period in those who have undergone cataract surgery and a reduction in visual acuity (sharpness). Patients on alpha-blockers or those who have severe kidney or liver impairment should not use Rapaflo.

QUESTION: How do I know when I need drug treatment for an enlarged prostate?

ANSWER: Your physician or urologist can help you determine if drug treatment is needed for an enlarged prostate gland or benign prostatic hyperplasia (BPH). In addition, the American Urological Association has developed a questionnaire to help men evaluate the severity of their symptoms from BPH. This self-administered test can help men determine what type of prostate treatment is needed, if any. The questionnaire involves answering the following 7 questions:

1. Over the past month, how often have you had the sensation of not emptying your bladder completely after you finished urinating?
2. Over the past month, how often have you had to urinate again less than two hours after you finished urinating?
3. Over the past month, how often have you found you stopped and started again several times when you urinated?
4. Over the past month, how often have you found it difficult to postpone urination?

5. Over the past month, how often have you had a weak urinary stream?
6. Over the past month, how often have you had to push or strain to begin urination?
7. Over the past month, how many times did you most typically get up to urinate from the time you went to bed at night until the time you got up in the morning?

For each question you must give a numerical answer using the following key:

Not at all=0
Less than 1 time in 5=1
Less than half the time=2
About half the time=3
More than half the time=4
Almost always=5

After answering all questions with a numerical score, the scores are added together for a total score. The total score can then be used to determine BPH severity as follows:

Total Score/BPH Severity
1-7 Mild BPH
8-19 Moderate BPH
20-35 Severe BPH

In general, no treatment is needed if symptoms are mild. Moderate symptoms usually call for some form of BPH treatment. Severe symptoms may indicate that surgery for BPH is needed. There are several types of drugs used to treat BPH, which I have reviewed in other columns. They help to improve urine flow, reduce symptoms, and provide for a better quality of life. However, they can also cause side effects in some people.

PROSTATE CANCER

QUESTION: What can you tell me about the new vaccine for prostate cancer?

ANSWER: The FDA recently approved Provenge, a new therapy for certain men with advanced prostate cancer that uses their own immune system to fight the disease. Actually, Provenge is not like a regular vaccine because it does not prevent prostate cancer, but instead helps to fight it. Unlike an everyday vaccine, Provenge is an individualized immune system therapy that is created by taking immune (white) blood cells from a patient, genetically engineering them in a laboratory, and then intravenously putting them back into the patient to help fight the cancer. This procedure is done 3 times in one month. The first treatment primes the patient's immune system and the other two treatments initiate an anticancer immune response. In a pivotal clinical study involving 512 men with advanced prostate cancer, treatment with Provenge was shown to increase the median survival by 4.1 months compared to men getting a "dummy" (placebo) treatment. The median survival time for patients receiving Provenge was 25.8 months, as compared to 21.7 months for those who did not receive the treatment. It should be noted, however, that patients with advanced prostate cancer have a life expectancy of about 2 years, so giving them 4 more months gives them about 20% more life. Also, since the 4.1 months is a median number, about half of the patients lived longer, while about half lived less than this time. Almost all of the patients who received Provenge in this study had some type of side effect. Common side effects reported included chills, fatigue, fever, back pain, nausea, joint ache, and headache. The majority of side effects were mild or moderate in severity. Serious side effects, reported in approximately one quarter of the patients receiving Provenge, included acute intravenous infusion reactions and stroke. More information about Provenge can be found at **www. provenge.com**.

QUESTION: I'm concerned about getting prostate cancer. What foods or supplements can help reduce my risk?

ANSWER: It has been estimated that one in four American men will develop prostate problems during their life, and one in six will be diagnosed with prostate cancer. It is now the most commonly occurring cancer and the second leading cause of death in men. Because of this, all men should see their doctor for regular prostate checkups. This won't reduce your risk, but regular checkups will provide for early detection if prostate cancer does develop.

Several nutrients found in certain foods have been linked with a lower risk of prostate cancer. These include: lycopene found in tomatoes or tomato products (sauces, ketchup, soup, juice), watermelon and papaya; omega-3 fatty acids or fish oils found in fatty fish like salmon or tuna; selenium found in foods like grains, fish, meats, or broccoli; and vitamin D from sunshine, or foods like milk, butter, cheese, fish, oysters, and fortified cereals. These nutrients are also available in numerous vitamin or supplement products. Several studies are currently being conducted to determine whether some of these nutrients can reduce prostate cancer risk in healthy men.

QUESTION: I heard the FDA is warning that some drugs may increase the risk of high-grade prostate cancer. What can you tell me about this?

ANSWER: In June of 2011 the FDA issued a Safety Announcement about drugs known as 5-alpha reductase inhibitors or 5-ARIs. Medications in this category include Proscar (finasteride), Propecia (finasteride), Avodart (dutasteride), and Jalyn (dutasteride plus tamsulosin). Proscar, Avodart, and Jalyn are used to improve symptoms of an enlarged prostate (benign prostatic hyperplasia or BPH) while Propecia is used to treat male pattern hair loss. All of these drugs work by blocking the production of a hormone that stimulates prostate growth. The Safety Announcement warns about an increased risk of being diagnosed with a more serious form of prostate cancer (high-grade) in men taking 5-ARI drugs. This risk appears to be low, but healthcare providers and patients should be aware of this information and product labeling will be changed to reflect this risk. The new safety information is based upon the FDA's review of two large studies that looked at these drugs to see if they could reduce or prevent prostate cancer in approximately 27,000 men over 50 years of age. Results from these studies, which lasted 4 to

7 years, showed an overall reduction in prostate cancer of 23% to 26% in men taking 5-ARI drugs. These reductions, however, were limited to men with lower-grade prostate cancers. Both studies showed an increase in high-grade forms of prostate cancer in men taking the 5-ARI drugs. The FDA Safety Announcement wants healthcare professionals and patients to be aware of this increased risk of high-grade prostate cancer in men taking these medications, and provides important guidance on the interpretation of prostate-specific antigen (PSA) tests in patients taking 5-ARI drugs.

QUESTION: Can hormone shots for prostate cancer increase the risk of osteoporosis?

ANSWER: Yes they can and this topic was recently reviewed in a Johns Hopkins Health Alert (**www.johnshopkinshealthalerts. com**, 2011). Also known as androgen deprivation therapy or ADT, hormone therapy for prostate cancer reduces the level of testosterone and estrogen, both of which help to maintain bone density in men. Although not all men getting androgen deprivation therapy will develop osteoporosis (bone loss), an estimated 50% will be affected by their fourth year of treatment, and more than 80% will be affected after 10 years. Using androgen deprivation therapy for a year or more increases fracture risk as well. A study in The New England Journal of Medicine reported that among men with prostate cancer who lived for at least five years after their diagnosis, the risk of a fracture was nearly 20% among androgen deprivation therapy users, compared with 13% for nonusers. As the use of long-term androgen deprivation therapy broadens to include some cancers confined to the prostate (not just those that have metastasized), even more men will be at increased risk for osteoporosis and broken bones-problems that can cause pain and loss of mobility, reduced quality of life and even death. The good news is that medication and lifestyle measures can help increase the strength of your bones, although you'll need to undergo periodic monitoring. When medication is required to halt bone loss in androgen deprivation therapy users with prostate cancer, bisphosphonates are the first-choice treatment. Bisphosphonates include alendronate (Fosamax), etidronate (Didronel), ibandronate (Boniva), pamidronate (Aredia), risedronate (Actonel), tiludronate (Skelid), and zoledronic acid (Zometa, Reclast).

Selective estrogen receptor modulators (SERMs) offer a second-line option (raloxifene, Evisa), and a new alternative called denosumab (Prolia), also holds great promise.

QUESTION: Can vitamin E protect against prostate cancer?

ANSWER: No, not according to the results of a large study recently reported in the Journal of the American Medical Association (2011). In fact, the study showed that men taking supplemental vitamin E may even be increasing their risk for prostate cancer by up to 17%. In this study, called the SELECT trial (Selenium and Vitamin E Cancer Prevention Trial), over 35,000 healthy men age 50 and older were divided into one of four treatment groups. One group received vitamin E (400 IU/day), a second group received the mineral supplement selenium (200 micrograms/day), a third group received both vitamin E and selenium, and the fourth group received placebos (dummy pills). After monitoring the men for up to 10 years, the study results showed that the men taking vitamin E by itself had a significantly increased risk of prostate cancer compared to those taking a placebo. Men in the study who were taking selenium alone or in combination with vitamin E also showed a smaller, but not significant increase in prostate cancer risk. Why vitamin E given alone might increase the risk for prostate cancer is not known, the researchers noted. It is estimated that more than 50% of men age 60 and older take supplements containing vitamin E and about one-quarter of them take as much as 400 IU/day despite the recommended daily dietary allowance of only approximately 22 IU/day. The SELECT study was funded by the National Cancer Institute and the National Center for Complementary and Alternative Medicine.

STATINS AND PROSTATE CANCER

QUESTION: Can statin drugs help prevent fatal prostate cancer?

ANSWER: There currently is not enough information available to say yes or no, but a recent study in the Journal Cancer (2011) suggests that perhaps statin use may be associated with protection against prostate cancer death. In this case-controlled study, researchers reviewed the medical records of 380 men who had died of prostate cancer and another 380 men of the same age and race without prostate cancer or with non-lethal prostate cancer. Most of the men were white and in their mid to late 60's. The researchers found that men who died of prostate cancer were about half as likely to have taken a statin drug compared to those who did not die of prostate cancer. When they accounted for whether or not men were overweight and other health problems and medications, it turned out that those with fatal cancers were 63% less likely to have ever taken a statin medication. In addition, the risk reduction was greater in men taking more potent statins. However, researchers point out that the use of statins to lower cholesterol may not be the reason for cancer death prevention, but perhaps other factors such as diet and exercise are involved. Clearly, more study is needed before any recommendation can be made to use statins for prostate cancer prevention.

According to the American Cancer Society, about 1 in every 6 men will be diagnosed with prostate cancer at some point, and 1 in every 36 men will die of the disease. There are currently seven statin drugs available: atorvastatin (Lipitor), fluvastatin (Lescol), lovastatin (Mevacor, Altoprev), pitavastatin (Livalo), pravastatin (Pravachol), rosuvastatin (Crestor), and simvastatin (Zocor). Atorvastatin, lovastatin, pravastatin, and simvastatin are also available as generic drugs.

LYCOPENE

QUESTION: Do you think lycopene can help prevent prostate cancer?

ANSWER: Yes, lycopene may be helpful in preventing prostate cancer and may even be useful in the treatment of prostate cancer. Prostate cancer is the most frequent type of cancer in American men. An estimated 189,000 new cases were diagnosed in the United States in 2002, and more than 30,000 men died of the disease. Approximately one in six American men will be diagnosed with prostate cancer during their life, and it is the second leading cause of death in men. Because of this, all men should see their doctor for regular prostate checkups.

Lycopene is a member of the carotenoid pigment family and is found in the blood and tissues of humans. It gives tomatoes, along with other fruits and vegetables a red color protecting them from the sun and helping in photosynthesis. Lycopene is found in high concentrations in tomatoes and tomato products, such as ketchup, tomato paste, and tomato sauce. Over 80% of the lycopene in American diets comes from tomato products. However, not all tomatoes contain the same amount of lycopene. Red tomatoes have 10 times more lycopene than yellow tomatoes, and other reddish foods such as watermelons, papaya, and pink grapefruit may contain lycopene but in smaller amounts than tomatoes. Tomato sauce and pizza are rich sources of lycopene, but strawberries, although red, do not contain lycopene. It appears that heating or cooking tomatoes releases the lycopene and tomato paste contains more lycopene than fresh tomatoes. Several studies have now shown that men who consume a higher amount of foods that contain lycopene have a lower risk of prostate cancer. A few studies and case reports have also shown that lycopene may be helpful in men with prostate cancer, but larger studies are needed to confirm this benefit. How lycopene works in affecting prostate health is not known, but it may inhibit tumor growth and provide antioxidant effects. It also affects insulin growth factor, which is linked to prostate cancer. The ideal "dose" of lycopene is not known, but 10 mg to 15 mg twice daily has been recommended. Fresh tomatoes contain about 30 mg to 70 mg of lycopene per 2 pounds whereas tomato paste contains about 300 mg per 2 pounds. Supplement products containing lycopene are also available. Lycopene is generally considered to be safe and very few adverse reactions have been reported.

PROPECIA AND PSA TESTS

QUESTION: I take Propecia for hair loss. Can it affect the PSA test for my prostate?

ANSWER: Yes it can, and you should let your physician know whenever you get a PSA test done. The reason for this concern was reviewed in a Johns Hopkins Health Alert (**www.johnshopkinshealthalerts.com**,

2009). The prostate-specific antigen (PSA) test measures an enzyme produced almost exclusively by the glandular cells of the prostate. It is secreted during ejaculation into the prostatic ducts that empty into the urethra. PSA liquefies semen after ejaculation, promoting the release of sperm. Normally only very small amounts of PSA are present in the blood, but an abnormality of the prostate can disrupt the normal architecture of the gland and create an opening for PSA to pass into the bloodstream. Thus, high blood levels of PSA can indicate prostate problems, including cancer. A blood test to measure levels of PSA was first approved by the U.S. Food and Drug Administration (FDA) in 1986 as a way to determine whether prostate cancer had been treated successfully and to monitor for its recurrence. Today, however, PSA tests are FDA approved for prostate cancer detection and are widely used to screen men for the disease. Now research suggests that the hair-growth medication Propecia (finasteride) significantly lowers a man's PSA level, producing misleading results and potentially masking the presence of prostate cancer. Propecia is the same medication as Proscar, which is used to control benign prostatic hyperplasia (BPH). The difference is the dosage—5 mg per day for Proscar vs. 1 mg for Propecia. Proscar is known to artificially lower PSA levels by about half, and doctors interpreting PSA results in these men compensate by doubling the PSA value. Propecia's impact on the PSA level has not been formally studied until now. Researchers in a study, which was reported in the journal Lancet Oncology, assigned 355 men age 40-60 to take either Propecia or a placebo (inactive pill) for 48 weeks. For analysis purposes, the men were grouped by age: 40-49 and 50-60. By the end of the study period, PSA levels among men in the younger group had dropped by an average of 40%; in the older group, PSA declined by an average of 50%. Among men taking the placebo, the PSA levels of the younger men had not changed, and the levels of the older men had risen by an average of 13%. So, if you use Propecia, be sure to let your physician know so that your PSA results can be adjusted accordingly.

FLOMAX AND
<u>CATARACT SURGERY</u>

<u>QUESTION</u>: Can Flomax interfere with cataract surgery?

<u>ANSWER</u>: It may, according to a large study recently reported in The Journal of the American Medical Association (JAMA). Flomax (tamsulosin) is commonly used to treat an enlarged prostate gland (benign prostatic hyperplasia or BPH), which affects nearly 3 out of 4 men by the age of 70. Flomax is classified as an alpha-blocker medication that helps to relieve urinary symptoms of BPH by relaxing smooth muscles in the prostate and neck of the bladder. However, it can also relax the smooth muscles in the iris of the eye, leading to a condition known as intraoperative floppy iris syndrome or IFIS, which can increase the risk of complications during cataract surgery. In the recent study published in JAMA, researchers looked at the medical records of over 96,000 men over the age of 65 who had cataract surgery between 2002 and 2007. Findings from this study showed that men who had prescriptions filled for Flomax within 14 days of the cataract surgery had more than double the risk of serious complications following the surgery than did men who were not prescribed Flomax, or those who received Flomax more than 15 days before the surgery, or those that were taking other alpha-blocking drugs for BPH or high blood pressure. Why other alpha-blockers were not associated with complications in this study is not clear, but it may be related to their lower specificity for relaxing smooth muscle. The serious surgical complications reported with Flomax use within 14 days of the cataract procedure included a lost lens or lens fragment, retinal detachment, and inflammation within or around the eye. Results from this study point out the importance of making sure that your physician performing cataract surgery is aware of all the medications you are taking prior to surgery so that the surgeon can plan and prepare accordingly.

CONDOMS

QUESTION: How do I use a condom correctly?

ANSWER: Condom-like devices have been used to sheath the male penis since antiquity. Condoms in their current forms have been marketed on a widespread basis virtually since the invention of latex rubber in the 1800s.

Condoms were once a source of embarrassment and humor. As the HIV/AIDS crisis worsened, however, they became important tools in the fight against sexually transmitted diseases. Many types of condoms are available at your local pharmacy. Proper usage is important to prevent pregnancy and the spread of infection.

After a condom is purchased, you must store it properly in a cool, dry place. Inside a car is not appropriate due to excess heat. Carrying condoms for a long period in your wallet is also not appropriate. Always check the expiration date of the condoms before purchase and before each use. If they have expired or were exposed to heat, discard them. Place the condom on the penis prior to any vaginal, oral, or anal contact. The uncircumcised male should pull the foreskin back before applying the condom. It is critical to identify the correct side of the condom by unrolling it a few turns to be sure which is the inside and which is the outside. If the condom is put on upside down, it will not unroll. Most men will then attempt to turn it over and unroll it correctly. This is a great mistake. When the penis is erect, it tends to leak a little ejaculate prior to full ejaculation. If the condom has been incorrectly placed, it usually has the ejaculate on it. If the male turns it over for correct placement, the male secretions that have already leaked onto the inside can reach his partner, causing transmission of STDs and increasing the chance of pregnancy. The condom should be unrolled completely to the base of the penis. If lubricant is needed beyond what was supplied in the condom, the correct type of lubricant must be chosen. It must not be oil-based, as with petrolatum or mineral oil. Instead, choose popular sexual lubricants such as K-Y or Replens. When the sexual act is finished, immediately withdraw the condom and penis by grasping the condom at the base of the penis. (Source: W.S. Pray, PhD, DPh: Recent developments in birth control and STD prevention for men. U.S. Pharmacist. August 2009: 12-15.)

QUESTION: I heard about a condom that helps you get an erection. What do you know about it?

ANSWER: A company in Britain is developing a product currently known as a "condom safety device" or CSD500. This condom, which has been called a "condom with a kick", contains an "erectogenic" chemical in its tip called glyceryl trinitrate or nitroglycerin. The principle action of nitroglycerin is vasodilation or expansion of the blood vessels. The idea behind the condom is that the nitroglycerin in the condom will be absorbed into the skin of the penis and cause blood vessels to dilate. This in turn increases blood flow into the penis to maintain an erection. However, unlike Viagra, Cialis, or Levitra, which are used for erectile dysfunction, this condom is meant for men who find themselves unable to maintain an erection while wearing a condom because of the loss of sensation. It is intended to help healthy men maintain a full erection during sexual intercourse, and reduce the risk of condom slippage, which occurs in at least 2% of condom users. By maintaining a man's performance throughout sexual intercourse, the CSD500 is designed to prevent unwanted accidents and may also help men who do not like using condoms more willing to practice safe sex. It has been estimated that about 13 billion condoms are used worldwide each year, so if 2% of these slip off, it could result in large numbers of unwanted pregnancies and sexually transmitted infections. Scientists at Futura Medical in Great Britain designed the CSD500. A market survey by the company showed that 88% of existing condom users would be interested in buying an erection-boosting condom and 49% of men who did not use condoms said that they would also consider using the CDS500. We might expect this new product to be available in Europe in the near future.

BREAST ENLARGEMENT

QUESTION: Can some drugs cause breast enlargement in males?

ANSWER: Breast enlargement in males, also known as "gynecomastia", can occur as a normal physiologic event at certain times in life or can be the result of several diseases or drug treatments. Growth of the breasts in men, as in women, is controlled by estrogen (female hormone) and hormonal imbalances can cause breast tissue to enlarge. One or both breasts may be affected. Gynecomastia is commonly seen in boys during puberty and nearly one-half of boys 12-16 years of age experience some breast enlargement. Although it is not usually a serious condition and often disappears without treatment, it can be very bothersome for these adolescents. Breast enlargement can also develop in a newborn baby due to exposure to the mother's hormones. In older men, gynecomastia can be a result of medical conditions such as liver or kidney disease, tumors, or hyperthyroidism. It can also be a side effect of certain medications. Drugs can cause breast enlargement in many different ways. For example, men taking estrogen for prostate cancer or transsexuals taking it in preparation for a sex-change operation can develop gynecomastia. Some medications can also increase the activity of estrogen in the body. In addition, drugs that block testosterone (male hormone) production can cause a hormonal imbalance resulting in gynecomastia. Still other drugs cause breast enlargement in unknown ways. While it is beyond the scope of this column to list all the drugs that can cause gynecomastia, I have listed some examples below. Please consult with your physician and pharmacist if you have any specific concerns about the medication that you are taking.

Some Drugs That Can Cause Gynecomastia
- ACE inhibitors (Captopril, Fosinopril, many others)
- Antiretroviral agents (many drugs used to treat HIV infection)
- Busulfan (Myleran)
- Calcium channel blockers (Nifedipine, Diltazem, many others)
- Chlorambucil (Leukeran)
- Cimetidine (Tagamet)
- Cisplatin (Platinol-AQ)
- Clomiphene (Clomid)
- Cyclophosphamide (Cytoxan)
- Diazepam (Valium)
- Digitalis (Digoxin, Lanoxin)
- Estramustine (Emcyt)
- Estrogens (Diethylstilbestrol)
- Finasteride (Proscar, Propecia)

- Flutamide (Eulexin)
- Isoniazid (Nydrazid)
- Ketocnoazole (Nizoral)
- Melphalan (Alkeran)
- Methyldopa
- Metoclopramide (Reglan)
- Metronidazole (Flagyl)
- Omeprazole (Prilosec)
- Penicillamine (Cupramine, Depen)
- Spironolactone (Aldactone)
- Tricyclic antidepressants (Amitriptyline, Imipramine, many others)

LOW TESTOSTERONE LEVELS

QUESTION: I heard about a new underarm prescription product for low testosterone levels in men. What can you tell me about it?

ANSWER: The FDA recently approved Axiron (testosterone topical solution) as a replacement therapy in men over 18 for certain conditions associated with a deficiency or absence of testosterone. Axiron is the first testosterone topical solution approved for application using an armpit (underarm) applicator. Other forms of testosterone replacement therapy include oral tablets, buccal tablets, subcutaneous pellets, transdermal patches, injections, and topical gels applied by the hands. Axiron solution is applied to the underarm once a day in the morning using a metered dose applicator. Men who use an antiperspirant or deodorant should apply it before using Axiron to avoid contamination of the deodorant. The most common side effects of Axiron include skin redness or irritation where the solution is applied, increased red blood cell count, headache, diarrhea, vomiting, and an increase in PSA blood levels (a test to screen for prostate cancer). Additional side effects can include more erections than are normal or prolonged erections. Other more serious side effects can also occur with Axiron and unintentional exposure of this product to women and children should be avoided.

Although the total number of men with testosterone deficiency is unknown, it has been estimated that up to 13 million men over 45 years of age in the U.S. may have symptoms associated with low testosterone. Symptoms of testosterone deficiency, also known as hypogonadadism or low testosterone, include erectile dysfunction, decreased sexual desire, fatigue and loss of energy, mood depression, regression of secondary sexual characteristics, and osteoporosis. Your doctor can determine if you may have testosterone deficiency and can order blood tests to measure testosterone levels to see if they are within the normal range. In a 4-month clinical trial with Axiron, approximately 84% of men who completed the study achieved average blood testosterone levels within the normal range when using this product.

IMPOTENCE
ERECTILE DYSFUNCTION (ED)

QUESTION: What can you tell me about the drug Viagra? Is it safe?

ANSWER: Everyone seems to be excited about Viagra, the drug for impotence, which can be taken orally. Many physicians are being bombarded with calls about this new medication and some doctors are actually using a rubber stamp for prescriptions. Viagra or sildenafil (sil-den-ah-phil) was first developed for the treatment of angina but was not found to be effective for this condition. However, some men taking the drug reported getting an erection as an unexpected side effect. It was then studied for use in men with "erectile dysfunction" (impotence). Impotence occurs in about half of all men between the ages of 40 and 70.

Viagra primes the penis to respond to sexual stimulation. It is thought to work by blocking an enzyme in the erectile tissue of the penis, which enhances the effect of a chemical known as nitric oxide. A reduced amount of nitric oxide appears to be a problem in men with impotence. Nitric oxide is a substance that causes blood vessels to expand in size, allowing more blood to flow to the penis. This increased blood flow causes the swelling and hardness of an erection, which reverses after ejaculation as the blood withdraws from the penis. The drug does not appear to produce these effects unless there is sexual stimulation and men with normal amounts of nitric oxide do not appear to benefit from taking it. Viagra should not be taken more frequently than once a day and should be taken about one hour before sexual activity.

Viagra was fairly well tolerated during its clinical studies. The most common side effects reported included headache, flushing, indigestion, nasal congestion, urinary tract infection, muscle aches, abnormal vision, diarrhea, dizziness, and rash. Another potential problem with using Viagra is in patients also taking nitrate medications. Viagra may cause serious low blood pressure in these people and it should not be used in combination with these drugs. Like all new drug products, a word of caution is in order. Remember that many side effects are not detected until a drug is used in very large numbers of people. For example, to have a good chance of identifying a side effect that only occurs in one person out of 1,000 who takes the drug, over 3,000 patients would have to be studied. No drug is perfectly safe and it has recently been reported that adverse reactions to drugs is the fourth largest cause of death in the U.S., right behind heart disease, cancer, and stroke. Recently identified heart valve problems with dieters using "fen-phen" is a case in point. Only time will tell if Viagra can live up to all its expectations.

QUESTION: My urologist recently prescribed Viagra for me and I was warned not to take any "nitrate medications" with it. What are "nitrate medications"?

ANSWER: As you know, Viagra or sildenafil (sil-den-ah-phil) is the very popular oral medication used to treat erectile dysfunction or impotence. It does, however, have its upside and downside. Viagra was fairly well tolerated during clinical studies, but numerous deaths have been reported since its approval and widespread use. Many of the patients that died were given or gave themselves a nitrate medication.

Viagra works to help blood vessels expand in size, allowing more blood flow to the penis, which causes the swelling and hardness of an erection. Unfortunately, the drug does not just work on blood vessels, which go to the penis, but elsewhere also. This expansion of blood vessels can cause low blood pressure or hypotension in some patients. Nitrates also cause blood vessels to expand and that is why they are useful in treating angina where not enough blood is getting to the heart, causing pain. When given together, Viagra and nitrate medications may work together to cause a serious lowering of the blood pressure, possibly leading to death or other events. Because of this, these medications should not be used together. Listed below are the trade and generic names of some commonly prescribed nitrate medications:

Some Commonly Prescribed Nitrate Medications
Generic Name
Some Trade Names

- **Isosorbide mononitrate**
    Monoket, ISMO, Imdur
- **Isosorbide dinitrate**
    Isordil, Sorbitrate, Dilatrate
- **Nitroglycerin**
    Nitrostat, Nitrolingual, Nitrogard, Nitro-time, NitroQuick, NitroTab
- **Nitroglycerin patches**
    Minitran, Nitro-Dur, Transderm-Nitro, Nitro-Dur, Deponit, Nitrek
- **Nitroglycerin ointment**
    Nitro-Bid

QUESTION: If I take Viagra at bedtime will it affect my sleep apnea?

ANSWER: Yes it may, according to a Johns Hopkins Health Alert (**www.johnshopkinshealthalerts.com**, 2007). Sleep apnea is a disorder characterized by repeated episodes of breathing cessation (apnea) during sleep. These episodes last from 10 seconds to nearly a minute, ending with a brief partial arousal. Episodes of sleep apnea can occur (and disrupt sleep) hundreds of times throughout one night. An estimated 18 million Americans have obstructive sleep apnea, yet 95% of them are undiagnosed and untreated. Sleep apnea is about twice as common among men as among women. Obstructive sleep apnea is caused by a blockage in the throat or upper airway. Recently, a report in a respected medical journal (Archives Internal Medicine) suggested that taking Viagra at bedtime may worsen severe obstructive sleep apnea. Viagra primes the penis to respond to sexual stimulation. It is thought to work by blocking an enzyme in the erectile tissue of the penis, which enhances the effect of a chemical known as nitric oxide. A reduced amount of nitric oxide appears to be a problem in men with impotence. Nitric oxide is a substance that causes blood vessels to expand in size, allowing more blood to flow to the penis. This increased blood flow causes the swelling and hardness of an erection, which reverses after ejaculation as the blood withdraws from the penis. The drug does not appear to produce these effects unless there is sexual stimulation and men with normal amounts of nitric oxide do not appear to benefit from taking it. However, Viagra also prolongs the action of nitric oxide, which promotes upper airway congestion, thereby contributing to sleep apnea. In the medical report referred to above, researchers studied 14 men with severe sleep apnea, who spent a night in a sleep lab having their breath and blood oxygen monitored after taking a single 50 mg dose of Viagra or a dummy pill (placebo). The men taking Viagra had a significantly lower level of oxygen in their blood and weren't getting as much oxygen as those taking the dummy pill. They also had more breathing pauses per hour. Based upon this information, if you have sleep apnea and take Viagra you should consult with your doctor about the risk of worsening your nighttime sleeping problems.

QUESTION: I saw a full-page ad about a new drug for impotence. Is it like Viagra?

ANSWER: The FDA recently approved Levitra (generic name vardenafil) for the treatment of impotence or erectile dysfunction. It is manufactured by Bayer and will be marketed by GlaxoSmithKline. This new drug works in a similar way and has side effects like Viagra. Levitra and Viagra prime the penis to respond to sexual stimulation. They are thought to work by blocking an enzyme in the erectile tissue of the penis, which enhances the effect of a chemical known as nitric oxide. A reduced amount of nitric oxide appears to be a problem in men with impotence. Nitric oxide is a substance that causes blood vessels to expand in size, allowing more blood to flow to the penis. This increased blood flow causes the swelling and hardness of an erection, which reverses after ejaculation as the blood withdraws from the penis. These drugs do not appear to produce these effects unless there is sexual stimulation and men with normal amounts of nitric oxide do not appear to benefit from taking these drugs. Like Viagra, Levitra should not be taken with nitrate medications (e.g. Imdur, ISMO, nitroglycerin, Isordil, Sorbitrate, etc.). It should also be avoided by people who take medicines called alpha-blockers, which are prescribed for high blood pressure or prostate problems (e.g., Hytrin, Prazosin, Minipres, Cardura, Doxazocin, etc.). These drugs can cause your blood pressure to go too low when taken with Levitra and you could get dizzy and faint. In addition, several other drugs can interact with Levitra so be sure that your doctor and pharmacist know all the medications that you take. In addition, Levitra should not be taken by men in whom sexual activity is inadvisable because of certain heart conditions. The most common side effects of Levitra are headache, flushing, stuffy or runny nose, indigestion, upset stomach, or dizziness. Levitra is taken one hour before sexual activity and should not be taken more than once a day. The manufacturer of Levitra is planning to widely advertise this new drug and has signed a 3-year sponsorship deal with the National Football League. A third product is also close to approval and is longer acting than either Viagra or Levitra. More information about Levitra can be obtained by calling 1-866-Levitra or on the Internet at **www. levitra.com**.

QUESTION: I heard about a new long-acting drug for erectile dysfunction. What can you tell me about it?

ANSWER: The FDA recently approved Cialis (See-Al-Iss) for the treatment of impotence or erectile dysfunction. Cialis (generic name tadenafil) was the third drug in its class to be approved for this use, the other two being Viagra and Levitra. All three of these drugs work in a similar way to increase blood flow to the penis, which helps men get and keep an erection satisfactory for sexual activity. Once the sexual activity is completed, blood flow to the penis decreases, and the erection goes away. Some form of sexual stimulation is also needed for an erection to occur with these drugs. The big difference between Cialis and Viagra or Levitra is that it stays in the body for a longer period of time. Studies have shown that its effects can last for up to 36 hours after taking the drug compared to 4 to5 hours for Viagra and Levitra. Because of its long duration of action, Cialis has been referred to in Europe as the "le weekender" with a Friday-night dose lasting until Sunday. Cialis can also be taken with a high-fat meal, which can be a problem with Viagra. Like Viagra and Levitra, Cialis should not be taken with nitrate medications (e.g., Imour, ISMO, Isordil, nitroglycerin, Sorbitrate, etc.). It should also be avoided by men who take alpha-blockers (other than Flomax), which are prescribed for high blood pressure or prostate problems (e.g., Hytrin, Prazosin, Minipress, Cardura, Doxazosin, Uroxatral, etc.). These drugs can cause the blood pressure to go too low, causing dizziness or fainting. Other drugs can also interact with Cialis, so be sure your doctor and pharmacist know all the medications that you are taking. Cialis should not be used more than once a day, and is not recommended for patients with low blood pressure, uncontrolled high blood pressure, angina, liver problems, retinal eye problems, or those who have had a stroke or heart attack in the past six months. In addition, those patients who have been advised by their doctor to avoid sexual activity due to cardiovascular conditions should not take the drug. The most common side effects of Cialis reported during drug testing were headache, indigestion, back pain, muscle aches, flushing, and stuffy or runny nose. Cialis is taken orally before expected sexual activity, but not more than once daily.

QUESTION: I heard that a new drug was approved for erectile dysfunction. What can you tell me about it?

ANSWER: In April 2012, the FDA approved Stendra (avanafil) to treat erectile dysfunction in men. It is the first new drug in a class of drugs call PDE5 inhibitors to be approved in a decade. All PDE5 inhibitors work by increasing blood flow to the penis and sexual stimulation is required to initiate an erection. Other drugs in this class include Viagra (sildenafil), Cialis (tadalafil), and Levitra or Staxyn (varadenafil). In clinical studies, Stendra was able to increase the rate of erections sufficient for sexual intercourse from less than 15% to as much as 57% compared to 27% with a "dummy pill" (placebo). One potential advantage of Stendra is that it may work in as little as 15 minutes, but direct comparisons with other similar drugs are not available. The recommended starting dose for Stendra is a 100 mg tablet taken approximately 30 minutes before sexual activity. Like other PDE5 inhibitors, Stendra should not be taken by men who take nitrates, commonly used to treat chest pain, because the combination can cause a sudden drop in blood pressure. The most common side effects of Stendra reported in more than 2% of patients during clinical studies included headache, redness of the face and other areas, nasal congestion, common cold-like symptoms, and back pain. In rare cases, some patients taking Stendra and other similar drugs may get an erection lasting longer than 4 hours, in which they should seek immediate medical care. ED occurs when a man has trouble getting or maintaining an erection, with an estimated 30 million American men affected by this problem. Its prevalence increases with age, and with various disease states such as diabetes, hypertension, and/or vascular disease.

QUESTION: Can Cialis be taken once a day for erectile dysfunction?

ANSWER. The FDA recently approved Cialis (2.5 mg and 5 mg) tablets for once daily dosing to treat erectile dysfunction (ED). When Cialis is taken once daily in these lower doses, men can attempt sexual activity at any time between doses. This low-dose daily treatment may be most appropriate for men with ED who anticipate more frequent sexual activity (e.g. twice weekly). For other men, Cialis (5 mg to 20 mg) taken as needed prior to anticipated sexual activity, may be the most appropriate dosage schedule. ED is defined as the consistent inability to attain and maintain an erection sufficient for sexual intercourse. Experts believe that 80-90% of ED cases are related to a physical or medical condition, such as diabetes, cardiovascular diseases, and prostate cancer treatment, while 10-20% are due to psychological causes. In many cases, however, both psychological and physical factors contribute to the condition. Cialis was first approved in the United States in 2003 for as-needed treatment of ED. It was the third drug in its class to be approved for this use, the other two being Viagra and Levitra. All three of these drugs work in a similar way to increase blood flow to the penis, which helps men get and keep an erection satisfactory for sexual activity. Once the sexual activity is completed, blood flow to the penis decreases, and the erection goes away. Some form of sexual stimulation is also needed for an erection to occur with these drugs. The big difference between Cialis and Viagra or Levitra is that it stays in the body for a longer period of time and studies have shown that its effects can last for up to 36 hours after taking the drug compared to 4 to 5 hours for Viagra and Levitra.

QUESTION: What prescription medicines should be avoided with Cialis?

ANSWER: Cialis (generic name tadalafil) is the newest drug approved for erectile dysfunction. Like Viagra and Levitra, Cialis helps to increase blood flow to the penis, which helps men get and keep an erection satisfactory for sexual activity. However, Cialis stays in the body for a longer period of time than Viagra or Levitra and its effects can last for up to 36 hours. It should be noted that some form of sexual stimulation is needed for an erection to occur with all of these drugs and numerous drug interactions can occur. The two most important types of drugs to avoid while taking Cialis are nitrates and most alpha-blockers. Both of these classes of drugs may cause a sudden, unsafe drop in blood pressure when used in combination with Cialis. Nitrates are commonly used to treat angina and include nitroglycerin (found in tablets, sprays, ointments, pastes, or patches), and isosorbide products (ISMO, Indur, Monoket, Isordil, Sorbitrate, Dilatrate-SR, Isoschron). Alpha-blockers are commonly used to treat prostate problems or high blood pressure and those that should not be used in combination with Cialis include Hytrin (terazosin), Cardura (doxazosin), Minipress (prazosin) or Uroxatral (alfluzosin). In addition to these medications, certain other drugs can interact with Cialis and a dosage adjustment may be needed. Some of these drugs include erythromycin (an antibiotic), ketoconozole (Nizoral) or Sporanox (antifungals), and Norvir or Crixivan (anti-AIDS drugs). Because many drug interactions can occur with Cialis, Viagra, and Levitra, always check with your doctor and pharmacist to avoid any problems with drug combinations. In addition, some non-prescription medicines can affect erectile dysfunction drugs, so be sure to let your doctor and pharmacist know about your use of these products also.

QUESTION: Why did the FDA take "True Man" and "Energy Max" off the market?

ANSWER: In May of 2007, the FDA issued a health risk alert advising consumers not to purchase or use "True Man" or "Energy Max" products sold as dietary supplements. These products are touted as sexual enhancement products and as treatment for erectile dysfunction. Both of these products are often advertised as "all natural" alternatives to approved prescription drugs for erectile dysfunction (Viagra, Levitra, Cialis) in advertisements appearing in newspapers, retail stores, and on the Internet. In November of 2007 the FDA requested a recall of these products. The reason for this health risk alert and recall is that these products contain ingredients very similar to approved prescription drugs. An FDA chemical analysis revealed that "Energy Max" contains a substance very similar to the active ingredient in Viagra and that "True Man" contains a substance very similar to the active ingredient in Levitra. Because these products were never approved by the FDA for effectiveness and safety, they are being recalled due to the risk they pose to the consumer. The risk of using these products is even more serious because consumers may not know that the ingredients can interact with other medications and dangerously lower their blood pressure. Of particular concern is the interaction of these products with nitrate medications. Nitrates are commonly used to treat angina and include nitroglycerin (found in tablets, sprays, ointments, pastes, or patches), and isosorbide products (ISMO, Indur, Monoket, Isordil, Sorbitrate, Dilatrate-SR, Isoschron). In view of these potential problems, the FDA recommends that consumers should discontinue use of these products and consult with their health care professional about approved treatments for erectile dysfunction.

QUESTION: I heard that the FDA is warning men not to use some dietary supplements to enhance sexual performance. What can you tell me about this?

ANSWER: The FDA recently issued warnings about two products, Man Up Now and Vigor-25, both marketed as natural dietary supplements to enhance male sexual performance. The reason for this warning is that these products have been found to contain the active drug ingredient (or similar iingredient) found in the prescription drug Viagra. This ingredient (sildenafil) may interact with other prescription drugs known as nitrates, including nitroglycerin, and can dangerously lower blood pressure. When blood pressure drops suddenly, the brain is deprived of an adequate blood supply that can lead to dizziness, lightheadedness, and other problems. The FDA is investigating the death of a 26-year-old man, possibly associated with the use of Vigor-25. The FDA feels that these products are dangerous to consumers because they claim to contain only natural or herbal ingredients when they actually are a prescription drug. Both of these products are sold on Internet sites, online marketplaces, and possibly in some retail outlets. The FDA advises consumers who have experienced any negative side effects from sexual enhancement products to stop using such products and consult a health care professional, and to safely discard the product. Adverse events or side effects from these and other products can be reported online at **www.fda.gov/MedWatch/report.htm**, or by calling 1-800-332-1088 to obtain a reporting form. Consumers are also urged to report suspected criminal activity regarding sexual enhancement products to the FDA's Office of Criminal Investigations by calling 1-800-551-3989 or by reporting it online at **www.fda.gov/OCI**.

QUESTION: Can some drugs prevent me from getting an erection?

ANSWER: Yes, there are numerous drugs that can cause a male to have difficulty in getting or sustaining an erection of the penis. This problem, which is also called erectile dysfunction or ED, has become a popular topic of discussion since the marketing of Viagra, the biggest blockbuster drug in pharmaceutical history. Before discussing the many different types of drugs that can interfere with the ability for a male to get an erection, let me briefly and simply review how an erection occurs. In the male, penile erection begins in the brain, which is stimulated by many different factors that affect sexual desire. Once stimulated the brain then sends impulses through the nervous system to the penis. This nerve stimulation leads to the production of chemicals including nitric oxide, which cause the relaxation of smooth muscles surrounding the penis. This relaxation produces a dilation or expansion of smooth muscle within blood vessels, which allows blood to flow into two chambers, which surround the penis called the copora cavernosa. These chambers then become engorged or full of blood, causing the penis to expand or become erect and rigid. This expansion of the penis also prevents blood from flowing out through the veins that carry blood from the penis and the blood is temporarily trapped. After an orgasm and ejaculation, the nervous system then causes the smooth muscle including blood vessels to again contract, which prevents blood from flowing into the chambers and promotes an emptying of blood from the chambers, which reverses the erection. Actually it's a very amazing process that involves the brain, nervous system, and circulation of blood within the blood vessels. Therefore, many different drugs affecting theses areas of the body may also affect the erection process. In the list that follows, I have summarized numerous types of drugs which can cause erectile dysfunction because of their ability to affect the brain, blood vessels, or nervous system. Please note that not all drugs that cause this problem are listed. If you have any questions regarding erectile dysfunction and a specific medication that you are taking, be sure to ask your doctor and pharmacist about it.

<u>Drugs That Can Cause Erectile Dysfunction</u>
Drug Type
Some Drug Examples (Generic Name, Trade Name)

Antihypertensives
- Clonidine (Catapres, Duraclon)
- Methyldopa (Aldomet)
- Beta-blockers:
  - Atenolol (Tenormin)
  - Labetalol (Normodyne)
  - Metoprolol (Lopressor)
  - Propranolol (Inderal, Betachron)
  - Pindolol (Visken)
- Thiazide diuretics:
  - Chlorthalidone (Hygroton)
  - Hydrochlorothiazide (Esidrex, Oretic, Hydrodiuril, Microzide)
- Indapamide (Lozol)
- Prazocin (Minipress)
- Amiloride (Midamor)
- Bepridil (Vascor)
- Reserpine

Anticholinergics
- Glycopyrrolate (Robinul)
- Hyoscyamine (Anaspaz, Levsin, Cytospaz)
- Propantheline (Norpanth, Pro-Banthine)
- Scopolamine (Isopto-Hyoscine, Transderm Scop)

Antidepressants

- Amoxapine (Asendin)
- Amitriptyline (Elavil, Endep)
- Desipramine (Norpramin)
- Fluoxetine (Prozac)
- Protriptyline (Vivactil)
- Clomipramine (Anafranil)
- Maprotiline (Ludiomil)
- Imipramine (Tofranil)
- Nefazodone (Serzone)
- Nortriptyline (Aventyl, Pamelor)
- Paroxetine (Paxil)
- Sertraline (Zoloft)
- Phenelzine (Nardil)
- Tranylcypromine (Parnate)
- Venlafaxine (Effexor)

Antipsychotics

- Fluphenazine (Prolixin)
- Haloperidol (Haldol)
- Thioridazine (Mellaril)
- Thiothixene (Navane)
- Chlorpromazine (Thorazine)
- Perphenazine (Trilafon)
- Resperidone (Risperdal)
- Trifluoperazine (Stelazine)

Tranquilizers

- Diazepam (Valium)
- Pentobarbital (Nembutal)
- Phenobarbital
- Secobarbital (Seconal)

Drugs of Habituation

- Alcohol
- Methadone
- Heroin
- Tobacco

Others

- Disulfiram (Antabuse)
- Cimetidine (Tagamet)
- Finasteride (Propecia, Proscar)
- Ketoconazole (Nizoral)
- Ranididine (Zantac)
- Spironolactone (Aldactone)
- Famotidine (Pepcid)
- Nizatidine (Axid)
- Carbamazepine (Tegretol)
- Digoxin (Lanoxin)
- Disopyramide (Norpace)
- Leuprolide (Lupron)
- Megestrol (Megace)
- Metoclopramide (Reglan)
- Phentermine (Adipex-P, Fastin, Ionamin)
- Phenytoin (Dilantin)
- Primidone (Mysoline)
- Prochlorperazine (Compazine)
- Promethazine (Phenergan)

QUESTION: Can drugs for erectile dysfunction cause hearing loss?

ANSWER: They may and the FDA is keeping an eye on this potential side effect. The FDA has received a total of 29 reports of sudden hearing loss, either partial or complete, in men taking erectile dysfunction (ED) drugs (Cialis, Levitra, and Viagra). This hearing loss may also be associated with ringing in the ears, vertigo, or dizziness and in most reported cases involved only one ear. In about one third of the cases, the event was temporary, but in the other two thirds the hearing loss was ongoing at the time of the report or the final outcome was not described. In view of these reports, the FDA has approved labeling changes for ED products to display more prominently the potential risk of sudden hearing loss. The FDA recommends that patients taking Cialis, Levitra, or Viagra who experience sudden hearing loss, should immediately stop taking the drug and seek prompt medical attention. It is important to also note that because some hearing loss is usually associated with the aging process, patients on these drugs may not think to talk to their doctor about it.

ED is the inability to obtain or maintain an erection and it occurs in about half of all men between the ages of 40 and 70. This problem increases with age, but other risk factors such as coronary artery disease, smoking, excess alcohol, diabetes, multiple sclerosis, high cholesterol, and high blood pressure can also be a factor.

HAIR LOSS

QUESTION: What drugs are available to help me grow hair?

ANSWER: Male pattern baldness is a very common condition. Hair loss in males may start in the late teens or early 20's and, by the age of 35 to 40, about 66% of male Caucasians will have some degree of hair loss. It is commonly found in the same family and is probably due to a person's genetic makeup and hormones produced. The hair loss usually begins in the front sides on the top of the head and may be extensive, depending on the person's age at the time it starts. It is now thought that hair loss is due to a hormone called DHT (di-hydro-tes-tos-stir-rone), which adversely affects the hair follicles where hair grows.

There are currently two drugs available in the United States that are approved by the FDA for the treatment of male pattern baldness or hair loss in men. The first product is called minoxidil (mi-noks-i-dil) or Rogaine solution, which is available in two strengths (2% and 5%) without a prescription. It is applied to the scalp twice a day. Exactly how this drug works to grow hair is not known, but it may increase blood flow to the scalp or stimulate the hair follicles. Regrowth of hair may start as early as two to four months after starting treatment. It can also be used to treat some types of hair loss in women. Some common side effects from using minoxidil include redness, itchiness, and dryness of the skin. Unfortunately this drug does not work in all people with hair loss, and if treatment is stopped any new hair will be lost within a few months. The second product available to treat hair loss in men is called finasteride (fi-nas-teer-ide) or Propecia. Finasteride in a higher strength is used to treat enlarged prostate glands and increased hair growth in these patients led to its use for hair loss. This prescription only drug is taken orally once a day and works in a different way compared to minoxidil. It blocks the action of an enzyme, which is needed to produce the hormone DHT, believed to cause hair loss. In some studies, about 83% of male patients with mild or moderate hair loss kept their hair or had grown more hair after taking this drug for one year. Some possible side effects from this medication include difficulty in getting an erection, a lower desire for sex and a decreased amount of semen produced. Propecia must also be used long-term. Although both of these drugs have never been directly studied with each other, it appears that about 50% of users report an increase in hair growth with either product.

QUESTION: I take Propecia for hair loss and have experienced some sexual side effects. If I stop taking the drug will these side effects go away?

ANSWER: Propecia (finasteride) taken as a 1 mg tablet once daily is approved to treat male pattern hair loss, also known as androgenic alopecia. Finasteride, the active ingredient in Propecia, is also approved to treat men with an enlarged prostate or BPH, but at a much higher dose. Finasteride works by blocking an enzyme that converts the hormone testosterone to a chemical known as dihydrotestosterone or DHT in the prostate gland, liver, and skin. This leads to a significant reduction in DHT in the scalp, which is believed to cause hair loss in men. Unfortunately, like all drugs, Propecia can cause adverse effects in some men including sexual side effects. These sexual side effects can include erectile dysfunction, libido disorders, ejaculation disorders, and orgasm disorders. Recently (2012), a study in The Journal of Sexual Medicine suggests that sexual dysfunction associated with Propecia use may last for many months or even years in some men, even after the medication is discontinued.

PROSTATE CANCER

QUESTION: Can aspirin help patients with prostate cancer?

ANSWER: According to a recent study in the Journal of Clinical Oncology (2012), men who have been treated for prostate cancer, either with surgery or radiation, could possibly benefit from taking aspirin. The finding of this observational study showed that the 10-year mortality rate from prostate cancer was significantly lower in patients taking aspirin (3% compared to 8% who did not take aspirin). The study looked at almost 6,000 men in the Cancer of the Prostate Strategic Urologic Research Endeavor nationwide database who had prostate cancer treated with surgery or radiotherapy. The results of this study suggests that aspirin prevents the growth of tumor cells in prostate cancer, especially in high-risk prostate cancer. This study supports other studies in patients with colorectal, prostate, or breast cancer which suggest daily aspirin use may help prevent cancer and have anti-cancer spreading effects. Exactly how aspirin may prevent or help treat cancer is not clearly understood because cancer and its spread (metastasis) is very complex, but it appears that aspirin's ability to prevent blood platelets from clumping together (aggregation) may be involved. However, in this study the dosage of aspirin therapy, duration and timing of aspirin use were not addressed in detail and further study is warranted. Before starting any aspirin therapy, patients should consult with their physician(s).

QUESTION: I heard that a new drug was approved for prostate cancer. What can you tell me about it?

ANSWER: The FDA recently (2012) approved Xtandi (enzalutamide) for the treatment of men with late-stage prostate cancer. Enzalutamide is known as an androgen receptor inhibitor, which works to decrease the growth and spread of prostate cancer cells. The approval of Xtandi was based upon a large clinical study involving almost 1,200 men with late-stage (metastatic castration-resistant) prostate cancer who had received prior treatment with the anti-cancer drug docetaxel. Results from this study showed that the men receiving Xtandi lived a median of 18.4 months or nearly 5 months longer than men receiving a "dummy" medication (placebo). The most common side effects observed in study participants taking Xtandi were weakness or fatigue, back pain, diarrhea, joint pain, hot flush, tissue swelling, musculoskeletal pain, headache, upper respiratory infections, dizziness, spinal cord compression and pain/numbness in the lower spine, muscular weakness, difficulty sleeping, lower respiratory infections, blood in urine, tingling sensation, anxiety, and high blood pressure. Seizures occurred in approximately 1% of those receiving Xtandi. Xandi is administered orally in capsule form once daily. In addition to docetaxel, other medications currently available to treat advanced prostate cancer include Jetvana and Provenge, which like docetaxel are administered intravenously and Zytiga which is given orally. According to the National Cancer Institute, an estimated 241,740 men will be diagnosed with prostate cancer and 28,170 will die from this disease in 2012.

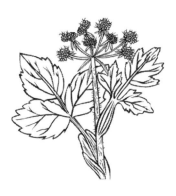

CHAPTER 4
HERBAL MEDICATIONS &
NUTRITIONAL SUPPLEMENTS

NUTRITIONAL SUPPLEMENTS

QUESTION: I heard about a number of herbal products and dietary supplements and their ability to cure medical problems. What can you tell me about them?

ANSWER: For thousands of years, Eastern and Western civilizations have reported numerous medical uses for plants and herbs. Over the years, using modern scientific methods, chemists have isolated many active plant ingredients and produced compounds to treat a variety of diseases. As the American public began to demand that drugs be proven safe and effective, it became difficult for manufacturers of herbal remedies to provide the required scientific data. Because of this, most herbal remedies disappeared from use early in the 20th century. However, during the past 20 years, Americans have been increasingly attracted to "all natural" products and this "back-to-nature" idea along with new health consciousness has resulted in renewed interest in herbal and natural therapies. The popularity of these so-called "alternative medicines" can also be traced to people's dissatisfaction with traditional medicine. In 1994, under pressure by lobbyists for the manufacturers of herbs and vitamins, the Food and Drug Administration (FDA) passed a law that deregulated these products. This new law (the Dietary Supplement Health & Education Act) redefined dietary supplements to include herbs, vitamins, minerals, and amino acids. The law also allows advertisements for dietary supplements in include information about the ways these products affect the human body. These health claims do not need to be approved by the FDA, but the advertisements must say that the product has not been evaluated by the FDA for treating, curing, or preventing any disease (such as "for treating arthritis"). However, other literature in the store where these products are sold can talk about health benefits as long as the literature is not produced by the store or manufacturer. Research into the safety and effectiveness of most of these supplements will probably never be done because of the high cost and because many of the products cannot be patented. In addition, a dietary supplement company does not have to report any injuries or illnesses that may be caused by their products, nor do they have to abide by strict procedures to prevent contaminants or impurities like pharmaceutical companies. Recent events, such as deaths from ephedrine-containing supplements or severe liver toxicity caused by herbal sedative tablets have now gotten the FDA concerned about these products and they may take steps in the future to ensure their safety. Meanwhile, consumers should be aware of the differences between approved prescription drugs, approved over-the-counter drug products and herbal or dietary supplements which do not have the blessing of the FDA. This is not to say that all these alternative medicine products are unsafe or ineffective, just that they are not regulated in the same way.

VITAMIN AND MINERAL DRUG INTERACTIONS

QUESTION: Can vitamins and minerals interact with medications?

ANSWER: Yes, there are several vitamin and mineral supplements that can interact with certain types of medications and lead to potential problems. To prevent these interactions it may be prudent to discontinue the supplement if the medication therapy is short term. In some situations, taking the medication and supplement at different times may prevent the interaction. If, however, the affected medication is needed for a chronic condition and the supplement is deemed necessary, then alternative therapy may be necessary. Below I have listed some of the vitamins and minerals that may interact with certain medications. Please note that this list does not show all potential interactions between medications and vitamin/mineral supplements. If you have any questions about the medication(s) and vitamin/mineral supplements that you take, please consult with your physician and pharmacist.

Drug Interactions With Vitamins & Minerals
Vitamin/Mineral Supplement
Affected Medication(s)
Potential Problem

- **Aluminum & Magnesium**
    Fluoroquinolones
    Tetracyclines
    Bisphosphonates (Fosamax, Didronel, Actonel, & others)
    Levothyroxine
    Decreased effectiveness
- **Calcium**
    Fluoroquinolones (Cipro, Floxin, & others)
    Tetracyclines (Doxycycline, Minocycline, & others)
    Levothyroxine (Synthroid, Levoxyl, & others)
    Decreased effectiveness
- **Iron**
    Fluoroquinolones
    Tetracyclines
    Digoxin (Lanoxin)
    Levothyroxine
    Decreased effectiveness
    Methyldopa
    Increased blood pressure
- **Niacin**
    Statins (Mevacor, Lipitor, Zocor, & others)
    Risk of muscle problems

- **Potassium (including salt substitutes)**
    ACE inhibitors (Lotensin, Capoten, Vasotec, Zestril, & others)
    ARB's (Cozaar, Diovan, Avapro, Atacand, & others)
    Digoxin (Lanoxin)
    Indomethacin (Indocin)
    Prescription potassium products
    Spironolactone (Aldactone)
    Triamterene (Dyrenium)
    Amiloride (Midamor)
    Increased levels of potassium in blood
- **Pyridoxine (Vitamin B-6)**
    Levodopa (Larodopa, Sinemet, & others)
    Decreased effectiveness
    Phenytoin (Dilantin)
    Risk of seizure
- **Vitamin A**
    Retinoids (Accutane, Soriatane)
    Increased risk of toxicity
- **Vitamin E**
    Warfarin (Coumadin)
    Risk of bleeding
- **Vitamin K**
    Warfarin (Coumadin)
    Decreased effectiveness

HAWTHORN

QUESTION: What can you tell me about hawthorn extract?

ANSWER: Hawthorn extract, also known as Crataegus, maybush, and whitehorn, has been used for many years as an oral treatment option for people with chronic heart failure. Hawthorn is a thorny, deciduous shrub up to five feet tall, found in the forests of North America, Europe, North Africa, and western Asia. The crude hawthorn drug extract is prepared from the leaves, white flowers, and berries of the shrub. In chronic heart failure, hawthorn extract is reported to improve not only the pumping ability of the heart but also to reduce the patient's susceptibility to angina. Hawthorn extract appears to have the ability to expand blood vessels and increase blood flow (vasodilation) and to improve the pumping effects of the heart. These effects help to relieve heart failure symptoms such as fatigue and shortness of breath. Reported side effects of hawthorn extract include dizziness/vertigo and gastrointestinal complaints. A recent review of hawthorn extract suggests that it may be useful when given together with approved prescription therapies for patients with chronic heart failure. However, it should be noted that hawthorn extract may interact with other medications and it should only be used under the direct supervision of a doctor who is familiar with the patient's medical history/medication regimen and who will be monitoring them closely.

PANTOTHENIC ACID & L-CYSTEINE

QUESTION: Is it safe to take pantothenic acid and L-cysteine together?

ANSWER: Probably, but there is no specific information about using this combination together that I could find. Pantothenic acid or vitamin B-5 is a water soluble vitamin that is used by the body to make proteins, metabolize fats and carbohydrates, manufacture key substances including hormones, red blood cells and chemicals needed to conduct nerve transmission. Some of its purported benefits include lowering of blood cholesterol and triglycerides; treatment of acne, osteoarthritis, and rheumatoid arthritis; prevention of gray hair; and weight loss. However, there is not a lot of scientific information available to support these claims. Deficiencies of pantothenic acid can cause irritability and restlessness, fatigue, headache, sleep disturbances, nausea, stomach cramps, vomiting, gas, and "burning feet". Pantothenic acid is found in a variety of foods including chicken, beef, oat cereals, egg yolks, tomato products, broccoli, potatoes and whole grains. It is also included in many vitamin B complex products. L-cysteine is a protein amino acid that contains sulfur. It is considered to be a non-essential amino acid, meaning that, under normal conditions, sufficient amounts of L-cysteine are made in the body. L-cysteine is involved in numerous chemical reactions in the body that produce a number of important compounds. It has been claimed that L-cysteine has anti-inflammatory properties, that it can protect against various toxins, and that it may be helpful in arthritis, but more research is needed before it can be recommended for any of these conditions. As I've noted many times before, no health claims for any dietary supplement products have been evaluated by the FDA, nor has the FDA approved any of these products to diagnose, cure, or prevent disease.

MILK THISTLE

QUESTION: What can you tell me about milk thistle?

ANSWER: Milk thistle is a herbal remedy that has been used for the prevention and treatment of a wide range of liver problems. The milk thistle plant is native to the Mediterranean, but is now grown in many areas, including Eastern Europe, Asia, the eastern United States, and California. The seeds of this plant and, to a lesser extent, the leaves and stems contain a group of active substances known as "silymarin". The liver-protecting and liver-repairing properties of silymarin are thought to be due to its ability to block damage causing toxins from getting into the liver (antioxidant) and by its ability to increase the production of proteins by liver cells leading to liver repair. Milk thistle has been used for chronic liver and gallbladder disorders, and for protection against liver damage caused by harmful drugs, chemicals, alcohol abuse, or hepatitis. It has also been used to treat poisoning from the death cup mushroom (Amanita phalloides). In Germany, the use of milk thistle has been endorsed as a nonprescription drug for chronic inflammatory liver disease and cirrhosis. It should be noted, however, that liver problems require a physician's attention and self-treatment is not advised. Milk thistle is marketed in the U.S. in the form of capsules or an oral liquid. The recommended dose of silymarin is 100 mg to 200 mg twice daily. Milk thistle appears to be well tolerated, but nausea, stomach fullness, and diarrhea can occur. Allergic reactions can also occur in some people. Like other dietary supplements, milk thistle products have not been approved by the FDA for use in the treatment of any disease.

ECHINACEA

QUESTION: What can you tell me about the herbal product Echinacea?

ANSWER: Echinacea, or purple coneflower, is a flowering herbal plant found in North America. The roots and above ground parts of Echinacea were used by Native American Indians for a variety of medical uses including the treatment of coughs, colds, insect stings and animal bites, as well as many types of skin diseases. Early physicians learned about this herb from the Native Americans around the mid-1800's and used it as a treatment for common colds and other infections before sulfa drugs became available in the 1930's.

Today, Echinacea is frequently used for the prevention and early treatment of the common cold and flu. Several active medicinal compounds have been identified in the roots and leaves of this plant, but these compounds do not have any significant bacteria killing ability. Instead, Echinacea appears to stimulate the immune system and several studies have shown that its use can reduce both the incidence of colds and flu as well as the severity and duration of these infections. This herb is very popular in Europe and many studies of Echinacea have been conducted in Germany. It is recommended that Echinacea be taken at the onset of viral symptoms and that its use be continued until 1-2 days after the symptoms go away.

Echinacea appears to be fairly safe to use. Its side effects can include allergic reactions (some serious) and people allergic to sunflower seeds or daisy plants should avoid its use. In addition, Echinacea should not be used by people who have severe systemic illness such as autoimmune disorders (rheumatoid arthritis, lupus, etc.) because of its ability to stimulate the immune system. It should also be avoided by people with tuberculosis, multiple sclerosis, and those that are HIV-positive, as Echinacea may aggravate these conditions.

In summary, Echinacea seems to be effective for the short-term, early treatment of viral upper-respiratory tract infections, where it acts as an immune system stimulant. It appears to be safe for use by most people. Like other herbal products, Echinacea has not been approved for use in the U.S. by the FDA.

QUESTION: Can Echinacea help in treating colds?

ANSWER: Echinacea may only have a small beneficial effect, if any, in reducing the severity and duration of the common cold according to a recent large study. The study, reported in the Annals of Internal Medicine journal (December 21, 2010), involved over 700 patients aged 12 to 80 years with a common cold. About half of the patients received Echinacea tablets and the other half received dummy tablets (placebos) for 5 days. Illness severity was assessed twice a day according to the patients' self-reporting their upper respiratory symptoms. Results from this study showed that patients taking Echinacea had only slightly milder symptoms and reduced their cold duration by only about a half-day compared to those taking the dummy tablets. These results were not statistically significant and could have occurred by chance alone. Echinacea is commonly used to treat colds, but its effectiveness continues to be debated and previous smaller studies have demonstrated mixed-results.

Echinacea, or purple coneflower, is a flowering herbal plant found in North America. The roots and above ground parts of Echinacea were used by Native American Indians for a variety of medical uses including the treatment of coughs, colds, insect stings and animal bites, as well as many types of skin diseases. Early physicians learned about this herb from the Native Americans around the mid-1800's and used it as a treatment for common colds and other infections before sulfa drugs became available in the 1930's. Echinacea can be prepared as a tea, pressed juice, tincture, or dried root.

CALCIUM SUPPLEMENTS

QUESTION: What is the difference between calcium supplements? Why is vitamin D needed?

ANSWER: There are numerous calcium supplement products available and they come in various types of tablet and liquid dosage forms. At least 11 different salt forms of calcium are available with calcium carbonate and calcium citrate being the most common form used in the U.S. Calcium is the fifth most abundant element in the body with about 99% of it found in the skeleton. It is a major component of bones and teeth. It is also needed for the function of nerve and muscle systems, for normal heart function, for cell membrane function, and for blood clotting. The usual daily dose of calcium as a dietary supplement is 500 mg to 2,000 mg (2 grams) per day. Calcium is recommended in doses of 1,500 mg/day for men over 65 and for postmenopausal women not taking estrogen replacement therapy. The recommended upper limit is 2,500 mg (2.5 grams) per day. These recommendations for calcium intake are based on the "elemental" calcium in the product and not the calcium salt. This can be misleading and confusing when selecting a calcium supplement. For example, calcium carbonate contains 40% "elemental" calcium, while calcium citrate contains 21%. "elemental" calcium, so be sure to read the label and look for "elemental" calcium in the product. The absorption of calcium from the gastrointestinal tract is similar for most of the calcium salts. The absorption of calcium can be improved by dividing the total daily dose into 2 to 3 doses daily. However, it should also be noted that calcium carbonate should be taken with meals to increase its absorption, but calcium citrate does not need to be taken with food. Most calcium carbonate in the U.S. comes from oyster shells. Calcium supplements can cause constipation and large doses can lead to kidney stones. Calcium supplements can interact with other drugs such as thiazide diuretics or certain antibiotics, so be sure to tell your pharmacist if you are taking calcium supplements. Vitamin D is involved in calcium absorption, but your ability to get enough vitamin D without taking supplements depends on where you live. Vitamin D is made in the skin from cholesterol when exposed to sunlight. People can get enough vitamin D to help with calcium absorption by spending about 10-15 minutes a day in the sun. People in northern climates may not get enough vitamin D from sunshine, especially in the winter, and may need to take a vitamin D supplement. However, it should be emphasized that the best source of calcium and vitamin D is foods. Good food sources for calcium include dairy products, sardines, clams, oysters, turnip greens, and mustard greens. Foods rich in vitamin D include vitamin-D-supplemented milk, egg yolk, liver, salmon, tuna, sardines, and milk fat.

PLEASE NOTE: Emerging clinical research has suggested that vitamin D may also be beneficial in patients with dementia, Parkinson's disease, multiple sclerosis, and depression. In December of 2010, the Institute of Medicine reported that most people up to age 70 need no more than 600 International Units (IUs) of vitamin D per day, and those 71 and older may need as much as 800 IUs per day. As for calcium, the Institute of Medicine report reommended already accepted levels to go along with your daily D—about 1,000 milligrams (mg) of calcium a day for most adults, 700 to 1,000 mg for young children, and 1,300 mg for teenagers and menopausal women. Too much calcium can cause kidney stones and this risk increases once people exceed 2,000 mg a day.

ST. JOHN'S WORT

QUESTION: I've heard a lot of people talk about Saint John's wort. What can you tell me about this product?

ANSWER: St. John's wort is a popular herbal remedy that is promoted for the treatment of depression, anxiety and difficulty in sleeping. It may also have antiviral and wound-healing properties, along with additional medicinal effects. Like other herbal remedies, this product is not regulated for safety and efficacy by the Food and Drug Administration. However, St. John's wort, unlike many other herbal preparations, has been studied and is widely used in Europe for the treatment of mild or moderate depression. It is currently proclaimed to be "nature's Prozac" and sales of St. John's wort in Germany outnumber all other antidepressants.

St. John's wort is a shrubby, perennial weed that grows along dry, gravelly roadsides, meadows, woods, hills, and hedges. It is cultivated worldwide, but grows quite well in Northern California and Southern Oregon. It blooms between June and September with the flowers forming brownish-black seeds contained within capsules. The plant is harvested and dried immediately to maintain its active ingredients. The active principles in St. John's wort are numerous, including tannins, hypericin, flavonoids, oils and other compounds.

This plant has been used since Greek and Roman times as a nerve tonic for mood and temperament. The origin of its name has an interesting history. One possible explanation for its name is the belief that the red spots on the leaves were the blood of St. John the Baptist and were thought to appear on the anniversary of the saint's beheading, said to be August 29. Another theory is that the plant blooms its brightest on June 24, which is considered the birthday of St. John the Baptist. Still another explanation is that the name resulted from the English tradition of throwing the flowers into a bonfire on the eve of St. John's Day. The name "wort" is derived from the Old English word for plant or herb.

Several research studies have shown that St. John's wort has antidepressant activity, but exactly how it works is not fully understood. Some of its ingredients may act to alter certain brain chemicals resulting in antidepressant effects. Approximately 50 to 80% of patients with mild or moderate depression have benefited from St. John's wort given three times daily in clinical studies. However, patients with self-diagnosed depression should seek medical attention before using St. John's wort. Like most antidepressant agents, maximum benefits are usually seen after 6 to 8 weeks of continued use. Other ingredients, including hypericin, have demonstrated antiviral activity. Because of this, it is being studied for its potential usefulness in the treatment of AIDS. The wound healing properties of St. John's wort may be due to the high content of tannins in the plant, which protect the skin. Several additional medicinal effects have also been purported for St. John's wort.

St. John's wort appears to be relatively safe to use. The most common side effects reported are emotional changes, tiredness, itching, restlessness, stomach upset, and weight gain. Dry mouth and dizziness may also occur. In addition, some people have developed sensitivity to sunlight after taking this plant product for a long period of time. Sensitivity reactions reported have included redness and inflammation of the skin. St. John's wort should probably not be used in combination with cheese, pickled meat, or alcohol. Several prescription medications including some antidepressants, narcotics, amphetamines and over the counter cold and flu medications should also be avoided when taking St. John's wort. It is also not recommended for use by pregnant women.

In summary, St. John's wort has a long history of use, especially in Europe. Several studies support its use for mild to moderate depression and side effects appear to be minimal. Additional studies are ongoing and will be needed to determine the overall medical value of this herbal product.

QUESTION: Are there any prescription drugs that can interact with St. John's wort?

ANSWER: Yes, there are several prescription medications that can interact with this herbal product. St. John's wort is a popular herbal remedy that is promoted for the treatment of depression, anxiety, and difficulty in sleeping. It may also have antiviral and wound-healing properties along with additional medicinal effects. However, like other herbal remedies, St. John's wort is not regulated for safety and effectiveness by the Food and Drug Administration. This plant has been used since Greek and Roman times as a nerve tonic for mood and temperament, and it was long believed to rid the body of evil spirits. Most recent research on St. John's wort has focused on its use in treating mild to moderate depression, and some studies have shown that it does have antidepressant activity. St. John's wort appears to be relatively safe to use with side effects such as upset stomach, dizziness, itching, dry mouth, restlessness, sleep problems, unusual tiredness, and increased blood pressure. It may also cause sensitivity reactions of the skin and is not recommended for use by pregnant women or while breastfeeding.

Several prescription drugs may interact with St. John's wort. For instance, breakthrough bleeding and a decrease in effectiveness has been observed in women taking birth control pills along with St. John's wort. This herbal product may also decrease the effectiveness of the heart medication Lanoxin (digoxin) and the blood thinner Coumadin (warfarin). The combined use of St. John's wort with other antidepressants known as MAO inhibitors or selective serotonin reuptake inhibitors (SSRI's) can likewise cause problems. In addition, St. John's wort may interact with levodopa used for Parkinson's disorder, with some immunosuppressive or anti-cancer drugs, and with certain drugs used to treat HIV infection. Please remember that there is still a need for more information and research in this area. Make sure you tell your doctor and pharmacist if you are taking St. John's wort so that dangerous drug interactions can be minimized.

CINNAMON

QUESTION: I heard that cinnamon could help people with diabetes. Is this true?

ANSWER: A study that was published in the journal Diabetes Care suggests that cinnamon may help to lower blood glucose (sugar) and also lower cholesterol levels in people with type 2 diabetes. In this study, which involved a total of 60 people with type 2 diabetes, subjects who were given 1, 3, or 6 grams of cinnamon per day for 40 days, reduced their blood glucose by 18-29%, lowered triglycerides by 23-30%, reduced total cholesterol by 12-26%, and lowered LDL (bad) cholesterol by 7-27%. There were no significant changes in HDL (good) cholesterol. These results were similar for all dose levels of cinnamon, which was given in divided doses 2 or 3 times daily. How cinnamon works to lower blood glucose and lipid levels is not known, but it appears to increase the body's sensitivity to insulin in some way. While this study was carried out in people with type 2 diabetes, the researchers suggest that the beneficial effects of cinnamon may be useful in other people as well. No adverse effects were associated with cinnamon use in this study. It should be pointed out, however, that this is just one fairly small study and more research is needed before definite recommendations for using cinnamon can be made.

Diabetes affects an estimated 16 million Americans and more than 140 million people worldwide. According to the World Health Organization, the incidence of diabetes is likely to more than double in the next 25 years. Over 90% of people with diabetes have type 2, which used to be called adult-onset or non-insulin dependent diabetes. When insulin cannot keep blood sugar (glucose) under control, many problems can develop such as kidney disease, cardiovascular disease, blindness, and nerve problems.

GOLDENSEAL

QUESTION: What can you tell me about Goldenseal?

ANSWER: Goldenseal is an herbal medicine that is also known as Yellow Root, Eye Root, Indian Turmeric, and Hydrastis. It is a native American plant that was introduced to early settlers by the Cherokee and Iroquois Indians. They used it as a yellow dye, as well as a wash for skin diseases and sore eyes, and a variety of other disorders. More recently it has been promoted for medicinal use in numerous situations including disorders of the gastrointestinal tract; congestion and chronic inflammation of the respiratory and urogenital tracts; colds and flu; diabetes; vaginal problems; middle-ear inflammation and congestion; as a rinse for throat, gum, and mouth inflammation or sores; and externally for lacerations, abrasions, boils, and other skin problems. One of the main ingredients in Goldenseal is a bitter tasting substance known as berberine. Berberine has been shown to have anti-infective and anti-inflammatory properties in laboratory studies. It is also known to lower blood sugar (glucose) and have anti-diarrheal effects. However, very little research and information is available regarding its clinical effectiveness in treating medical problems and like all other herbal preparations it has not been approved for safety and effectiveness by the FDA. Goldenseal in very large doses may cause convulsions and overstimulation of the nervous system. It can also cause an upset stomach, diarrhea, and vomiting. Goldenseal should not be used by pregnant or breast-feeding women or by people with high blood pressure. It should also not be taken together with vitamin B or heparin (a blood thinner). Goldenseal is available as a dried root, in tablet or capsule form, as a liquid extract, and as a tincture. Its dosage depends upon the form used and the condition being treated.

GINKGO BILOBA

QUESTION: What can you tell me about Ginkgo? Can I take aspirin with it?

ANSWER: Ginkgo biloba is a very popular herbal product that is sold in the U.S. as a dietary supplement. The active ingredients in this herbal medicine are extracted from the fan-shaped leaves of the ginkgo biloba tree. The leaves are double, or bi-lobed; hence the name "biloba". The ginkgo is the world's oldest living tree and can be traced back more than 200 million years to the Permian period. The tree can live for 1,000 years and grow to a massive height of 100 to 125 feet with a trunk 3 to 4 feet in diameter. As a testimony to its hardiness, a single ginkgo tree is reported to have survived the atomic blast in Hiroshima, sprouting from its base after its trunk was completely destroyed.

Ginkgo has been used for a wide variety of medical disorders throughout history. Even today it is among the leading prescriptions in Germany and France. To keep up with the worldwide demand for ginkgo, plantations containing more than 25 million trees have been established in Sumter, South Carolina and near the Atlantic coast of France. Ginkgo produces a number of effects in the body. It can improve blood circulation and can reduce the risk of blood clots. It also appears to have antioxidant properties that protect cells and may help to relieve wheezing and other respiratory complaints. In view of these effects, ginkgo has been used for a number of medical conditions including Alzheimer's disease (AD) and dementia, diabetes, depression, leg cramps, impotence, prevention of heart attacks or strokes, dizziness, ringing in the ears, headaches, and asthma. In Germany the Federal Health Authorities (an FDA-like authority that reviews and approves herbal products) have declared ginkgo to be effective for the treatment of cerebral disturbances or dementia that result in disturbance of concentration, ringing in the ears, vertigo, weakened memory, and mood swings accompanied by anxiety. They also believe that ginkgo is effective for leg cramping and pain due to poor circulation. A number of studies suggest that ginkgo can improve blood flow to the brain and to the legs.

Only standardized products that contain ginkgo biloba extract (GBE) should be used. As a general memory booster and for poor circulation a daily dose of 120 mg of GBE divided into 2 or 3 doses can be used. Beneficial effects may take from 1 to 2 months to appear. Side effects from GBE are usually few and mild. Infrequently irritability, restlessness, diarrhea, nausea, vomiting, headache and allergic skin reactions can occur. Since ginkgo can prevent the blood from clotting, it may be of concern to people already taking anticoagulants (like Coumadin or aspirin). In this case there may be a greater possibility of bleeding, so be sure to check with your doctor and pharmacist.

PLEASE NOTE: A 6-year study recently published in the Journal of the American Medical Association (2009) concluded that ginko biloba in a dose of 120 mg twice daily did not prevent dementia or Alzheimer's disease in the elderly nor did it slow age-related mental decline.

SAW PALMETTO

QUESTION: Is saw palmetto any good for an enlarged prostate?

ANSWER: Possibly, but remember that it hasn't been approved by the FDA for this use. An enlarged prostate gland (benign prostatic hypertrophy or BPH) is the most common benign tumor in men, affecting their ability to urinate. By age 55, 25% of men complain of a decrease in the force of their urinary stream and this rises to 50% by age 75. Typical symptoms of BPH include weak urine stream, hesitancy in initiating urination, dribbling, sensation of not emptying the bladder completely, frequency of urination, need to urinate during the night, and urgency to urinate. It is important to have a physician evaluate theses symptoms because other medical problems such as urinary tract infection and bladder or prostate cancer can produce the same effects.

The saw palmetto is a low, scrubby fan-palm that grows from South Carolina to Florida. It was once widely used for a variety of ailments including urogenital disorders, but after World War II, physicians in the U.S. began to question its effectiveness and it disappeared from use. European scientists, however, continued to study saw palmetto and recognized that an extract made from its blue-black berries produced an increase in urine flow, increased the ease in urinating, and decreased the frequency of urination in men with BPH. It is not exactly clear how this herb works, but it seems to block the effects of male hormones and to reduce inflammation. Although there have not been any long-term studies using saw palmetto, it appears to be safe. Side effects have included headache, nausea, dizziness, and diarrhea in high doses.

Another potential problem is that this herbal remedy for BPH may also lower PSA levels and mask prostate cancer. Since these side effects are fairly mild, saw palmetto has become very popular because many of the commonly prescribed medications for BPH have the potential for producing impotence, lightheadedness, or other undesirable effects. Its dosage is usually 160 mg taken twice a day. (Please see next question).

QUESTION: I heard that saw palmetto doesn't help with prostate problems. Is that true?

ANSWER: It is estimated that saw palmetto is used by over 2 million Americans for the treatment of an enlarged prostate (benign prostatic hypertrophy or BPH). However, studies that have shown saw palmetto to be effective are limited by the small number of men participating and their short duration. Recently, results from a large well-controlled study involving 225 men older than age 49 with BPH who were treated with saw palmetto was reported in a very respected medical journal (The New England Journal of Medicine). Men in this study were treated with saw palmetto extract (160 mg twice a day) or with a placebo (dummy pill) for one year. After one year of treatment, the study concluded that saw palmetto did not improve symptoms or other measures of BPH such as prostate size, urinary flow, residual urine after urinating, PSA levels, or quality of life. In addition, men taking saw palmetto had similar side effects compared to those taking a placebo. While this was a very good study, it is possible that other saw palmetto preparations or a different dose may have been effective. Until additional studies and information become available, the effectiveness of saw palmetto for treating BPH is still unproven and it is not approved by the FDA for this use.

QUESTION: What's the latest information about saw palmetto and urinary problems from an enlarged prostate?

ANSWER: Recently, results from a large well-controlled study involving 369 men older than age 45 with BPH who were treated with saw palmetto was reported in the Journal of the American Medical Association (2011). Men in this study were treated with increasing doses of saw palmetto fruit extract or a placebo (dummy medication) for up to 72 weeks. Results from this study showed that treatment with saw palmetto did not significantly improve urinary tract symptoms of BPH even when used in up to 3 times the standard dose (320 mg/day). The researchers also observed no adverse effects that could be attributed to saw palmetto. Until additional studies and information become available, the effectiveness of saw palmetto for treating BPH is still unproven and it is not approved by the FDA for this use.

ALOE

QUESTION: Would you please comment on the use of aloe gel for the treatment of burns?

ANSWER: Aloe gel (or aloe vera gel) is a mucilaginous substance that is obtained from the inner portion (center) of the aloe plant's leaf. It should not be confused with aloe latex, which is the bitter juice found just under the outer skin of the aloe leaf. A dried form of this latex or juice has been used orally as a stimulant laxative, but may cause abdominal cramping, bloody diarrhea, rupture of the colon, kidney damage, electrolyte disturbances, and even death.

Aloe gel, however, is one of the most widely used herbal preparations for the treatment of various skin conditions. The use of this gel in medicine dates back to as early as 1500 B.C. It was even used by the Seminole Indians, who applied the gel to injuries and wounds to promote healing. Today the gel is used by itself and is also contained in a wide variety of ointments, creams, lotions, and shampoos. When the gel was chemically analyzed, it was shown to contain water, amino acids, fatty substances, enzymes and sugars. Topical aloe gel has been shown to reduce inflammation, act as a skin protectant, and stimulate wound healing. A 1993 study showed that the gel also has possible therapeutic value in burns and a wide variety of soft tissue injuries. The researchers found that aloe gel penetrates injured tissue, relieves pain, reduces inflammation, and acts to increase the blood supply to the injury. Other studies have not shown a beneficial effect for topical aloe gel. Use of the fresh gel is generally recommended, since many of the active ingredients appear to deteriorate upon storage. The external use of aloe gel is considered safe but allergic reactions can occur, especially in people allergic to plants like garlic, onion, or tulips. It should also be noted that the use of aloe gel has not been approved by the FDA.

YOHIMBINE

QUESTION: My doctor has prescribed yohimbine to improve my sex life. What can you tell me about this drug?

ANSWER: Yohimbine has been promoted as an aphrodisiac for a long time. It is a herb that comes from the bark of the West African yohimbine tree, and some studies have shown that it may be helpful in the treatment of impotence. Impotence (or erectile dysfunction) is the inability of a male to attain or maintain penile erection in order to complete sexual intercourse. Impotence occurs in about half of all men between the ages of 40 and 70. It can be caused by a variety of medical problems or psychological factors, such as sexual anxieties, guilt, fear, feelings of inadequacy and the like. Exactly how the drug works for impotence is not entirely known. However, an erection is linked to an increase in blood flow to the penis and/or a decrease in blood outflow from the penis. Yohimbine may have some effect on blood flow to the penis, but it also exerts a stimulating effect on one's mood, which may be helpful in males with psychological causes of impotence. Side effects can occur with yohimbine and therefore it should be used under the care of a physician. Possible side effects include elevated blood pressure and heart rate, anxiety, nervousness, irritability, tremor, inability to sleep, dizziness, headache, skin flushing, low blood pressure, nausea, and vomiting. You should notify your doctor of any side effects if they occur. Yohimbine should also not be used in geriatric patients, females, or in people with psychiatric disorders, kidney disease, or patients with a history of gastric or duodenal ulcer. Like many drugs, serious drug interactions can occur between yohimbine and other medications such as antidepressants, antihypertensives, and stimulants. Make sure you tell your doctor and pharmacist about all your medications—prescription, non-prescription, herbals, etc. when any new drug is used. The usual dose of yohimbine for impotence is one tablet (5.4 mg) three times a day. If minor side effects occur, the dosage should be reduced to ½ tablet three times a day. Response to the drug may take days or weeks, but it should not be used for more than 10 weeks without a positive response.

ANDROSTENEDIONE

QUESTION: My teenage son wants to start taking "andro" to make him stronger. What do you think about this?

ANSWER: Sales of androstenedione (andro-steen-die-onn) or "andro" supplements have skyrocketed since a famous baseball player admitted using this product. Androstenedione is a "pre-hormone" drug that is converted by the body to the male hormone testosterone (tes-tos-ter-onn) when taken as a supplement. Since this product actually leads to the production of testosterone, the main concern is of testosterone's effect on the body. Testosterone is known as an anabolic and androgenic steroid that produces a large number of effects, including an increase in the manufacture of proteins by the body leading to more muscle mass and increased strength. It also has numerous masculinizing properties such as development of the male sex organs, growth of a beard and other body hair, deepening of the voice, and other changes associated with puberty. In short, it is a hormone with numerous biological effects, many of which are still not known or are poorly understood.

A major concern with growing adolescents is that the increased levels of testosterone may actually stunt their growth. A teenager taking this steroid may fool his body into thinking it is older and shut off bone growth and stunt height. Increases in testosterone can also cause harm to the liver, heart, and sex organs and even produce psychological effects including uncontrolled anger or aggression. Additional adverse effects of this steroid in boys are the production of acne, balding, and enlarged breasts. Numerous adverse effects may not even show up until many years later. You may recall the death of an NFL football star who attributed his brain cancer to the abuse of steroids like testosterone. In view of the potential harm associated with using this supplement in teenagers (male or female) who are going through changes and with their bodies still growing, I would not recommend its use. There are just too many unanswered questions and more scientific study is needed. Also, remember that these supplements are not governed by the FDA like other drug products.

<u>COENZYME Q10</u>

<u>QUESTION</u>: What can you tell me about coenzyme Q10?

<u>ANSWER</u>: Coenzyme Q10 (also known as coenzyme Q, ubiquinone, and ubiquinone-Q10) is marketed as a dietary supplement and can be found in many health food stores and pharmacies. It is a vitamin-like substance that is produced in the body and participates in a variety of chemical functions within body cells. It is also present in dietary meat and poultry. High amounts of coenzyme Q10 can be found in the heart, liver, kidney, and pancreas. Although its exact functions in the body are not completely understood, coenzyme Q10 appears to protect cellular membranes and to act as an antioxidant like some other vitamins. A deficiency of coenzyme Q10 has been suggested as a cause of many diseases including cardiovascular disease, cancer, and even periodontal (gum) disease. Because of this, coenzyme Q10 has been studied for its use in numerous disorders such as angina, congestive heart failure, several types of cancer, and high blood pressure. Results from these limited numbers of studies have shown varying degrees of effectiveness, but more study will be needed to better determine its beneficial effects. The dose of coenzyme Q10 depends upon the condition being treated with small doses for gum disease and higher doses for heart disease. Side effects from coenzyme Q10 appear to be minimal with nausea, loss of appetite, diarrhea, and skin rash occurring in less than 1% of people taking it. Like other dietary supplements, none of the coenzyme Q10 products have been approved by the FDA for use in the treatment of any disease.

<u>QUESTION</u>: Why did my doctor tell me to take coenzyme Q10 while I'm on a statin drug to lower my cholesterol?

ANSWER: Probably because your doctor is concerned about the effect of statin drugs in reducing the amount of coenzyme Q10 that your body makes. There are currently seven statin drugs available: atorvastatin (Lipitor), fluvastatin (Lescol), lovastatin (Mevacor, Altoprev), pitavastatin (Livalo), pravastatin (Pravachol), rosuvastatin (Crestor), and simvastatin (Zocor). Atorvastatin, lovastatin, pravastatin, and simvastatin are also available as generic drugs. Coenzyme Q10 (also known as CoQ10, coenzyme Q, ubiquinone, or ubiquinone-Q10) is a vitamin-like substance that is produced in the body and participates in a variety of chemical functions within body cells. It is also present in dietary meat and poultry. High amounts of coenzyme Q10 can be found in the heart, liver, kidney, and pancreas. Although its exact functions in the body are not completely understood, coenzyme Q10 appears to protect cellular membranes and to act as an antioxidant like some other vitamins. Coenzyme Q10 also plays a critical role in energy production within cells. A deficiency of coenzyme Q10 has been suggested as a cause of many diseases including cardiovascular disease, cancer, and even periodontal (gum) disease. Statin drugs are very effective in lowering cholesterol levels, but unfortunately in doing so, they also block the production of coenzyme Q10. The depletion of this essential compound may be especially important in people with cardiovascular problems, such as congestive heart failure (CHF) or angina. In view of this, many physicians will recommend supplements of coenzyme Q10 to be taken while receiving statin drugs. Daily doses of 100 mg-200 mg taken in two or three divided doses have been recommended. However, like other dietary supplements, none of the coenzyme Q10 products have been approved by the FDA for use in the treatment of any disease.

DHEA

QUESTION: What can you tell me about DHEA?

ANSWER: Dihydroepiandrosterone or DHEA is a hormone produced mainly in the adrenal glands (which sit on top of the kidneys) of both men and women. It is sold as a dietary supplement and has been promoted as a "fountain of youth" or "anti-aging hormone". The reason for this is that its production in our bodies peaks at about age 25 and then begins to decline as we get older. By age 70, production falls to as low as one-twentieth of what it was at age 25. DHEA is produced in the body from cholesterol and it then can be converted to testosterone (male hormone) or estrogen (female hormone). Some of the proposed benefits of DHEA include more energy, reduced heart disease, fat loss, better memory, and improved immune system. However, research studies with DHEA are very limited and most involve only lab animals like rodents, which are very different than people. Results from studies in humans have been confusing thus far. Serious side effects of DHEA are also possible and include liver damage and a higher risk of breast cancer in postmenopausal women. In addition, other side effects related to testosterone and estrogen may occur. Use of DHEA by athletes is banned by both the NCAA (National Collegiate Athletic Association) and the USOC (United States Olympic Committee). In my opinion, DHEA is a very potent, complex, and poorly understood hormone with many effects on the body—both known and unknown. Because of this, its use is risky business until more information becomes available. Also remember that DHEA is sold as a dietary supplement so that clinical testing and purity standards do not have to be met like FDA approved products.

GREEN TEA

QUESTION: What can you tell me about green tea?

ANSWER: Green tea is prepared from the leaves and leaf buds of an evergreen shrub native to the mountainous regions of Southeast Asia. The Chinese have used the leaves to prepare beverages for over 4,000 years, believing that the tea can cure or prevent a number of diseases. Green tea has also been used to flavor food and the oil from the leaves has been used in perfumes and cosmetics. Green tea is mainly consumed in Japan and China, where it has evolved into a cultural habit and a part of everyday life. The active ingredients in green tea are thought to be chemicals known as polyphenols, flavonoids, or catechins. Green tea also contains caffeine, theobromine, theophylline, B-vitamins, and vitamin C. Some of the potential medicinal actions of green tea include lowering of cholesterol levels, antimicrobial activity, antioxidant activity, and anti-cancer activity. Although most research studies with green tea involve animals, there are some studies in humans that support its beneficial effects. In one large study carried out in Japan from 1990 to 1995, the use of green tea (over 7 cups/day) appeared to reduce the risk of stomach cancer and another study in women revealed that drinking 5-10 cups or more of green tea daily delayed cancer onset or recurrence. In addition, the antibacterial effects of green tea against bacteria found in the mouth and gastrointestinal tract has been well documented. Another Japanese study suggests that regular green tea consumption may contribute to an extended life span. In addition, the use of green tea is also being studied for neuroprotection in Parkinson's disease. However, these studies are limited and more research is needed. It appears that the moderate consumption of green tea is safe, but over consumption may produce effects associated with excessive caffeine use such as insomnia, nervousness, and rapid heart beat. Precaution is also needed in patients who are taking anticoagulants like Coumadin because green tea may antagonize its effect. People with high blood pressure, sleep problems, asthma, heart conditions, or elevated cholesterol should check with their doctor before becoming a regular green tea drinker.

FISH OIL

QUESTION: I've heard that fish oil is good for you. What do you think?

ANSWER: Interest in fish oils or omega-3 fatty acids goes back to the 1920's, when researcher's found that coronary heart disease was uncommon in the Greenland Eskimos who consumed a lot of fish. Certain fish, such as mackerel, herring, salmon, trout, halibut, tuna, and shrimp are rich in compounds thought to have important health benefits. Fish oil is being studied for a number of beneficial cardiovascular effects including abnormal heart rhythm, coronary artery disease, high blood pressure, stroke, and high triglyceride levels. It appears that fish rich in the omega-3 fatty acids EPA (eicosapentaenoic acid) and DHA (docosahexaenoic acid) may be helpful for people at early risk of heart disease. The FDA has also approved a qualified health claim for EPA and DHA omega-3 fatty acids in dietary supplements. Dietary supplements containing EPA and DHA can state that "consumption of omega-3 fatty acids may reduce the risk of coronary heart disease-but the scientific evidence supporting this claim is not conclusive". Some fish oil products containing EPA and DHA include Sea-Omega, Super EPA, Promega Pearls, Cardi-Omega 3 Capsules, Marine Lipid concentrated Softgels, Carlson Super Omega-3 Fish Oils, and Twin EPA Extra Strength Fish Oil concentrate. A dose of approximately 1-2 grams (total EPA plus DHA) per day is probably adequate. However, it should be noted that with many dietary supplements, the amount of EPA and DHA noted on the label may not be the actual amount found in the product. In addition, fish oil supplements may potentially interact with other drugs or herbal products and your doctor and pharmacist should be consulted when using these products. Furthermore, fish oil products should be used with caution in people with diabetes or those taking anticoagulants or aspirin and should not be used during pregnancy or in children.

QUESTION: Can fish oil help to alleviate depression?

ANSWER: The fatty oil found in salmon, cod, and other fish has been touted for its effectiveness in a number of diseases including heart disease, rheumatoid arthritis, cancer, dermatitis, dementia, high blood pressure, psoriasis, colitis, and depression. Cold water fish oils contain large amounts of omega-3 fatty acids (EPA and DHA) which are also known as essential fatty acids. These essential fatty acids have been shown to have a large number of biochemical effects in the body and have therefore been studied for their potential usefulness in many different disorders. The theory behind the use of fatty acids found in fish oil to treat depression is based upon the idea that people with depression may not have enough essential fatty acids (especially DHA) in their diet. It is thought that these fatty acids are involved in a number of hormonal and neurotransmitter activities in the body, which can affect chemicals in the brain producing depression. This theory is supported by the observation that the incidence of depression has sharply increased in the U.S. since the beginning of the century, and this coincides with a decrease in our dietary intake of essential fatty acids from fish and other sources. In contrast, countries that have a large dietary intake of these fatty acids such as Japan, China, and Taiwan have lower rates of depression. These fatty acids may boost levels of the brain chemical known as serotonin, which is similar to the activity of many antidepressant drugs. Currently, however, there does not appear to be sufficient clinical research data available to say for sure if fish oil is effective for depression or not and additional study is needed. More information is available related to the potential benefit of fish oil in heart disease. The American Heart Association recommends consumption of fish, but does not find justification for fish oil capsule supplementation. Side effects of fish oil capsules can include diarrhea, abdominal pain, and bloating. Caution should be observed in patients taking anticoagulants or aspirin and in patients with diabetes. Like all dietary supplements, fish oil capsules have not been approved by the FDA.

QUESTION: Is fish oil helpful in treating multiple sclerosis?

ANSWER: Probably not according to a study recently reported in the online journal Archives of Neurology (2012). In this Norwegian study, 92 patients with relapsing-remitting multiple sclerosis (MS) were treated with fish oil supplements containing the oega-3 fatty acids eicosapentaenoic acid (EPA) and docosahexaenoic acid (DHA) or a "dummy pill" (placebo). After the first 6 months, all patients were also given interferon injections, which are commonly used to treat MS. The researchers in this study found that after 7 months and 24 months of treatment there were no differences in the number of brain lesions seen on MRI testing, functionality, fatigue, or quality of life measurements between those taking the fish oil supplements or a placebo. Overall, they concluded that these fish oil supplements have no beneficial effects on MS disease activity. Some smaller studies have suggested a potential benefit of fish oil in treating MS because of their anti-inflammatory and potential neuroprotective properties, but this larger and better designed study did not.

MS affects about 400,000 people in the United States. There are four basic presentations of MS, the most common being the relapsing form. The exact cause of MS is unknown, but what is known is that the myelin sheath, an insulating cover surrounding nerve axons, is damaged by an immune action leading to damage to the brain and spinal cord. This damage, which can be seen on MRI scans as a lesion, leads to visual disturbances, muscle weakness, coordination difficulties, and memory and cognition problems. It most commonly occurs in people ages 20-40, and affects women 2 to 3 times more often than men. Common complaints include weakness, fatigue, pain, bladder and bowel problems, as well as balance, visual, and other sensory disturbances. There is no cure for MS. The strategies for treating MS include: reducing the number of attacks, reducing the number of lesions observed in MRI scans, slowing the progression of disability, and improving the speed of recovery.

VITAMIN C

QUESTION: How much is too much vitamin C? A friend said they heard something on the radio about side effects but could not remember what they were.

ANSWER: Vitamin C (also known as ascorbic acid or ascorbate) is a water-soluble antioxidant vitamin that is needed for many chemical reactions. It must be ingested since it is not produced in the body and is necessary for the formation of connective tissue (the tissue that holds the body's structures together). Vitamin C also helps the body to absorb iron, protects against cell damage, and helps to maintain vision and immunity. It may also help to prevent heart disease and stroke, and possibly lower the risk of some cancers. The use of large doses of vitamin C to prevent colds is not supported by research, but it may reduce the duration of a cold. A deficiency of this vitamin can cause weakness, fatigue, swollen or bleeding gums, bruising, joint pain, impaired healing, and bone problems. Vitamin C supplementation may be of particular importance in people who may be susceptible to a deficiency such as smokers, the elderly, women taking birth control pills, people who regularly use aspirin, and those that exercise excessively.

Vitamin C has been called the "fresh-food" vitamin, and most of the daily dietary intake comes from fruits and vegetables. Foods that contain high amounts of vitamin C include citrus fruits, papaya, strawberries, sweet peppers, broccoli, tomatoes, collard greens, spinach, and potatoes. The recommended daily allowance (RDA) or dose of vitamin C for most adults is 60-100 mg per day. A normal diet containing fresh fruits and vegetables contains many times this amount, but cooking may decrease the amounts ingested. About 200 mg of vitamin C per day will saturate the body, and since it is water soluble, most doses above this amount will be excreted in the urine. Doses higher than 1,000 mg a day can cause diarrhea or kidney stones in some people. Excessive vitamin C may also produce changes in the menstrual cycle and cause too much iron to be absorbed by the body. It should also be noted that vitamin C can interact with some medications such as warfarin (Coumadin) and may interfere with certain lab test results, so be sure to let your health care provider know if you are taking vitamin C supplements.

VITAMIN D

QUESTION: Can vitamin D prevent prostate cancer and can it help the heart?

ANSWER: Vitamin D (also known as the "sunshine vitamin") is known to have a number of beneficial effects and is required for bone strengthening, growth and repair. Vitamin D is found in many foods including fortified milk and cereals, fatty fish, fish liver oils, and egg yolk. It is also formed in the skin when the skin is exposed to sunlight. In addition to its effects on bone, vitamin D is thought to play a key role in many other medical conditions including prostate cancer and cardiovascular disease, as outlined in a Johns Hopkins Health Alert (**www.johnshopkinshealthalerts.com**, 2009). During the past decade, there's been a surge in research into the association between vitamin D and prostate cancer. Multiple studies have reported a link between sub-optimal levels of vitamin D and an increased risk of developing various cancers including prostate cancer, although not all studies have been confirmatory. While these findings are encouraging and could eventually lead to widespread screening for and treatment of vitamin D deficiencies, we still need a large, randomized, placebo-controlled trial to demonstrate whether vitamin D supplementation can actually prevent prostate cancer. Vitamin D was first isolated by Adolf Windaus, who was awarded the Nobel Prize in 1928 for his work. Vitamin D is not actually a vitamin, it's a hormone. A vitamin is a substance you have to get from food. Vitamin D, however, is manufactured in the body—the definition of a hormone. While researchers are still working to determine the effects of vitamin D on the prostate, here are some of the heart benefits of this vitamin:

- **Blood pressure regulation**. While there is no direct evidence that vitamin D supplementation will lower blood pressure, people with high blood pressure generally have low blood levels of vitamin D.
- **Heart attack, stroke, heart failure reduction**. A recent study in Circulation reported that events such as heart attacks, strokes, and heart failure were anywhere from 53% to 80% higher in people with low levels of vitamin D in their blood. That risk increased even more in people with high blood pressure. Low blood levels of vitamin D may increase the risk of heart disease and stroke, especially for people with high blood pressure, according to researchers with the Framingham Heart Study. The scientists followed 1,739 men and women for more than five years and reported that participants with low blood levels of vitamin D were 62% more likely to develop cardiovascular disease than those with higher levels. For those with low vitamin D levels and high blood pressure, cardiovascular risk doubled.
- **Helps reduce inflammation**. Researchers speculate that more vitamin D could lead to less inflammation in the arteries. Until recently, most researchers believed that heart disease was essentially a "plumbing" problem caused by an accumulation of hardened fat and cholesterol in the coronary arteries, known as plaque. However, an increasing body of evidence now shows that this accumulation of plaque is actually the result of chronic, low-grade inflammation in the coronary arteries. Researchers also believe that in the battle

against heart disease, damping down this inflammation is nearly as important as lowering cholesterol.

PLEASE NOTE: Emerging clinical research has suggested that vitamin D may also be beneficial in patients with dementia, Parkinson's disease, multiple sclerosis, and depression. December of 2010, the Institute of Medicine reported that most people up to age 70 need no more than 600 International Units (IUs) of vitamin D per day, and those 71 and older may need as much as 800 IUs per day. As for calcium, the Institute of Medicine report reommended already accepted levels to go along with your daily D—about 1,000 milligrams (mg) of calcium a day for most adults, 700 to 1,000 mg for young children, and 1,300 mg for teenagers and menopausal women. Too much calcium can cause kidney stones and this risk increases once people exceed 2,000 mg a day.

VITAMIN E

QUESTION: I enjoyed your column about vitamin C a couple of weeks ago. What can you tell me about vitamin E?

ANSWER: Vitamin E is actually a group of eight compounds known as tocopherols that protect the body's cells against damage by reactive chemicals known as free radicals. It is a fat-soluble antioxidant vitamin that also helps to protect red blood cells from rupture and it is needed for a number of chemical reactions in the body. There is some evidence that vitamin E improves the immune system and may protect against some forms of cancer, Alzheimer's disease (AD), and cataracts. In addition, some newer research suggests that vitamin E may be helpful in reducing the complications from diabetes. Vitamin E has also been promoted for a variety of other medical problems, such as heart disease, macular degeneration, acne, sexual dysfunction, arthritis, fibrocystic breast disease, gout, and PMS, but scientific findings are inconclusive. A deficiency of vitamin E in humans is extremely rare because adequate amounts are supplied in the normal diet. Good food sources of vitamin E include vegetable oils, margarine, whole grain cereals, wheat germ, green leafy vegetables, sunflower seeds, and nuts. Meats, fruits, and milk contain very little vitamin E. Because there are several different forms of vitamin E, its dosage or potency is usually standardized in International Units (IU). The recommended dietary allowance (RDA) is approximately 15 IU. Recent study data suggests that high doses of vitamin E may actually increase one's overall risk of dying, and doses greater than 150 IU/day are not recommended. Patients taking oral anticoagulants (blood thinners) such as Coumadin (warfarin) or aspirin should notify their doctor if they take high doses of vitamin E because it can interfere with blood clotting. In addition, iron supplements should not be taken at the same time as vitamin E because they may interfere with each other.

VITAMIN B-12

QUESTION: My husband has been getting B-12 shots for 8 months and doesn't feel any different. Would over-the-counter B-12 vitamins help?

ANSWER: Vitamin B-12, also known as cyanocobalamin, is found in liver, meat, fish, and dairy products like milk or cheese. It is not present in plant foods, thus vegetarians are at risk of developing a deficiency of this vitamin. Vitamin B-12 deficiency can lead to anemia, nerve damage, sore tongue, loss of appetite, and neurological symptoms. The use of vitamin B-12 has been purported to help anemia, prevent heart disease, ease dementia, and fight fatigue. In healthy people who do not have restricted diets, the body maintains vitamin B-12 levels and a deficiency is not usually a problem. However, some people have trouble absorbing vitamin B-12, which can lead to a deficiency. For vitamin B-12 to be absorbed into the blood it must first combine with a protein in the stomach known as the "intrinsic factor" which carries the vitamin through the intestinal tract. People who don't produce the "intrinsic factor" can develop a type of anemia known as "pernicious anemia". Vitamin B-12 shots are given to people with this disorder to correct the deficiency and the anemia. Other possible causes of vitamin B-12 deficiency include abnormal bacterial growth in the intestinal tract, certain diseases, or surgery that removes part of the stomach or intestine. In addition, aging produces changes in the gastrointestinal tract, and about 10-30% of Americans over age 60 have difficulty in absorbing vitamin B-12. Some medications such as metformin (Glucophage) can also interfere with the absorption of vitamin B-12. Because of the possibility of vitamin B-12 deficiency, many people take vitamin B-12 supplements. Vitamin B-12 shots are useful for people who may have trouble absorbing the vitamin, but oral products are effective if there are no gastrointestinal problems. It appears that excessive intake of vitamin B-12 will not cause any problems.

QUESTION: I am 70 years old and get vitamin B-12 shots each month for anemia. What can you tell me about "No Shot" vitamin B-12 tablets?

ANSWER: Anemia, or a low number of red blood cells, can have many causes in older people, including abnormal bleeding or chronic disorders and needs to be evaluated by a physician. Anemia can also be caused by a deficiency of vitamin B-12, iron, or folic acid. These nutrients are needed by the bone marrow to produce red blood cells. Red blood cells are very important because they contain hemoglobin, which enables them to carry oxygen from the lungs and deliver it to the body's tissues. All cells in the body need this oxygen to produce energy for the cell's activities. When energy is produced, carbon dioxide is released and is carried back by red blood cells to the lungs and breathed out. Vitamin B-12, also known as cyanocobalamin, is found in liver, meat, fish, and dairy products like milk or cheese. It is not present in plant foods, and vegetarians are at risk of developing a deficiency of this vitamin. In addition, aging can lead to changes in the gastrointestinal tract that prevents vitamin B-12 from being absorbed leading to a deficiency. It is estimated that 10-30% of people over 50 years of age have difficulty in absorbing this vitamin. In view of this, vitamin B-12 injections may be used to correct a deficiency of this vitamin. Nonprescription oral vitamin B-12 products are available, but are only effective if there are no gastrointestinal problems preventing their absorption. A nasal vitamin B-12 product is also available (Nascobal), but requires a prescription. I am not too familiar with the

No-Shot vitamin B-12 supplement product, but it is promoted for use by vegetarians, for maintaining a healthy nervous system, and to help promote natural energy. This product utilizes sublingual (under the tongue) tablets, which the company claims to provide for efficient absorption of vitamin B-12. However, it should be noted that like all supplement products, this product has not been evaluated or approved by the FDA for the treatment of any condition.

NEW VITAMIN DISCOVERED

QUESTION: I heard that a new vitamin has been discovered. What is it?

ANSWER: Japanese scientists have discovered a new vitamin that seems to play an important fertility role in mice, and may have a similar function in humans. The vitamin is known as pyrroloquinoline quinone or PQQ substance and is the first new vitamin discovered in 55 years. During experiments, mice deprived of PQQ suffered from reduced fertility and roughened fur. The best sources of PQQ appear to be "natto"—a pungent Japanese dish of fermented soybeans, parsley, green tea, green peppers, kiwi fruit and papaya. PQQ is not generally included in multivitamin products currently on the market. This new vitamin is believed to belong to the vitamin B group, which includes vitamin B-1 (thiamine), vitamin B-2 (riboflavin), vitamin B-6 (pyroidoxine), and vitamin B-12 (cyanocobalamin).

Vitamins are essential micronutrients required by the body in small amounts for growth, development, and function. They are not sources of energy like proteins, carbohydrates, or fats, but some are needed for the release of energy from food while others are needed to make important compounds used by the body. Most vitamins cannot be formed in the body, and must be obtained from outside sources. Someone who consumes too little of certain vitamins may develop a nutritional deficiency. A variety of conditions can also increase the need for vitamins such as lactation, pregnancy, use of certain drugs, excessive alcohol or tobacco use, and some illnesses. Vitamins are either fat soluble (dissolve in fat) like vitamins A, D, E, and K or are water soluble (dissolve in water) like the B vitamins, pantothenic acid, niacin, biotin, and folic acid. Some vitamins can be harmful when taken in very high doses such as vitamin A, D, niacin, B-6, and C. Some vitamins can also interfere with certain drugs. If you have any questions about vitamins, be sure to ask your doctor or pharmacist.

MULTIPLE SUPPLEMENTS

QUESTION: I take several non-prescription products including folic acid, baby aspirin, and Caltrate 600 plus soy. Are these drugs compatible?

ANSWER: Let me first briefly review the use of these over-the-counter (OTC) medications. Folic acid is a water-soluble vitamin found in fresh leafy green vegetables, fruits, liver and other organ meats, dried beans, peas, lentils, and whole-wheat products. It is necessary for the production of normal red blood cells and its use as a dietary supplement has also been promoted for the prevention of heart disease and other disorders. Low levels of folic acid may be associated with high levels of homocysteine, which has been implicated in the development of clogged arteries and heart attacks. Aspirin in low doses is also promoted for its beneficial effects in the prevention of heart attacks due to its anticoagulant effect on the blood. It prevents platelets in the blood from sticking to each other, which occurs during the formation of a blood clot. Caltrate 600 is a high potency calcium supplement, which contains 600 mg of calcium. An adequate supply of calcium in adults over age 40 is important to help prevent osteoporosis. The ingredients in many plant derivatives including soya beans and other legumes contain "phytoestrogens" or "isoflavonoids" which have estrogen-like activity. Because of this, products containing soy substances are being promoted for the treatment of problems associated with menopause—but remember that the FDA has not approved them for this use. Regarding the compatibility of these particular nonprescription products, I cannot think of any significant potential problems. However, there are many drug interactions that can occur between each of these OTC medications and numerous prescription drugs. In view of this, be sure to advise your doctor and pharmacist of your use of these nonprescription drugs whenever a prescription drug is ordered. With all the herbal products and other supplements now available, this communication with your doctor and pharmacist is very important to prevent medication-related problems.

NONI JUICE

QUESTION: A friend of mine takes noni juice for her arthritis. What can you tell me about this juice?

ANSWER: Noni juice (also called mengkudu juice and other names) is made from the fruit of the noni tree (Morinda citrifolia), found in the South Pacific Islands of Tahiti or Fiji and more recently Hawaii. It is a smelly, slightly sweet juice that has been touted as a cure for numerous ailments including arthritis, high blood pressure, menstrual cramps, infections, pain, diabetes, ulcers, sprains, depression, sexual dysfunction, senility, heart disease, and many others. Noni juice appears to contain a mixture of vitamins, minerals, organic acids, and substances known as anthraquinones. Sales of this juice have been estimated to be over 23 million dollars per month in the United States alone. It is available as a liquid juice or in capsule form.

I will not argue with anyone who claims that noni juice helps them. However, there does not appear to be any significant scientific data to support the use of noni juice for any particular medical condition. Side effects of noni juice can include diarrhea and allergic reactions. Some products can also contain high amounts of sugar, which could pose a problem for patients with diabetes. In addition, since noni juice may also contain high amounts of potassium, its use could be a problem in patients with kidney disease who need to restrict their potassium intake. Until more scientific information is available, I would not recommend the use of noni juice for the treatment of any medical problem. Also, keep in mind that the FDA has not approved the use of noni juice for the treatment of any medical disorder.

SAM-E

QUESTION: What can you tell me about the food supplement called SAM-e?

ANSWER: S-adenosylmethionine or SAM-e for short has been touted as an over-the-counter "miracle" product. It is among the 25 top selling dietary supplements in the U.S. and is mainly promoted for the treatment of depression, osteoarthritis, and to enhance liver function. Discovered in 1952, SAM-e is produced naturally in the body from the amino acid methionine, and adenosine triphosphate (ATP) which supplies energy for chemical reactions. Folic acid and vitamin B12 are also needed for its production. Its exact functions in the body are not entirely known. Manufacturers of SAM-e claim that it improves joint health and mobility for people with osteoarthritis. They also claim that it is beneficial for the improvement of mood and emotional well being. Some clinical trials do support these claims but more information and additional studies are needed. In a small number of studies in people with osteoarthritis the effectiveness of SAM-e was comparable to Naprosyn (naproxen), Motrin (ibuprofen), Indocin (indomethacin), and Feldene (piroxicam) in reducing pain and morning stiffness and in improving joint movement. Other studies have shown that SAM-e may also be comparable to some antidepressant drugs like Elavil (amitriptyline) or Tofranil (imipramine) for the treatment of depression. Likewise, some research has shown beneficial effects in the treatment of various forms of chronic liver disease. Side effects associated with SAM-e include nausea, vomiting, diarrhea, headache, dizziness, insomnia, restlessness, and anxiety. It may also interact with other medications including prescription antidepressants so consult your doctor and pharmacist before using this product. The usual starting dose of SAM-e is 200 mg once or twice daily. Higher doses may be needed for some disorders. Also, remember that like other nutritional products, SAM-e has not been approved for the treatment of any disorder by the FDA.

PLEASE NOTE: A recent study in the Am J of Psychiatry (2010) suggests that SAM-e can be an effective adjunctive treatment for patients with major depressive disorder who have not responded to other anti-depressant drugs known as selective serotonin reuptake inhibitors (SSRIs).

KAVA

QUESTION: I take the herb kava when I can't sleep. What can you tell me about this herbal product?

ANSWER: Kava (also called kava-kava, ava, and awa) is an herbal product that is prepared from the roots of a pepper plant (Piper methylysticum) that is grown in many South Pacific islands. The drinking of a beverage made from Kava predates recorded history and it has been used as a ceremonial beverage in welcoming important visitors, in marriages, in settling disputes, and in preserving the good graces of kings and chiefs. Kava bars offer the beverage on various Pacific islands, where the muddy looking liquid is drunk from coconut shells. This beverage causes a numbing effect in the mouth followed by a relaxed sociable state in which fatigue and anxiety are lessened.

The use of kava has been rapidly gaining popularity in the United States and Europe for its anti-anxiety and sedative effects. In Germany it has been approved for conditions of nervous anxiety, stress, and restlessness. Kava is also believed to improve the quality of sleep in humans. Exactly how this herb works is not understood, but its affects are very similar to tranquilizer drugs known as benzodiazepines that act on the central nervous system. A few small short-term clinical studies have shown that kava can help people with certain anxiety disorders.

When used in low doses, side effects from kava appear to be minimal. However, gastrointestinal problems and visual problems can occur at higher doses and kava use has been implicated in Europe in at least 25 cases of serious liver problems including hepatitis, cirrhosis, and liver failure. In view of this, it is advisable to avoid Kava altogether. In addition, very high doses can cause muscle problems and a skin problem known as "kava dermopathy". This side effect produces a swollen face, bloodshot eyes, yellow discoloration of the skin and fish scale like lesions on the skin. The legend behind this skin problem is that kava grew from the grave of a girl named Kava'onau, a leper who was sacrificed by her parents for their king. The South Pacific islanders feel that the dermopathy is a symbol of the girl's leper lesions.

Because of its effect on the nervous system, kava should not be used by people who must drive or operate heavy machinery. It should also be avoided by patients with Parkinson's disease, depression, or during pregnancy and breast-feeding. Furthermore, many drug interacions are possible (especially with alcohol or sedatives) and caution must be exercised when using kava with other medications. Be sure to consult with your physician and pharmacist before using any kava product.

Several kava products are available including capsules, tablets, liquids, and powder formulations. Usually one capsule two to four times per day is used for anxiety and one capsule taken one hour before bedtime may enhance the quality of sleep. Also keep in mind that like other herbal products, kava has not been approved for use by the FDA.

QUESTION: Should people be concerned about taking kava products?

ANSWER: Yes, the popular herbal supplement kava may cause potentially severe liver damage, according to a new FDA warning. Products containing kava have been implicated in liver-related injuries such as hepatitis, cirrhosis, and liver failure in more than 25 events reported in Europe and Canada. These cases include liver failure resulting in six liver transplants and three deaths. In view of this, the FDA is warning physicians to check their patients who use kava supplements or teas for possible symptoms of liver damage after similar reports in the United States. The FDA also urges any person taking kava who experiences symptoms of serious liver damage (jaundice, brown urine, nausea, vomiting, light-colored stools, unusual tiredness, weakness, stomach pain, loss of appetite, etc.) to consult their doctor. Furthermore, anyone with a history of liver problems should talk with their doctor before using supplements that contain kava. Kava is a common ingredient found in many herbal supplements promoted for relaxation, sleeplessness, menopausal symptoms, and other uses. The kava plant is native to the South Pacific where it has been used for many, many years to make a ceremonial beverage in welcoming important visitors, in marriages, in settling disputes, and in preserving the good graces of kings and chiefs. Other frequently-used names for kava includes ava, awa, kava root, kava kava, Piper methysticum, rauschpfeffer, kava pepper, kew, sakau, tonga, wurzelstolk, and yangona. I believe that kava products are now banned in Germany and the U.K. Under U.S. federal law, dietary supplements do not have to be proven safe or effective before they can be sold, and the FDA has not determined whether kava dietary supplements provide the benefits for which they are promoted. Kava can also interact with a number of other medications and alcohol, which I have discussed in previous columns. To report any possible adverse effects of kava, contact the FDA at (800)332-1088 or on the internet at **www.fda.gov/medwatch**.

VALERIAN

QUESTION: I have trouble sleeping and saw an ad on TV for a product called Alluna Sleep. Do you think it will help?

ANSWER: You're certainly not alone when it comes to insomnia, or the inability to attain restful sleep. Approximately one-third to one-half of the population suffers from occasional difficulty in sleeping. Chronic sleep difficulties affect nearly 20% of the population. Insomnia tends to be worse in women, but sleep difficulties increase with age in both men and women. Sleep difficulty can include trouble falling asleep, frequent awakenings after falling asleep, or early awakenings with an inability to go back to sleep. The causes of insomnia are numerous. Short-term insomnia (a week or less) can often result from sudden changes in daily routine, like a change in work schedule or from stress in one's life, such as marital difficulties, financial worries, or a death in the family. Large evening meals, evening exercise, or excessive TV watching prior to sleep can cause sleep difficulties. Certain medical problems such as arthritis, heart disease, lung disease, stomach ulcers, sleep apnea, and psychiatric conditions like depression can also cause insomnia. In addition, medications like decongestants, diuretics, steroids, antihypertensive, or antidepressants can cause difficulty in sleeping. The use of alcohol, smoking, and caffeine consumption could also lead to sleep problems.

The herbal sleep aid, Alluna Sleep, has been heavily advertised on TV and radio, and in several national magazines. It contains the roots of a tall perennial herb known as valerian. Although the active chemicals in valerian have not been identified, it has long been used for treating insomnia. Exactly how valerian works is not known, but it appears to affect a chemical in the brain known as GABA, which aids in relaxation. It seems to be modestly effective as a sedative-hypnotic medication. An FDA-like group in Germany has approved valerian as a calmative and sleep-promoting agent useful in treating states of unrest and anxiety—produced sleep disturbances. It appears to be safe to use, but remember that like all herbal products, it has not been evaluated by the FDA.

GARLIC

QUESTION: My husband takes garlic tablets every day to help lower his cholesterol. He may need to have surgery and I wonder if the garlic supplement could be a problem?

ANSWER: Yes it may be a problem. Garlic supplements may increase the risk of bleeding and it is recommended that they be discontinued at least seven days before surgery. Many people don't realize that popular herbal and dietary supplements can affect the way their body reacts to medications or surgery. Although there is not a lot of information available about this topic, earlier this year an article in The Journal of The American Medical Association provided some guidelines for discontinuing certain supplements or herbs prior to surgery. I have outlined their recommendations below and on the next page.

Herb/Supplement: Echinacea
Possible Risk During Surgery: Decreased effectiveness of immuno-suppressive therapies
Recommendation: Discontinue as far in advance of surgery as possible.

Herb/Supplement: Ephedra (ma huang)

Possible Risk During Surgery: Increase in blood pressure and heart rate, stroke, or abnormal heart rhythm
Recommendation: Discontinue at least 24 hours before surgery

Herb/Supplement: Garlic
Possible Risk During Surgery: Increased risk of bleeding, especially if taken with blood thinners like Coumadin (warfarin) or aspirin
Recommendation: Discontinue at least 7 days before surgery.

Herb/Supplement: Gingko
Possible Risk During Surgery: Increased risk of bleeding, especially if taken with blood thinners like Coumadin (warfarin) or aspirin
Recommendation: Discontinue at least 36 hours before surgery.

Herb/Supplement: Ginseng
Possible Risk During Surgery: May lower blood sugar, increase blood pressure, or increase risk of bleeding
Recommendation: Discontinue at least 7 days before surgery.

Herb/Supplement: Kava
Possible Risk During Surgery: May increase the sedative effects of anesthetics and other drugs used during surgery
Recommendation: Discontinue at least 24 hours before surgery.

Herb/Supplement: St. John's wort
Possible Risk During Surgery: May affect the metabolism of other drugs
Recommendation: Discontinue at least 5 days before surgery.

GLUCOSAMINE

QUESTION: I've seen new ads on TV showing that glucosamine can rebuild your cartilage if you have osteoarthritis. Can it really do this?

ANSWER: Osteoarthritis or "wear and tear" arthritis is a very common medical problem that probably affects almost everyone over the age of

60 to some extent. Unlike rheumatoid arthritis, which usually begins at an earlier age and has a different cause, osteoarthritis is caused by the breakdown of joint cartilage—the cushion between bones that works like a shock absorber. As the cartilage breaks down, the bones begin to rub together, causing pain and loss of movement. It usually affects the hands and weight-bearing joints, such as the knees, hips, feet, and back.

A good treatment program for osteoarthritis can help to reduce pain and stiffness, and improve joint movement and function. This may include joint protection, exercise, heat and cold treatment, weight reduction, surgery in some situations, and numerous medications. Medications for osteoarthritis include various anti-inflammatory drugs such as acetaminophen (Tylenol), aspirin, ibuprofen (Motrin), or the newer more expensive non-steroidal anti-inflammatory drugs (NSAIDs) like Vioxx and Celebrex. Topically applied preparations containing capsaicin may also be helpful in relieving the pain of osteoarthritis for some patients. Another potential treatment for osteoarthritis of the knees is the injection of a fluid known as sodium hyaluronate into the knee joint to help lubricate it and act as a shock absorber.

The dietary supplement glucosamine and chondroitin sulfate has also been widely used for osteoarthritis. Glucosamine, which occurs naturally in the human body, is said to play an important role in the maintenance and repair of cartilage. Chondroitin is said to prevent certain chemicals from breaking down cartilage in joints. They are known as "chondroprotective" agents and are used in an attempt to actually stop the breakdown of cartilage and rebuild it. Does it really work? In the past couple of years, American researchers have studied if glucosamine and chondroitin can help in osteoarthritis. In one clinical study involving 93 patients with osteoarthritis of the knees, glucosamine and chondroitin were found to be significantly more effective than a placebo (dummy pill) for the management of joint pain and movement. In a review of 15 other studies focusing on osteoarthritis of the knee or hip, researchers also found that glucosamine and chondroitin had moderate to large beneficial effects but, another recent study of 98 patients with osteoarthritis of the knee showed that glucosamine alone was not any more helpful than a placebo for knee pain. Results from another study showed that the long-term use of glucosamine may actually prevent changes in joint structure and significantly improve symptoms in patients with knee osteoarthritis. In this three year study involving 212 patients, researchers found progressive joint-space narrowing in the knees of patients taking glucosamine once a day—but not in those taking a placebo. In other words, it appeared that glucosamine actually helped to slow down the degenerative osteoarthritis process and not just help with pain relief. Although the results were not as dramatic as those portrayed in the TV ad you refer to, it was a very important study. Additional studies are ongoing. It should also be kept in mind that even though glucosamine is widely available as a nutritional supplement, it can have side effects. For example, there is some information available that glucosamine can make glucose control more difficult in patients with diabetes. It can also cause gastrointestinal problems, insomnia, headaches, and a tired feeling.

QUESTION: Does glucosamine and/or chondroitin help with osteoarthritis?

ANSWER: I have a number of fellow senior softball players with osteoarthritis or joint pain that swear by glucosamine/chondroitin to relieve their pain and improve joint function. In the past I have also written several columns about glucosamine/chondroitin supplements, basically surmising that study results have been mixed and that more study is needed to evaluate these products. Recent study results, however, from the National Institutes of Health (NIH) have concluded that these supplements do not really help with osteoarthritis. In 2006, the NIH conducted a study named the Glucosamine/Chondroitin Arthritis Intervention Trial (GAIT). This study included 1,600 participants with osteoarthritis of the knee. It was the first large-scale study that tested whether glucosamine and chondroitin used separately or in combination reduced pain in these individuals. Results from this 6-month study, which cost $12.5 million to conduct, showed that, overall, these supplements were no more effective than a dummy pill (placebo) at relieving pain. However, among a small group of study participants with moderate to severe knee pain, those taking the combination supplement reported greater pain relief than taking a placebo, but this group was too small for researchers to say for sure that the supplement works. Because of this, a second study (GAIT-Part 2) was carried out. This second GAIT study, which involved 572 individuals from the original study, utilized x-rays to measure if daily glucosamine/ chondroitin supplements over a period of 18 more months prevented a loss of joint space (loss of cartilage) between the ends of the knee bones. Results from this study in late 2008 showed that glucosamine and/or chondroitin did no better than placebo in slowing structural damage (loss of cartilage) in these people with knee osteoarthritis. In spite of these study results it is hard to argue with success, and many people will probably continue to take supplements.

An estimated 27 million adults in the United States live with osteoarthritis—the most common type of arthritis. Osteoarthritis, also called degenerative joint disease, is caused by the breakdown of cartilage, which is the connective tissue that cushions the ends of bones within the joint. Osteoarthritis is characterized by pain, joint damage, and limited motion. The disease generally occurs late in life, and most commonly affects the hands and large weight-bearing joints, such as the knees. Age, female gender, and obesity are risk factors for this condition.

More information about osteoarthritis and these supplements can be found at **www.nccam.nih.gov/news/2008**.

ACAI BERRY

QUESTION: What can you tell me about acai berry?

ANSWER: The acai (pronounced a-sigh-EE) berry is a grape size reddish-purple fruit that comes from the acai palm tree, which is native to Central and South America. It is a relative of the blueberry, cranberry, and other dark purple fruits. Acai is a popular food source in southern Brazil where it is consumed in a bowl mixed with granola and as an ice cream flavor or juice. The acai berry contains several substances called anthocyanins and flavonoids, which are powerful antioxidants that may protect against life's stressors. Acai has been widely marketed in the U.S. as a dietary supplement and companies sell acai berry products in the form of tablets, juice, smoothies, instant drink powder, and whole fruit. This berry is also available in some cosmetics and beauty products. Marketers of acai products claim that it provides increased energy levels, improves sexual performance, improves digestion, promotes weight loss, provides detoxification, improves skin appearance, improves heart health, and improves sleep, along with other claims. Unfortunately, there does not appear to be any good scientifically controlled studies to prove these claims and the FDA has not evaluated these acai supplement products. People with pollen allergies or a known hypersensitivity to acai or similar berries should avoid this fruit, but when consumed in moderate amounts, acai appears to be safe.

Body Building Supplements

QUESTION: What can you tell me about the FDA warning concerning the use of body building products?

ANSWER: The FDA recently issued a Public Health Advisory warning consumers to stop using any body building products that are represented to contain steroids or steroid-like substances. Many of these products are marketed as dietary supplements but instead are unapproved and misbranded drugs because they contain synthetic steroid or steroid-like ingredients. These products are frequently marketed as alternatives to anabolic (promoting muscle building) steroids for increasing muscle mass and strength and are sold online and in some retail stores. They are often promoted to athletes to improve sports performance and to aid in recovery from training and sporting events. The FDA has received reports of serious adverse events associated with the use of these products including liver injury, stroke, kidney failure, and pulmonary embolism (blockage of an artery in the lung). Acute liver injury is known to be a possible harmful effect of using anabolic steroid-containing products. In addition, anabolic steroids may cause other serious long-term side effects including shrinkage of the testes and male infertility, masculinization of women, breast enlargement in males, short stature in children, adverse effects on blood lipid levels, and increased risk of heart attack and stroke. Along with this Public Health Advisory, the FDA has also sent a Warning Letter to a manufacturer of body building supplements that contain synthetic steroids. The products named in the Warning Letter are marketed by American Cellular Laboratories and include "Tren-Xtreme", "MASS

Xtreme", "ESTRO Xtreme", AH-89-Xtreme", "HMG Xtreme", "MMA-3 Xtreme", "VNS-9 Xtreme", and "TT-40-Xtreme". Due to the potentially serious health risks associated with using these types of products, the FDA recommends that consumers immediately stop using all body building products that claim to contain steroids or steroid-like substances. Furthermore, consumers should consult their health care professional if they are experiencing symptoms possibly associated with these products such as nausea, weakness or fatigue, fever, abdominal pain, chest pain, shortness of breath, jaundice (yellowing of the skin or whites of the eyes) or brown/discolored urine. The FDA also recommends that consumers talk with their health care professional about any body building supplements they are taking or plan to take, particularly if they are uncertain about a product's ingredients.

BLACK COHOSH

QUESTION: What can you tell me about the herb called Black Cohosh?

ANSWER: Black Cohosh (also known as Black Snakeroot, Squaw Root, Rattle Root, and Bugbane) has been used for treating "female complaints" since before colonial times. This perennial plant is native to the Eastern United States growing 3 to 9 feet tall and producing small white flowers in July through September. The name "Cohosh" comes from an Algonquin word meaning "rough" which refers to the plant's lumpy black roots. The English name "Bugbane" comes from the belief that the plant's strong odor repels insects.

Many uses have been reported for this herb, including the treatment of menstrual pain and cramps, absence of menstruation, rheumatoid pain, headache, cough, and inflammation. It has also been used by native Americans to aid in labor. Black Cohosh was an ingredient in Lydia Pinkham's Vegetable Compound, a popular patent remedy for "female complaints" that was sold earlier in this century. Active ingredients in Black Cohosh appear to produce numerous effects in the body including estrogen-like activity. Some clinical studies have shown Black Cohosh to be effective for the treatment of PMS and painful menstruation. It has also been found to be useful in relieving the uncomfortable symptoms of menopause, such as hot flashes, sweating, headache, etc. Side effects of Black Cohosh are usually mild and can include stomach upset, weight gain, and dizziness. Due to its hormonal effects, Black Cohosh should not be taken during pregnancy or while breast feeding and it should not be used for longer than six months. The dose of Black Cohosh is usually 40 mg twice a day. For PMS symptoms it should be taken about a week to 10 days before your period. Remember that like all herbal products, Black Cohosh has not been approved by the FDA and if you have any questions, be sure to talk to your doctor and pharmacist.

PLEASE NOTE: A recent study in the journal Menopause (2009) concluded that Black Cohosh did not reduce the number of hot flashed and night sweats in menopausal women.

NATURAL DIET AIDS

QUESTION: Are there any "natural" supplements that can help with weight control? What about "tummy roll" in seniors?

ANSWER: Numerous herbal and other dietary supplement products are being promoted as "natural" diet aids. Despite their many claims, most of these products are probably not only ineffective but can produce serious side effects in some people. A summary of some of the "active" ingredients in these preparations are listed below.

Ingredient
Some Possible Side Effects
Comments
- **Chromium picolinate**
  Kidney problems
  Also called a "fat burner".
- **Citrus aurantium**
  Unknown
  Often combined with St. John's wort. Also called "bitter oranges" or "herbal phen-fen".

- **Ephedra or mahung**
  Dizziness, high blood pressure, headaches, seizures, stroke, heart attack, nervousness, inability to sleep
  Also called "legalized speed", or "herbal phen-fen". Often combined with St. John's wort.
- **Garcinia**
  Unknown
  More information is needed
- **Guarana**
  Stimulant like caffeine in coffee. When used with ephedra may cause high blood pressure or stroke
  Also called a "fat burner".
- **Pyruvate**
  Unknown
  More information is needed
- **Senna**
  Colon and electrolyte problems with long term use
  Decrease in weight due to water loss. Also used as a laxative.
- **St. John's wort**
  Dizziness, dry mouth, increased sensitivity to light, gastrointestinal distress
  May be useful in treating mild depression.
- **5-hydroxytryptophan**
  Heart or lung problems
  More information is needed

In addition, a variety of other herbs (e.g., uva ursi, chickweed, ginseng, etc.) have been touted as diet aids but appear to be ineffective for this use. Check with your doctor before using any of these weight loss products and remember that none of them have been approved by the FDA for this use. As I've noted before, the best treatment of obesity involves a combination of reduced intake of calories, nutritional counseling, exercise, and behavior modification. For the "tummy roll", abdominal exercises like sit-ups, stomach crunches and obliques, and leg raises can be helpful.

HERBAL PRODUCTS
AND DRUG INTERACTIONS

QUESTION: Why don't herbal products include information on their labels about interactions with other medications?

ANSWER: Good question. Herbal products should be treated like other medicines because many of them contain potent drugs. This shouldn't come as a surprise since about one-third of all current prescription medications are derived from plants and other natural sources. However, since the FDA does not regulate the standardization, effectiveness, safety, and drug interactions of these products, their labeling does not require important information for consumers. Wouldn't it make sense to include information about patients who shouldn't use the product, side effects, and potential drug interactions on the labels of these preparations? This lack of consumer information problem goes back to 1994 when Congress passed the Dietary and Supplement Health Education Act (DSHEA). This act classifies herbal remedies as dietary supplements and thereby excludes them from the labeling requirements for both nonprescription and prescription medications. In spite of this lack of consumer information, however, herbal medicine sales increased 59% in 1997 and they are becoming increasingly popular. It has been estimated that about one-third of all Americans use herbal products. In addition to information about side effects and drug interactions, standardization of these products is also a cause for concern. A recent study tested 20 herbal dietary supplements containing the active ingredient ephedra and found that half of the products tested did not contain the amount ephedra claimed on the label. These differences were greater than 20%. Until the current labeling situation for herbal products changes, it is important for consumers to seek the advice of their pharmacist and physician who now have to "be the label". Many of these products do cause side effects and can interact dangerously with other medications—but don't look for their labeling to help you.

QUESTION: Some time ago you talked about herbal products and drug interactions. What herbs can interfere with Coumadin?

ANSWER: It is very important to know what may interfere with Coumadin (warfarin) therapy because increasing its effect may cause bleeding and decreasing its effect may cause blood clots to form. Several herbs may have the potential to interfere with Coumadin therapy, but not a lot of detailed scientific information is available. Some herbs actually may contain warfarin or have anticoagulant properties, which could lead to bleeding problems. Others may decrease the effects of Coumadin. In addition to herbal products, some dietary supplements may interfere with Coumadin therapy. In the list on the next page I have listed a number of herbs and a few dietary supplements which have the potential for interactions with Coumadin. Please remember, however, that the list may not be all-inclusive and that more scientific study and information is needed. Also note that patients receiving Coumadin must be monitored closely for signs and symptoms of bleeding and their blood needs to be monitored on a regular basis.

Potential Increase In Risk Of Bleeding With Coumadin

Angelica root
Arnica flower
Anise
Asafoetida
Bogbean
Borage seed oil
Bromelain
Capsicum
Celery
Chamomile
Clove
Danshen
Devil's claw
Dong quai
Fenugreek
Feverfew
Garlic
Ginger

Ginkgo
Horse chestnut
Licorice root
Lovage root
Meadowsweet
Onion
Papain
Parsley
Passionflower herb
Poplar
Quassia
Red clover
Rue
Sweet clover
Turmeric
Vitamin E
Willow bark

Potential Decrease In Coumadin Effects

Coenzyme Q10
Ginseng
Green tea

QUESTION: Is it OK to take herbal products with other medications?

ANSWER: Numerous herbal products may cause problems when used in combination with either prescription or nonprescription medications. However, there is only very limited information available regarding drug interactions with natural products like herbal remedies. You should always consult with your doctor and pharmacist if you are taking any medications and would like to use a herbal product. Some of the known drug interactions that are possible with commonly used herbs are listed below. But please remember that very little information is known about this topic and not all drug interactions or herbs are included in this list.

Some Commonly Used Herbs
Medication(s) That May Interact

- **Feverfew**
  Aspirin
  Dipyridamole (Persantine)
  Warfarin (Coumadin)
- **Garlic**
  Aspirin
  Clopidogrel (Plavix)
  Dipyridamole (Persantine)
  Sanquinavir (Invirase)
  Warfarin (Coumadin)
- **Ginger**
  Aspirin
  Dipyridamole (Persantine)
  Warfarin (Coumadin)
- **Ginkgo biloba**
  Aspirin
  Clopidogrel (Plavix)
  Dipyridamole (Persantine)
  Warfarin (Coumadin)
- **Ginseng (American, Korean, Asian)**
  Anti-diabetic drugs
  Aspirin
  Clopidogrel (Plavix)
  Furosemide (Lasix)
  Phenelzine (Nardil)
  Warfarin (Coumadin)
- **Ginseng (Siberian, Eleuthero)**
  Digoxin (Lanoxin)
- **Kava** kava
  Alcohol; Sedatives
- **St. Johns wort**
  Antidepressants (Many products)
  Cyclosporine
  Dextromethorphan (Many cold products)
  Digoxin (Lanoxin)
  Ephedrine

Lithium (Many products)
Meperidine (Demerol)
Pseudoephedrine (Sudafed, other decongestant products)
Sanquinavir (Invirase)
Selegiline (Eldepryl)
Warfarin (Coumadin)
Yohimbine (Many products)

QUESTION: Can herbal dietary supplements interact with prescription medications?

ANSWER: Yes, and I've noted this several times in earlier columns. A John's Hopkins Health Alert (**www.johnshopkinshealthalerts.com**, 2008) provided the following information, which was excerpted from their Special Report, "When Herbs and Prescription Drugs Don't Mix".

Many herbal dietary supplements are considered safe when used as directed, with no serious side effects reported—yet. But problems with herbal products have been identified. It's important to tell your doctor what supplements you use, to avoid interactions with any prescription drugs you may need to take.

Herbal supplements contain biologically active compounds that should not be considered safe just because they are sold over the counter or come from "natural" sources such as plants. When trying a new herbal supplement, ask your doctor or pharmacist whether there are known safety issues associated with the herbal supplement, especially interactions with other medications.

A fundamental problem in assessing either the efficacy or the side effects of herbal products is the lack of strict manufacturing quality standards, allowing substantial variability of products between different manufacturers and even between different batches of one product from the same manufacturer. As a consequence, firm conclusions on these compounds are difficult to reach.

Be especially cautious before going in for surgery. Some herbal remedies appear to increase the risk of bleeding. Others may interfere with drugs commonly used before, during, and after surgery, including anesthetics. It is probably most reasonable to stop taking any dietary supplements at least a week before surgery, to give them time to "wash out" of your system.

Here are some of the more popular herbal remedies thought to interact with certain prescription drugs.

Herbal Supplement 1—Ginkgo

Ginkgo inhibits the action of platelets in the blood, thus interfering with blood coagulation. Don't use ginkgo if you are taking the blood thinner warfarin (Coumadin) or antiplatelet drugs such as clopidogrel (Plavix). Ginkgo may lower blood sugar, so don't use it if you are already taking drugs for diabetes.

Herbal Supplement 2—Garlic

Chemical compounds in garlic may inhibit blood clotting. Don't use garlic supplements if you are already taking anticoagulants or antiplatelet drugs. Garlic can also interfere with the action of the antiviral drug saquinavir (Invirase), which is used to treat HIV infection.

Herbal Supplement 3—Licorice Root

Taking large amounts of licorice may cause high blood pressure and retention of water and salt. It can also deplete potassium in the body, leading to abnormal heart rhythms or symptoms of weakness or fatigue. Licorice would have the tendency to counteract the effect of some diuretics (water pills), drugs that are commonly prescribed for heart disease and high blood pressure.

Herbal Supplement 4—Kava

Kava appears to be toxic to the liver, so it is advisable to avoid kava altogether.

Herbal Supplement 5—Asian Ginseng

Asian ginseng may lower your blood sugar. Don't use it if you are already taking diabetes drugs to lower your blood sugar. Asian ginseng may also inhibit blood clotting. Don't use ginseng if you are already taking anticoagulants or antiplatelet drugs.

Herbal Supplement 6—St. John's Wort

The problem of St. John's wort interfering with the metabolism of many drugs is probably the best defined of all herbal interactions with other drugs. St. John's wort can interact with a variety of prescription drugs, either increasing or decreasing their effect. These drugs include the antiviral drug Invirase, the anti-rejection drug cyclosporine, the cardiac drug digoxin, the blood thinner Coumadin, antidepressants, and some cancer medications.

Please note that the examples listed above are just some of the potential interactions that can occur between herbal supplements and prescription medications. Many others are possible, so be sure to let your physician and pharmacist know what herbal supplements you are taking to try and prevent any potential drug interaction problems.

UNSAFE HERBALS

QUESTION: Are there any herbal products that can be harmful to use?

ANSWER: Yes. "Natural" does not necessarily mean safe and there are many herbal remedies that are risky to use. Below I have listed a number (but not all) of herbs that can be unsafe to use and their potential health hazards.

Some Potentially Unsafe Herbs
Possible Health Problems
- **Aconite**
  Nausea, vomiting, heart rhythm disorders, respiratory system paralysis
- **Bitter orange**
  Fainting, heart rhythm disorder, heart attack, stroke
- **Chaparral**
  Liver & kidney damage
- **Coltsfoot**
  Cancer, liver damage
- **Comfrey**
  Liver damage, cancer
- **Country mallow**
  Heart attack, arrhythmia, stroke

- **Ephedra** (Ma-Huang)
  High blood pressure, irregular heartbeat, nerve damage, heart attack, stroke, headaches, seizures, inability to sleep, tremors
- **Germander**
  Liver disease
- **Germanium**
  Kidney damage
- **Greater celandine**
  Liver damage
- **Jin bu huan**
  Liver damage
- **Kava**
  Liver damage
- **Licorice**
  When used in high doses for long periods may cause headache, water retention, low potassium, high blood pressure, heart problems
- **Lobelia**
  Breathing problems, sweating, rapid heartbeat, low blood pressure, coma
- **Magnolia-Stephania**
  Kidney disease
- **Pennyroyal**
  Liver damage
- **Poke root**
  Overdose can cause vomiting. May be fatal in children
- **Sassafras**
  Liver damage
- **Willow Bark**
  Reye's syndrome in children. Allergic reactions in adults
- **Wormwood**
  Nerve problems, mental problems, paralysis
- **Yohimbine**
  High or low blood pressure, anxiety, rapid heart rate, heart problems

"FAT BURNERS"

QUESTION: I tried a "fat burner" for three days and had difficulty urinating, terrible heartburn, and felt like I was "high" on drugs. What is in this nonprescription product that could cause these side effects?

ANSWER: According to the label you sent me this so-called "fat burner" product contains at least 25 different ingredients including various herbs, vitamins, and minerals. As you discovered, even these "natural supplements" can cause serious side effects in some people. "Natural" does not mean "safe". Remember poisonous mushrooms are also "natural". If you had a large magnifying glass you may have seen the Warning at the bottom of this dietary supplement's label. It warns you to not use this product if you are pregnant, or if you have heart disease, thyroid disease, certain psychiatric conditions, glaucoma, difficulty in urinating, enlarged prostate, or a seizure disorder. It also warns you to avoid this product if you are taking other medications like MAO inhibitors or over-the-counter (OTC) products containing ephedrine, pseudoephedrine, or phenylpropanolamine. The label further warns that this product is not appropriate for everyone, which you can attest to.

The side effects you experienced could be caused by several of the ingredients listed on the product label. At least four of the ingredients (Guarana which contains caffeine, Ma Huang which contains ephedrine, Goldenseal, and Nettles) can cause gastrointestinal problems such as nausea, vomiting, diarrhea, or stomach pain. The ephedrine in Ma Huang can also cause urinary retention and that is why it should not be used by men with enlarged prostate glands. As for the "high" you experienced, likely culprits include: caffeine from Guarana seed; Goldenseal; Ginseng; and the ephedrine in Ma Huang. These compounds stimulate the central nervous system, raise blood pressure, can cause increased or irregular heart rates, and produce irritability or nervousness.

As I've noted many times before, none of these dietary supplements have been approved by the FDA for safety and effectiveness like drug products. People who use these supplements should always read product labels and take notice of all warnings. They should also let their physician and pharmacist know that they are taking them because of potential side effects and possible interactions with prescribed or OTC medications. Supplement users who suffer harmful effects that they think are related to a supplement can report them to the FDA by calling 1-800-FDA-1088.

LEMONGRASS

QUESTION: What can you tell me about lemongrass?

ANSWER: Lemongrass (cymbopogon) is a tall, aromatic, perennial grass, which grows up to two feet in height and is native to Southern Europe and North Africa, but is cultivated around the world in warm temperate and tropical regions. It is widely used as an herb in Asian and Caribbean cooking, but also has been used for medicinal purposes. The main constituent of lemongrass oil is citral, which makes up about 80% of the total components. As a folk medicine, lemongrass has been used as an antispasmodic, analgesic, for the management of nervous and gastrointestinal disorders, to treat fevers, to treat nausea and vomiting, to treat inflammation, to help with urination and water retention, and to treat bacterial and fungal infections. In addition, there is some laboratory evidence that citral can induce programmed cell death (apoptosis) in some cancer cells. However, it should be noted that there is insufficient information available to recommend the use of lemongrass or citral for any of these conditions nor has the FDA approved its use for any medical condition. In fact, the FDA recently issued a "Warning Letter" to at least one manufacturer/distributor of citral advising the company to review its web site, product labels, and other labeling and promotional materials to ensure that they do not make unsubstantiated treatment claims. Lemongrass is considered to be of low toxicity but should not be used in women who are pregnant. Citral has also been shown to cause benign prostate enlargement in rats. You should consult with your physcian(s) before using any lemongrass or citral product.

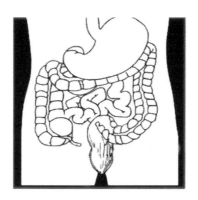

CHAPTER 5
GASTROINTESTINAL
PROBLEMS

HEARTBURN

QUESTION: I recently received a free sample of Pepcid AC. How does this medicine prevent heartburn and how does it compare to other nonprescription medications for heartburn?

ANSWER: We have all been bombarded with advertisements for the numerous over-the-counter (OTC) products now available to treat or prevent heartburn, acid indigestion, and sour stomach. Certainly, this has created confusion amongst consumers who want to choose the most effective product. Besides Pepcid AC, there are 3 other similar products currently available without a prescription: Tagamet-HB 200; Zantac-75; and Axid AR. While these products are similar, they contain a different active ingredient. The AC stands for acid controller, the HB for heartburn and AR for acid reducer. The 75 in Zantac-75 stands for the dosage in each tablet (75 mg) and the 200 stands for the dosage in each Tagamet-HB 200 tablet. All of these products are categorized as "H2-(histamine) receptor antagonists". Histamine is a substance produced by the body and has many different functions, depending upon what type of "receptor" it acts on. For example, H1 receptors are important in allergic disorders and antihistamines that block these receptors such as Benadryl help to relieve allergic reactions. On the other hand, H2 receptors are responsible for the production of stomach acid to help with digestion and H2 receptor antagonists block histamine's effect on the stomach's ability to produce acid. Hence, these drugs are useful in treating or preventing the heartburn, indigestion, and sour stomach caused by foods that lead to excessive acid in the stomach. They are a "specialized" type of antihistamine. Basically, all of these products do the same thing—prevent you from producing too much stomach acid. The only real differences between these products are the dosage used and possibly the potential to interfere with other medications that may be taken along with them. To treat heartburn, acid indigestion, or sour stomach these drugs are taken as needed up to twice a day. For prevention of these problems, they should be taken 1 hour before eating a meal expected to cause these problems. All of these products are relatively safe to take and have been used by millions of people with an overall incidence of side effects less than 3%. The most common side effects from these products are headache, drowsiness, constipation, diarrhea, nausea, vomiting, and abdominal pain or discomfort. One possibly important difference between these products is the potential for their interaction with other drugs. Tagamet-HB 200 can increase the blood levels of other drugs such as Dilantin (phenytoin), Coumadin (warfarin), and theophylline containing medications. Therefore, it may be wise to avoid Tagamet-HB 200 if you are taking these other drugs. In addition, all of these products can possibly reduce the effectiveness of certain antibiotics, such as Penetrex, Vantin, Sporanox, and Nizoral, and probably should be avoided if taking these drugs. You should also keep in mind that higher doses of the H2 antagonists, such as those found in prescription only products, can lead to more drug interactions or side effects and therefore the recommended dose should not be exceeded. In conclusion, all of these OTC products are equally effective in treating or preventing heartburn, acid indigestion, or sour stomach and the least expensive product should be used. However, if you are also taking one of the other medications noted above, then Tagamet-HB 200 should be avoided. Furthermore, if you want rapid relief of stomach symptoms, then antacid products may be preferred because they provide immediate relief while the H2 antagonists take 1-2 hours to work. Many antacid products are also much less expensive.

QUESTION: I regularly use Zantac for heartburn. Can I drink alcohol while on this medication?

ANSWER: No, it is not a good idea to mix Zantac (generic name ranitidine) and alcohol for a variety of reasons. Heartburn, also known as GERD (gastroesophageal reflux disease), is a common disorder that approximately 10% to 20% of the U.S. population treats with various medications. The burning sensation of heartburn is usually caused by a backward movement of acidic stomach contents into the esophagus or swallowing tube. This back flow of stomach contents is usually prevented by a muscle in the esophagus (sphincter), which can become weak and lose its tone. Some risk factors for developing GERD or heartburn include obesity, pregnancy, hiatal hernia, certain foods, tobacco use, and alcohol. Alcohol use can increase the secretion of stomach acids, lower the muscle tone in the esophagus, and can also directly irritate the stomach and esophagus. Medications used to treat heartburn commonly include nonprescription antacids or histamine-2 blocking drugs (H2-blockers) like Zantac. Unlike antacids that neutralize acids that are present in the stomach, H-2 blockers actually prevent the production of acids by the stomach. Recently, studies have shown that Zantac can interfere with the breakdown (metabolism) of alcohol, causing blood alcohol levels to reach dangerously high levels, even with light to moderate drinking. This interaction can even impair the driving ability of social drinkers and should be avoided. Blood alcohol levels in people who drink while taking Zantac are not only higher but remain high for longer periods of time. Therefore, going back to your original question, the effects of alcohol may actually lead to or aggravate heartburn or GERD and in addition can result in higher and more sustained blood levels, affecting driving ability when mixed with Zantac.

QUESTION: I heard that they have taken the medicine that I use for heartburn (Propulsid) off the market. Why and what can I use instead?

ANSWER: The manufacturer of Propulsid, Janssen Pharmaceutica, stopped marketing this product in the United States because it was associated with a number of serious heart problems. Propulsid was reported to have caused numerous heartbeat problems (cardiac arrhythmias) that led to at least 80 deaths being reported to the FDA by the end of 1999. These heart problems were thought to be caused by the drug itself in susceptible patients or when it was combined with certain other medications such as antiarrhythmics, antipsychotics, antidepressants, or some anti-infectives. Many of these drugs interacted with Propulsid and caused its level in the blood to increase to dangerous levels. Propulsid, which was approved in 1993, will still be available to patients who do not respond to other drugs through a special limited access program, but the patient's doctor must document that other therapies do not work. In addition an electrocardiogram (EKG) must be completed prior to treatment with Propulsid and doctors must verify that no interacting drugs are also being used.

Other drugs that can be used for heartburn or gastroesophageal reflux disease (GERD) include antacids, and acid-reducing agents such as Tagamet, Axid, Zantac, Pepcid, Prilosec, or Prevacid. Other new drugs are also being developed that might be useful alternatives to Propulsid. Lifestyle changes such as avoiding alcohol, quitting smoking, and avoiding fatty, chocolate, caffeinated, or citrus foods may also be helpful in preventing heartburn. You should talk to your doctor about these alternatives and what would be best for you.

QUESTION: My wife frequently gets heartburn, especially after eating. What can she do to prevent this?

ANSWER: Heartburn is caused by a "backup" of stomach contents into the esophagus or swallowing tube. In technical terms it is called gastroesophageal reflux disease or GERD. It is a very common disorder that affects millions of Americans. In fact, approximately 36% of people in the U.S. have heartburn at least once a month and 7% report daily symptoms. Normally the esophagus acts to move food and liquids from the mouth into the stomach and has a circular muscle (sphincter) at its lower end to prevent stomach contents from backing up. Sometimes this muscle loosens up and allows some of the stomach contents (which are acidic) back up into the esophagus causing a burning sensation in the lower chest, commonly called heartburn. Most patients complain of heartburn after a meal and upon lying down at bedtime. Heartburn may also occur when the patient bends or stoops over and after some types of exercise. Some patients complain of an acid, burning, bitter taste, or "sour" stomach. Heartburn appears to be more common in the elderly and the pain is sometimes difficult to distinguish from angina. If not treated properly, GERD may lead to complications such as bleeding from ulcers in the esophagus or a narrowing of the esophagus. Cough, bronchitis, and pneumonia can also occur.

Depending upon the severity of GERD, many different treatments are available. Some helpful non-drug measures that can be taken include not eating at least 3 hours before going to bed, losing weight if needed and avoiding tight fitting clothes. Dietary suggestions for prevention of GERD are to avoid foods that may cause the esophageal sphincter muscle to loosen (e.g., chocolate, mints, fats), avoid food that irritates the GI tract (e.g., citrus juice, tomato products, spicy foods, coffee), and reducing the size of meals. Patients with GERD should also try not to smoke and limit their alcohol consumption.

The drug treatment for GERD is primarily aimed at reducing the amount of stomach acid produced, neutralizing the stomach acid produced, and preventing the contact of stomach acid with the esophagus. These treatments can help to relieve the heartburn symptoms, help healing when needed, and prevent the possible complications noted earlier. Antacid products (Tums, Maalox, Mylanta, etc.) have been used for a long time to treat GERD. These products counteract or "neutralize" stomach acids so that they cannot damage the esophagus. They are fast acting (5-15 minutes) but only work for a short period of time (1-3 hours) and therefore must be taken frequently. More recently, newer drugs called H-2 antagonists have become available in both prescription and non-prescription products (e.g., Zantac, Tagamet, Pepcid, Axid, etc.). These drugs block the production of gastric acid by antagonizing histamine receptors in the stomach, which help to make the acid. These drugs do not act as fast as antacids, but work for a longer period of time, usually allowing a twice a day dosing schedule. More potent inhibitors of stomach acid production are also available by prescription and can be used in severe types of GERD (e.g., Prilosec, Prevacid). Likewise, medications that stimulate the activity of the GI tract can be helpful and may be prescribed for some patients with GERD (e.g., Reglan). Patients can usually use non-prescription products to prevent or treat mild heartburn effectively. However, non-prescription medications should not be used for more than 14 days without an evaluation by a physician.

PLEASE NOTE: Prilosec and Prevacid are now available over-the-counter.

QUESTION: I recently heard that the "little purple pill" for heartburn will be switched from a prescription to an over-the-counter (OTC) medication. Is this true?

ANSWER: Yes Prilosec, commonly called the "little purple pill", could soon become available as a nonprescription medication. Prilosec (generic name omeprazole) is one of the world's best-selling prescription drugs for the treatment of heartburn. Recently an FDA Gastrointestional Drugs Advisory Committee voted to recommend the approval of Prilosec for over-the-counter use in its full prescription strength for the prevention of frequent heartburn symptoms. The FDA is not required to follow the recommendations of its advisory committees, but it usually does. If approved, the maker of Prilosec will be required to make various labeling changes so that the OTC drug is used correctly by consumers.

Prilosec is a potent inhibitor of stomach acid production, which can produce heartburn. Unlike antacids like Tums or Rolaids, which are fast acting, Prilosec takes a few days to inhibit acid production and relieve heartburn symptoms. Heartburn is caused by a "backup" of stomach contents into the esophagus or swallowing tube. In technical terms it is called gastroesophageal reflux disease or GERD. Prilosec is generally well tolerated but, along with other side effects, it can cause headache in about 7% of patients and diarrhea, stomach pain, or nausea in 2-3% of patients. Drug interactions with Prilosec are also possible and product labeling should be carefully read prior to its use.

PLEASE NOTE: Prilosec is now available over-the-counter.

QUESTION: Now that non-prescription Prilosec and Prevacid are available, how do I know when to use antacids or other products for heartburn?

ANSWER: Heartburn is caused by a "back up" of stomach contents into the esophagus or swallowing tube. It is a symptom of a medical condition known as gastroesophageal reflux disease or GERD. It is a very common disorder that affects millions of Americans. Normally the esophagus acts to move food and liquids from the mouth into the stomach and has a circular muscle (sphincter) at its lower end to prevent stomach contents form backing up (reflux). Sometimes this muscle loosens up and allows some of the acidic stomach contents to back up into the esophagus causing a burning sensation in the lower chest, commonly called heartburn. If not properly treated, GERD can lead to complications such as bleeding from ulcers in the esophagus or a narrowing of the esophagus. A number of non-drug measures can be taken to reduce the incidence of GERD. These include not eating at least 3 hours before going to bed, losing weight if needed, quitting smoking, and avoiding tight-fitting clothes. Changes in diet can also be helpful, such as avoiding foods and beverages that aggravate GERD (e.g., alcohol, citrus, and tomato juices, coffee, tea, cola, chocolate, fatty or greasy foods, garlic, onions, peppermint, spearmint, spicy foods). Reducing fat intake and cutting down on food portion size can also be beneficial.

The nonprescription drug treatment of GERD is primarily aimed at reducing the amount of stomach acid produced, neutralizing the stomach acid produced, and preventing the contact of stomach acid with the esophagus. Antacid products (Tums, Maalox, Mylanta, etc.) counteract or "neutralize" stomach acids so that they cannot damage the esophagus. They are fast acting (5-15 minutes) but only work for a short period of time (1-3 hours) and therefore must be taken frequently. Other nonprescription products such as Zantac, Tagamet, Pepcid AC, Axid AR, etc. are known as H-2 antagonists. These drugs block the production of gastric acid by antagonizing histamine receptors in the stomach, which help to make the acid. These drugs do not act as fast as antacids, but work for a longer period of time, usually allowing a twice a day dosing schedule. Antacids and H-2 blockers are usually taken while you are having heartburn, and can also be taken 30-60 minutes before you eat a meal that you suspect will cause heartburn. Prilosec OTC on the other hand, is primarily used to treat frequent heartburn—2 or more days each week for about 1 month. Frequent heartburn is reported by 45% of people with heartburn. Prilosec

OTC is known as a proton pump inhibitor, or PPI for short. It acts by stopping the flow of acid into the stomach. Prilosec does not start working as fast as antacids or H-2 antagonists, but a single daily dose is effective for 24 hours or longer. The dosage regimen for Prilosec OTC in treating frequent heartburn is one 20 mg tablet daily with a full glass of water before eating the first meal of the day for 14 consecutive days. This regimen will be effective in about half of patients who can go for several months with no or milder symptoms. This regimen can be repeated after 4 months have elapsed, but nonprescription treatment beyond 14 days is not recommended. People whose symptoms return more quickly should see their physician to discuss the need for long-term therapy and monitoring. The most common side effects of Prilosec OTC are diarrhea, headache, nausea, stomach pain, and rash. It can also interact with some prescription drugs, so be sure that your pharmacist and doctor are aware of all the medications (prescription and nonprescription) that you take.

QUESTION: Can some drugs for heartburn increase the risk of fractures?

ANSWER: Yes, the FDA is revising the labeling for both prescription and non-prescription drugs called proton pump inhibitors (PPIs) to include new safety information about a possible increased risk of fractures of the hip, wrist, and spine when using these medications. These drugs work by reducing the amount of acid in the stomach and include popular medications such as Nexium, Prilosec, Zegerid, Prevacid, Protonix, and Aciphex. The new safety information is based on the FDA's review of several studies that reported an increased risk of fractures of the hip, wrist, and spine with proton pump inhibitor use. Some studies found that those at greatest risk for these fractures received high doses of proton pump inhibitors or used them for one year or more. The majority of the studies evaluated individuals 50 years of age or older and the increased risk of fracture primarily was observed in this age group. While the greatest increased risk for fractures in these studies involved people who had been taking prescription proton pump inhibitors for at least one year or who had been taking high doses of the prescription medications (not available over-the-counter), as a precaution, the "Drug Facts" label on the OTC proton pump inhibitors (indicated for 14 days of continuous use) also is being revised to include information about this risk. Healthcare professionals and users of proton pump inhibitors should be aware of the possible increased risk of fractures of the hip, wrist, and spine with the use of proton pump inhibitors, and weigh the known benefits against the potential risks when deciding to use them. The FDA also notes that proton pump inhibitors are effective in treating a variety of gastrointestinal disorders, and people should not stop taking their proton pump inhibitor unless told to do so by their healthcare professional.

QUESTION: Why is the FDA warning people about using drugs for heartburn?

ANSWER: On February 8, 2012 the FDA issued a Safety Announcement that the use of stomach acid reducing drugs known as proton pump inhibitors (PPIs) may be associated with an increased risk of Clostridium Difficile-associated diarrhea (CDAD). Clostridium difficile (C. difficile) is a bacterium that can cause diarrhea that does not improve. Symptoms include watery stool, abdominal pain, and fever, and patients may go on to develop more serious intestinal conditions. The disease can also be spread in the hospital. Factors that may predispose an individual to developing CDAD include advanced age, certain chronic medical conditions, and taking broad spectrum antibiotics. Treatment for CDAD includes the replacement of fluids and electrolytes and the use of special antibiotics. The FDA is working with manufacturers to include information about the increased risk of CDAD with use of PPIs in the drug labels. Prescription PPIs are used to treat conditions such as gastroesophageal reflux disease (GERD), stomach and small intestine ulcers, and inflammation of the esophagus.

Prescription Proton Pump Inhibitor (PPI) Drugs
Generic Name/Found In Brand Name(s)
- dexlansoprazole/Dexilant
- esomeprazole magnesium/Nexium
- esomeprazole magnesium and naproxen/Vimovo
- lansoprazole/Prevacid
- omeprazole/Prilosec
- omeprazole and Sodium bicarbonate/Zegerid

- pantoprazole sodium/Protonix
- rabeprazole sodium/AcipHex

Over-the-counter (OTC) PPIs are used to treat frequent heartburn.

Over-the-Counter Proton Pump Inhibitor (PPI) Drugs
Generic Name/Found In Brand Name(s)
- lansoprazole/Prevacid 24HR
- omeprazole magnesium/Prilosec OTC
- omeprazole and sodium bicarbonate/Zegerid OTC
- omeprazole/Omeprazole

The FDA is informing patients who use a PPI of the following:
- Seek immediate care if you use PPIs and develop diarrhea that does not improve. This may be a sign of Clostridium difficile-associated diarrhea (CDAD).
- Your healthcare professional may order laboratory tests to check if you have CDAD.
- Do not stop taking your prescription PPI drug without talking to your healthcare professional.
- Discuss any questions or concerns about your PPI drug with your healthcare professional.
- If you take an OTC PPI drug, follow the directions on the package carefully.

Meanwhile, the FDA is also reviewing the risk of CDAD in users of histamine H2 receptor blockers. H2 receptor blockers are used to treat conditions such as gastroesophageal reflux disease (GERD), stomach and small intestine ulcers, and heartburn. H2 receptor blockers are marketed under various brand and generic drug names as prescription and OTC products. A table of prescription and OTC H2 receptor blockers is found below:

Prescription H2 Receptor Blocker Drugs
Generic Name/Found In Brand Name(s)
- cimetidine/Tagamet
- famotidine/Pepcid, Duexis
- nizatidine/Axid, Nizatidine

- ranitidine/Zantac, Tritec

Over-the-Counter (OTC) H2 Receptor Blocker Drugs
Generic Name/Found In Brand Name(s)
- cimetidine/Tagamet HB
- famotidine/Pepcid Complete, Pepcid AC
- nizatidine/Axid AR
- ranitidine/Zantac

GAS PROBLEMS

QUESTION: I seem to "pass gas" a lot. What can I do about it?

ANSWER: This is one of the most frequent and embarrassing complaints that people have relating to their gastrointestinal system. Some people are fearful of passing gas with others present, while others experience discomfort due to excessive gas and worry that they may have some dangerous disease. Studies have shown that both men and women pass gas an average of 10 to 14 times a day in varying amounts. In addition, approximately 20% of people aged 65-93 years experience stomach discomfort, often due to gaseous buildup. Intestinal gas is made up of carbon dioxide, methane, nitrogen, oxygen, and hydrogen.

Excessive gas in the gastrointestinal tract (also known as flatulence) can be caused by a number of different factors. A major source of gas is a diet consisting of complex carbohydrates that cannot be easily digested. Instead they are fermented by intestinal bacteria, which produces gas. Foods such as beans, broccoli, cabbage, brussels sprouts and cauliflower fall into this group. Sugar-free foods which contain sorbitol or fructose can also produce excessive gas. Another common cause of gas buildup is swallowed air. Unless this swallowed air is released by belching, it will be eliminated as intestinal gas. Some causes of air swallowing include eating while lying down, eating too fast, poorly fitting dentures, nasal congestion, chewing gum, sucking on hard candies, and smoking a cigar or pipe. Carbonated drinks and beer can also cause gaseousness, since they contain a great deal of gas. Likewise, antacids containing sodium bicarbonate can also produce gas and should be avoided. Still another cause of excessive gas in some people is the inability to digest lactose found in milk and dairy products.

The treatment and prevention of excessive gas depends upon the cause or causes. If diet is a factor, eliminating problem foods or drinks will be helpful. Swallowed air can be reduced by not eating too fast, chewing food thoroughly, and sitting up while eating. Properly fitting dentures or a nasal decongestant can also be helpful in some people. In those individuals who cannot digest milk and dairy foods, a product known as Lactaid or Dairy Ease taken with these foods can be beneficial. Other products containing simethicone may also allow easier elimination of gas. Finally, a product called Beano can be taken with foods that are hard to digest to prevent gas. Beano contains an enzyme that helps digestion of complex carbohydrates before they can cause gas. If none of these measures helps, a physician should be consulted to determine the cause of excessive gas and its proper treatment.

IRRITABLE BOWEL SYNDROME

QUESTION: I heard about a new drug for irritable bowel disease. What can you tell me about it?

ANSWER: You're probably talking about Lotronex, which the FDA recently re-approved for restricted use. Lotronex was originally approved by the FDA for the treatment of irritable bowel syndrome in women during February of 2000, but was withdrawn from the market in November of 2000 due to serious side effects. The drug has been associated with over 80 cases of ischemic colitis, where the blood flow to the colon is cut off, and over 100 cases of severe constipation. At least 4 deaths have been attributed to its use. However, it can be an effective treatment for some women with chronic diarrhea caused by irritable bowel syndrome who do not respond to other therapy. Under the restricted use program, Lotronex can only be prescribed by certain physicians, who must promise to report all side effects and to educate patients on the risks and benefits of treatment. Patients who receive the restricted drug must also read and sign a form agreeing to Lotronex treatment and they must return to the doctor for every refill.

In addition, pharmacists must provide patients with an FDA-approved Medication Guide when the drug is dispensed.

Irritable Bowel Syndrome (IBS) is a very common gastrointestinal problem that affects up to 20% of the U.S. population and occurs in three times as many women as men. People with IBS have chronic or recurrent abdominal pain and discomfort and irregular bowel movements such as diarrhea, constipation, or both. Health care professionals used to think that IBS was caused by the emotional state of the patient (psychosomatic), but recent research suggests that there may be a chemical or physiologic basis for this disorder. The chemical involved is thought to be a substance known as serotonin, which causes an overstimulation of the gastrointestinal tract causing the symptoms of IBS. Lotronex works by blocking this chemical (serotonin) and preventing it from over stimulating the GI tract. Lotronex was only approved for use in women with IBS who have diarrhea—not constipation, because the most common side effect of the drug is constipation, which occurs in about 28% of patients taking it. It is estimated that about 5% or less of female patients with IBC who failed other drug treatments should receive Lotronex under the new restricted use program.

QUESTION: What can I do to treat irritable bowel syndrome without a prescription?

ANSWER: Physician visits for IBS is second in number only to office visits for the common cold. In the past, IBS was referred to as a spastic colon or nervous stomach but these descriptions are no longer considered to be appropriate. Symptoms of IBS include lower abdominal pain, disturbances in bowel movements (diarrhea and/or constipation), and bloating. The average patient experiences symptoms about 5 to 7 days each month and the onset of IBS occurs between the ages of 30 and 50 in over one-half of patients. Although the cause of IBS is not fully understood, it appears that the symptoms are caused by abnormal motility (movement) of the gastrointestinal (GI) tract and a greater sensitivity to pain in the GI tract. Many different chemicals (neurotransmitters) are needed to regulate GI function along with pain sensitivity and they may be involved in the development of IBS. Emotional state, stress, prior GI infection, antibiotic use, or food sensitivity may also be associated with the development of IBS. Many types of medications and certain foods can aggravate IBS. Medications that affect bowel habits and cause diarrhea or constipation, such as antibiotics and certain antacids, can imitate symptoms of IBS. Foods or drinks that can exacerbate IBS include alcohol, caffeine, chocolate, high-fat foods, apple or grape juice, bananas, broccoli, cabbage, and dairy products.

The treatment of IBS depends upon the patient's symptoms and their severity. Many patients with mild IBS will benefit from education about the disorder, reassurance, and dietary and lifestyle changes. The identification and elimination of aggravating foods, relaxation techniques, and mild exercise may also be useful. The use of heating pads, hot baths, or warm drinks can slow GI contractions and help with abdominal pain. Not too many non-prescription medications are available to treat IBS. OTC antidiarrheal agents like loperamide (Imodium) may be useful in patients with diarrhea-predominant IBS. Patients with constipation as the main symptom may benefit from increased dietary fiber intake or the use of fiber supplements or bulk-forming laxatives like psyllium or methycellulose. Sometimes a stool softener like docusate or a stimulant laxative containing senna or bisacodyl may also be helpful for constipation-predominant IBS. It should be noted that numerous prescription medications are also available to treat IBS.

QUESTION: I heard about a new drug for people with irritable bowel syndrome with constipation. What can you tell me about it?

ANSWER: The FDA recently approved Zelnorm (generic name tegaserod) for the short-term (4-6 weeks) treatment of women with irritable bowel syndrome (IBS) whose primary bowel symptom is constipation. It is the first drug to be approved for this type of IBS. Zelnorm does not cure IBS, but improves patient symptoms such as stomach pain, bloating, and constipation. It does this by increasing the movement of stools (fecal matter) through the bowels by stimulating certain chemicals in the gastrointestinal tract. The most common side effects of Zelnorm include headache, stomach pain, diarrhea, nausea, gas, and back pain. It is not to be used for women with diarrhea and IBS and is not approved for use in men with IBS.

Health care professionals used to think that IBS was caused by the emotional state of the patient (psychosomatic), but recent research suggests that there is a chemical or physiologic basis for this disorder. The chemical involved is thought to be a substance known as serotonin, which causes overstimulation of the gastrointestinal tract and producing the symptoms of IBS. Zelnorm appears to reduce the symptoms by affecting this chemical. Zelnorm is taken twice daily, but is not effective in all women with this disorder.

PLEASE NOTE: On March 30, 2007 the manufacturer (Novartis) suspended its U.S. marketing and sales of Zelnorm at the request of the FDA, because a safety analysis found a higher chance of heart attack, stroke, and unstable angina (heart/chest pain) in patients treated with Zelnorm compared to treatment with an inactive substance (placebo). The manufacturer will continue to supply Zelnorm only for emergency use.

QUESTION: I heard about an antibiotic that may be useful for irritable bowel syndrome (IBS). What can you tell me about it?

ANSWER: While the exact cause(s) of IBS are not known, some researchers say that one of its possible causes is an overgrowth of bacteria in the small intestine. They suggest that when a person with IBS eats, these bacteria compete with food being digested producing a gas that causes the bloating and a feeling of stomach pressure or fullness. These researchers have been able to use a breath test (lactulose breath test) to detect the type of gases that are produced by people with IBS compared to people without IBS. They have also investigated the use of an antibiotic, called Xifaxin (rifaximin) as a potential treatment for IBS and found that it greatly improved symptoms in patients taking the drug. Xifaxin is an antibiotic that is not absorbed when taken orally, so it remains in the small intestine to hopefully kill off the unwanted bacteria. However, much additional research is needed and Xifaxin is not approved for the treatment of IBS. Currently, Xifaxin has only been approved for the treatment of certain types of traveler's diarrhea. In addition to its potential benefits in treating IBS, Xifaxin is also being studied for its use in other conditions such as Crohns disease and certain liver problems.

CROHN'S DISEASE

QUESTION: I have Crohn's disease and heard about a new treatment. What can you tell me about it?

ANSWER: Crohn's disease is a chronic inflammatory disorder of the gastrointestinal tract first described by Dr. Crohn in 1932. The cause of Crohn's disease is unknown, but it occurs more frequently in whites than in blacks and orientals, with a 3 to 6 times greater incidence in Jews compared with non-Jews. It affects approximately 1 million people in the U.S. and Europe and usually occurs between the ages of 15 and 35, but can occur at any age. While the cause of Crohn's disease is unknown, heredity, infection, the immune system, and stress may be involved in this disorder. Symptoms of Crohn's disease can include fever, rectal bleeding, stomach pain, diarrhea, fatigue, and weight loss. Complications such as obstruction of the intestine and the formation of abnormal passages (fistulae) from the gastrointestinal tract that may allow fluids to drain out or cause infection can develop.

The treatment of mild to moderate forms of Crohns disease includes anti-inflammatory drugs, known as aminosalicylates (sulfasalazine, mesalamine, or olsalazine). Steroids like prednisone or hydrocortisone are used for moderate to severe forms of this disease. And up to now, drugs that block the immune system (such as azathioprine, mercaptopurine, cyclosporine, or methotrexate) are used if the disease gets worse. About 15% to 40% of patients with Crohn's disease do not respond to these treatments. However, a new drug has recently been approved for use in these patients who do not respond. The drug is named Remicade (generic name, infliximab) and is the first biotech drug approved for this use. Remicade works by blocking the activity of a substance called tumor necrosis factor (TNF), which is involved in the inflammation process. Remicade must be given by injection and studies have shown that about 80% of patients respond after 4 weeks of treatment, with approximately 50% going into clinical remission. Remicade can also help to close the abnormal passages (fistulae) discussed earlier. Side effects of Remicade appear to be mild and the drug is also being tested for use in rheumatoid arthritis.

PLEASE NOTE: The FDA has recently warned that patients taking Cimzia, Enbrel, Humira, or Remicade (also known as tumor necrosis factor (TNF) blockers) should be aware that they are more susceptible to serious fungal infections. Patients taking these drugs who develop a persistent fever, cough, shortness of breath, and fatigue should promptly seek medical attention.

QUESTION: I heard about a new oral medication for Crohn's disease. What can you tell me about it?

ANSWER: The new oral medication that you heard about to treat Crohn's disease is called Entocort EC. Its generic name is budesonide, which is also marketed for inhalation use to treat asthma and allergies. Budesonide is a steroid drug that helps in the treatment of Crohn's disease by reducing inflammation and suppressing the immune system. Entocort EC is a specially formulated capsule that is designed to slowly release the active ingredient, budesonide, only after it reaches the intestine. Because of this it primarily acts in the intestine and produces fewer steroid side effects. It is taken orally as 3 capsules once a day. During clinical studies, Entocort EC improved symptoms in 48% to 69% of patients with Crohn's disease after two months of use. The most common side effects of Entocort EC in clinical studies were headache, respiratory infection, nausea, and some steroid side effects such as acne and facial swelling. The management of Crohns disease can be very difficult and Entocort EC provides a new treatment alternative for some patients.

QUESTION: I heard that a new drug was approved for Crohn's disease. What can you tell me about it?

ANSWER: The FDA recently approved Tysabri (natalizumab) for the treatment of moderate-to-severe Crohn's disease (CD) in patients with evidence of inflammation who have had an inadequate response to, or are unable to tolerate other Crohn's disease therapies. Actually, Tysabri was first approved in 2004 for the for the treatment of relapsing forms of multiple sclerosis (MS), but the manufacturer took the drug of the market in 2005 due to a potentially rare and frequently fatal side effect known as PML (progressive multifocal leukoencephalopathy).

However, in 2006, the FDA allowed Tysabri to be made available in a restricted-distribution system called TOUCH (Tysabri Outreach Unified Commitment to Health) for the treatment of relapsing forms of MS. Crohn's disease patients using Tysabri must also be enrolled in a special restricted drug distribution program called CD TOUCH. Tysabri is known as a monoclonal antibody that has been shown to reduce inflammation and induce remission among patients with moderately to severely active CD. It is administered intravenously by trained professionals at infusion centers. In addition to PML, other serious side effects of Tysabri include hypersensitivity reactions, such as anaphylaxis and liver injury. Serious infections have also been observed in patients receiving immunosuppressants while on Tysabri. Common side effects include headache, fatigue, infusion reactions, urinary tract infections, joint and limb pain, and rash.

PLEASE NOTE: In February 2010, the FDA warned the public that the risk of developing progressive multifocal leukoencephalopathy (PML), a rare but serious brain infection associated with the use of Tysabri (natalizumab), increases with the number of Tysabri infusions received. This new safety information, based on reports of 31 confirmed cases of PML received by the FDA as of January 21, 2010, will now be included in the Tysabri drug label and patient Medication Guide.

QUESTION: What can you tell me about a new treatment for Crohn's disease?

ANSWER: Recently, the FDA approved Cimzia (certolizumab pegol) for the treatment of patients with moderate to severe active Crohns disease who have not responded to conventional therapies. Cimzia works by blocking the activity of a substance known as tumor necrosis factor (TNF), which is involved in the inflammation process. It is administered by injection subcutaneously as an initial dose and at Weeks 2 and 4. In patients who obtain a clinical response, the recommended maintenance regimen is 400 mg subcutaneously every 4 weeks. During clinical study, the most common side effects of Cimzia were upper respiratory infection, urinary tract infection, and joint pain. However, other serious adverse reactions can occur and patients need to be closely monitored. Cimzia is also being studied for its potential use in rheumatoid arthritis and psoriasis.

PLEASE NOTE: The FDA has recently warned that patients taking Cimzia, Enbrel, Humira, or Remicade (also known as tumor necrosis factor (TNF) blockers) should be aware that they are more susceptible to serious fungal infections. Patients taking these drugs who develop a persistent fever, cough, shortness of breath, and fatigue should promptly seek medical attention.

CONSTIPATION

QUESTION: I have constipation and my stool comes out in a cluster of round balls (illustration enclosed). I take a mild vegetable laxative but I'm not getting the right solid smooth waste outgo. What do you think?

ANSWER: Thank you for your letter and illustration. Stools are often classified into 7 types based upon the Bristol Stool Scale, which was developed at the University of Bristol, United Kingdom in 1997. This scale is based upon how much time the stool spends in the colon with Type 1 being in the colon the most time and Type 7 being in the colon the shortest time. According to the Bristol Stool Form Scale the 7 types of stool according to their appearance in the toilet water are as follows:

- Type 1: Separate hard lumps, like nuts (hard to pass)
- Type 2: Sausage-shaped, but lumpy
- Type 3: Like a sausage but with cracks on its surface
- Type 4: Like a sausage or snake, smooth and soft
- Type 5: Soft blobs with clear cut edges (passed easily)
- Type 6: Fluffy pieces with ragged edges, a mushy stool
- Type 7: Watery, no solid pieces (entirely liquid)

Constipation is the most common digestion-related complaint in the U.S. It is usually described as a condition in which a person has uncomfortable or infrequent bowel movements. Many people think that they should have a bowel movement at least once a day. In general, however, as many as three bowel movements per day to as few as three per week is considered "normal". Although constipation can affect people of all ages, there appears to be an increased prevalence among people 65 years and older. The incidence of constipation is about 5% in people aged 65 to 74, and it rises to about 10% in those over 75. Adult women are also more likely to suffer from constipation than men. The average weight of a stool is about 3-1/2 ounces, but it varies a lot. About 75% of the stool is water, but most of this water is locked up inside of bacteria and undigested plant cells. Half to two-thirds of the stool is bacteria and the rest is mainly undigested residues of plant foods (fiber). Please discuss your stool concerns with your doctor to determine if any additional tests or treatment is necessary.

QUESTION: What non-prescription medications are good for constipation?

ANSWER: There are numerous causes of constipation. Lifestyle causes of constipation include travel, inadequate fluid or dietary fiber intake, and inadequate exercise. Several medical conditions such as cancer, irritable bowel syndrome, multiple sclerosis, diabetes, depression, dementia, kidney problems, or Parkinsons disease are also associated with constipation. Because of this, referral to a physician for evaluation may be necessary. In addition, many drugs can induce constipation such as certain pain relievers, antacids, antihistamines, diuretics (water pills), cholesterol-lowering drugs, anti-hypertensives, tranquilizers, and many others.

There are numerous nonprescription medications available for treating constipation. However, in many cases constipation can be alleviated with lifestyle changes such as increased fiber in the diet, adequate fluid intake, and exercise. Some of the most common nonprescription medications for treating constipation are bulk-forming laxatives, stool softeners, and stimulant laxatives. Bulk forming laxatives dissolve or swell in the fluids of the digestive tract, promoting an increase in stool size and frequency. Some product examples are Citrucel, Fiber Con, Metamucil, Perdiem, and Serutan. These products need to be taken with adequate amounts of water and should not be used by people with partial bowel obstruction, fecal impaction, difficult swallowing, gastrointestinal strictures, or throat problems. Stool softeners or emollient laxatives act as "surface-active" agents or surfactants and work to soften a firm stool mass making it easier to pass. Stool softeners should be avoided if nausea, vomiting, or abdominal pain is present. Some product examples are Colace, Dialose, and Surfak. Stimulant laxatives as their name implies contain ingredients that irritate the intestinal tract causing it to increase its motility, promoting a bowel movement. Stimulant laxatives should not be used by pregnant women, or when rectal bleeding, intestinal obstruction, or appendicitis is suspected. Product examples include Dulcolax, Carters, Ex-Lax, Correctol, Feen-A-Mint, Senokot, X-Prep, and Neoloid Emulsified Castor Oil. Stimulant laxatives can cause many side effects including severe abdominal cramping, electrolyte abnormalities, dehydration, vomiting, etc. and should not be used for more than one week. Many other types of nonprescription laxatives are also available along with numerous generic products. Make certain that you read all package labeling for laxatives including warnings, and follow the directions exactly. If you have additional questions regarding constipation or laxative use, be sure to consult with your physician and pharmacist.

QUESTION: I heard that a new prescription drug was approved for chronic constipation. What can you tell me about it?

ANSWER: Chronic constipation is characterized by decreased frequency of bowel movements, persistent symptoms of straining, lumpy or hard stools and feelings of blockage or incomplete bowel evacuation. It is one of the most common disorders suffered by Americans and is prevalent in about 4.4 million people. This condition affects women more often than men and also affects those over the age of 65 more frequently. Current treatment options include dietary changes such as eating more fiber and drinking more fluids along with an increase in physical activity. If these measures fail, various nonprescription laxatives and prescription medications can be tried. Recently, the FDA approved a new type of prescription medication to treat constipation when the cause is unknown. This new drug is named Amitiza (lubiprostone) and it works in a different way than other medications to relieve constipation. Amitiza is taken orally twice a day where it works on the lining of the small intestines to increase the amount of intestinal fluids, which softens the stool and promotes bowel movements providing relief from abdominal bloating and discomfort. The most common side effects of Amitiza include nausea, headache, and diarrhea. You should consult with your physician to determine if this new medication is appropriate for you.

CONSTIPATION & IRRITABLE BOWEL SYNDROME

QUESTION: I heard a new drug was approved to treat irritable bowel syndrome and constipation. What can you tell me about it?

ANSWER: The FDA recently (2012) approved Linzess (linaclotide) to treat adults with chronic idiopathic constipation (CIC) and to treat irritable bowel syndrome with constipation (IBS-C). Linzess is a capsule taken once daily on an empty stomach, at least 30 minutes before the first meal of the day. Linzess helps relieve constipation by helping bowel movements occur more often. In IBS-C, it may also help ease abdominal pain. During clinical studies involving over 1,600 patients with IBS-C, patients taking Linzess experienced a reduction in the amount of abdominal pain and more complete spontaneous bowel movements than those taking a "dummy" pill (placebo). In addition, in clinical studies involving over 1,200 patients with CIC, patients taking Linzess also experienced more complete spontaneous bowel movements than those taking a placebo. The most common side effect reported during the clinical studies was diarrhea. Linzess should not be used in patients 16 years of age and younger. According to the National Institutes of Health, an estimated 63 million people are affected by chronic constipation. Chronic idiopathic constipation is a diagnosis given to those who experience persistent constipation and do not respond to standard treatment. Additionally, an estimated 15.3 million people are affected by IBS. IBS-C is a subtype characterized mainly by abdominal pain and by hard or lumpy stools at least 25% of the time and loose or watery stools less than 25% of the time.

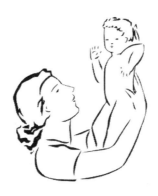

CHAPTER 6
MOM AND THE KIDS

FLUORIDE DROPS

QUESTION: We just had a prescription for fluoride drops filled for our 9-month-old son. On the prescription label it said to avoid dairy products when giving this medication—why?

ANSWER: The ingestion of fluoride (actually sodium fluoride) during the period of tooth development can significantly reduce the amount of dental decay. Sodium fluoride either given by mouth or applied topically can actually increase the resistance of teeth to dental caries. It is thought that fluoride may "toughen" dental enamel and also may interfere with the bacteria causing decay. Besides the reduction of dental caries in children, benefits of fluoridation extend through adulthood, resulting in fewer decayed, missing, or filled teeth, and greater tooth retention. Therefore, in communities without fluoridated water, fluoride supplements are recommended in children from 6 months to 16 years of age. The problem with dairy products such as milk or cheese is that they contain calcium and it can bind with fluoride to produce calcium fluoride, which is not readily absorbed by the gastrointestinal tract like sodium fluoride is. Because of this, dairy products should not be taken at the same time as the fluoride drops. The drops can be given to your baby undiluted, or mixed with fluids or food—but not dairy foods. Furthermore, if you move to a community with fluoridated water, then the fluoride drops should be discontinued.

INFANT FORMULA

QUESTION: I have decided not to breastfeed my baby. What can you tell me about using infant formula products?

ANSWER: Although breastfeeding is considered to be the best way to feed an infant, infant formulas do provide another choice for mothers who decide not to. Infant formula products are patterned after breast milk and they offer balanced nutrition for infants. Most infant formulas use cow's milk as their protein source, with carbohydrates, fats, vitamins, and minerals added so that they are very similar to human milk. Although numerous regular infant formula products are available, there are few nutritional differences between them. Some infants, however, have problems with milk based products and require special product formulas. For example, some babies develop excess gas or diarrhea while on formula because they have a milk protein allergy making it difficult for them to digest cow's milk protein. These infants need to be switched to a soy protein formula such as Prosobee, Nursoy, or Isomil. Additional specialty infant formulas are available for children with lactose intolerance and for firming loose, watery stools in infants older than six months. Premature babies and those born with certain diseases also need special formulas. Your baby's pediatrician can help you select the product which is best for you.

Once you have selected a particular formula, a wide variety of product types can be used. Powders are usually the least expensive, but can be time consuming to prepare. Concentrated liquids are also economical, but like powders they need to be mixed with sterilized water. The most convenient (but also the most expensive) products are the ready-to-feed formulas. They come in four and eight ounce single-serve bottles that need only a sterilized nipple.

It is also important to use proper sanitation when bottle feeding. All bottles, nipples, and rings must be cleaned and sterilized properly before they are used. Some recommendations for good bottle feeding are listed below:

- Some experts suggest that moms always hold the baby when feeding to encourage social interaction.
- Bottles should be held by the person feeding the baby because infants too young to hold their own bottle are at risk of choking if the bottle is propped.
- Babies should be burped once or twice during the feeding and once afterward to help remove swallowed air.
- Always check the expiration date on formula and do not use dented, leaky, or damaged containers.
- Store unopened infant formula at room temperature.
- Always wash your hands thoroughly before handling formula.
- Before opening containers wash, rinse and dry the tops of formula cans and use a clean can opener.
- Cover opened cans of concentrated or ready-to-feed formula with aluminum foil or plastic and store in the refrigerator. Use within 48 hours.
- Store opened cans of powder formula in a cool, dry place. Use within one month of opening.
- Check directions and follow instructions precisely when preparing formula.
- Never reuse leftover formula in a bottle, as it can breed bacteria.
- Never use a microwave oven to warm formula. The formula can heat unevenly and burn the baby.
- Never freeze infant formula, as freezing can cause the formula to become grainy or cause the fat to separate out.

BREASTFEEDING AND DRUG USE

QUESTION: I am planning to breastfeed my infant. What advice can you give me about using medications while I am breastfeeding?

ANSWER: Breast milk has been shown to possess better nutritional and immunity improving properties compared to infant formulas, and the American Academy of Pediatrics recommends breastfeeding during the first six months of life. In view of this, the number of American mothers breastfeeding their infants have increased from 22 percent in 1971 to over 60 percent today. Since many of these mothers may want or need to take medication during the breastfeeding period your question is very appropriate. Human milk is a mixture of water (95-97 percent) containing proteins, minerals, carbohydrates and fat (3-5 percent). Most drug products do pass into the breast milk, but generally the amounts that pass are small and may not post a risk to the infant. Some non-prescription medications considered to be safe to use during breastfeeding include: acetaminophen (Tylenol) or ibuprofen (Motrin) for pain; psyllium (Metamucil) or docusate (Colace) for constipation; oxymetazoline (Afrin) nasal spray or drops for congestion; and kaolin-pectin (Kaopectate) for diarrhea. On the other hand, some medications can be harmful and should be avoided while breastfeeding if possible. For instance, any antihistamines and nicotine-containing smoking cessation products along with numerous prescription drugs should be avoided. You need to consult with your doctor and pharmacist about all prescription and non-prescription medications to be used while breastfeeding. Some suggestions to try and minimize your infant's exposure to drugs while breastfeeding are listed below:

• If you really don't need a medication (such as for cold or headache symptoms) don't take it, or delay taking it if possible.
• Use locally applied medications when feasible. For example, utilize creams, ointments, nose drops or sprays, etc. This will minimize the amount of drug getting into the breast milk.
• Avoid nursing approximately one to three hours after taking an oral medication, because this is usually the time that there are highest amounts of the drug getting into the breast milk.
• Take medication before the infant's longest sleep period. This may be especially useful for long-acting drugs given once a day.
• Temporarily withhold breast-feeding during short-term medication use. Perhaps milk saved prior to the medication or formula can be used during this period.
• Discontinue nursing if a toxic medication has to be taken.

BREAST MILK

QUESTION: I want to use a breast pump and store the milk. What can you tell me about storing and using breast milk?

ANSWER: As I've noted before, breast milk has been shown to possess better nutritional and immunity improving properties compared to infant formulas. Recently (2012), the FDA provided the following advice regarding the storage and usage of breast milk.

How To Store Breast Milk

- Make sure your hands are clean and dry before handling pumped breast milk.
- If your breast pump does not collect milk in a clean storage container, begin by pouring your milk into a container designed for storing milk in the refrigerator or freezer. Try not to touch the insides of the storage container.
- You may want to store milk in single-serving sizes of 2 to 4 ounces.
- Seal the container with a solid lid and label each container with the date the milk was pumped.
- Breast milk that will be frozen should have at least one inch between the milk and the container lid. Frozen milk expands as it freezes.
- Store milk in the main refrigerator or freezer compartment, away from the door, to avoid changes in temperature that may compromise the milk.
- Use milk that has been in the refrigerator or freezer the longest first.

How Long Breast Milk Can Be Stored
At Room Temperature

Temperature / Storage Time
60° F / 24 hours
66° F to 72° F / 10 hours
79° F / 4 to 6 hours
86° F to 100° F / 4 hours

In The Refrigerator
Temperature / Storage Time
32° F to 39° F / Up to 8 days

In The Freezer
Type / Storage Time
Compartment (contained within a refrigerator) / Up to 2 weeks
Self-Contained (bottom, top mount, side-by-side, or stand alone freezer) / 3 to 4 months
Deep Freezer (with a constant 0° F temperature) / 6 to 12 months

How To Thaw And Use Breast Milk
- Always make sure to check the date on the milk's container before using. Do not use undated milk, or milk that has been stored too long.
- Thaw frozen milk in the refrigerator or under cool, running water.
- Heat the milk under warm, running water and gently swirl the container to mix the milk.
- If warm water is not available, heat a pan of water on the stove. Once the water is warm, not boiling, remove the pan from the stove and place the milk container in the pan. Never warm the milk container directly on the stove.
- Never microwave breast milk because microwaves can cause dangerous hot spots that could burn you or a baby.
- Always test the temperature of the milk on the inside of your wrist before feeding it to a baby. The milk should feel warm, not hot.
- After thawing, milk should be stored in the refrigerator for no more than 24 hours.
- Never refreeze thawed milk. Throw away previously frozen milk that is not used within 24 hours.

How To Transport Breast Milk
If you are transporting milk, such as from work to home, pack it in a cooler filled with ice. Do not leave the milk in a cooler for more than 24 hours.

NURSING AND CODEINE

QUESTION: Why is the FDA warning nursing mothers about using codeine?

ANSWER: The FDA recently issued a warning to healthcare providers and nursing mothers about a potential serious side effect in nursing infants whose mothers are taking codeine. Codeine is a narcotic ingredient found in many prescription pain relievers and over-the-counter cough syrups. It has been used safely by nursing mothers for many years. However, last year a medical journal described a healthy 13-day-old breast fed baby who died from a morphine overdose. Laboratory tests showed high levels of morphine in the baby's blood and further testing showed that the baby's mother had a genetic trait that made her body metabolize codeine much faster and completely than most other people. When codeine enters the body, some of it is changed (metabolized) in the liver to morphine. Since morphine stays in the body much longer than codeine, someone who is a rapid metabolizer of codeine will accumulate more morphine in their body which will also pass into the breast milk, potentially leading to an overdose in the infant. The potential for a morphine overdose also depends upon how much codeine the mother is taking, how much is changed to morphine and gets into the breast milk, and how much breast milk the baby drinks each day. It is estimated that the number of people who are "ultra-rapid metabolizers" of codeine ranges from <1% to 28%, depending upon the population group. The only way to find out is with a genetic test. Signs of morphine overdose in infants include increased sleepiness, difficulty breastfeeding, breathing difficulties, and limpness in the baby. If a nursing baby shows these signs, the baby's doctor should be contacted right away. If the doctor cannot be reached right away, the baby should be taken to an emergency room or 911 should be called. Signs of morphine overdose in a nursing mother include sleepiness and constipation. Nursing mothers should talk to their doctors about taking codeine and if codeine needs to be taken, the lowest dose should be used for the shortest amount of time possible to relieve pain or cough. The FDA is now requiring manufacturers of prescription codeine products to include information about differences in codeine metabolism and concerns with breastfeeding in the drug label.

FOLIC ACID IN PREGNANCY

QUESTION: I am planning on starting a family and a friend said that I should start taking folic acid. Why?

ANSWER: Folic acid is a B vitamin that can help to prevent birth defects of the brain and spinal cord, called "neural tube defects" (NTDs), when taken before pregnancy and in the early weeks of pregnancy. About 2,500 babies are born with neural tube defects (NTD's) each year. These defects include spina bifida, which could mean the baby will never be able to walk, and anencephaly which means the baby's brain and skull do not develop fully, resulting in death. Folic acid may also help to prevent other birth defects, such as cleft lip and palate. It is not well understood how folic acid prevents NTDs, but some studies suggest that it may correct a nutritional deficiency or may help the way some people process or "metabolize" substances in the body. Some people have a deficiency of folic acid even it they are eating the right foods, because of the way their body handles these foods. Since NTDs begin in the first month of pregnancy, it is important for women to have enough folic acid in their system before pregnancy. Therefore, folic acid is recommended for all women of childbearing age, as 50% of pregnancies in this country are unplanned. The recommended dose of folic acid is 400 micrograms (0.4 milligram) daily, in addition to eating a healthy diet including foods rich in folic acid. Foods that are rich in folic acid include fortified breakfast cereals, orange juice, other citrus fruits and juices, leafy green vegetables, beans, peanuts, broccoli, asparagus, peas, and lentils. Cooking can destroy some of the folic acid found in foods. Some authorities recommend that women should increase their intake of folic acid to 600 micrograms (0.6 milligram) daily once their pregnancy is confirmed. However, women should not take more than 1,000 micrograms (1 milligram) without their doctor's advice. Recent studies suggest that folic acid may also help to prevent heart disease and stroke, along with colon and cervical cancers. Therefore many people, besides women of childbearing age, may benefit from taking folic acid.

NON-PRESCRIPTION
DRUGS AND PREGNANCY

QUESTION: What non-prescription medications can I take during my pregnancy?

ANSWER: In general, it is best to avoid using any drug during pregnancy unless it is absolutely necessary. The reason for this is that most drugs cross the placenta to some extent and a mother who takes a drug might expose her developing baby to it. The first three months of pregnancy is usually considered the period of time when a drug can cause the most harm to the baby, but taking some drugs anytime during a pregnancy can be potentially dangerous. However, drug therapy during pregnancy may be needed to treat medical conditions and pregnancy itself can produce a number of discomforts such as heartburn, constipation, and hemorrhoids.

Some non-prescription drugs can be safely taken during pregnancy, but pregnant women should always consult a healthcare provider before taking any medication. For pain relief or fever control, the short-term use of acetaminophen (Tylenol) is frequently recommended since the drug appears to be safe for the baby and the mother. Aspirin and other pain relievers like ibuprofen or naproxen are not a good choice during pregnancy, as they can cause complications in labor and delivery when taken late in the pregnancy. Aspirin can also increase the risk of bleeding in the mother and the newborn. For the treatment of allergy and cold symptoms, the use of a humidifier or a saline nasal spray can be helpful. The antihistamine chlorpheniramine has also been used safely during pregnancy. Many pregnant women will experience constipation, which can be helped by drinking plenty of water or juice and eating high-fiber foods. If this is not effective, bulk-forming laxatives such as Metamucil or Fiberall, which are not absorbed into the system, are safe to use. Stimulant laxatives should not be used because they can trigger uterine contractions. Likewise, the use of mineral oil should be avoided because it can interfere with the absorption of important vitamins. For hemorrhoids, topical preparations are available which are safer than suppositories. The occasional use of a product like Tums can be helpful for heartburn and indigestion. Very little is known about the safety of the many newer heartburn medications during pregnancy. In addition, the safety and effectiveness of homeopathic and herbal remedies in pregnancy have not been established and should be avoided.

DRUGS AND PREGNANCY

QUESTION: Where can I get information about using drugs during pregnancy?

ANSWER: Generally speaking, all drugs should be avoided during pregnancy unless they are absolutely necessary. In spite of this, it is estimated that more than 90% of pregnant women take prescription or nonprescription drugs or use social drugs such as tobacco and alcohol, or illicit drugs at some time during their pregnancy. About 2 to 3% of all birth defects are due to the use of drugs during pregnancy. However, in many women who have chronic medical conditions such as asthma, diabetes, or high blood pressure, the risk of not taking their medications during pregnancy may outweigh the risks of taking prescribed drugs. In these situations, the drugs should be taken under a doctor's supervision, and at the lowest dose needed. To help determine the risks of taking prescription medications during pregnancy the FDA has developed 5 risk categories for drugs as follows:

Category A
Controlled studies in women fail to demonstrate a risk to the fetus in the first trimester (and there is no evidence of a risk in later trimesters), and the possibility of fetal harm appears remote.

Category B
Either animal-reproduction studies have not demonstrated a fetal risk but there are no controlled studies in pregnant women, or animal-reproduction studies have shown an adverse effect (other than a decrease in fertility) that was not confirmed in controlled studies in women in the first trimester (and there is no evidence of a risk in later trimesters).

Category C

Either studies in animals have revealed adverse effects on the fetus (teratogenic or embryocidal or other) and there are no controlled studies in women, or studies in women and animals are not available. Drugs should be given only if the potential benefit justifies the potential risk to the fetus.

Category D

There is positive evidence of human fetal risk, but the benefits from use in pregnant women may be acceptable despite the risk (e.g., if the drug is needed in a life-threatening situation or for a serious disease for which safer drugs cannot be used or are ineffective.

Category X

Studies in animals or human beings have demonstrated fetal abnormalities, or there is evidence of fetal risk based on human experience or both, and the risk of the use of the drug in pregnant women clearly outweighs any possible benefit. The drug is contraindicated in women who are or may become pregnant.

Please note that the FDA does not categorize over-the-counter drugs but requires them to carry at least this warning: "If pregnant or breast-feeding, ask a healthcare professional before use".

In order to help determine if a medication should be taken during pregnancy or lactation, an Internet web site is available for information. This web site is **www.SafeFetus.com** and it is maintained by a team of physicians and pharmacists. Using this site, you type in the name of the medication (brand name or generic name) in the search box, or click on a letter in the alphabet and look for the drug manually. The site will then provide you with the medication's fetal risk category and breast-feeding precautions. By placing your mouse cursor over the words that are boldface in the text, a simple explanation of that word will come up. In addition to using this source of information, pregnant or breast-feeding women should always check with their physician and pharmacist before taking any prescription or nonprescription drugs.

URINARY TRACT INFECTIONS AND PREGNANCY

QUESTION: Is it OK to take an antibiotic for a urinary tract infection during pregnancy?

ANSWER: Urinary tract infections in pregnant women are a common problem and can result in premature delivery and low-birth-weight infants. While many antibiotics are considered safe to use during pregnancy, others are not. Common classes of antibiotics that are generally considered safe to use during pregnancy include penicillins (amoxicillin, ampicillin, and others), cephalosporins (such as cephalexin, and others), and erythromycin. However, other types of antibiotics such as tetracycline (minocycline, oxytetracycline, doxycycline, and others), quinolones (such as ciprofloxacin, levofloxacin, moxifloxacin, ofloxacin, and others) should be avoided if possible. In addition, a recent study in the journal Archives of Pediatrics and Adolescent Medicine reported that sulfa drugs (such as trimethoprim and sufamethoxazole-Bactrim or Septra) and nitrofurantoins (such as Macrobid) may not be safe to use during pregnancy. This study showed that birth defects such as rare brain and heart problems or shortened limbs may be linked to the use of sulfa drugs while heart problems and cleft palate may be linked to using nitrofurantoins, but the study authors noted that it's unclear whether the birth defects were caused by the drugs or by the underlying infections being treated. Anyone who is pregnant or thinks they may be pregnant should make sure that their physician and pharmacist know this information to try and prevent any potential problems when a drug is prescribed.

SEROQUEL DURING PREGNANCY

QUESTION: I take Seroquel for bipolar disorder. Can this drug pose a risk when taken during pregnancy?

ANSWER: Seroquel (quetiapine) is an antipsychotic medication that is used to treat bipolar disorder and other conditions. Recently, the FDA has issued a safety notice requiring labeling changes for all antipsychotic drugs to show potential side effects to children born to mothers taking these medications during the third trimester. Antipsychotic drugs may cause abnormal muscle movements and withdrawal symptoms in newborns including tremor, sleepiness, and difficulty with breathing or feeding. The FDA has received at least 69 reports of abnormal muscle movement or withdrawal among newborns whose mother took antipsychotic drugs during their last 3 months of pregnancy. In their safety notice, the FDA advises patients taking antipsychotic medication to:

• Notify your healthcare professional if you become pregnant or intend to become pregnant while taking an antipsychotic medication.
• Do not stop taking your antipsychotic medication if you become pregnant without first talking to your healthcare professional. Abruptly stopping antipsychotic medication can cause significant complications in your treatment.
• Talk to your healthcare professional if you have concerns about any treatment you are receiving during pregnancy.

Antipsychotic medications include the following (Not all drugs are listed):

Brand Name/Generic Name
• Abilify/aripiprazole
• Clozaril/clozapine
• FazaClo ODT/clozapine
• Fanapt/iloperidone
• Geodon/ziprasidone
• Haldol/haloperidol
• Invega/paliperidone
• Invega Sustenna/paliperidone
• Loxitane/loxapine
• Moban/molindone
• Navane/thiothixene
• Orap/pimozide
• Risperdal/risperidone
• Risperdal Consta/risperidone

- Saphris/asenapine
- Seroquel/quetiapine
- Seroquel XR/quetiapine
- Stelazine/trifluoperazine
- Thorazine/chlorpromazine
- Zyprexa/olanzapine
- Zyprexa Relprevv/olanzapine
- Zyprexa Zydis/olanzapine
- Symbyax/olanzapine and fluoxetine
- No Current Brand Name/fluphenazine
- No Current Brand Name/perphenazine
- No Current Brand Name/perphenazine and amitriptyline
- No Current Brand Name/prochlorperazine
- No Current Brand Name/thioridazine

HERBAL USE & PREGNANCY/BREASTFEEDING

QUESTION: What herbal medications should be avoided during pregnancy or while breastfeeding?

ANSWER: Although there is very little information available about the safety of using herbal medications during pregnancy or while breastfeeding, some herbal products should be avoided. For example, herbs or herbal ingredients that affect uterine contraction, such as rue, tansy, black cohosh, or pennyroyal, are not recommended during pregnancy. Likewise, cathartic laxative herbs like senna can cause potential problems. In addition, some herbs that are commonly found in foods such as sage, tumeric, ginger, and garlic can be a cause for concern during pregnancy when taken in very large doses or in concentrated forms. Similarly, some herbal medications that are excreted in breast milk and passed on to the baby can be a problem for women who breastfeed. For example, herbs that affect the central nervous system, cathartic laxatives, or herbal products that contain potentially toxic ingredients should be avoided when breastfeeding. Again, however, I must emphasize that very little information is currently available about this topic. A recent article pertaining to this subject lists the following common herbs that should be avoided during pregnancy or while breastfeeding.

Common Herbs To Avoid During Pregnancy

- Aloe
- Black cohosh
- Buckthorn
- Cascara segrada
- Chamomile, Roman
- Chaste tree berry
- Feverview
- Garlic (high doses)
- Ginger (high doses)
- Goldenseal
- Gotu kola
- Guggul
- Horehund
- Horseradish (fresh)
- Kava kava
- Licorice
- Mahuang
- Pennyroyal
- Rue
- Sage
- Senna
- St. John's wort
- Tansy
- Tumeric (high doses)
- Wormwood
- Yarrow

Common Herbs To Avoid While Breastfeeding

- Aloe
- Black cohosh
- Buckthorn
- Cocoa
- Coffee

- Kava kava
- Ma huang
- Sage
- Senna
- Tea
- Wintergreen

MEDICINE CABINET CONTENTS

QUESTION: You recently wrote about the contents of a medicine cabinet. I'm expecting a new baby and would like to know what I should stock in the medicine cabinet for my new arrival?

ANSWER: Stocking some basic nonprescription medications and supplies in the medicine cabinet is a good idea to help you deal quickly with common ailments during the baby's first year. The following items may be very useful to you:

- **Saline nasal drops and a bulb aspirator.** Saline nasal drops can be helpful for colds in children younger than 2 years old. Infants cannot blow their nose to remove nasal secretions and the accumulation of thick mucus can interfere with their ability to eat or sleep. Saline nose drops help to liquefy these secretions so that they can be gently suctioned with a nasal bulb aspirator.
- **Topical protectants for diaper rash.** Although topical protectants are not a replacement for good diaper hygiene, they can help to prevent and treat diaper rash (dermatitis). Most of these creams or ointments contain zinc oxide and/or petrolatum and provide a physical barrier between the skin and external irritants. They also help to lubricate the skin, and either absorb moisture or prevent it from coming into contact with the skin.
- **Simethicone drops.** Excessive crying in infants is often due to discomfort from intestinal gas. Excessive gas may also cause colic, irritability, or fussing. Simethicone helps to break up the gas bubbles in the GI tract and allow the gas to be expelled more easily.

- **Thermometer.** The use of digital rectal thermometers are usually recommended for infants. Under the arm (auxiliary) temperature reading using an oral thermometer may also be used for screening purposes in infants younger than 3 months to detect a fever. Digital electronic pacifier thermometers may be a useful alternative.
- **Adhesive bandages, cotton balls, and swabs.**
- **Antibiotic ointment.**
- **Child-safe sunscreen lotion** (for infants over 6 months old).
- **Hydrocortisone 0.5% cream or ointment** (for minor skin rashes, insect bites, etc.).
- **Hydrogen peroxide** (topical antiseptic).
- **Medicine dropper or oral syringe.**
- **Petrolatum jelly.**
- **Rubbing alcohol.**
- **A list of emergency phone numbers** including the National Poison Hotline (1-800-222-1222).

In addition, you should periodically check the expiration dates of all products that you store and discard those that are outdated. Also, remove any products that have been taken off the market and discard them. Please read all product labeling carefully to determine proper storage conditions, directions for use, and expiration dates.

SEXUAL DYSFUNCTION

QUESTION: Do any medications cause sexual problems in women?

ANSWER: Yes, there are numerous medications that can cause sexual dysfunction in women. It has been estimated that about two out of three women experience one or another form of sexual dysfunction and that one in four women between the ages of 21 and 30 have a low sex drive. There are four basic categories of sexual dysfunction in women: desire disorders, arousal disorders, orgasmic disorders, and sex pain disorders. Some women can have a combination of these disorders. Desire disorders are characterized by a lack of interest in intercourse while arousal disorders are characterized as an inability to feel or maintain sexual excitement.

Women with orgasmic disorders have an inability to reach an orgasm or the climax of sexual excitement. Sex pain disorders may include pain during sexual intercourse (dyspareunia) or an involuntary contraction of the muscles around the opening of the vagina (vaginismus) that makes sexual intercourse painful or impossible. While there are many causes of female sexual dysfunction, medications may be involved in disorders of sexual desire, sexual arousal, and orgasmic dysfunction. It is beyond the scope of this column to list all the medications that can cause female sexual dysfunction, but I have listed some of the types of medications that may be involved in the lists below:

Medications That May Cause Sexual Desire Disorders
- Anticonvulsants
- Antidepressants
- Anti-fungal drugs
- Antipsychotics
- Barbiturates
- Blood pressure medications
- Cholesterol medications
- Heart medications
- Oral contraceptives
- Stomach medications
- Tranquilizers

Medications That May Cause Sexual Arousal Disorders
- Antidepressants
- Antihistamines
- Anti-Parkinson medications
- Blood pressure medications
- Stomach medications
- Tranquilizers

Medications That Can Cause Orgasmic Dysfunction
- Antidepressants
- Narcotics
- Tranquilizers

Please note that these lists do not list all possible types of medications that may cause sexual dysfunction in women, nor do all drugs in each category produce these effects. If you have a specific question about any medications that you may be taking, please consult with your doctor and pharmacist.

BIRTH CONTROL

QUESTION: I heard that a new birth control product was approved that stops your periods. What can you tell me about it?

ANSWER: The FDA recently approved Lybrel (to symbolize "liberty") a new low dose combination oral contraceptive. Unlike most other oral contraceptives that are taken for 21 days followed by 7 days off, Lybrel is taken every day or 365 days a year. Studies have shown that Lybrel is just as effective in preventing pregnancy as other oral contraceptives, but because there is no drug-free interval, monthly periods are stopped. Lybrel is intended for women who are seeking contraception and who are interested in putting their menstrual cycle on hold. During clinical study, 59% of women taking Lybrel achieved amenorrhea (absence of all bleeding and spotting), 20% experienced spotting only-not requiring any sanitary protection, and 21% required sanitary protection due to breakthrough bleeding. In view of this, women considering using Lybrel must weigh the convenience of having no periods against the inconvenience of unscheduled bleeding or spotting. The occurrence of unscheduled bleeding decreases over time in most women who continue to take Lybrel for a full year. The risks of using Lybrel are similar to the risks of other oral contraceptives and include an increased risk of blood clots, heart attacks, and strokes, especially in cigarette smokers. Because Lybrel users will eliminate their regular periods, it may be difficult for women to recognize if they become pregnant and they should take a pregnancy test if they think they are pregnant. Some people have also expressed concerns about whether blocking periods is safe or natural, but many doctors appear to think otherwise.

QUESTION: I heard about some new birth control products. What can you tell me about them?

ANSWER: The FDA has recently approved two new types of birth control products, a skin patch and a vaginal ring. The skin patch product is marketed as Ortho Evra and contains a combination of estrogen and progestin hormones. It is used to prevent pregnancy and is the first hormonal skin patch approved for this use. During clinical studies, pregnancy rates were about 1 per 100 women-years of use. However, the patch may be less effective in women weighing more than 198 pounds. A patch is worn continuously for 1 week and then replaced with a new patch on the same day of the week for 3 weeks. The fourth week is patch-free to allow time for a menstrual period. The patch can be worn on the lower abdomen, buttocks, or upper body, but not on the breasts. If a patch becomes partially or completely detached for more than 1 day, the woman should start a new contraceptive cycle by applying a new patch immediately. Side effects of this patch reported during studies included breast symptoms, headache, skin reactions at the application site, nausea, upper respiratory tract infection, menstrual cramps, and stomach pain.

The vaginal ring product is marketed as NuvaRing, which also contains a combination of estrogen and progestin hormones. It is inserted into the vagina by the woman, and is the first hormonal vaginal contraceptive ring approved by the FDA. In clinical studies use of this ring was associated with 1-2 pregnancies per 100 women years of use. The vaginal ring is about 2 inches in diameter and should remain in place continuously for 3 weeks. It is then removed, allowing for a menstrual period. A new ring must then be inserted exactly 1 week after removal of the previous ring even if menstrual bleeding is not finished. If the ring is out of the vagina for more than 3 hours, an additional method of contraception, such as male condoms or spermicide, must be used until the ring has been in place continuously for 7 days. Common side effects reported in clinical studies with the vaginal ring included vaginitis, headache, upper respiratory tract infection, vaginal discharge, sinusitis, weight gain, and nausea. It should also be noted that the risks of using either of these products are similar to birth control pills including blood clots, heart attack, and stroke, particularly in cigarette smokers.

QUESTION: I heard about a new birth control pill that produces fewer periods. What can you tell me about it?

ANSWER: A new oral contraceptive (birth control pill) was recently approved that reduces a woman's periods from every month to 4 per year. This new prescription product is named Seasonale and comes in an extended-cycle tablet dispenser that contains a 3-month supply of tablets (84 pink tablets and 7 white tablets). One pink tablet that contains the active ingredients (estrogen plus progestin) is taken each day for 84 consecutive days, followed by 7 days of white (inactive) tablets. Withdrawal bleeding (period) should occur after the active pink tablets are all taken and during the 7 days of inactive white tablets. This cycle is then repeated 4 times per year. Seasonale works like other oral contraceptives to prevent pregnancy and is similar in effectiveness, but is taken for a longer duration (3 months instead of 1 month). This new product provides convenient packaging and may be attractive to women who experience severe cramping, heavy bleeding, and other menstrual-related symptoms. However, while women have fewer periods when using Seasonale, they also have a greater risk of unexpected "breakthrough" bleeding between periods compared to women taking monthly oral contraceptives. Some people have expressed a concern about whether or not 4 periods per year are enough over a long period of time or will this adversely affect the uterus. It should also be noted that the risks of using Seasonale are similar to other birth control pills including blood clots, heart attacks, and strokes, particularly in cigarette smokers.

QUESTION: I heard about an implantable contraceptive that is effective for 3 years. What can you tell me about it?

ANSWER: The FDA recently approved Implanon, a long-lasting implantable contraceptive. Implanon is a matchstick-sized rod that is implanted under the skin of a woman's upper arm and releases a continuous low dose of a progestin hormone (etonogestrel) over a 3-year period. It is the only implantable birth control method approved in the United States, but it has been used by about 2.5 million women in other countries since 1998. During clinical studies involving more than 900 women, Implanon was 99% effective in preventing pregnancy over a 3-year period. The implant can be removed at any time if a woman wants to get pregnant, and fertility appears to return to normal. However, Implanon must be removed at the end of the third year and be replaced by a new implant if continued contraceptive protection is desired. Some of the more common side effects of Implanon reported during clinical studies included headache, vaginitis, weight increase, acne, and breast pain. In addition 11% of the women discontinued the implant because of irregular menstrual bleeding. The manufacturer of Implanon (Organon) will be conducting a national clinical training program on the insertion and removal of Implanon, and only healthcare professionals completing this program will be able to prescribe this implant for their patients. Organon also makes a vaginal contraceptive ring product (Nuvaring) that contains the same active progestin ingredients as Implanon (etonogestrel).

PLAN B

QUESTION: What can you tell me about Over-The-Counter Plan B?

ANSWER: The FDA recently approved Over-The-Counter (OTC) access for Plan B for women 17 years of age and older. It remains a prescription only product for women aged 16 and under. Plan B is an emergency contraceptive or so-called "morning after pill" used to prevent pregnancy after unprotected sex or a known or suspected contraceptive failure. It is supplied in a package containing two tablets of levonorgestrel, a synthetic hormone used at lower doses in birth control pills for over 35 years. One tablet is taken orally as soon as possible within 72 hours of unprotected sex and the second tablet should be taken 12 hours after the first dose. Plan B primarily prevents pregnancy by stopping the release of an egg from the ovary (ovulation) or by preventing the union of sperm and egg (fertilization). It may also inhibit implantation of a fertilized egg in the uterus, but is not effective once the process of implantation has begun. Plan B is not for routine contraceptive use and is not effective if the woman is already pregnant. Clinical studies have shown that when used correctly, Plan B can reduce the expected number of pregnancies by 89%.

The most common side effects of Plan B are nausea, stomach pain, fatigue, headache, menstrual changes, dizziness, and breast tenderness. OTC Plan B will be made available in a program known as CARE (Convenient Access, Responsible Education). This program is designed to limit the availability of Plan B only to pharmacies and clinics with professional healthcare supervision, to educate healthcare professionals and consumers regarding the availability and responsible use of Plan B, and to monitor the effectiveness of the age restriction and safe distribution of Plan B. OTC Plan B will be for sale in pharmacies behind the prescription counter and personal identification showing proof of age (18) will be required. It will not be sold at gas stations or convenience stores. According to some sources, widespread use of emergency contraception like Plan B could potentially prevent an estimated 1.5 million unintended pregnancies and 800,000 abortions each year in the United States.

ELLA

QUESTION: What can you tell me about the new 5-day morning-after pill?

ANSWER: The FDA recently approved Ella (ulipristal), a new prescription product for emergency contraception. It was approved to prevent pregnancy when taken orally within 120 hours (5 days) after unprotected sex or contraceptive failure. Ella should not be used as a routine method of contraception. Unlike Plan B (levonorgestrel), which is sold without a prescription for women aged 17 and older and must be taken within 72 hours (3 days) of unprotected sex, Ella is a prescription-only product and may be taken within 5 days of unprotected sex. In a large clinical study, Ella was shown to significantly reduce the pregnancy rate, from an expected rate of 5.5% to an observed rate of 2.2% when a single dose was taken within 48 to 120 hours after unprotected sex. Results from a comparative study between Ella and Plan B also showed that women who received Ella within 72 hours of unprotected sex had a pregnancy rate of 1.9% compared to 2.6% in women taking Plan B within 72 hours of unprotected sex. Ella works by blocking or delaying the release of an egg from the ovary (ovulation) and may also change the lining of the uterus in a way that affects implantation of a fertilized egg. The most common side effects of Ella during clinical studies were headache, abdominal pain, nausea, pain or discomfort during menstruation, fatigue, and dizziness. It is estimated that approximately 3 million unintended pregnancies occur each year and nearly half of these unintended pregnancies are among women using regular methods of birth control where a failure occurred.

NON-PRESCRIPTION
WATER TABLETS

QUESTION: Are there any non-prescription or herbal diuretic (water pill) products available?

ANSWER: Non-prescription diuretic products are marketed for the relief of menstrual discomfort such as excess water weight, bloating, swelling, painful breasts, cramps, and tension. They are usually taken about 5 to 6 days before the beginning of menses to help relieve the symptoms caused by excess water retention. The active ingredients in these over-the-counter (OTC) products are ammonium chloride and/or caffeine, which promote diuresis (urination). Ammonium chloride can cause nausea and vomiting, headache, rapid breathing, drowsiness, and confusion. It should not be used by people with kidney or liver problems. Caffeine can cause stomach irritation, nervousness, and difficulty in sleeping when taken close to bedtime. Also, other caffeine containing products like coffee, tea, hot chocolate, and colas can produce additive effects with non-prescription caffeine containing diuretics. OTC diuretic products include Aqua-Ban, Aqua-Ban Plus, and Maximum Strength Aqua-Ban.

Herbal products that affect the kidneys are not really considered to be diuretics and are usually referred to instead as "aquaretics". These herbal preparations do not work in the body in the same way as diuretic drugs. They tend to produce greater blood flow to the kidneys and are promoted for use in some minor kidney disorders or to prevent kidney stones. However, more information is needed before they can be recommended for these uses. Some herbal "aquaretics" include goldenrod, parsley, dandelion, juniper, birch leaves, and lovage root. Remember that OTC drugs and herbals can produce side effects, so check with your doctor and pharmacist before using these products.

FACIAL HAIR

QUESTION: What can I do to get rid of unwanted facial hair?

ANSWER: Unwanted facial hair is a common problem that affects over 41 million American women. Unwanted facial hair is not a medical problem, but in our society it is usually not considered to be cosmetically acceptable. There are many possible causes including the natural aging process, heredity, hormonal changes during puberty or menopause, certain medical conditions, and the use of some medications such as birth control pills, testosterone and other male hormones, steroids, and minoxidil (Rogaine). Numerous treatment options exist for removing unwanted facial hair which can include the use of nonprescription and prescription medications, bleaching, shaving, plucking, waxing, electrolysis, and laser therapy. Nonprescription medications used for the removal of unwanted hair are known as depilatories. Depilatories contain chemicals that actually dissolve hair, which can then be easily removed from the skin. They are applied in the form of gels, lotions, creams, aerosols, or roll-ons. These products are efficient, but can cause skin irritation or chemical burns. Because of this, depilatory products should only be used on sites listed in their labeling and should not be applied to the eyebrows or any other area around the eyes or to inflamed or broken skin. Various waxing products are also available for removing unwanted hair and are often used by women for eyebrows, the chin, and upper lip. Hot or cold wax products pull hair from the skin, which can be quite painful. Waxes should not be used by people with diabetes or circulatory problems, as they may irritate the skin and cause infection. In addition, they should not be applied to the eyelashes, inside the nose, or ears. Recently, the first prescription cream for the management of unwanted facial hair was approved by the FDA. This cream, Vaniqua, does not actually remove hair, but slows hair growth. Studies have shown that it can slow the growth of unwanted facial hair in areas around the lips and under the chin. It is applied twice a day and complements other methods of hair removal such as waxing, shaving, or bleaching. Some women may experience minor and temporary skin irritations with Vaniqua such as redness, stinging, burning, tingling, or rash. It is not a quick fix and may take two or more months before results become visible.

BREAST CANCER RESEARCH

QUESTION: I heard that the FDA might let women try new drugs for breast cancer earlier. What can you tell me about this?

ANSWER: Yes, the FDA is planning to try an innovative approach in testing new drugs for breast cancer in the hopes of giving more women with aggressive, early-stage cancers the chance to try promising drugs while they have the best chance at a cure. In June 2012 the FDA issued a new guidance document, which would allow drug companies to test their promising medications for a few months on women with highly aggressive breast cancers before they have surgery, with the hope that this therapy would be a cure. Traditionally, by the time experimental drugs are tried on women with earlier-stage disease they have been tested in thousands of women with more advanced disease, for whom the risk of trying the drug is balanced with its potential for prolonging their lives. The new FDA treatment guidance document will apply to women with an especially deadly form of breast cancer called "triple-negative" breast cancers. Most breast tumors are called estrogen-receptor positive, because they are fueled by the hormone estrogen. Other breast tumors are HER2-positive, because a protein called HER2 is involved. A third type is driven by the hormone progesterone. These types of breast cancer have good treatments, but "triple-negative" tumors tend to grow and spread more quickly, occurring more often in younger or African-American women. The proposed early treatment approach is termed "neoadjuvant" therapy in which women are treated with either approved chemotherapy or approved chemotherapy plus an experimental drug for a few months prior to surgery. If women in the experimental drug group achieve a substantial improvement compared to the other group, the new drug would be given a provisional type of FDA approval called "accelerated approval". The researchers would then continue to follow women receiving the drug for several years to see if the treatment is safe and if their cancers come back. If treated women continue to be disease-free without serious side effects the drug could then get full FDA approval. This novel treatment approach could potentially speed access to new breast cancer drugs. Breast cancer is the second-leading cause of death in women, exceeded only by lung cancer, according to the American Cancer Society.

BREAST CANCER

QUESTION: I heard that a new drug was approved for late-stage breast cancer. What can you tell me about it?

ANSWER: In June 2012 the FDA approved Perjeta (pertuzumab) injection as a new therapy, to treat patients with HER2-positive late stage (metastatic) breast cancer. Dr. Gandhi provided an excellent review about exciting new drugs to treat breast cancer in the Chronicle a couple of weeks ago and Perjeta is one of them. Approximately 20% of breast cancers have increased amounts of a protein called HER2, which contributes to cancer cell growth. Perjeta is a new drug that targets the HER2 protein and is given in combination with another anti-HER2 drug named Herceptin (trastuzumab) along with a type of chemotherapy drug known as Taxotere (docetaxel). Because Herceptin and Perjeta work against HER2 in different ways, in combination they have a more potent effect against this type of breast cancer. During clinical studies involving over 800 women with HER2-positive metastatic breast cancer, the combination of Perjeta, Herceptin, and Taxotere increased the progression-free survival by about 6 months, compared to the combination of Herceptin and Taxotere by themselves. The 3-drug combination appeared to be fairly well-tolerated by patients. Breast cancer is the second leading cause of cancer-related death among women. This year an estimated 226,870 women will be diagnosed with breast cancer, and 39,510 will die from the disease. Much more promising research is underway to treat this disease.

ASPIRIN AND BREAST CANCER

QUESTION: Can aspirin be helpful for women with breast cancer?

ANSWER: The results of a recent study reported in the Journal of Clinical oncology found that women with breast cancer who take aspirin on a regular basis at least 2 days a week may have a lower risk of dying from breast cancer or having their breast cancer spread to other parts of the body (metastasis). This observational study involved 4,164 female registered nurses who were diagnosed with breast cancer between 1976 and 2002 and were followed until they died or until June 2006, whichever came first. The study results showed that breast cancer survivors taking aspirin at least 2 days a week had a nearly 50% lower risk of breast cancer death and risk of distant metastasis compared to those who did not take aspirin. The study did not look at the dose of aspirin used, but most regular use was likely for heart disease prevention at the 81 mg/day level, the researchers suggested. Results from this study, however, did not find an association between aspirin use and the incidence of breast cancer. It is not known how aspirin may affect cancer growth, but aspirin does have anti-inflammatory effects and also blocks an enzyme known as cyclooxygenase, which could play a role in blocking breast cancer growth by decreasing the amount of estrogen produced. It should be noted that in spite of the positive findings from this study, more research is needed to confirm any benefits. Experts point out that this was an observational study and was limited by the use of self-reporting by patients. The study's authors caution women who are undergoing breast cancer treatment to talk to their doctors before taking aspirin because it can cause serious gastrointestinal bleeding and can interact with other medications.

DRUGS TO PREVENT
BREAST CANCER

QUESTION: What drugs are approved to prevent breast cancer?

ANSWER: There are two drugs that have been approved by the FDA to lower the risk of breast cancer in women who are considered to be at high risk of developing this disease. These anti-estrogen drugs are tamoxifen and raloxifene (Evista). Tamoxifen, which has been available for many years to treat breast cancer, is also approved for the reduction of breast cancer risk in premenopausal and postmenopausal women who are at increased risk of breast cancer. Raloxifene, which is used to treat and prevent osteoporosis in postmenopausal women, is additionally approved to reduce the risk of invasive breast cancer in postmenopausal high-risk women. In recent years, these drugs were compared in one of the largest breast cancer prevention studies ever, known as the STAR Study (Study of Tamoxifen And Raloxifene). This research study involved almost 20,000 postmenopausal women who were at increased risk of breast cancer. Initial results of the STAR study showed that both raloxifene and tamoxifen reduced the risk of developing invasive breast cancer by about 50% after almost 4 years. Longer-term study results showed that as women completed 5 years of taking the drug and stopped taking it, tamoxifen continued to reduce the risk for both invasive and non-invasive breast cancer by about 50% while raloxifene reduced the risk by about 38%. However, it should also be noted that women taking raloxifene had fewer serious side effects than women taking tamoxifen including less uterine cancers, blood clots, and cataracts. Much more information about the STAR Study can be found at the National Cancer Institute's web site (www. cancer.gov, search STAR). In addition to tamoxifen and raloxifene, another type of drugs known as aromatase inhibitors that stop the production of estrogen have also shown great promise in preventing breast cancer in high-risk women and may provide an additional preventative treatment option.

MENOPAUSE AND AT-HOME TESTS

QUESTION: I'm approaching menopause and may want to take estrogens. Is there a home-test kit available to check my hormone levels?

ANSWER: Yes. The FDA recently approved a home test that women can use to detect perimenopause, early menopause, and menopause. As you know, menopause or "change of life" is the time in a women's life when the cyclic function of the ovaries and menstrual periods cease. The average age at which menopause occurs is about age 50, but menopause may occur naturally in women as young as age 40 or as late as age 60. Regular menstrual cycles may continue up to menopause, but usually the last periods tend to vary in duration and amount of flow. Perimenopause is the phase prior to the onset of menopause during which the periods become irregular. Symptoms of perimenopause, which can begin as early as age 35, include irregular menstrual cycles, hot flashes, short-term memory loss, mood swings, depression, and disturbed sleep. With age, a woman's ovaries become progressively less responsive to hormones with smaller amounts of estrogen and progesterone produced, and egg release (ovulation) eventually stops. The Menopause Home Test is similar to an at-home pregnancy test. It is an easy-to-use test that measures the amount of a hormone (follicle stimulating hormone or FSH) in the urine. According to the manufacturer, results of the test are fast and extremely accurate. This use at home self-test can help a woman determine whether menstrual period changes are being cause by menopause, allowing them to seek a physician's guidance to determine appropriate therapy. The manufacturer of the home test product recommends two tests (1-2 weeks apart) every 6 to 12 months when the symptoms of menopause occur. However, women should talk to their physicians about using the test and how often. At this time, the Menopause Home Test is not available in stores and can only be ordered from Physicians Laboratories online at **www.menopausehometest.com** or by calling 1-800-500-2055. The web site also contains a variety of educational health-related material for both women and men.

QUESTION: I heard about a new at-home test for menopause. What can you tell me about it?

ANSWER: Menopause is a normal and natural part of a woman's life. It occurs with a decrease in the production of estrogen and progesterone and an increase in the production of follicle stimulating hormone (FSH). Estrogen and progesterone are the hormones that control the monthly cycle of egg release (ovulation), and as women approach menopause egg release slows down and eventually stops. In response to these decreased levels of estrogen and progesterone, the body increases the production of FSH to try and normalize hormone levels. Menopause is defined as the absence of a menstrual cycle for 12 consecutive months. Perimenopause is the transitional phase that occurs before menopause when hormone levels widely fluctuate. In the United States the average age at which menopause occurs is about 50, but may occur in women as young as age 40 or as late as age 60. In order to help women determine their menopausal status, the FDA has approved an at-home diagnostic test named MenoCheck. This test measures the level of FSH in the morning's urine. Two consecutive MenoCheck tests taken seven days apart can determine whether FSH levels are elevated, indicating the onset of menopause. Women using this product must follow product instructions carefully for proper testing and should consult with their physician to discuss the results. MenoCheck is designed to offer women privacy, convenience, and ease of use. By knowing their menopausal status women, along with their physicians, can make more informed decisions regarding any appropriate treatment. MenoCheck does not require a prescription and is available at many local retail pharmacies. More information about MenoCheck can be found on the Internet at **www.menocheck.com**.

SOY SUPPLEMENTS & MENOPAUSE

QUESTION: Do soy supplements help menopause symptoms?

ANSWER: Probably not, according to a recent study published in the medical journal Archives of Internal Medicine. This study, which was funded by the U.S. National Institutes of Health (NIH), evaluated

248 women between the ages of 45 to 60 who were within 5 years of the start of menopause. Most of the women reported one or more menopausal symptoms such as hot flashes, night sweats, insomnia, loss of sex drive, or vaginal dryness. About one-half of the women were given soy isoflavone supplements and about one-half were given a placebo (dummy pill). After two years, the researchers measured the women's bone mineral density to screen for bone loss and they looked at their reports of menopausal symptoms. Results showed that the two groups showed no significant differences in bone mineral density of the lumbar spine, hip, or thigh bone. In addition, the two groups of women showed no differences in any of the menopausal symptoms at the end of the study, except for hot flashes, which were actually higher in those taking soy supplements (48% versus about 32% in the placebo group). The interest in soy supplements, which are very weak estrogens, was greatly increased after the Women's Health Initiative Study was halted in 2002, after finding an increased risk of strokes, heart attacks, and breast cancer in women who took combination hormone therapy using estrogen and progesterone.

MENOPAUSE AND HORMONAL REPLACEMENT THERAPY (HRT)

QUESTION: I heard about a new skin spray for hot flashes due to menopause. What can you tell me about it?

ANSWER: The FDA recently approved Evamist (estradiol transdermal spray) for the treatment of moderate to severe vasomotor symptoms (hot flashes) due to menopause. It is the first approved transdermal spray containing an estrogen hormone. Approximately two million American women naturally enter into menopause between the age of 45 and 55. Menopausal symptoms occur when a woman's ovaries stop producing estrogen and may include hot flashes, discomfort or pain during sexual intercourse due to vaginal atrophy (thinning of the vagina), and changes in skin and hair. Evamist contains the estrogen estradiol in a metered-dose spray pump that is designed to deliver estradiol into the bloodstream following topical application. The starting dose of

Evamist is one spray daily to the inner surface of the arm between the elbow and the wrist. This dosage can be increased to two or three sprays daily depending upon the patient's clinical response. During clinical study, Evamist reduced the number of hot flashes in postmenopausal women by about 2 to 3 per day and also reduced their severity. The most common side effects of Evamist were headache, breast tenderness and nipple pain, nausea, back pain, and inflammation of the nose and throat. However, as I've noted before, the use of estrogens may increase the risk of getting heart attacks, strokes, breast cancer, uterine cancer, endometrial cancer, blood clots, and dementia. Because of this, the use of estrogens should always be at the lowest dose and for the shortest duration consistent with treatment goals and a woman's individual risks. Your physician can determine if the use of Evamist or another estrogen product is right for you.

QUESTION: What's your opinion regarding hormone replacement therapy for menopausal women?

ANSWER: As you may know, menopause is the time in a women's life when the cyclic function of the ovaries and menstrual periods stop. As you approach menopause the ovaries produce smaller and smaller amounts of the hormones estrogen and progesterone, and egg release (ovulation) eventually stops. Women may or may not experience any symptoms during menopause, and if symptoms do occur, they can be mild, moderate, or severe. Symptoms of menopause can include hot flashes (flushes) which can affect up to 75-85% of women, psychological and emotional symptoms, night sweats, dizziness, tingling sensations, loss of bladder control, vaginal dryness, and other effects. Osteoporosis is also a problem during menopause and cardiovascular disease progresses more rapidly after menopause. The treatment of menopause with estrogens is known as hormonal replacement therapy or HRT. Until recently, there have been hundreds of studies that provided conflicting evidence about the benefits of hormone replacement therapy, such as controlling hot flashes or night sweats, and preventing osteoporosis or heart disease. However, in July 2002, findings from the Heart and Estrogen/Progestin Replacement Study showed that the long-term use of a combination of estrogen and progestin (Prempro) may significantly increase a women's risk of breast cancer, stroke, and heart attack. In addition, a second report indicated that the long-term treatment with estrogen and progestin in women with heart disease may increase the risk of blood clots and biliary tract surgery. Results from a third study also concluded that, overall, the health risks from the use of combination HRT exceed the benefits. In view of this new information, the decision to use HRT should be made very carefully based upon the advice of your physician(s). For younger menopausal women with severe symptoms such as hot flashes and night sweats, HRT may be an effective treatment to reduce the severity of symptoms—but the risk to benefit ratio must be weighed on an individual basis. In addition, it is recommended that all products containing estrogen alone or in combination with a progestin for use in postmenopausal women should only be used at the lowest effective dose and for the shortest duration consistent with treatment goals and risks for the individual woman. In light of the new findings, women taking HRT to reduce the risk of heart attacks, strokes, or osteoporosis should ask their physician about other medications that could be used for these purposes. Furthermore, women who are discontinuing HRT should taper the medication because stopping quickly may produce an increase in menopausal symptoms, such as hot flashes or night sweats.

QUESTION: I heard about a new skin patch for "hot flashes" that is applied only once a week. What is it?

ANSWER: The FDA recently approved a low dose estrogen/progestin skin patch for the treatment of menopausal symptoms such as hot flashes and night sweats. This prescription-only patch is named Climara Pro and is applied to the lower abdomen once a week. During clinical studies this patch was shown to reduce hot flashes by up to 80% after 3 months of treatment in menopausal women who have not had their uterus removed. In addition to a convenient once-weekly application schedule, another advantage of the skin patch over oral hormonal therapy is a very low rate of nausea and gastrointestinal complaints. The most common side effects of Climara Pro are skin reactions to the patch, vaginal bleeding, and breast pain. Like other estrogen/progestin combination products, Climara Pro should not be used by women with known or suspected pregnancy, or those with certain types of cancer such as breast cancer or uterine cancer. Women with unusual vaginal bleeding, blood clots, or those who have had a stroke or heart attack in the past year should also avoid it. As I've noted before, the long-term use of estrogen with progestin may significantly increase a women's risk of breast cancer, stroke, heart attack, and blood clots. Because of this, the use of estrogen alone or in combination with a progestin, should always be limited to the lowest effective dose and for the shortest period of time consistent with the treatment goals and risks for each individual woman.

QUESTION: Is the FDA going to take Premarin and Prempro off the market?

ANSWER: The FDA is not planning to take Premarin and Prempro off the market at this time. However, the FDA is requiring new safety information to be included in the labeling of all estrogen and estrogen plus progestin products for use by postmenopausal women. These labeling changes are based upon the results from a recent large study conducted by the Women's Health Initiative (WHI) and sponsored by the National Institutes of Health (NIH). Results from this study have shown that postmenopausal women taking estrogen plus progestin have an increased risk of heart attack, stroke, breast cancer, and blood clots. In addition, the risk of dementia is increased in women over the age of 65. It is estimated that about 10 million postmenopausal women in the United States currently use estrogen and combination estrogen plus progestin products for relief of menopausal symptoms such as hot flashes, night sweats, or vaginal dryness, and for the prevention of osteoporosis (weak bones). The new product labeling emphasizes that these products should only be used when the benefits clearly outweigh the risks. In addition, they should be used at the lowest dose and for the shortest duration for individual women. Women who choose these therapies after discussing their treatment with their doctor should also have yearly breast exams by a healthcare provider, perform monthly breast self-exams, and receive periodic mammography exams. It is also recommended that when these products are being used solely for vaginal dryness that topical vaginal products should be considered. Likewise, when being prescribed solely for the prevention of postmenopausal osteoarthritis that other non-estrogen treatments should be considered. Estrogens and progestins should not be used to prevent heart disease, heart attacks, or strokes. These new labeling changes will probably influence how these products are prescribed in the future. Postmenopausal women who are currently using estrogen or estrogen plus progestin products or thinking about their use should talk to their physician to determine which therapy is best for them. Further information about this new product labeling is available online at **www.fda.gov/cder/ drug/infopage/estrogens_progestins/ default.htm**.

QUESTION: I heard about a new prescription lotion to treat hot flashes. What can you tell me about it?

ANSWER: The FDA recently approved Estrasorb, a topical emulsion (lotion) for the treatment of hot flashes associated with menopause. It contains the estrogen, estradiol, and is the first topical emulsion (lotion) approved for this use. The lotion, which is packaged in foil pouches, is rubbed into the skin on the thighs and calves once a day. It is believed that many women may prefer this type of estrogen therapy compared to oral tablets, skin patches, or the new vaginal ring. Studies have shown that this estrogen lotion reduces the number of hot flashes by about 9 to 11 per day and also lessens their severity. During clinical studies, the most common side effects of Estrasorb were breast pain, headache, sinusitis, itching, infection, and disorders involving the lining of the uterus. However, estrogens, even when applied as a lotion, may increase the risk of endometrial or breast cancer and cardiovascular problems such as heart attacks, strokes, and blood clots. Because of this, estrogens should only be used in the lowest effective dose and for the shortest duration consistent with treatment goals and risks for the individual woman. You should consult with your doctor to determine if this new estrogen lotion is appropriate for you.

Hot flashes are a common complaint of women who are postmenopausal, but their cause is not well understood. A hot flash is described as a sudden burning or hot sensation that begins in the head and neck and passes down the body in waves. Hot flashes have been associated with anxiety, warm temperatures, caffeine, alcohol, spicy food, and physical contact. It is also thought that a reduction in estrogen levels during menopause leads to a reduction in a chemical known as serotonin that helps to regulate the body's temperature, causing hot flashes.

QUESTION: Since there is so much concern about using estrogens for hot flashes, what other medications can be used for this problem?

ANSWER: Many women are concerned about using hormonal replacement therapy or HRT (estrogen plus progestin) for postmenopausal hot flashes. The Women's Health Initiative Study was stopped early in July of 2002, because it showed that hormonal therapy led to a higher incidence of heart attacks, strokes, blood clots, and breast cancer. During this study, there was a 112% higher risk of blood clots, a 38% greater risk of strokes, a 23% higher risk of heart attacks, and a 26% increase in breast cancer in women taking these drugs. On the flip side, the study demonstrated that hormonal therapy decreased the incidence of colorectal cancer, endometrial cancer, and hip fractures. Because of this the FDA has mandated changes in product labeling for these hormonal products, and lower dose estrogens products are being utilized more frequently.

It is thought that a reduction in estrogen levels during menopause leads to a reduction in a chemical known as serotonin that helps to regulate the body's temperature, causing hot flashes. In view of this, several non-hormonal drugs that increase serotonin blood levels have been used for the shot-term management of hot flashes. These drugs include the antidepressants Effexor, Paxil, and Prozac. The anticonvulsant Neurontin, which affects body temperature, has also been tried for the short-term treatment of hot flashes with some success. In addition, some alternative medicines such as soy or black cohosh may be useful for the short-term relief of hot flashes. It should be noted, however, that none of these non-hormonal medicines have been approved for the treatment of hot flashes and your physician should be consulted to determine your best therapeutic option.

QUESTION: I heard that a new lower-dose of Prempro has been approved for symptoms of menopause. Is it as effective as the higher dose?

ANSWER: Yes, results from a large study of postmenopausal women have shown that a new lower-dose of Prempro is similar in effectiveness to the higher dose product for the treatment of moderate to severe symptoms of menopause such as hot flashes and vaginal or vulvar atrophy (severe dryness, itching, and burning in or around the vagina). Prempro is a combination product that contains both conjugated estrogens and the progestin medroxyprogesterone acetate or MPA. The progestin is used in combination with the estrogens because it helps to protect against endometrial cancer in postmenopausal women with a uterus. In the study I referred to, both the low and high doses of Prempro reduced the number of hot flashes by about 11 per day compared to a reduction of about 6 per day for women getting a "dummy" (placebo) pill. The FDA approved the lower-dose Prempro product after concerns arose regarding the potential risks associated with higher doses of the combination product such as cancer and cardiovascular problems such as heart attacks, strokes, and blood clots. However, the lower-dose Prempro is not approved for the prevention of postmenopausal osteoporosis. An even lower dose product is also being developed by the maker of Prempro. Common side effects of Prempro include headache, breast pain, irregular vaginal bleeding or spotting, stomach/abdominal cramps or bloating, nausea and vomiting, and hair loss. Many other side effects are possible and you should consult with your doctor to see if Prempro is appropriate for you. The FDA recommends that estrogens and progestins be used at the lowest effective dose and for the shortest duration consistent with treatment goals and risks for the individual woman. They also advise doctors to consider topical preparations such as vaginal creams when treating vaginal or vulvar atrophy by itself.

QUESTION: I heard about a new vaginal estrogen product for menopause. What can you tell me about it?

ANSWER: A new vaginal ring that contains estrogen (estradiol acetate) was recently approved for the treatment of moderate to severe symptoms associated with menopause such as hot flashes and vaginal or vulvar atrophy (severe dryness, itching, and burning in or around the vagina). An estimated 10 million postmenopausal women in the U.S. currently use estrogens to ease menopausal symptoms and to prevent osteoporosis. Estrogens are hormones made by a woman's ovaries. The ovaries normally stop making estrogens when a woman is between 45 to 55 years old. This drop in body estrogen levels is known as the "change of life" or menopause and produces very uncomfortable symptoms in some women such as "hot flashes", "hot flushes", or vaginal dryness and itching. This new vaginal ring (Femring) is a soft, flexible ring that releases estrogen into the vagina and into the bloodstream over a 3-month period. Once inserted into the vagina the Femring should remain in place for 3 months and then be replaced by a new Femring. Common side effects of Femring include headache, breast pain, irregular vaginal bleeding or spotting, stomach/abdominal cramps or bloating, nausea and vomiting, and hair loss. Other side effects can also occur including high blood pressure, liver problems, high blood sugar, fluid retention, enlargement of fibroid tumors and vaginal yeast infections. In addition, estrogens can increase the risk of endometrial or breast cancer and cardiovascular problems such as heart attacks, strokes, and blood clots. Because of this, estrogens should only be used in the lowest effective dose and for the shortest duration consistent with treatment goals and risks for the individual woman. The FDA also advises doctors to consider topical preparations such as vaginal creams when treating vaginal or vulvar atrophy by itself. You should consult with your healthcare provider to determine if the Femring is appropriate for you.

QUESTION: I heard about a new prescription product for treating menopausal symptoms that may cause less water retention. What can you tell me about it?

ANSWER: The FDA recently approved Angeliq for the treatment of menopausal symptoms such as hot flashes, night sweats, and vaginal dryness. This new oral tablet, which is taken once daily, contains estradiol (estrogen) and drospirenone (progestin). Drospirenone is somewhat different from other progestins used in hormonal replacement therapy (HRT) because it can counter the excess water and sodium retention sometimes caused by taking estrogen. It also has anti-male hormone (antiandrogenic) properties, which may be helpful in treating postmenopausal women with acne or excessive body or facial hair (hirsutism) who need HRT. However, Angeliq can also increase potassium levels in the blood and this needs close monitoring in women taking this therapy. It should be noted that the FDA now requires new safety information to be included in the labeling of all estrogen and estrogen plus progestin products based upon results from the Women's Health Initiative (WHI) study. This study showed that postmenopausal women taking estrogen plus progestin have an increased risk of heart attack, stroke, breast cancer, and blood clots. In addition, the risk of dementia is increased in women over the age of 65. These products should only be used when the benefits clearly outweigh the risks, and should be used at the lowest dose and for the shortest duration for individual women. It is recommended that when these medications are being used solely for vaginal dryness that topical vaginal products should be considered. Your physician can determine if HRT is appropriate and what product is most suitable for you.

PREMENSTRUAL SYNDROME

QUESTION: What can I do for PMS without a prescription?

ANSWER: PMS or premenstrual syndrome is a group of physical and psychological symptoms that occur before a menstrual period. Approximately 40% to 90% of females are affected by PMS, but the type and intensity of symptoms vary from woman to woman and from month to month in the same woman. In addition, about 5% of American women of reproductive age have a severe form of PMS called premenstrual dysphoric disorder or PMDD, which can cause major disruption in their daily life. While the cause of PMS is not completely understood, it may occur in part due to changes in hormonal levels during the menstrual cycle. Symptoms of PMS generally fall into three categories: mood disruptions, behavior disorders, and changes in physical function. Mood disruptions can include mood swings, irritability, hostility, depression, anxiety, nervousness, forgetfulness, confusion, and difficulty in sleeping. Behavioral problems can include sweet cravings, increased food intake, crying, impaired concentration, increased sensitivity to noises, and changes in alcohol tolerance. Changes in physical function can include weight gain, headache, awareness of heart beat, fatigue, joint or muscle pain, dizziness, bloating, abdominal cramping, breast tenderness and swelling, constipation, or diarrhea. Symptoms of PMS may begin a few hours before or up to 14 days before a menstrual period, and they usually disappear after the period begins. However, women who are approaching menopause may have symptoms that continue through and after the menstrual period. The self-treatment of PMS can involve a number of different strategies to relieve the uncomfortable symptoms. A reduction in salt and sugar intake along with the elimination of caffeine and alcohol may help to relieve fluid retention, irritability, and bloating. Exercise and stress reduction methods such as meditation or relaxation techniques can also help relieve nervousness and agitation. Heat therapy using a heating pad, hot water bottle, or the ThermaCare heat wrap can also help to relieve painful abdominal cramping. Taking over-the-counter pain relievers like acetaminophen (Tylenol) or nonsteroidal anti-inflammatory drugs such as ibuprofen (Motrin) or naproxen (Aleve) can be useful for headaches, pain due to abdominal cramps, and joint pain or muscle pain due to PMS. In addition, nonprescription water tablets (diuretics) such as pamabrom (Aqua-Ban) may help to relieve symptoms related to water retention. Various vitamins, supplements, and herbal remedies have also been promoted for PMS symptoms, but the effectiveness of these products has not been proven. Women with more severe PMS symptoms or those with PMDD should consult with their physician for appropriate treatment.

OSTEOPOROSIS

QUESTION: I heard about a new type of drug for osteoporosis. What can you tell me about it?

ANSWER: Osteoporosis is a bone disorder that can lead to fractures affecting about 10 million Americans, 80% of whom are women. Another 18 million people have a condition known as low bone mass, which puts them at high risk for osteoporosis. As the population ages, osteoporosis will become much more common. This disease produces a loss of bone mass throughout the skeleton, making the bones more fragile which increases the risk of fractures, particularly in the hip, spine, and wrist. Osteoporosis is caused by an imbalance between the formation of new bone and bone breakdown due to hormone deficiencies, aging, medication, or other causes. Some of the risk factors for osteoporosis and fractures include the following:

- Advanced age
- Dementia
- Being female
- Personal or family history of fracture
- White or Asian race
- Alcoholism
- Cigarette smoking
- Estrogen or testosterone deficiency
- Inadequate calcium, vitamin D, and vitamin K in diet
- Physical inactivity
- Low body weight or small body build

Osteoporosis, like high blood pressure, is often called a "silent disease" because bone loss occurs without symptoms, and may go undetected until a fracture occurs. Preventative measures for people of all ages are very important and should include adequate intake of calcium and vitamin D, along with regular weight-bearing exercise, smoking cessation, and moderation in alcohol intake. But even with enough dietary calcium intake and a healthy lifestyle, many postmenopausal women and others at risk of osteoporosis can continue to lose bone. The most commonly used tool to diagnose osteoporosis and predict fracture risk is a test for bone mineral density (BMD).

The newly approved drug for osteoporosis is Forteo (generic name teriparatide). Unlike previously available drugs that slow down the breakdown of old bone, Forteo is the first available drug that actually stimulates new bone formation. It increases bone mineral density (BMD) and bone strength. Clinical studies have shown that Forteo can significantly reduce the incidence of fractures of the spine and other bones in postmenopausal women with osteoporosis. Common side effects of Forteo include dizziness and leg cramps. However, there is some concern that it may cause a type of bone tumor and this is being studied further. Forteo needs to be given by injection once a day. It is injected subcutaneously into the thigh or abdominal wall using a prefilled pen device. Currently, it is only recommended for postmenopausal women with osteoporosis who are at high risk of fracture or who can't take other medications.

BACTERIAL VAGINOSIS

QUESTION: I heard about a new vaginal prescription treatment for bacterial vaginosis that only requires a single dose. What can you tell me about it?

ANSWER: The FDA recently approved Clindesse (clindamycin vaginal cream) for the single dose treatment of bacterial vaginosis or BV. Bacterial vaginosis is a leading cause of vaginal complaints in the U.S. and is twice as common as yeast infections. It is really not an infection, but an imbalance in the bacteria normally found in the vagina (normal vaginal flora). One or more types of bacteria overgrow and displace the others (lactobacilli) causing an imbalance, which leads to symptoms. The large numbers of overgrown bacteria cause a heavy discharge and change the acid-base balance of the vagina to alkaline (increased pH). Symptoms of BV include an increased amount of vaginal discharge; thick, milky, yellowish discharge; and discharge with a "fishy" or ammonia-like odor which may smell worse after sexual intercourse. However, many women with BV have no symptoms and it is possible for teens and young girls to get it also. It is important that the vaginal environment is in balance to help keep the lining of the vagina healthy and prevent infections or other disorders, such as pelvic inflammatory disease or endometritis (an inflammation of the uterine lining). In addition, BV has been associated with delivery complications in pregnant women. Until the arrival of Clindesse, vaginal treatments for BV usually required 3 to 7 days of treatment, depending upon the medication utilized. Oral treatments are also available, but these may cause more side effects or interact with other drugs or alcohol. Clindesse cream is the only approved vaginal medication for BV that can be given as a single-dose. The active ingredient in Clindesse kills the overgrown bacteria and helps to bring the vaginal pH back into balance. It comes in a single-dose pre-filled disposable applicator that is administered intravaginally once at any time of the day. It should not be used by anyone who has a history of hypersensitivity to its ingredients. In addition, it should be noted that the cream contains mineral oil which may weaken latex or rubber products such as condoms or diaphragms and their use is not recommended with Clindesse cream for 5 days after treatment.

REPHRESH

QUESTION: What can you tell me about the vaginal product RepHresh?

ANSWER: RepHresh is a nonprescription clear vaginal gel that is used to help women maintain a healthy vaginal acidity or pH value. In chemistry, the acidity or alkalinity of a substance is expressed in pH values with a pH value of 7 being neutral, a pH value less than 7 being acidic, and a pH value over 7 being basic or alkaline. For example, stomach acid has a pH of about 1 to 5 while lye (sodium hydroxide) may have a pH of 11 to 14. In the vagina, a normal pH of about 4.5 (acidic) is important for maintaining good vaginal health. In women, anything that reduces the acidity (increases the pH) of the vagina can increase the likelihood of vaginal infections, bacterial vaginosis, or other problems. The acidity of the vagina may be reduced by hormonal changes shortly before and during menstrual periods or during pregnancy. Frequent douching, use of spermicides, and semen can also reduce vaginal acidity. In addition, aging and sexual activity can affect vaginal pH. In a normal vagina, the acidity of vaginal secretions is maintained by lactic acid, which is produced by bacteria called lactobacilli. When one or more types of vaginal bacteria overgrow and displace the number of protective lactobacilli, the pH of the vagina increases and problem infections or bacterial vaginosis can occur.

RepHresh is a clear vaginal gel available over-the-counter that is administered with an applicator once every 3 days. It contains two acidic polymers, polycarbophil and carbomer. When applied to the vagina, these polymers stick to the vaginal epithelial cells until they turnover with new cells (3-5 days) and help to restore vaginal secretions to an optimal pH of 4.5 which prevents non-protective bacteria and yeasts from overpopulating. The use of RepHresh may be useful during times when women are more susceptible to higher pH levels, such as after their period, after unprotected sex, during pregnancy, or after a hysterectomy. It may also be of benefit in women who experience regular vaginal odor, irritation, discomfort, or infections. Side effects of RepHresh appear to be minimal, but some women may notice a residue after its initial use caused by the elimination of dry vaginal cells. Women considering using RepHresh should consult with their physician or gynecologist to determine if this product would be appropriate for them.

QUESTION: What can you tell me about RepHresh Brilliant pH tampons?

ANSWER: RepHresh Brilliant pH tampons are different from traditional tampons because they contain 2 ingredients (L-lactide and citric acid) that help to reduce the usual increase in vaginal pH that occurs during a woman's menstrual period. In chemistry, the acidity or alkalinity of a substance is expressed in pH values with a pH value of 7 being neutral, a pH value less than 7 being acidic, and a pH value over 7 being basic or alkaline. For example, stomach acid has a pH of about 1 to 5 while lye (sodium hydroxide) may have a pH of 11 to 14. In the vagina, a normal pH of about 4.5 (acidic) is important for maintaining good vaginal health. In women, anything that reduces the acidity (increases the pH) of the vagina can increase the likelihood of vaginal infections, bacterial vaginosis, or other problems. The acidity of the vagina may be reduced by hormonal changes shortly before and during menstrual periods or during pregnancy. Frequent douching, use of spermicides, and semen can also reduce vaginal acidity. In addition, aging and sexual activity can affect vaginal pH. In a normal vagina, the acidity of vaginal secretions is maintained by lactic acid, which is produced by bacteria called lactobacilli. When one or more types of vaginal bacteria overgrow and displace the number of protective lactobacilli, the pH of the vagina increases and problem infections or bacterial vaginosis can occur. During a woman's period the high pH of blood (7.4) causes vaginal pH to increase beyond the normal range, and tampons retain the fluids that cause pH to increase. When tampons were first invented in 1929, they were designed for leak protection, comfort, and convenience. The RepHresh Brilliant pH tampons may also help to reduce the risk of vaginosis and perhaps other types of vaginitis.

Tampon Use Basics

- Use tampons only during menstruation.
- Change your tampon at least every 4 to 8 hours.
- You can wear a tampon overnight for up to 8 hours. Before going to bed, insert a new tampon and replace it immediately upon waking.
- Always remove your used tampon before inserting a new one.
- Be sure to remove the last tampon you use at the end of your period.

VIAGRA

QUESTION: My husband has been taking Viagra for about 2 years and it works well for us. However, I seem to develop vaginal itching and wonder if Viagra could be the cause?

ANSWER: Probably not. Viagra, the popular impotence drug, works to help blood vessels expand in size, allowing more blood flow to the penis which causes the swelling and hardness of an erection. This expansion of the penis also prevents blood from flowing out through the veins that carry blood from the penis and the blood is temporarily trapped. After an orgasm and ejaculation, the nervous system then causes the blood vessels to contract, which prevents blood from flowing to the penis, which reverses the erection. Unfortunately, Viagra's effect does not just work on blood vessels that go to the penis, but elsewhere also, which can cause low blood pressure or hypotension in some patients. Some other possible side effects with Viagra include headache, flushing, indigestion, nasal congestion, urinary tract infection, muscle aches, abnormal vision, diarrhea, dizziness, and rash. In regards to your vaginal itching, the amount of Viagra found in the semen of patients taking the drug is very small (less than one-tenth of one percent). Because of this, I don't think that it is the cause. Vaginal irritation and itching is a fairly common symptom in females, especially postmenopausal women. The causes of vaginal itching and irritation may be difficult to determine but may include allergy to topically applied vaginal products or infection, especially if there is a vaginal discharge. In the absence of an infection, hydrocortisone cream (Gynecort) or over-the-counter products containing povidone-iodine may be helpful. However, you should talk to your physician(s) about this problem and should not self-treat this condition if it lasts for more than a week.

VAGINAL DRYNESS

QUESTION: What can I use for vaginal dryness?

ANSWER: Vaginal dryness or atrophic vaginitis is a common complaint in up to 40% of postmenopausal women. It is caused by inflammation of the vaginal tissues, which may become thin and dry from decreased estrogen levels. Estrogen helps to keep vaginal tissue healthy and protect it from infection. The most common cause of atrophic vaginitis is a decrease in estrogen production due to menopause, but it can also occur after surgical removal of the ovaries, following childbirth, during breast-feeding, or from certain drugs. Symptoms of this disorder include vaginal irritation, dryness, burning, itching or vaginal discharge. Sexual intercourse may be painful and may be followed by light bleeding. Urinary tract symptoms, including frequency and painful urination, may also accompany this condition. Treatment for atrophic vaginitis is aimed at reducing the discomfort of vaginal dryness during everyday activities and in restoring lubrication during intercourse. Because this condition is caused by lower levels of estrogen, the most effective therapy is an estrogen supplement. Many doctors prefer vaginal estrogen products including creams, tablets, or a vaginal ring that releases estrogen once in place. These topical products reduce the side effects of systemic estrogen replacement therapy such as oral tablets and skin patches. The type of estrogen to use, its dose, frequency, and time needed to treat each patient is different and must be determined by your physician. Nonprescription water-soluble vaginal lubricants such as K-Y jelly, Replens, and many others may be useful to help relieve dryness and pain during intercourse. Your pharmacist can help you select an appropriate water-soluble product. Vaseline should not be used because it is difficult to remove from the vagina. In addition, products that may aggravate vaginal symptoms such as powders, scented soaps, perfumes, spermicides, and pantyliners should be avoided.

QUESTION: Can Replens help with vaginal dryness due to menopause?

ANSWER: Nearly all women will experience vaginal dryness at some time in their life. This dryness can be caused by childbirth, breastfeeding, menopause, intense exercise, stress, and even some medications. Vaginal dryness can also occur when douching, using tampons, or at the end of the menstrual cycle. Vaginal dryness during menopause is a result of estrogen deficiency, which leads to a reduction in the elasticity and thickness of the vaginal wall along with a reduced blood flow and secretions in the vagina. These changes can produce itching, dryness, burning, and painful sexual intercourse. Replens is a polycarbophil-based non-prescription, long-lasting vaginal moisturizer with bioadhesiveness. Bioadhesiveness is a property that allows a compound to adhere to the surface of the body's mucous membranes, like the vagina. This product does not contain estrogen or spermacides, and can be inserted into the vagina using the supplied applicator anytime during the day or night. For best results, most women should use the moisturizer every three days. As the cells of the vaginal wall are regenerated, dry cells are cleared and the moisturizing ingredients in Replens are eliminated naturally. Clinical study has shown that using Replens can improve the quality of life for many menopausal women and help to relieve vaginal burning, itching, and painful intercourse. Replens is available in most pharmacies and comes in a 14 application package with a reusable vaginal applicator or an 8 count package of pre-filled applicators.

EYELASH ENHANCER

QUESTION: I heard that a new prescription product increases the length, thickness, and darkness of eyelashes. What can you tell me about this?

ANSWER: The FDA recently approved Latisse (bimatoprost ophthalmic solution) as a novel prescription treatment for hypotrichosis of the eyelashes. Eyelash hypotrichosis is another name for having inadequate or not enough eyelashes. This product is the first treatment approved by the FDA to enhance eyelash prominence as measured by increases in length, thickness, and darkness of eyelashes. While it is not known exactly how Latisse works, it appears to bind to receptors involved in the development and regrowth of the hair follicle. Latisse comes as a solution that is applied to the base of the upper eyelashes once daily with a disposable applicator. Latisse users can expect to experience longer, fuller, and darker eyelashes in about 8 to 16 weeks. However, to maintain these effects, continued treatment is required. If the use of Latisse is discontinued, eyelashes will gradually return to where they were prior to treatment over a period of weeks to months, which is the average eyelash hair cycle. Common side effects of Latisse include eye redness, itchy eyes, and increased skin pigmentation. The active ingredient in Latisse, bimatoprost, was first approved by the FDA in 2001 as an eye drop used to lower intraocular pressure in people with open-angle glaucoma or ocular hypertension. Patients treated with this eye drop experienced eyelash growth as a side effect, hence its development for this use. The FDA has also recommended that the manufacturer of Latisse study the use of this product in younger people and in post-chemotherapy patients with loss of eyelashes.

MENSTRUAL CRAMPS

QUESTION: I have a lot of pain and cramping during my period. What nonprescription medication can I use for this problem?

ANSWER: Pain or discomfort which occurs during menstruation is known as "dysmenorrhea" and is a very common complaint occurring in 40%-70% of all women of reproductive age. It is especially common in adolescent females with as many as 90% of high school females experiencing this problem. It has been reported that 25% of female students miss class because of dysmenorrhea, and 55% of students report that cramps interfere with their school work. Some women suffer from this problem throughout their fertile years, but most find that it subsides gradually by their mid-20's or after pregnancy. Some types of dysmenorrhea (secondary) are caused by other medical problems such as pelvic inflammatory disease, uterine polyps or fibroids, ovarian cysts, etc. and therefore an evaluation by a physician is needed. If the pain and discomfort is not due to other medical problems, then it is called "primary dysmenorrhea". Primary dysmenorrhea is thought to be caused by chemicals known as prostaglandins that are released during menstruation. These prostaglandins produce strong contractions of the uterus to help expel the menstrual discharge, but they also cause the cramping pain. The most commonly used nonprescription medications for dysmenorrhea are pain relievers (analgesics) and water tablets (diuretics). The most effective OTC analgesics for dysmenorrhea are the non-steroidal anti-inflammatory drugs (NSAIDs). These include ibuprofen (Motrin IB, Advil, Midol IB, etc.), naproxen (Aleve), and ketoprofen (Orudis KT, Actron). They work to prevent the production of prostaglandins that cause the pain and cramping and should all be taken with food. Nonprescription diuretics may be effective for the temporary water weight gain, bloating, and swelling that can occur during the menstrual period. Useful products include Aqua-Ban, which contains ammonium chloride and Maximum-Strength Aqua-Ban, which contains the diuretic pamabrom. Make sure that you read all of the labeling for these products, including their precautions and proper dosage. Finally, some herbal products have been promoted for the treatment of dysmenorrhea including Black Cohosh and Chaste Tree Berry, but they have not been approved by the FDA for this use.

QUESTION: I heard that a new drug was approved to treat heavy menstrual bleeding. What can you tell me about it?

ANSWER: The FDA recently approved Lysteda (tranexamic acid) tablets for the treatment of heavy menstrual bleeding. It is the first non-hormonal product cleared to treat heavy menstrual bleeding (menorrhagia). Heavy menstrual bleeding is reported each year by about 3 million U.S. women of reproductive age. Women with uterine fibroids may experience heavy menstrual periods, but in most cases, there is no underlying health condition associated with the condition. Heavy menstrual periods can cause pain, mood swings, and disruptions to work and family life. Use of Lysteda in clinical studies resulted in a significant reduction in menstrual blood loss in women. However, the use of Lysteda while taking hormonal contraceptives may increase the risk of blood clots, stroke, or heart attack. In view of this, women using hormonal contraception should take Lysteda only if there is strong medical need, and if the benefit of treatment will outweigh the potential increased risk. Lysteda is administered as two 650 mg tablets three times a day for a maximum of 5 days during monthly menstruation. The most common side effects of Lysteda during clinical trials included headache, sinus and nasal symptoms, back pain, abdominal pain, muscle and joint pain, muscle cramps, anemia, and fatigue. Women interested in this product should consult with their personal physician to see if Lysteda is appropriate for them.

POISON-PROOFING

QUESTION: I have a young child at home who likes to get into everything. Do you have any tips to protect him from accidental poisoning from medications or other hazardous products?

ANSWER: Accidental poisoning in children occurs much too often. As a concerned parent you can take several measures to prevent these mishaps and to "poison-proof" your home. First of all, teach your child to ask first before putting anything into his mouth. It is also important to never call medicines or vitamins candy, because to small children many medicines look like candy. If you are called to the door or phone, take any open or available medicines or other potentially harmful products or your child with you. You should also use child-proof containers for medications whenever possible and dispose of old medicines by flushing them down the toilet.

To help you "poison-proof" your home a number of measures can be taken. All medicines, cigarettes, alcohol, cleaning products and other harmful chemicals should be stored out of reach and sight of children. Never store them in the same cabinets with food. Installing safety latches on cabinets and drawers is another good idea to protect your child. Insecticide products or garden chemicals that require leaving a powder or pellets in areas where pets or children may go should also be avoided. Some houseplants are also poisonous, such as poinsettias and mistletoe and should not be used in households where children can get at them.

Finally, every household with children should have Syrup of Ipecac available (one ounce per child is recommended), which can be used to induce vomiting if poisoning occurs. However, Syrup of Ipecac should never be used without the advice of a physician or a Poison Control Center. The reason for this is that some poisons can cause more harm to the child if they are vomited up.

If a potential poisoning does occur in your household, contact the Florida Poison Information Network at 1-800-282-3171, the National Poison Information Network at 1-800-222-1222, or if the situation is life threatening, call 911.

IPECAC SYRUP FOR POISONING

QUESTION: Should I keep syrup of ipecac in the house in case my child swallows something he or she shouldn't?

ANSWER: It is probably a good idea for every household with children to consider keeping a small bottle of syrup of ipecac (one ounce per child) in their medicine cabinet, which can be used to induce vomiting if poisoning occurs. However, syrup of ipecac should never be used without the advice of a physician or a Poison Control Center. The reason for this is that some poisons can cause more harm to the child if they are vomited up. For example, some corrosive substances like drain or oven cleaner can cause damage to the swallowing tube (esophagus) going down and more damage when it goes back up when vomiting is induced. Another potential problem with using syrup of ipecac is that vomiting may interfere with other treatment. For instance, many emergency room doctors often give activated charcoal to patients who have swallowed a poison. The charcoal works to prevent the poison from being absorbed into the bloodstream, but if the patient is vomiting the charcoal cannot be given and valuable time is wasted. Syrup of ipecac should also not be given to someone who is drowsy or is losing consciousness because they might inhale (aspirate) the vomited material or choke on it. Some cases where ipecac syrup may be useful include a child who has ingested a large amount of noncorrosive materials such as poisonous mushrooms, lead paint chips, or aspirin. When ipecac syrup is used it should be given as soon as possible after being told to do so by a Poison Control Center or doctor. The usual dose for children 1-12 years of age is one-half ounce (15 ml) orally followed by 1 to 2 glasses of water. This can be repeated one more time if vomiting does not occur within 20 to 30 minutes. Use only water after administering ipecac syrup and do not use milk or carbonated beverages. If a potential poisoning does occur in your household, contact the Florida Poison Information Network at 1-800-282-3171 or if the situation is life-threatening, call 911. A national toll-free number is also available which will route your call to the nearest Poison Control Center (1-800-222-1222). Please keep these phone numbers handy by the telephone.

ATTENTION DEFICIT HYPERACTIVITY DISORDER (ADHD)

QUESTION: My son was put on Ritalin for attention deficit hyperactivity disorder. What can you tell me about this medication?

ANSWER: Attention deficit hyperactivity disorder or ADHD is a neurobiological disorder that primarily affects children and adolescents but also may persist into adulthood. While some estimates are much higher, the National Institute of Health believes that 3% to 5% of American school-age children have ADHD. It is much more common in males than females. ADHD is characterized by hyperactivity, inability to control impulses, and difficulty in paying attention. Individuals with this disorder often fail to pay close attention to details, make careless mistakes, and are easily distracted which makes it difficult to complete tasks. They may also find it difficult to sit still or be patient. As a result, academic problems are common in children with ADHD and this may be the first sign of any problem. The cause of ADHD is not known but there is some evidence that there may be genetic or environmental risk factors for its development. The symptoms may lessen during the teen years and adulthood or may continue.

Ritalin or methylphenidate (MPH) is not a cure for ADHD but helps to control the symptoms. How it works is still unclear, but it is a stimulant that works in the brain and affects a number of chemicals involved in alertness, behavior, and activity. Studies indicate that the use of MPH can improve attentiveness and academic performance, improve behavior and impulse control, decrease aggressive behavior, and improve peer relations. It works best when combined with non-drug therapies such as counseling, techniques to modify behavior, and special planning in the school classroom. The most common side effects of MPH include sleeping difficulty, decreased appetite, irritability, stomach pain, dizziness, and headaches. An increase in heart rate and blood pressure can also occur. Concern about the long-term use of MPH and its effect on children's growth has also been expressed. Medication "holidays" during the summer months may help to allay this concern. It should also be noted that MPH is a drug abused on the street, particularly by teenagers who refer to it as vitamin R. It is taken by mouth, inhaled, or injected for its stimulant effect. Therefore, the handling and storage of this medication needs to be tightly controlled. For the treatment of ADHD, MPH is usually taken 2 or 3 times daily but if it is taken near bedtime it may interfere with sleep. Recently, a once-daily controlled-release preparation with the tradename Concerta was also approved by the FDA. Other longer-acting products including a 24-hour skin patch of MPH are under development and may be available in the future. Finally, an organization that you might find helpful is CHADD (Children and Adults with Attention Deficit Disorders) 1-800-233-4050 or 1-954-587-3700.

QUESTION: I heard about a new drug for treating attention-deficit/ hyperactivity disorder (ADHD). What can you tell me about it?

ANSWER: The newly approved drug for ADHD is Strattera (generic name-atomoxetine). It is not entirely clear how this new drug works, but it is known to block a chemical in the nervous system know as norepinephrine. In numerous studies involving children, adolescents, and adults with ADHD, Strattera was found to be effective in reducing the symptoms of ADHD such as lack of attention and hyperactivity/ impulsiveness and improved social and family functioning. Strattera appears to be similar in effectiveness to other drugs used to treat ADHD such as Ritalin (generic name-methylphenidate). However, Strattera is not a stimulant drug and is not classified as a controlled substance. Because of this, it is not subject to rigid prescribing, dispensing, or advertising rules. It is also less likely to be diverted and abused. Common side effects of Strattera include decreased appetite, nausea, vomiting, tiredness, and upset stomach. However, severe liver injury can also occur in some patients. Strattera is taken once a day in the morning as a single dose, or in divided doses in the morning and late afternoon or early evening. An organization that you might find helpful is CHADD (Children and Adults with Attention Deficit Disorders) 1-800-233-4050 or 1-954-587-3700.

QUESTION: I heard about a new skin patch used to treat attention deficit hyperactivity disorder. What can you tell me about it?

ANSWER: The new skin patch used to treat ADHD is named Daytrana and it contains methylphenidate (Ritalin), which has been used orally for many years to treat ADHD. Methylphenidate is not a cure for ADHD but helps to control symptoms. It is unclear how this drug works, but it is a mild central nervous system stimulant that affects a number of brain chemicals involved in alertness, behavior, and activity. The skin patch is applied to the hip area in the morning and is worn for approximately 9 hours then removed. It can be removed earlier if a shorter duration of effect is desired or if late day side effects appear. When applied to the skin, the patch releases the methylphenidate, which flows through the skin and into the bloodstream. During clinical studies, the most common side effects of Daytrana were decreased appetite, sleeplessness, sadness/crying, twitching, weight loss, nausea, nasal congestion, inflammation of the nasal passages, and irritation (redness, itching) at the site of patch application. Daytrana should not be used by some people with ADHD and it can interact with other medications. You should consult with your doctor to determine if Daytrana would be a useful ADHD treatment alternative for your child.

QUESTION: I heard that children with ADHD should have a heart exam before being treated with medication. Why is this?

ANSWER: The American Heart Association (AHA) recently issued a recommendation that children with attention deficit hyperactivity disorder (ADHD) should have a thorough heart workup, including an electrocardiogram (ECG), before taking stimulant-type medications used to treat this disorder. The reason for this is that these medications which include Ritalin, Daytrana, Concerta, Methylin, Metadate, others (methylphenidate), Adderall (amphetamine mixed salts), and Strattera (atomoxetine) can increase heart rate and blood pressure, which could lead to serious problems in some children with heart problems. It has been reported that over two dozen children taking these drugs died suddenly between 1992 and 2005, which led to warnings in drug labeling information. According to the AHA, an ECG is painless and only takes 10 minutes. If children are found to have heart defects or other heart problems they can then be treated and monitored appropriately.

QUESTION: I heard about a new drug for treating attention-deficit/hyperactivity disorder (ADHD). What can you tell me about it?

ANSWER: The newly approved drug for ADHD is Intuniv (generic name-guanfacine). It is not entirely clear how this new drug works, but it is known to act on chemical receptors in the front of the brain, which is an area that has been linked to ADHD. During clinical studies in children and adolescents aged 6 to 17 years, Intuniv was found to be effective in reducing the symptoms of ADHD such as lack of attention and hyperactivity/impulsiveness, and improved social and family functioning. Unlike other drugs like Ritalin used to treat ADHD, Intuniv is not a stimulant and is not classified as a controlled substance. Because of this, it is not subject to rigid prescribing, dispensing, or advertising rules. It is also less likely to be diverted and abused. Common side effects of Intuniv include sleepiness, headache, fatigue, and upper abdominal pain.

QUESTION: I heard that a new drug for treating attention deficit hyperactivity disorder (ADHD) was approved. What can you tell me about it?

ANSWER: The FDA recently approved Kapvay (clonidine extended-release tablets) for the treatment of children and adolescents aged 6 to 17 with ADHD. Kapvay can be used by itself to treat ADHD or can be used in combination with a stimulant medication like Ritalin (methylphenidate) or amphetamine. While it is not known exactly how Kapvay works to improve the symptoms of ADHD, it is believed to act in an area of the brain that regulates attention and plays a critical role in impulse control, working memory and executive function. In clinical studies, Kapvay was shown to significantly improve the core symptoms of ADHD, such as inattention, hyperactivity, and impulsivity. The most common side effects of Kapvay include sleepiness, fatigue, upper respiratory infection (cough, rhinitis, sneezing), irritability, throat pain, insomnia, nightmares, emotional disorder, constipation, nasal congestion, increased body temperature, dry mouth, and ear pain. Kapvay is a non-stimulant medication and is taken twice a day.

CORRECT USE OF NONPRESCRIPTION MEDICATIONS IN CHILDREN

QUESTION: What can I do to make sure that non-prescription (OTC) medicines for my children are used correctly?

ANSWER: Great question. The National Council on Patient Information and Education (NCPIE) has developed the following 10 tips to be "medwise" (**www.bemedwise.org**, 2009):

- **When in doubt, ask first**. Your child's health is too important for guesswork. So any time you have a question about which OTC medicine is best for your child or how and when to give the medicine, ask your doctor or pharmacist first.
- **Make sure the pediatrician knows about all the OTC medicines your child takes before he or she writes a new prescription**. Similarly, if your child takes prescription medicines, check with your pediatrician or pharmacist before giving your child an OTC product.
- **Know your child's weight so you can give the proper dose of the medicine as recommended on the product label**. Most pediatricians and pharmacists agree that the child's weight is the best way to determine the correct dose. For this reason, health professionals often recommend that parents keep an accurate scale in the house so that they can check the child's weight before giving OTC medicines.
- **Follow the directions on the label carefully**. Because OTC drugs are serious medicines that can do harm if taken incorrectly, always read the entire label information before giving a child any OTC product. In this way, you will be certain that you have selected the right product, understand the dosing instructions, and are aware of any warnings or precautions that could apply.
- **Use the specific dropper, dosing cup or other device that comes packaged with your child's medicine**. Because kitchen spoons and other household utensils vary in size and are not accurate enough to measure doses of medicines, using them can result in giving your child either too large or too small a dose of the medication. The same thing can happen when you use a dosing device from another children's medicine.
- **If using multiple OTC medicines, you have to watch for both duplicate ingredients and usage**. First check the active ingredient(s) used in each OTC medicine and make sure that you are not giving your child more than one product with the same active ingredient without first checking with a healthcare professional. Because many cough and cold preparations contain the same active ingredient as pain relievers, it is possible to give a child two different products that contain the same active ingredient without realizing it. Second, check for usage duplication. For example, two cold medicines may

contain different active ingredients, but both of those ingredients act as fever reducers. That's usage duplication, and it should also be avoided. To play it safe, read the "Drug Facts" label and compare. Don't be hesitant to ask your pediatrician or pharmacist for advice on product selection.

- **Give babies and children only those medicines that are especially formulated for their weight and age.** Cutting adult strength tablets in half or trying to estimate a child's dose of an adult-strength liquid can result in an accidental overdose. Similarly, giving older children liquid medicines that are especially formulated for babies can also lead to dosing errors.
- **Keep in mind that most OTC medicines are for temporary relief of minor symptoms.** If the condition persists or gets worse contact your pediatrician or other healthcare professional.
- **Don't give medicines in the dark.** This is often a problem because children get sick at night, and the parents can make a mistake reading the dosing device if they can't see well.
- **Teach children that OTC medicines are not candy and they should not touch, sniff, or taste them on their own.** Only let children take OTC medicines from a responsible adult. Keep all medicines and household products out of children's reach.

FEVER IN CHILDREN

QUESTION: What can I give my child for fever?

ANSWER: Fever is the most common symptom of disease in children. About 20-30% of calls from parents to pediatricians are about fever, and it is the most frequent reason for office visits by children under two years of age. It should be noted that a child's skin may feel warm to the touch, but touch is not a reliable method for detecting fever. Body temperature should be measured orally, rectally, or in the arm pit or ear. Rectal temperature measurements are usually preferred for children less than about three years of age, since young children have difficulty forming a tight seal around a thermometer with their lips. In general, fever is considered "mild" if it is between about 100 degrees F and

102 degrees F, and "high" when it reaches 104 degrees F. In pediatric patients, an oral temperature up to 99 degrees F or a rectal temperature up to 100 degrees F is considered "normal". However, "normal" body temperature varies with age, time of day, physical activity, temperature of the surrounding area, and the amount of clothing worn. The American Academy of pediatrics recommends that a pediatrician be contacted before attempting home treatment of fever in a child 3 to 6 months old with a fever of 101 degrees F or greater and in a child older than 6 months with fever of 103 degrees F or higher. They also recommend that a pediatrician should be immediately contacted if their child has a fever and:

- Is 2 months of age or younger with a rectal temperature of 100.2 degrees F or higher
- Looks very ill, is unusually drowsy, or is very fussy.
- Has additional symptoms, such as a stiff neck, severe headache, severe sore throat, severe ear pain, an unexplained rash, or repeated vomiting or diarrhea.
- Has a condition that suppresses immune responses, such as sickle-cell disease, or cancer or is taking steroids.
- Has had a seizure.

Either acetaminophen (Tylenol, Tempra, Liquiprin, Panadol, etc.) or ibuprofen (Advil, Motrin, etc.) are both effective nonprescription products for treating fever in children. The use of aspirin in children and adolescents with fever has been associated with the development of Reye's syndrome and is not recommended. Unfortunately acetaminophen and ibuprofen are also among the most commonly misused nonprescription medications. The reason for this is that many parents give their children incorrect doses of these medications, because they are confused with the many different types of products available and have trouble giving accurate doses. For example, these products are available in concentrated oral drops for infants, in oral liquids for children, and chewable tablets—all with different dosing instructions. Because of the potential for confusion and errors when using these products be sure to follow the directions on the package labeling very carefully. You should use the specific dropper, oral syringe, dosing cup, or other device that comes packaged with the product, since kitchen spoons can vary in size. Also be sure to know your child's weight so that you can give the proper dose and don't measure or give these medications in the dark. In addition, other medications also may contain acetaminophen or ibuprofen and if given together can lead to overdosing. Finally, if you have any questions about the proper product to use for your child or dosing instructions, make certain that you "Ask The Pharmacist" for advice. Please read column below regarding the use of liquid acetaminophen.

LIQUID ACETAMINOPHEN

QUESTION: What should I know about giving liquid acetaminophen to my infant?

ANSWER: Several liquid acetaminophen products for infants are now available including concentrated infant drops in a concentration of 80 mg/0.8 mL and 80 mg/1.0 mL which are sold with droppers for administration, and a less concentrated formulation which contains 160 mg/5 mL which is sold with an oral syringe for proper dosing. In view of the potential for dosing errors with these products, the FDFA recently issued a Safety Communication to help avoid confusion and avoid dosing problems.

The Food and Drug Administration (FDA) is urging consumers to carefully read the labels of liquid acetaminophen marketed for infants to avoid giving the wrong dose to their children. A less concentrated form of the popular medication is arriving on store shelves, and giving the wrong dose of acetaminophen can cause the medication to be ineffective if too little is given or cause serious side effects and, possibly, death if too much is given. Before giving the medication, parents and caregivers need to know whether they have the less concentrated version or the older, more concentrated medication. The FDA is concerned that infants could be given too much or too little of the medicine if the different concentrations of acetaminophen are confused. Parents need to be very careful when giving their infant liquid acetaminophen and should do the following:

- Read the Drug Facts label on the package very carefully to identify the concentration of the liquid acetaminophen, the correct dosage, and the directions for use.
- Do not depend on a banner proclaiming that the product is "new." Some medicines with the old concentration also have this headline on their packaging.
- Use only the dosing device provided with the purchased product in order to correctly measure the right amount of liquid acetaminophen.
- Consult your pediatrician before giving this medication and make sure you're both talking about the same concentration.
- Adding to the confusion is the fact that that the box and the bottle may look much the same for both old and new versions of the medication. Read the Drug Facts label to tell the difference between the two liquid acetaminophen products:
- Look for the "Active ingredient" section of the Drug Facts label usually printed on the back of an over-the-counter (OTC) medication package.
- If the package says "160 mg per 5 mL" or "160 mg (in each 5 mL)", then this is the less concentrated liquid acetaminophen. This medication should come with an oral syringe to help you measure the dose.
- If the package says "80 mg per 0.8 mL" or "80 mg per 1 mL," then this is the more concentrated liquid acetaminophen. This product may come with a dropper.

If the dosing instructions provided by your healthcare provider differ from what is on the label, check with a healthcare professional before administering the medication. Do not rely on dosing information provided from other sources such as the Internet, old dosing charts, or family members. It is important to understand that there is no dosing amount specified for children younger than 2 years of age. If you have an infant or child younger than 2 years old, always check with your healthcare provider for dosing instructions. Acetaminophen is marketed for infants under brand names such as Tylenol, Little Fevers Infant Fever/Pain Reliever, Pedia Care Fever Reducer Pain Reliever and Triaminic Infants' Syrup Fever Reducer Pain Reliever. There are also store brands (e.g., Rite Aid, CVS, Walgreens brand, etc.) on the shelves.

Richard P. Hoffmann, RPh, PharmD

BENZOCAINE
PRODUCTS FOR TEETHING

QUESTION: Why is the FDA warning about the use of benzocaine products for teething?

ANSWER: The U.S. Food and Drug Administration (FDA) is warning the public that the use of benzocaine, the main ingredient in over-the-counter (OTC) gels and liquids applied to the gums or mouth to reduce pain, is associated with a rare, but serious condition. This condition is called methemoglobinemia and results in the amount of oxygen carried through the blood stream being greatly reduced. In the most severe cases, methemoglobinemia can result in death.

Benzocaine gels and liquids are sold OTC under different brand names such as Anbesol, Hurricaine, Orajel, Baby Orajel, Orabase, and store brands. Benzocaine is also sold in other forms such as lozenges and spray solutions. These products are used to relieve pain from a variety of conditions, such as teething, canker sores, and irritation of the mouth and gums. Methemoglobinemia has been reported with all strengths of benzocaine gels and liquids, including concentrations as low as 7.5%. The cases occurred mainly in children aged two years or younger who were treated with benzocaine gel for teething. People who develop methemoglobinemia may experience pale, gray or blue colored skin, lips, and nail beds; shortness of breath; fatigue; confusion; headache; lightheadedness; and rapid heart rate. In some cases, symptoms of methemoglobinemia may not always be evident or attributed to the condition. The signs and symptoms usually appear within minutes to hours of applying benzocaine and may occur with the first application of benzocaine or after additional use. If you or your child has any of these symptoms after taking benzocaine, seek medical attention immediately. Benzocaine products should not be used on children less than two years of age, except under the advice and supervision of a healthcare professional. Healthcare professionals and consumers are advised to consider the American Academy of Pediatrics' recommendations for treating teething pain instead of using the benzocaine teething products:

- Give the child a teething ring chilled in the refrigerator.
- Gently rub or massage the child's gums with your finger to relieve the symptoms of teething in children.

If these methods do not provide relief from teething pain, consumers should talk to a healthcare professional to identify other treatments. Adult consumers who use benzocaine gels or liquids to relieve pain in the mouth should follow the recommendations in the product label. Consumers should store benzocaine products out of reach of children. FDA encourages consumers to talk to their healthcare professional about using benzocaine.

Additional Information for Consumers and Caregivers

- Labels of marketed benzocaine products currently do not as of yet contain warnings about the risk of methemoglobinemia, even though the use of benzocaine can cause this serious condition.
- Benzocaine products should not be used on children less than two (2) years of age, except under the advice and supervision of a healthcare professional.
- Store benzocaine products out of reach of children.
- If benzocaine products are used, watch for signs and symptoms of methemoglobinemia, including pale, gray or blue colored skin, lips, and nail beds; shortness of breath; fatigue; confusion; headache; lightheadedness; and rapid heart rate. If you or your child has any of these symptoms after taking benzocaine, seek medical attention immediately.
- Signs and symptoms of methemoglobinemia may appear within minutes to one or two hours after using benzocaine. Symptoms may occur after using benzocaine for the first time, as well as after several uses.
- The development of methemoglobinemia after treatment with benzocaine gels and liquids has been reported to occur following a single administration of the product.
- Benzocaine gels and liquids should be used sparingly and only when needed, but not more than four (4) times a day. If pain persists despite using the product as labeled, contact your healthcare professional for further evaluation and treatment recommendations.

TONSILLITIS

QUESTION: My seven-year-old son has a sore throat and painful swollen glands in the upper neck. What can I do to help?

ANSWER: It sounds like your son may have tonsillitis and you should have him examined by a physician. Symptoms of tonsillitis include a sore throat, usually made worse by swallowing, and pain sometimes felt in the ears. Young children may also have fever, headache, loss of appetite, vomiting, bad breath, swollen and tender lymph glands, a hoarse voice, and feel tired. Sometimes they may have difficulty swallowing or breathing if the tonsils are enlarged. The tonsils are located on the sides of the back of the throat and they help to defend against infection. Tonsillitis or inflamed tonsils is a common problem in children and is most often caused by bacteria or viruses. Infected tonsils are usually red and swollen and may have pits or crevices filled with pus. A throat swab of the infected area can help to determine if it is caused by a bacteria or a virus.

The treatment for tonsillitis includes plenty of fluids and bed rest. Acetaminophen (Tylenol) or ibuprofen (Advil, Motrin) can be used for treating pain and fever. Aspirin should not be used in young children because it can lead to the development of Reye's syndrome. Gargling with warm salt water or sucking on a throat lozenge may help to relieve the sore throat pain. If the tonsillitis is caused by a virus, antibiotics are not useful. However, if the throat culture done by a physician shows that the tonsillitis is caused by bacteria, then an antibiotic will need to be prescribed. If this is the case, make sure that your son takes the entire prescription even if he feels better in order to prevent a reoccurrence of the infection. Some children can develop chronic recurring infections of the tonsils. In the past surgical removal of the tonsils was commonly performed to prevent this problem, but today this is not routinely done.

ASTHMA

QUESTION: My 12 year-old son has asthma. What can you tell me about asthma in children?

ANSWER: The incidence of asthma in children is rising and the FDA recently (2012) provided a consumer information update about this lung problem that affects breathing. Asthma is a chronic lung disease that inflames and narrows the airways. In the past the stereotypical asthmatic child was frail and inactive, relying on an inhaler to breathe. The good news is that better treatment options are now available, allowing children with asthma to live active, independent lives. The Food and Drug Administration (FDA) works to make sure that the drugs and devices used to treat asthma are safe and effective.

The bad news is that the number of reported cases of asthma in children has been rising. In 2010, there were 7 million children with asthma, 9.4% of Americans under 18, according to the Centers for Disease Control and Prevention, up from 6.5 million, or 8.9%, in 2005. One reason may be that doctors are diagnosing more kids as asthmatic. Illnesses once known as bronchitis or a croupy cough are now being recognized as asthma. Its symptoms may include coughing, wheezing (a whistling sound when you breathe), chest tightness and shortness of breath, according to the National Heart, Lung and Blood Institute (NHLBI). Uncontrolled asthma can lead to chronic lung disease and a poor quality of life, and may slow growth. It is recommended that parents work with a pediatrician, and an allergist or pulmonologist (lung specialist) if needed, to develop and follow an asthma action plan that details the treatment options when certain symptoms occur. The things that make asthma worse are known as "triggers". They include:

• Season and climate changes
• High levels of air pollutants
• Tobacco smoke
• Mold
• Mites, roaches
• Plant pollen
• Pet dander
• Strong scents, like perfumes

In addition, certain factors may increase a child's risk of developing asthma:

• Family history of asthma

- Multiple episodes of wheezing before age 2
- Living in crowded housing
- A family member who smokes
- Obesity

While asthma is never "cured", a variety of FDA-approved medications can help manage symptoms.

- For quick relief of severe symptoms, doctors will prescribe "rescue" medications, such as albuterol, which open up the bronchial tubes in the lungs. The goal is not to use it, but have it available at home, school, etc. just in case it is needed.
- To stabilize chronic and persistent symptoms, doctors will prescribe "controller" medications. The most common, safe and effective controller medications are the inhaled corticosteroids (ICS). With regular treatment, they improve lung function and prevent symptoms and flare-ups, reducing the need for rescue medications.
- Children whose asthma is triggered by airborne allergens (allergy-causing substances), or who cannot or will not use ICSs, might take a type of drug called a leukotriene modifier. These come in tablet and chewable forms, though for many people they tend to be less effective than ICSs, especially for more severe asthma.
- For more severe cases that are not controlled with ICSs or leukotriene modifiers alone, adding long-acting beta agonists (LABAs) such as salmeterol or formoterol might be recommended. the FDA cautions against using LABAs alone without an ICS, and recommends that if one must be used, it should be for the shortest time possible.

Most asthma medications are inhaled. Babies and toddlers use a nebulizer, a machine that delivers liquid medication as a fine mist through a tube attached to a face mask. Older children can use a metered dose inhaler or dry-powder inhaler. To ensure that the proper dose of medication gets into a child's lungs, doctors might also prescribe a device called a spacer, or holding chamber which attaches to the inhaler. Spacers are helpful in younger children who have difficulty with the timing and coordination needed to use an inhaler.

5-IN-1 PEDIATRIC VACCINE

QUESTION: I heard about a new pediatric vaccine that reduces the number of shots my child may need. What can you tell me about it?

ANSWER: The FDA recently approved the first 5-in-1 pediatric combination vaccine for protection against diphtheria, tetanus, pertussis, poliomyelitis, and Haemophilus influenzae type b. Diphtheria is a contagious, sometimes, fatal, infection of the upper respiratory tract. Tetanus (lockjaw) is a disease caused by a bacterial neurotoxin that produces severe muscle spasms. Pertussis (whooping cough) is a highly contagious bacterial infection, which results in fits of coughing that usually end in a prolonged, high-pitched, deeply indrawn breath (the whoop). Polio is also a highly contagious, sometimes fatal, viral infection that affects nerves and can produce permanent muscle weakness, paralysis, and other symptoms. Haemophilus influenzae type b can cause serious disease such as meningitis and infection in the bloodstream. The new vaccine, Pentacel, was approved for use in infants and children 6 weeks through 4 years of age (prior to fifth birthday). The vaccine is administered as a four-dose series at 2, 4, 6, and 15-18 months of age. According to the current Recommended Childhood Immunization Schedule of the U.S. Centers for Disease Control and Prevention (CDC), up to 23 injections are needed by the time a child reaches 18 months of age with single vaccines. The use of Pentacel vaccine could reduce the number of shots by seven. The most common side effects of Pentacel include injection site redness, swelling, and tenderness; fever; fussiness and crying.

VACCINE FOR INFECTIONS

QUESTION: I heard about a new vaccine that helps prevent infections in children. What can you tell me about it?

ANSWER: The recently approved vaccine is named Prevar and it will help to prevent a number of infections in young children. It is not used to treat infections, only to prevent them. This new vaccine contains seven different substances (antigens) from bacteria called Streptococcus pneumoniae, which stimulate the children to produce antibodies to fight off infections. The safety and effectiveness of Prevar was demonstrated in several clinical studies, including one involving over 38,000 children. In this large study, the vaccine was found to be 100% effective in preventing infections caused by bacteria that it was designed to prevent (pneumococcal bacteria). These bacteria can cause many well known infections including pneumonia, upper respiratory tract infections, blood stream infections, and meningitis. Children under five years old are very susceptible to these infections, which can cause severe complications and even death. It is hoped that this new vaccine will not only prevent serious infections, but may also cut down on the spread of bacteria that become resistant to antibiotic treatment. It may also reduce the incidence of recurring ear infections in children and reduce the need for ear tubes to treat chronic infections. Because of its effectiveness in preventing infections, the Center for Disease Control & Prevention recommends that Prevar be used in all infants up to 23 months in age. They also recommend its use in certain older children (ages 2 to 5) who may be at higher risk for infection. For infants, the vaccine immunization requires a series of four shots, given at approximately 2 months, 4 months, 6 months, and 12 to 15 months of age. The most common side effects of Prevar include pain and swelling at the site of injection, fever, irritability, drowsiness, restless sleep, and decreased appetite.

ZINGO

QUESTION: I heard about a new product that prevents pain in children requiring a needle insertion procedure. What can you tell me about it?

ANSWER: The FDA recently approved Zingo, a new and innovative product to reduce pain associated with needle insertion procedures in children. Zingo provides rapid, topical, local analgesia to reduce the pain associated with intravenous insertions or blood draws, in children ages 3 to 18. It contains the local anesthetic lidocaine, which numbs the skin within one to three minutes after use. Zingo is a needle-free system that uses compressed gas to speed the delivery of lidocaine into the skin. Currently available local anesthetics commonly take 20 minutes or longer to numb the insertion area. In clinical trials, children treated with Zingo prior to needle insertion had significantly less pain than children who did not receive Zingo. During these studies, Zingo was also well tolerated and was associated with a low incidence of skin reactions such as redness, swelling, and itching. Intravenous insertions and blood draws are among the most common interventions performed at a hospital, with more than 18 million pediatric needle insertion procedures done in the United States each year. Needlesticks are also a source of deep anxiety in children. A recent survey found that 70% of children experience fear and stress during a visit to the doctor or hospital that involves a needlestick procedure, and more than half of all children cry during these procedures. This problem is compounded in children with chronic illnesses who must undergo frequent intravenous insertions. The manufacturer of Zingo is also studying its use in adults. In the future there may also be opportunities to use this needle-free delivery system for other drugs such as insulin.

COUGH, COLD, AND FLU PRODUCTS

QUESTION: Why did the FDA recommend that nonprescription cough and cold products not be used in children under 2 years of age?

ANSWER: The FDA recently issued a Public Health Advisory for parents and caregivers strongly recommending that over-the-counter (OTC) cough and cold products should not be used to treat infants and children less than 2 years of age, because serious and potentially life-threatening side effects can occur from such use. These OTC cough and cold products include decongestants, expectorants, antihistamines, and cough suppressants for the treatment of colds. There are a wide variety of rare, serious adverse events reported with cough and cold products including death, convulsions, rapid heart rates, and decreased levels of consciousness. In view of these potential side effects, OTC cough and cold products are not considered safe or effective in children under 2. This FDA announcement does not include a final recommendation for using these products in children 2 to 11 years of age, which is under review. The FDA plans to issue its recommendations on using OTC cough and cold medicines in children 2 to 11 years of age as soon as the review is complete. Meanwhile, it is recommended that parents and caregivers that choose to use these products in children 2 to 11 years of age should do the following:

- Follow the dosing directions on the label of any OTC medication,
- Understand that these drugs will NOT cure or shorten the duration of the common cold,
- Check the "Drug Facts" label to learn what active ingredients are in the products because many OTC cough and cold products contain multiple active ingredients, and
- Only use measuring spoons or cups that come with the medicine or those made specially for measuring drugs

QUESTION: Why were baby cold medications pulled from the market?

ANSWER: Recently, the makers of infant nonprescription cough and cold products voluntarily recalled certain medicines for infants and toddlers under the age of 2. The products removed from the market contain antihistamines, decongestants, expectorants, or antitussives that can cause serious side effects or even death if not dosed correctly. In addition, many say that there is little evidence that these medicines are effective in young children. Last month the FDA released a lengthy report that suggested the use of some of the medications had been linked to serious side effects and some deaths in children, many of whom were under the age of 2 and received an unintentional overdose. The American Academy of Pediatrics has also warned that kids' cough and cold products are not safe or effective for kids under 6. Products involved in this recall include: Concentrated Infants' Tylenol Drops Plus Cold; Concentrated Infants' Tylenol Drops Plus Cold & Cough; Pediacare Infant Drops Decongestant; Pediacare Infant Drops Decongestant & Cough; Pediacare Infant Dropper Decongestant; Pediacare Infant Dropper Long-Acting Cough; Pediacare Infant

Dropper Decongestant & Cough; Dimetapp Decongestant Plus Cough Infant Drops; Dimetapp Decongestant Infant Drops; Little Colds Decongestant Plus Cough; Little Colds Multi-Symptom Cold Formula; Robitussin Infant Cough DM Drops; Triaminic Infant & Toddler Thin Strips Decongestant; and Triaminic Infant & Toddler Thin Strips Decongestant Plus Cough. CVS Caremark Corporation also said it would end its sales of the CVS-brand equivalent products. The recall does not affect products intended and labeled for use in children age 2 and older. The FDA is, however, considering banning the use of over-the-counter cold medications in children under age 6.

QUESTION: What can you tell me about new warnings for kids taking flu drugs?

ANSWER: Recently the FDA's Pediatric Advisory Committee recommended that stronger warnings be placed on labels of the antiviral flu medicines, Tamiflu and Relenza, due to concerns about potential psychiatric side effects in children. About 700 cases (mostly in Japan) of psychiatric side effects such as delirium, delusions, or hallucinations have been reported with these drugs. While no fatalities have been reported for Relenza, 25 cases of pediatric deaths were reported for Tamiflu, with 3 of the deaths occurring in the United States. In Japan, 5 children died after falling from windows or balconies, or running into traffic according to the FDA. In view of these reports, FDA advisers have recommended a stronger warning label for Tamiflu to note the patient deaths. For Relenza, addition of a warning about hallucinations and delirium is recommended. The manufacturers of these flu medications are opposed to the label changes because it is very difficult to tell if the side effects are due to the drugs or the flu itself. Approximately 48 million people worldwide have taken Tamiflu since it was approved in 1999. Relenza has been used by about 4 million people since it was marketed in 1999. Relenza is an inhaled product that delivers the antiviral medication to the lungs, and Tamiflu is given orally. The flu virus is a major cause of death and illness the United States. Complications from the illness kill about 36,000 Americans a year, with children and the elderly especially at risk.

RINGWORM

<u>QUESTION</u>: My child has a ringworm infection on his upper arm. What can I use to treat it?

<u>ANSWER</u>: Ringworm is not caused by a worm, but is actually an infection of the skin caused by a fungus called tinea. If the infection involves the body (usually the trunk, face, and upper extremities) it is named "tinea corporis", and if it involves the scalp it is named "tinea capitis". These infections often appear as a round or oval shaped lesion with an outer red margin. The inside of the lesion frequently appears to be healthy skin, while the outer margin is inflamed, red, and scaly, The circular lesion gives the appearance that a worm is circling beneath the skin, hence the name "ringworm". When the skin is broken down by moisture and friction it's prone to infection from fungi, thus there is a higher incidence of this infection among people living in humid climates. Ringworm of the body can be contracted by contact with an infected animal, infected soil or infected person. This infection is more common in people who participate in activities such as gardening, contact sports, and grooming pets. Children can contract the fungus by playing with a stray cat or dog. Person to person infection is more likely to occur whenever people are in close proximity to one another, like in families or in day care centers. Outbreaks have also occurred in athletic teams, such as wrestlers, where the infection involves the arms, trunk, head, and neck where closest contact occurs. When infection spreads this way in athletes, it's nicknamed "tinea corporis gladiatorum". The number of itchy skin lesions in people infected with ringworm of the body may be one to twenty or more.

While ringworm of the body can be stubborn and difficult to get rid of, a number of effective nonprescription antifungal products are available for use. Some antifungal products include:

Product (Active Antifungal Ingredient)
* Desenex (undecylenic acid and zinc undecylenate)
* Cruex (undecylenic acid and zinc undecylenate)
* Tinactin (tolnaftate)
* Aftate (tolnaftate)
* Mycelex OTC (clotrimazole)

- Lotrimin AF Clotrimazole)
- Micatin (miconazole)

Antifungal products should be applied in the morning and at night, ideally after a shower or bath. Reapply the product after activities such as swimming or exercising. If the condition fails to clear up in four weeks, a physician should be consulted. These products should be only used as directed on their labels and should not be used on children younger than two years of age. Some people will notice that their symptoms (itching, pain, cracked skin) may go away after several days and stop using the product. However, ringworm infections may reoccur if they are not treated long enough (four to six weeks). Various other treatments for ringworm are also available upon prescription by a doctor.

HEAD LICE

QUESTION: I heard about a new prescription treatment for head lice. What can you tell me about it?

ANSWER: The FDA recently (2012) approved Sklice Topical Lotion (ivermectin) for the treatment of head lice in patients 6 months of age and older. Sklice contains an antiparasitic agent that binds with certain channels carrying chloride ions into the nerve and muscle cells of the head lice, leading to paralysis and death of the parasite. During clinical studies, a single 10-minute application of Sklice Topical Lotion eliminated head lice in about 75% of people treated without the need for nit combing in most patients. The most common side effects of Sklice Topical Lotion are inflammation of the eyelids, redness in the eye, eye irritation, dandruff, dry skin, and a skin-burning sensation.

Head lice (Pediculus capitis) is a very common problem with 6 to 12 million people becoming infested with head lice in the U.S. each year. The vast majority of these cases involve children 1-12 years of age. Outbreaks are common in crowded places such as schools, day care centers, and nursing homes. Anyone with hair can get it. Head lice is easy to get but can be difficult to get rid of, making it a real hassle for parents. Lice are tiny parasites that bite the scalp and suck the victim's blood causing irritation and itching, usually in the hair around the ears or nape of the neck-but it can occur anywhere on the head. If left untreated, infections and inflammation can occur. Potential ways of getting head lice include the following:

- Close personal contact (head to head)
- Sharing head phones, helmets, hats, hair ribbons, hair brushes or combs
- Switching headrests, movie seats, or car seats
- Sharing pillows or beds
- Sharing towels

If you would like more information you can contact the National Pediculosis Association, P.O. Box 610189, Newton, MA 02161; (617)449-NITS. Or, if you're on the Internet: **www.headlice.org** or **// kidshealth.org/parent/healthy/infection.html**

QUESTION: I heard about a new prescription treatment for head lice. What can you tell me about it?

ANSWER: The FDA recently approved Natroba (spinosad) topical suspension for the treatment of head lice in patients 4 years of age and older. Natroba works to kill head lice in an interesting way. It causes muscle contractions and excites the central nervous system in insects, which results in paralysis and death of the parasites that cause head lice. During clinical studies, Natroba eliminated head lice in about 85% of people treated. Natroba is easily applied to the scalp and scalp hair and is left on for ten minutes prior to rinsing with warm water. Once Natroba is rinsed off, a fine-tooth comb may be used to remove dead lice and nits from the hair and scalp, but combing is not required. If live lice are seen one week (7 days) after the first application, Natroba should be used again. The most common side effect of Natroba is redness at the site of application.

QUESTION: My 8-year old son was sent home from school because of head lice. What can I do to get rid of it?

ANSWER: The treatment of head lice involves 3 steps. Step 1 is to kill existing lice in the hair. Several good non-prescription products are available for this use including Rid, Pronto, A-200, and Nix. All of these products kill lice by getting into their pores and attacking their nervous system leading to death. However, lice pores will close when wet and so shampoo products must be applied to dry hair to be effective. In addition, freshly laid lice eggs known as "nits" will not be killed because their nervous system is not developed. Because of this, a second shampooing process 7 to 10 days after the first treatment may be necessary to kill this group of mature nits. You should carefully follow the directions for use with each product. Some general instructions for shampoo products are to remove your son's shirt and use a towel to cover his eyes. The shampoo should be applied beginning at the roots of the hair and progress out to the tips. Make sure all hair is saturated, then massage the shampoo into the scalp. After the recommended time (usually about 10 minutes), add enough warm water to produce lathering and rinse thoroughly. Any lice should be combed out along with tangles using a comb.

Step 2 involves removing the nits, which can be a tedious and time consuming job. The nits are attached to the hair with a cement-like substance and therefore must be removed using a special fine-toothed comb, which comes with many of the treatment products. Hair should be combed in small sections, beginning at the scalp at the top of the head, working with about a half inch of hair at a time and keeping the teeth of the nit comb deep in the hair to increase effectiveness.

Step 3 is to avoid reinfestation by cleansing the home environment. Lice can live without a blood meal for about 2 days (nits up to 10 days), living in upholstery, bed pillows, carpets, clothes or even car seats. Any item that is washable should be washed in hot water for at least 15 minutes. Upholstery and car seats should be thoroughly vacuumed and the vacuum bag carefully thrown away. Exposing items to sunlight for several hours can also help to kill surviving lice and nits. Any hair accessories should be soaked in hot water for at least 15 minutes or thrown away. Toys or items that cannot be washed should be placed in a sealed plastic bag and stored outside the home for 2 weeks. Parents should check the hair for lice daily and avoiding the types of contacts noted earlier must be followed.

If you would like more information you can contact the National Pediculosis Association, P.O. Box 610189, Newton, MA 02161; (617)449-NITS. Or, if you're on the Internet :**www.headlice.org** or **// kidshealth.org/parent/healthy/infection.html**

QUESTION: I heard that a new prescription drug was approved for head lice. What can you tell me about it?

ANSWER: The FDA recently approved benzyl alcohol lotion 5% (Ulesfia) for the topical treatment of head lice infestation in people 6 months of age and older. It is a unique prescription product that kills head lice by asphyxiation. In order to survive, lice breathe through sophisticated spiracles that close upon contact with most liquids, allowing the lice to go into suspended animation and survive for hours without breathing. This new lotion prevents lice from closing their spiracles, thereby asphyxiating them within 10 minutes and causing their death. In clinical studies, 75% of people treated with benzyl alcohol lotion were lice free 2 weeks after the final treatment. Benzyl alcohol lotion is applied to dry hair, using enough to completely saturate the scalp and hair. It is rinsed off with water after 10 minutes and the treatment is repeated in 7 days. Once the lotion is washed off, a fine-tooth comb may be used to remove treated lice and nits from the hair and scalp. All personal items exposed to the hair or lice should be washed in hot soap or dry-cleaned. Common side effects of this medication include irritations of the skin, scalp, and eye, and numbness at the site of application. Benzyl alcohol lotion appears to be an effective first line treatment for head lice and does not have the potential to produce neurotoxic side effects of some other lice medications.

IMPETIGO

QUESTION: I heard about a new prescription drug for impetigo. What can you tell me about it?

ANSWER: The FDA recently approved Altabax, a new antibiotic ointment for the topical treatment of impetigo in adults and pediatric patients at least nine months of age. Impetigo is a common and highly contagious skin infection caused by bacteria. The infection leads to the formation of scabby, yellow-crusted itchy sores and, sometimes, small blisters filled with yellow fluid. Impetigo is most common among infants and children ages 2 to 6 years. Children are especially susceptible to infections because their immune systems are still developing. The itching caused by impetigo often leads to extensive scratching, especially in children, which helps to spread the infection. The infection can spread easily in schools and childcare settings, as well as anywhere groups of people are in close contact. Altabax ointment is the first new type of topical antibiotic to be approved by the FDA in almost 20 years. It is applied to affected areas of the skin twice a day for 5 days. During clinical study Altabax ointment was found to be effective in treating impetigo in about 86% of patients with this infection. Because Altabax ointment contains a new type of antibiotic that works against bacteria in a different way than other antibiotics, it may have a lower potential for antibiotic resistance, which has become a major public health concern. Resistance occurs when bacteria change in a way that reduces or prevents effective treatment with antibiotics. Over the past decade, almost all types of bacteria have become stronger and less responsive to antibiotics.

CHICKENPOX

QUESTION: My eight-year-old son has chickenpox. What can be used for treatment?

ANSWER: Chickenpox is a common and highly contagious disease caused by a virus called the varicella-zoster virus, which strikes most often in children between the ages of five and nine. This same virus can also cause a very painful skin condition later in life known as herpes zoster or shingles. If one child develops chickenpox, about 90% of others in the household who have never had the disease will develop it. About 95% of adults in the U.S. have had chickenpox. Most cases of chickenpox occur between January and May, often during epidemics that go through schools or neighborhoods. Chickenpox is highly contagious and can be spread by direct contact, droplets or through the air. It is usually mild but can cause serious problems. The rash from chickenpox is very itchy and can become infected if scratched. It usually takes about 11 to 21 days for the rash to occur after exposure to the virus. Children are contagious from about two days before the rash appears until scabs are produced, which normally takes 4-6 days. Once children have had chickenpox they are immune to getting it again. However, as I noted earlier, the virus can become active again later in life after a stressful event and cause shingles. About 24 hours before the rash appears, a child may develop a low fever, lose his or her appetite and feel tired. When the rash appears, it quickly spreads from a flat red rash to clear blisters that look like "tear drops". After about 24 hours, these blisters turn from clear to cloudy, then easily break open and a dry scab opens. New groups of the rash appear over the next 3 to 4 days with the rash usually spreading from the body to the face and scalp.

The treatment of chickenpox includes lowering any fever and controlling the itch to prevent infection. To treat a child's fever only non-aspirin products, such as acetaminophen (Tylenol), should be used. Oral antihistamines, such as Benadryl, given every 4-6 hours as needed, can help the itching. Topical drying agents such as calamine lotion can also be applied. In young children, keeping the fingernails short and using mittens at bedtime may also help to reduce scratching. Clothes and bed linens should be changed daily, and frequent baths using a drying agent, such as colloidal oatmeal, may have a soothing effect. The prescription of an antiviral agent called acyclovir may also be needed in some cases. The best treatment is avoiding exposure to someone with chickenpox. A new varicella virus vaccine is also available and is recommended for children aged 12 months through 12 years who have never had chickenpox.

TNF BLOCKERS & CANCER IN CHILDREN

QUESTION: I heard that some arthritis drugs can raise the cancer risk in children. What can you tell me about this?

ANSWER: The FDA recently issued an Alert that it is requiring stronger warnings regarding the risk for cancer in children and adolescents who are taking drugs known as tumor necrosis factor (TNF) blockers for the treatment of juvenile rheumatoid arthritis, Crohns disease, and other inflammatory diseases. These drugs block the overproduction of a protein, which can cause inflammation and damage to bones, cartilage, and tissue. TNF blockers are given by injection and include Remicade, Enbrel, Humira, Cimzia, and Simponi. The FDA's Alert was based upon an analysis of U.S. reports of cancer in children and adolescents treated with TNF blockers that showed an increased risk of cancer, occurring after an average of 30 months of treatment. About half of the cancers were lymphomas, a type of cancer involving the immune system and some of the reported cancers were fatal. Psoriasis is also associated with the use of TNF blockers, and this information will be incorporated into the updated prescribing information. The FDA issued the following information for patients receiving TNF blockers:

- Be aware that taking TNF blockers may increase the risk of developing lymphoma, leukemia, and other cancers.
- Be aware that taking TNF blockers may increase the risk of developing psoriasis and may worsen pre-existing psoriasis.
- Review the Medication Guide that accompanies TNF blockers.
- Do not stop or change medicines that have been prescribed without first talking with a knowledgeable healthcare professional.
- Pay close attention for any signs or symptoms of cancer such as unexplained weight loss or fatigue, swollen lymph nodes in the neck, underarms or groin, or easy bruising or bleeding. Promptly discuss any signs and symptoms with a healthcare professional.
- Pay close attention for any signs or symptoms of new onset psoriasis or worsening psoriasis such as red scaly patches or raised bumps on the skin that are filled with pus.

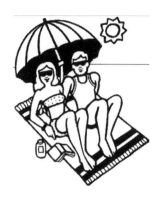

CHAPTER 7
SKIN CARE

BURNS

<u>QUESTION</u>: I occasionally burn my hand on the stove. What should I do when this happens?

<u>ANSWER</u>: The treatment of any burn is based upon how severe the burn is. First degree burns are the least serious and only affect the outermost layer of skin. These burns produce skin redness, mild swelling, tenderness, and pain. A common example of a first degree burn is sunburn. Cooling the skin is the fastest and best way to stop the burning and reduce damage to the skin. For first degree burns that do not involve a large area of the body (like your hand), pain can be relieved by placing the burned area in cold water or by applying a wet, cold cloth. If cold water is not available, any cold liquid clean enough to drink can be used. This cooling treatment should be continued until the burn is pain free in and out of the water (usually 10 to 45 minutes). Other tips to keep in mind for minor burns are:

- In order to avoid frostbite, do not use an ice pack or put ice on the burned area.

314

- Antibiotic ointments like bacitracin can be used once the pain has gone away, but do not cover the burn with a dressing.
- Do not apply any type of unsterile ointments or balms to the burn.
- Use aspirin or ibuprofen for pain relief.
- Drink plenty of liquids, since burns can cause a loss of water.

Second degree burns are more serious because they involve both the outer and inner layer of skin. These burns produce blisters, swelling, weeping of fluids, and severe pain. Like first degree burns, the therapy for second degree burns involves cold treatment as noted earlier. In addition, keep these tips in mind:

- Do not attempt to break blisters—they are nature's burn dressing. If blisters break open, apply a thin layer of antibiotic ointment and a dry nonstick sterile dressing.
- Never use plastic to cover a burn because it traps moisture and can lead to infection.
- Wash the area gently with lukewarm water and a mild soap. Change the dressing once or twice a day.
- Keep burned arms or legs elevated to reduce swelling.

Third degree burns affect all skin layers and can damage fat and muscle under the skin. They are severe burns and always require medical attention. If the burned skin looks leathery, charred, or pearly gray, it is a third degree burn. In addition, if nerves are damaged by the burn, pain may not be present. Remember, only first degree and some second degree burns should be treated at home.

DERMATITIS/INCONTINENCE

QUESTION: My husband has to wear adult diapers and sometimes gets a rash. What can I do for this problem?

ANSWER: Diaper rash (also called dermatitis) is usually only thought of as a problem with infants. However, more than 12 million adults are incontinent and are also at risk from diaper rash. The cause of this problem is the same in infants and adults. The occlusive nature of a diaper prevents the evaporation of moisture from the surface of the skin, which causes softening and leads to a breakdown of the skin. Wet skin breaks down easier than dry skin when there is friction caused by a diaper rubbing against the skin. In addition, moist skin makes it easier for bacteria to grow. Since feces contain over 10 billion bacteria per milligram (a very small amount) of dried stool, the opportunity for infection in the damaged skin is very great. Feces also contain enzymes that can damage the skin and urine can further irritate the skin. All areas of skin that are in close contact with the diaper are likely to develop a rash. Thus, the buttocks, upper thighs, lower abdomen and genitalia are commonly affected. Mild cases of diaper rash appear as shiny patches of red skin, while more severe cases can result in eroded areas of skin and infection.

The prevention of diaper rash primarily involves keeping the skin dry and keeping urine and feces from mixing together. The best preventative is frequent diaper changes especially as soon as possible after urination or a bowel movement. The area covered by the diaper should be cleansed with mild soap and water and allowed to air dry before applying the next diaper. Skin protectants are the safest method for treating diaper rash. These products include ingredients such as allantoin, calamine, cod liver oil, dimethicone, kaolin, lanolin, mineral oil, petrolatum, talc, cornstarch, white petrolatum, and zinc oxide. Many other compounds have been used to treat diaper rash but their safety or effectiveness have not been proven. Your pharmacist can assist you in selecting an appropriate product containing one or more of these ingredients. Powders containing kaolin, cornstarch or talc should not be used on broken skin. Broken skin is more likely to be infected with bacteria or fungi and proper treatment requires a physician. Most commercial diaper wipes should be avoided during an active case of diaper rash, because they may contain soap or other chemicals that irritate the skin.

The second most common reason for institutionalizing elderly patients is incontinence. Men are found to be more likely than women to develop incontinence-related skin irritations, probably because women are more likely than men to use preparations to prevent such problems. More information on incontinence and its prevention can be obtained from: The National Association for Continence (P.O. Box 8310, Spartanburg, SC 29305—1-800-BLADDER) or The Simon Foundation for Continence (P.O. Box 815, Wilmette, IL 60091—1-800-12SIMON)

SEBORRHEIC DERMATITIS

QUESTION: I heard about a new prescription medication used to treat seborrheic dermatitis. What can you tell me about it?

ANSWER: Seborrheic dermatitis is a common inflammatory skin disease characterized by a red, scaly, itchy rash that primarily occurs on the face, scalp, hairline, eyebrows, and trunk. Approximately 8.5 million people in the United States suffer from this condition that often recurs. This skin disorder usually begins gradually, causing dry or greasy scaling of the scalp (dandruff), sometimes with itching but not hair loss. In more severe cases, yellowish to reddish scaly pimples appear along the hairline, behind the ears, in the ear canal, on the eyebrows, on the bridge of the nose, around the nose, on the chest, and on the upper back. Seborrheic dermatitis is common in infants and affects 2-5% of adults, more commonly men. It is usually more severe in winter and is commonly found in people with Parkinson's disease, zinc deficiency, and people with AIDS. The cause of seborrheic dermatitis is not well understood, but there is evidence that a yeast like fungus may be involved.

There is no way to prevent or cure seborrheic dermatitis, but it can be controlled. In adults, the scalp can be treated with a shampoo containing one or more of these ingredients: pyrithione zinc; selenium sulfide; sulfur; an antifungal drug; salicyclic acid; or coal tar. The scalp should be shampooed several times per week. Topical mild corticosteroids like hydrocortisone 0.5% to 1% cream or lotion can also be used effectively on the head and other affected areas. The use of topical hydrocortisone, however, should not exceed 7 days. The new prescription product that you heard about to treat seborrheic dermatitis in adults and children over 12 is Xolegel. It is a topical gel that contains the antifungal drug ketoconazole. In a large clinical study, Xolegel applied once daily was effective in treating patients with moderate to severe seborrheic dermatitis. Results from this study showed that about 25% of patients treated with Xolegel were cleared or almost cleared of seborrheic dermatitis after 14 days, compared to about 14% of patients not treated. Xolegel also improved skin redness, scaling, and reduced itching. Your physician or dermatologist can determine which treatment is best for you.

DRUGS AND PHOTOSENSITIVITY

<u>QUESTION</u>: My heart medication, Cordarone, makes me sensitive to the sun and I seem to burn even with sunscreen. Is there any medication comparable to Cordarone that does not have this side effect?

<u>ANSWER</u>: Cordarone (generic name amiodarone—pronounced a mee oh da rone) is an antiarrhythmic drug that is used to treat various types of abnormal heart rhythms. There are many different types of drugs that are used to treat abnormal heart rhythms, which result from a disturbance in the electrical impulses that spread through the heart. Antiarrhythmic drugs are grouped into four different classes depending upon how they work. Cordarone is called a class 3 antiarrhythmic because it mainly works on the heart in between beats to affect its rhythm. As you noted, one of the side effects of this drug is that it increases your sensitivity to sunlight (photosensitivity). This side effect occurs in about 10% of people taking the drug. Individuals who experience this effect seem to be particularly sensitive to long wave ultraviolet-A (UVA) light, and may get sunburned even through glass windows and/or cotton clothing. Sunscreens will not prevent this effect unless they absorb UVA light. Opaquing sunscreens that produce a physical barrier to the sun will, however, provide adequate protection. These screens usually contain zinc oxide or titanium dioxide. A couple of examples of products with these ingredients are RVPaque and Hawaiian Tropic Protective Tanning. Avoidance of exposure to the sun and protective clothing should be used to help prevent this side effect. If taken over a long period of time, Cordarone may also infrequently produce a blue-gray skin discoloration, which may be more likely to

occur in people with fair skin, or those with frequent, unprotected exposure to sunlight. This effect may go away slowly when the drug is stopped. A new class 3 antiarrhythmic drug named Stedicor (generic name azimilide) should be available in the near future, but I'm not sure if it causes photosensitivity or if it would be the right medication for you. Be sure to discuss this problem with your cardiologist.

QUESTION: A few weeks ago a reader asked about a drug that made her more sensitive to the sun. What other drugs can do this?

ANSWER: Numerous medications can make a person more sensitive to the sun causing sunburn, a side effect known as photosensitivity. A listing of some of the more commonly used oral medications that can cause this side effect can be found on the following pages.

Some Medications That Can Cause Photosensitivity
Generic Name (Trade Name(s))
Acetazolamide (Diamox)
Acetohexamide (Dymelor)
Acitretin (Soriatane)
Amantadine (Symmetrel)
Amiodarone (Cordarone)
Amitriptyline (Elavil, Endep)
Amoxapine (Asendin)
Azithromycin (Zithromax)
Butabarbital (Butisol, Buticaps)
Captopril (Capoten)
Carbamazepine (Carbatrol, Tegretol)
Chloroquine (Aralen)
Chlorpromazine (Thorazine)
Chlorpropamide (Diabinese)
Chlorthalidone (Hygroton)
Ciprofloxacin (Cipro)
Clomipramine (Anafranil)
Co-trimoxazole (Bactrim, Septra)
Danazol (Danocrine)
Dantrolene (Dantrium)
Demeclocycline (Declomycin)

Desipramine (Norpramin)
Diflunisal (Dolobid)
Diphenhydramine (Benadryl)
Doxepin (Sinequan)
Doxycycline (Atridox, Doryx, Doxy, Monodox, Periostat, Vibramycin)
Ethinyl Estradiol or Norethindrone (Numerous birth control products)
Felbamate (Felbatol)
Flucytosine (Ancobon)
Fluphenazine (Prolixin)
Flurbiprofen (Ansaid, Ocufen)
Flutamide (Eulexin)
Furosemide (Lasix)
Glipizide (Glucotrol, Glucotrol XL)
Glyburide (DiaBeta, Glynase, Micronase)
Griseofulvin (Fulvicin P/G, Fluvicin U/F, Grifulvin V, Grisactin, Gris-PEG)
Haloperidol (Haldol)
Hydrochlorothiazide (Esidrex, HydroDIURIL, Microzide, Oretic)
Ibuprofen (Advil, Motrin, Nuprin, Rufen)
Imipramine (Tofranil)
Indapamide (Lozol)
Isotretinoin (Accutane)
Ketoprofen (Actron, Orudis, Oruvail)
Levofloxacin (Levaquin)
Lomefloxacin (Maxaquin)
Loxapine (Loxitane)
Maprotiline (Ludiomil)
Methotrexate (Rheumatrex)
Methyldopa (Aldomet)
Metolazone (Mykrox, Zaroxolyn)
Minocycline (Minocin)
Nabumetone (Relafen)
Naproxen (Aleve, Anaprox, Naprelan, Napron X, Naprosyn)
Nifedipine (Procardia, Procardia XL, Adalat CC)
Norfloxacin (Noroxin)
Nortriptyline (Aventyl, Pamelor)
Ofloxacin (Floxin, Ocuflox)

Oxaprozin (Daypro)
Perphenazine (Trilafon)
Phenelzine (Nardil)
Phenobarbital
Piroxicam (Feldene)
Prochlorperazine (Compazine)
Promethazine (Phenergan)
Protriptyline (Vivactil)
Quinidine (Cardioquin, Quinidex, Quinaglute)
Risperidone (Risperdal)
Secobarbital (Seconal)
Sulfamethoxazole (Gantanol)
Sulfasalazine (Azulfidine)
Sulfisoxazole (Gantrisin)
Tetracycline (Sumycin, Topicycline)
Thiethylperazine (Torecan)
Thioridazine (Mellaril)
Thiothixene (Navane)
Tolazamide (Tolinase)
Tolbutamide (Orinase)
Trazodone (Desyrel)
Triamterene (Dyrenium)
Trifluoperazine (Stelazine)
Trimethoprim (Proloprim, Primsol)
Valproic Acid (Depakene, Depakote

SUNSCREENS

QUESTION: I love going to the beach but I worry about too much sun exposure and use various sunscreen products. What's the difference between these products and what does "SPF" mean?

ANSWER: I too love the sun and that is a big reason why my wife and I moved to Florida, the Sunshine State. Skin cancer, however, is definitely a concern with too much sun exposure. In the United States, the incidence of skin cancer has more than doubled in the past 20 years, making it the most common of all cancers. Non-melanoma skin cancers, including squamous cell and basal cell carcinoma, occur most frequently but when diagnosed at an early stage can almost always be cured. Malignant melanomas are far more serious and their incidence has been increasing at a startling rate. In the U.S., the lifetime risk of developing malignant melanoma is 1 in 1,500 for those born in 1935 compared to 1 in 105 for those born in 1991. These figures should get everyone's attention. Fair skinned people with red, blonde, or brown hair, light colored eyes, and freckles, who always burn and never tan are at a higher risk for skin cancer than others. A history of severe blistering sunburns during childhood and adolescence may also make a person more likely to get skin cancer.

Sunlight consists of many types of radiation, but ultraviolet (UV) light rays are responsible for most of the harmful effects on the skin, including skin wrinkling, cataracts, and skin cancer. Two types of UV sunlight reach the earth, A and B (UVA and UVB). About 5% to 10% is UVB and 90% to 95% is UVA but both can increase the risk of skin cancer. In addition, artificial sources of UV light can also cause skin damage. In order to decrease the risk of skin cancer, people should stay out of the sun, wear protective clothing, and use sunscreen products. In the U.S., the ABCs of sun protection are Away from sun, Block the sun, and Cover up. In Australia they are promoting a skin cancer prevention campaign called SLIP, SLOP, and SLAP—slip on clothing, slop on sunscreen, and slap on a hat.

Sunscreen products contain substances that either absorb, reflect, or scatter UV radiation and prevent it from entering the skin. There are two basic types—chemical sunscreens and physical sunscreens. Chemical sunscreens block UV radiation (UVA, UVB, or both) by absorbing the radiation. Numerous chemical ingredients are used in these products such as PABA (para-aminobenzoic acid), cinnamic acid derivatives, salicylic acid derivatives, benophenone derivatives, and many others. Physical sunscreen products on the other hand do not absorb UV radiation but instead reflect or scatter the light. One of their advantages is that they may not cause skin sensitivity reactions like chemical sunscreens. However, they may cause acne or heat rash, are messy, and are not cosmetically appealing. They are very useful for limited sun-sensitive areas like the nose, ears, and lips. Commonly used ingredients in these products are zinc oxide, titanium dioxide, talc, kaolin, red petrolatum, and many others. The sun protection factor or SPF indicates the amount of protection for a given product. This number basically tells how much longer than usual a person can stay in the sun without burning. For example, if someone can stay in the sun unprotected without burning for 15 minutes, a sunscreen product with SPF 4 extends this time period to 1 hour. A sunscreen product with an SPF of 15 blocks about 93% of UV radiation, while an SPF 30 sunscreen blocks 97%, and an SPF 60 sunscreen blocks 98%. Most "water-resistant" products will retain their protective effect for at least 40 minutes in water and most "waterproof" sunscreens remain effective for at least 80 minutes in water. It is recommended that sunscreen should be applied generously to all exposed areas 30 minutes before skin exposure and reapplied every 2 to 3 hours and after swimming or sweating. Remember to SLIP, SLOP and SLAP when enjoying the sun.

QUESTION: I heard about a new type of sunscreen product. What can you tell me about it?

ANSWER: The FDA recently approved Anthelios SX, a sunscreen made by L'Oreal, that offers protection from both ultraviolet A (UVA) and ultraviolet B (UVB). It will be sold over-the-counter as a daily moisturizing cream with sunscreen. What is new about this product is that it contains an ingredient called ecamsule that shields skin from the UVA radiation, which penetrates deeper into the skin than UVB. According to some experts, UVB causes sunburn and skin cancer, while UVA causes aging (wrinkles) in addition to some skin cancers. Furthermore, ecampsule does not break down quickly in the sun like some other sunscreens and provides longer protection against UVA. However no sunscreen completely protects people against UVA and UVB radiation and the FDA continues to recognize that in addition to using a sunscreen, consumers should protect themselves from sun exposure by limiting time in the sun and wearing protective clothing. Anthelios SX contains two additional sunscreens (avobenzone and octocrylene) and has a sun protection factor (SPF) of 15, which primarily measures UVB protection. The SPF number basically tells how much longer than usual a person can stay in the sun without burning. A comparable index to protection from UVA radiation has yet to be developed. The safety and effectiveness of Anthelios SX included information from 28 studies in over 2,500 people, ranging in age from six months to over 65 years old. The most common side effects of this product during clinical studies included acne, dermatitis, dry skin, eczema, abnormal redness, itching skin discomfort, and sunburn. This new sunscreen has not previously been marketed in the U.S., but has been available in Europe and Canada as Mexoryl SX since 1993. Anthelios SX has also been shown to be more effective in protecting against irregular pigmentation caused by sun exposure. Some dermatologists say that people with darker skin, including African Americans and Latinos, will experience a more even skin tone and fewer lines with the new sunscreen. Anthelios SX is expected to cost about twice as much as traditional sunscreens. Your dermatologist can help determine whether this new sunscreen is the best choice for you. Skin cancer is the most common of all cancers. Melanoma accounts for only 4% of skin cancer cases but the most cancer deaths, and the number of new melanoma cases is on the rise. This year there will be about 62,000 new cases of melanoma nationwide, and nearly 8,000 people will die from this disease, according to the American Cancer Society.

DRY SKIN

QUESTION: What can I do for dry skin?

ANSWER: Dry skin can usually be related to occupational or environmental factors. Work-related dry skin involves mostly the hands or other parts of the body directly involved in the occupation. On the other hand, environmental dry skin can be associated with taking long, hot showers or not drinking enough water. Dry skin is more common in older people because the skin becomes thinner, which produces a roughened skin surface and hormonal changes result in lowered skin lubrication. Dry skin is more common during the winter months and is often referred to as "winter itch". It may also occur due to prolonged detergent use, malnutrition, hypothyroidism, dehydration, or physical damage to the skin. A common cause of dry skin is frequent or prolonged bathing or showering with hot water as well as excessive use of soap, both of which can increase dryness of the skin. In addition, low humidity and dry air can cause the skin to lose moisture, become less flexible, and crack when flexed, which leads to an increased rate of moisture loss. Healthy skin has a water content of 10% to 20%. Once the skin's water content drops below 10%, skin becomes dry, flaky and itchy. A key to preventing dry skin is to maintain skin hydration by avoiding long hot baths and consuming enough fluids. Nonprescription products such as bath oils, emollients/moisturizers, and oatmeal products can also be helpful. Some useful over-the-counter products for dry skin include Cetaphil Liquid, Lubriderm Bath and Shower Oil, Alpha Keri Oil/ Lotion, Aveeno Moisturizing Cream/Lotion, Corn Huskers Lotion, and Neutrogena Body Oil or Cream. Lotions and creams containing alpha hydroxy acids such as Am Lactin may be useful for patients with extremely rough, dry skin. The use of humidifiers may also help to alleviate problems caused by dry air.

WRINKLES

QUESTION: What can I do for wrinkles on my face?

ANSWER: Many years of exposure to the sun is believed to be responsible for the visible signs of aging skin and wrinkles. Overexposure to the sun increases the production of enzymes that break down the connective tissue known as collagen found under the skin. This breakdown causes premature aging of the skin along with wrinkles and yellow discoloration. Sunlight also thins the skin and may lead to precancerous growths known as actinic keratoses, or solar keratoses. The market for antiaging products is greatly increasing as wrinkles are occurring in the baby boom generation. These antiaging products usually contain ingredients known as alpha hydroxy acids (AHAs) and are often referred to as "cosmeceuticals". AHAs have become very popular and are found in many nonprescription skin care products, from cleansers to night creams. These acids are derived from a variety of sources such as fruits, sugar cane, and milk. They work on the skin to help remove (exfoliate) the dry, outermost layers of the skin while moisturizing the skin layers underneath. This helps to give the dull, flaky skin a new glow and reduce signs of aging. Some of these products contain glycolic acid (from sugar cane plants), which is also used in "chemical peels". Lactic acid, the same type that comes from sour milk, is commonly found in skin moisturizers because it has water holding properties which may be the reasoning behind the old "milk bath" treatments. Other alpha hydroxy acids include malic acid (from apples), citric acid (from oranges and lemons), and tartaric acid (from grapes). Vitamin C has also been promoted as an antiaging compound due to its antioxidant effects. Vitamin C is thought to help strengthen the skin. The vitamin A derivative, tretinoin, is contained in Retin-A and has been approved by the FDA for prescription use since 1995 to improve the appearance of photoaged skin. Renova, which also contains tretinoin, is the first prescription cream on the market to be approved for reducing fine facial wrinkles and lines. This product contains a rich skin softening cream that was developed specifically to treat fine lines, wrinkles, brown spots, and skin surface roughness. Tretinoin acts on epidermal skin cells affecting their growth, but exactly how it works is not known. Up to six months treatment with Renova may be required before the effects are seen. When using either nonprescription products containing AHAs or prescription tretinoin, patients may experience some redness, itching, dryness, or flaking, due to irritation. In addition, consumers using these products should limit their exposure to the sun and sun lamps, and should always use a sunscreen with a SPF rating no lower than 15. Care should also be taken not to get the product into the eyes. Although these anti-aging products have become very popular, very little evidence is available that deep wrinkles can be smoothed out permanently or that skin damage can be reversed.

QUESTION: What can you tell me about Botox?

ANSWER: There has been a lot of media attention given to Botox since it was recently approved by the FDA for cosmetic use. It is now approved for the temporary improvement of certain lines (wrinkles) on the face associated with facial muscle activity in adults 65 years old or younger. Previously, Botox had been approved for the treatment of cervical dystonia in adults, a disorder that causes neck muscles to contract on their own resulting in an awkward positioning of the head or causing spasms or jerks of the neck. Botox had also been approved to treat a squinting disorder of the eye known as strabismus and eye twitching called blepharospasm. Botox is actually a neurotoxin produced by a type of bacteria known as Clostridium botulinum, which causes botulism, a severe form of food poisoning. Botulinum toxins block muscle contraction by interfering with a chemical (acetylcholine) needed for muscle function. It reduces wrinkles by preventing facial muscles from contracting. Botox Cosmetic is injected into the muscles between the eyebrows using a small needle. Injections are usually given into specific facial muscles at five sites. Patients may report feeling minor to moderate discomfort, somewhat like a pinch during the injection treatments. Results can be seen within a few days, with the maximum effect in about one week. These effects usually last up to four months. Botox Cosmetic should not be used when there is an infection at the injection site and it should be used with caution in people with certain muscle disorders. Other drugs may also interfere with its use including certain antibiotics (aminoglycosides), quinidine, and magnesium. In addition, Botox Cosmetic is not recommended for use during pregnancy or when breastfeeding. Common side effects of Botox Cosmetic include headache, respiratory infection, flu syndrome, drooping of the upper eyelid, and nausea. Botox Cosmetic treatments may have to be repeated within two to four months to maintain the effect.

SCARS

QUESTION: I have a couple of unsightly scars on my skin. Are there any over-the-counter (OTC) products available that can improve the appearance of these scars?

ANSWER: Most of us have some types of scars, which can be unsightly and make us self-conscious and embarrassed. These scars develop because of cuts, scrapes, accidents, or surgeries which cause damage to the skin. Scaring is a part of the body's normal healing process following an injury to the skin. Unfortunately, scar tissue is not the same as normal skin. Scar tissue may lack hair follicles or sweat glands, and may be less stretchable due to a decrease in elastic skin fibers.

Scar tissue may also lack cells that give color to skin and may contain other cells that produce itching in the area of the scar. In addition, there are many different types of scars. Flat scars are the most common type, which may be red or dark and raised after the wound has healed, but become paler and flatter over time. Raised scars are caused by an imbalance of protein substances that are produced during the healing process. They are usually red or dark and raised and may be itchy or painful. Sunken scars that are recessed into the skin can occur and may result from acne or chickenpox. Stretch marks can also develop when the skin is stretched rapidly during pregnancy or adolescent growth spurts resulting in red marks that become paler with time.

Although no scar can be removed completely, surgery or other techniques can help modify the scar in some cases, and some topical treatments may help to improve the appearance and texture of a scar. Over the years, many OTC treatments for scars have been tried. Ancient Egyptians used calamine dressings (zinc oxide) for scars and several other preparations including cocoa butter or vitamin E products have been tried with limited amounts of success. Any improvement from these remedies probably results from the massaging and pressure during their application with the oil or butter bases helping to soften the scarred skin. A potential problem with using vitamin E topically is that it can cause a skin rash in some people. More recently, however, two additional OTC products became available that appear to be more effective. One of them is an onion extract/allantoin gel preparation with the tradename Mederma. This gel is thought to work by reducing the formation of irritating chemicals and a substance that makes up a part of the scar. It also has antibacterial properties. The use of Mederma has shown effectiveness in reducing the size of the scar, fading red scars, and making various types of scars appear softer and smoother. This greaseless, odorless, clear gel absorbs into the skin and should be massaged into the scar three to four times a day for several weeks or months to maximize its effectiveness. The second product is a silicone sheeting known by the tradename Rejuveness. How it works is not known, but it may help to generate static electricity that works to flatten out the scar and cause it to lighten. These silicone sheets are applied to the scar area and are held in place by tape. It should be noted that both of these products should only be used after wounds heal completely. Patients using these preparations should monitor the scar's flexibility, color changes and feeling, including itching, burning, and pain to determine its effectiveness.

ACNE

QUESTION: I read about the 15 year old boy who crashed his plane into a Tampa skyscraper. Supposedly he had a prescription for a medication that can lead to suicide attempts. What can you tell me about this medication?

ANSWER: The prescription medication you are referring to is called Accutane or isotretinon. This medication is taken orally for the treatment of severe cases of acne. Acne, also called acne vulgaris, is a very common skin condition in teenagers. It occurs when the skin pores become clogged, leading to the development of pimples, whiteheads, blackheads, and in its most severe form may cause disfiguring cysts and abscesses, which can result in scarring. Acne tends to develop in teenagers because of an interaction among hormones, skin oils, and bacteria that live on the skin and in the hair. What starts acne is not known, but during puberty, the sebaceous glands within hair follicles of the skin become more active and produce excessive oil (sebum). Often, dried sebum, flaked skin, and bacteria collect in the skin pores and block sebum from flowing up through the pores causing pimples, blackheads, etc. The treatment of mild superficial acne can include nonprescription products containing benzoyl peroxide, salicylic acid, or sulfur/resorcinol combinations. Moderate types of acne are usually treated with either topical or oral antibiotics that require a prescription. Severe cases of acne, however, may require the use of other medications such as Accutane. Accutane is a vitamin A derivative and is known as a "retinoid". Exactly how Accutane works is not known, but it does inhibit the production of sebum by the sebaceous glands. It is a potent medication that must not be taken by women who are pregnant or may become pregnant since it has an extremely high risk of producing birth defects. Numerous other serious side effects are associated with the use of Accutane, including psychiatric disorders. Product labeling states that Accutane may cause depression, psychosis, and rarely, suicidal ideation, suicide attempts, and suicide. The reason for these psychiatric side effects is unknown, and more study is needed. Like all medications, the potential risk of side effects needs to be weighed against the potential benefits of the drug.

ECZEMA

QUESTION: I heard about a new non-steroid treatment for eczema. What can you tell me about it?

ANSWER: Protopic (generic name tacrolimus) ointment is the first new prescription treatment approved in over 40 years for atopic dermatitis, commonly known as eczema. Atopic dermatitis is an inflammatory skin disease with a chronically relapsing course that is characterized by episodes of intense itching, skin redness, and severely dry skin. It occurs primarily in infants, children, and young adults, but can also affect older people. This skin condition is not contagious but it is known to be genetically linked. If one parent has the condition, the child has greater than a 25% chance of developing it also and if both parents have it, the child has a 50% chance of developing it. Atopic dermatitis can also be aggravated by various factors such as skin irritants, allergens, changes in temperature and humidity, emotional stress, and skin infections.

Until Protopic recently became available, the use of topical corticosteroids were the main treatment of this skin condition. However, topical corticosteroids when used for long periods of time can cause thinning of the skin and in some cases serious side effects when they are absorbed through the skin. Protopic ointment is not a steroid drug, but is actually a type of antibiotic that works on the patient's immune system in the skin to improve the condition. The ointment is applied to the affected skin areas twice a day with treatment continued for one week after skin clearing. Common side effects of Protopic include temporary stinging or burning sensations in up to 60% of patients. This problem appears to decrease as the skin heals. Patients using Protopic should also avoid sunlight and tanning beds, because it affects the skin's immune system, which may increase the risk of skin cancer.

In conclusion, this new treatment for atopic dermatitis or eczema is not a cure, but represents a valuable alternative treatment for patients with this skin disorder who cannot tolerate or who don't respond to other therapies.

PSORIASIS

QUESTION: I heard about a new drug for severe psoriasis. What can you tell me about it?

ANSWER: Psoriasis is a chronic skin disorder that affects about 7 million people in the United States. It is a recurring disease that produces silvery scaling bumps and various-sized plaques (raised patches) on the skin. Psoriasis can occur at any age, but it is more common in people 16 to 22 years of age and those 57 to 60 years of age. The condition often runs in families and typically involves the scalp, elbows, knees, back, and buttocks. The eyebrows, armpits, navel, and groin may also be affected. An abnormally high rate of growth and turnover of skin cells causes the scaling. The cause of this rapid skin cell growth is not known, but the immune system is thought to play a role in the development of psoriasis. Most people with limited psoriasis have few problems beyond the flaking skin, but the skin's appearance can be embarrassing. However, some people have extensive psoriasis or may develop a painful and debilitating condition known as psoriatic arthritis.

The goals of treating psoriasis are to suppress symptoms and to reduce the severity and extent of disease. Patients with mild to moderate psoriasis are usually treated with various ointments and creams. Patients with more severe psoriasis usually require stronger agents that are taken orally or require injection. Ultraviolet light therapy can also be helpful in some patients. The newly approved drug that you heard about is named Amevive and must be given by injection once a week. It has been found to be useful for treating adult patients with moderate to severe chronic plaque psoriasis and works by suppressing the patient's immune system.

QUESTION: I heard that the FDA has issued a warning about a drug used to treat psoriasis. What can you tell me about it?

ANSWER: The FDA recently announced labeling changes, including a serious "Black-Box Warning", to highlight the potential risk of life-threatening infections in people receiving the drug Raptiva for psoriasis. In addition to this warning, the manufacturer of Raptiva will be required to include a Medication Guide for patients receiving this medication. This new product labeling will warn about the risk of bacterial blood infections, viral meningitis, serious fungal infections, and a rare brain inflammation known as progressive multifocal leukoencephalopathy or PML. Patients receiving Raptiva should be educated about recognizing the signs and symptoms of infection. Raptiva is a once-weekly injection approved for adults with moderate to severe psoriasis. It works by suppressing the patient's immune system to reduce psoriasis flare-ups, however, by suppressing the body's natural defense system, it can also increase the risk of serious infections and malignancies in some patients.

ROSACEA

QUESTION: I heard about a new prescription product used to treat rosacea. What can you tell me about it?

ANSWER: Rosacea (sometimes called adult acne) is a persistent skin disorder that produces redness, tiny pimples, and broken blood vessels, usually on the central area of the face. In advanced cases the skin may thicken, especially around the nose, making it look red and swollen. This is called bulbous nose rosacea or rhinophyma. The cause of rosacea is not known, but it usually occurs during or after middle age and is most common in people with fair complexions. It is more prevalent in women, but usually more severe in men. People with rosacea blush easily and the disorder appears to run in families. Anything that makes the face red will aggravate rosacea and should be avoided if possible. For example, foods or beverages that cause the blood vessels in the skin to expand (dilate) such as spicy foods, alcohol, coffee and other caffeine containing drinks should be avoided. Stress or embarrassment, strenuous exercises, and hot flashes caused by menopause can also trigger rosacea. Non-prescription acne preparations that contain alcohol, acetone, witch hazel, menthol, peppermint, eucalyptus oil, or clove oil should also be avoided. Likewise, products containing niacin (which can cause flushing) and topical corticosteroids (like hydrocortisone and many others) can worsen rosacea and should not be used. Men with this condition should use an electric shaver and not use an after-shave lotion that stings or burns.

Although there is no cure for this disorder, several drugs can be used to improve the symptoms and appearance in rosacea sufferers. Oral antibiotics such as tetracycline, doxycycline, or minocycline are effective medications. If you can't take these drugs, erythromycin or ampicillin are alternative treatments. In addition, the topical prescription anti-infectives metronidazole or clindamycin (lotion, cream, or gel) can be very useful to treat rosacea. Two newly approved topical treatments are also available. The first one is Finacea, which contains azelaic acid in a gel form. It is applied twice daily and has been shown to be effective for the topical treatment of the inflammatory papules and pustules of mild to moderate rosacea. The second product is Rosula lotion, which contains the long-standing ingredients sodium sulfacetamide (a sulfa drug) and sulfur along with urea to help moisturize the skin. It is applied 1 to 3 times daily and has demonstrated effectiveness in the treatment of acne, acne rosacea, and seborrheic dermatitis.

The most recently approved product for adults with rosacea is Oracea. It is the first FDA-approved oral medication for treating this condition. Oracea capsules contain a low dose (40 mg) of the antibiotic doxycycline and is taken once-daily. In low doses, doxycycline reduces inflammation and it is these anti-inflammatory properties that are thought to be beneficial in treating this condition. During clinical studies, Oracea taken once a day was shown to significantly reduce inflammatory skin lesions in patients with rosacea and many of these patients were clear or almost clear of these lesions after treatment.

It should be noted that severe cases of rosacea with rhinophyma may require surgery. Your physician or dermatologist can determine which therapy is best for you.

VITILIGO

QUESTION: What drugs or other treatments are used for vitiligo?

ANSWER: Vitiligo is a condition in which a loss of pigment producing cells (melanocytes) in the skin results in smooth, whitish patches of skin. In some people, only one or two patches of hypopigmented skin appear, while in others there may be whitish patches over a large part of the body. The condition is more common in the tropics and among blacks. The whitish patches of skin are very prone to sunburn and the skin affected by vitiligo may also produce white hair because the melanocytes are lost from the hair. The cause of vitiligo is not known, but it may occur after physical trauma, especially head injury. It may also be associated with other diseases such as Addison's disease (underactive adrenal glands), diabetes, certain types of anemia, thyroid disease, and other disorders. Because of its appearances, vitiligo can be very bothersome psychologically to some people.

There is no known cure for vitiligo, but several types of treatments may be helpful to some individuals. Small areas of affected skin can be camouflaged with various dyes that won't soil clothing and can last for several days. The use of light-sensitive drugs known as psoralens in combination with ultraviolet A light can be effective in some people, but this treatment must be continued for a long time. Topical corticosteroids are also sometimes effective at causing skin repigmentation. In addition, several other types of topical and oral drugs that increase skin pigmentation may be beneficial in some patients with vitiligo. Sunscreen products should be used on affected skin areas to protect against sunburn. You should consult with a dermatologist to determine what specific therapy would be best for you.

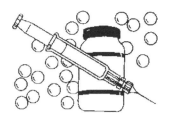

CHAPTER 8
DIABETES

TYPE 2 DIABETES AND INSULIN

<u>QUESTION</u>: I have type 2 diabetes and worry that I will need to use insulin. What can you tell me about insulin and type 2 diabetes?

<u>ANSWER</u>: Approximately 26 million Americans have type 1 and type 2 diabetes. Type 2 diabetes is the most common type, accounting for an estimated 95% of all diabetes cases. Diabetes is a chronic disease that occurs when the body either does not produce, or use, the hormone insulin, which controls blood sugar (glucose). People with type 2 diabetes require regular monitoring and ongoing treatment to maintain normal or near normal blood sugar levels. Treatment includes lifestyle modifications, self-care measures and medications. Most people who are newly diagnosed with type 2 diabetes are usually treated with a combination of diet, exercise, and oral medication(s). However, some people will need to add insulin because their blood sugar levels are not well controlled. You should not be afraid to use insulin because it can help to prevent many complications of the disease. This topic was recently reviewed in a JohnsHopkins Health Alert (**www.johnshopkinshealthalerts.com**, 2011).

Research shows that when started earlier, insulin can help prevent many complications of diabetes including heart and kidney disease. But the idea of taking insulin makes many people with type 2 diabetes uncomfortable, even scared. Insulin has traditionally been viewed as a last resort for treating type 2 diabetes, but it is increasingly recommended earlier in therapy. If your hemoglobin A1c (A1c) level is above 10% your doctor may start you on insulin right away. It could be for a brief period before returning to oral medication, or it could be permanent depending on your particular circumstance. Below are two common concerns you may have about insulin treatment:

- **"I feel like a failure. I should have been able to control my diabetes with diet and exercise."** For most people, type 2 diabetes is a progressive disease. Initially, you may be able to control it with lifestyle modifications, but over time the body gradually produces less and less of its own insulin. If diet and exercise do not bring your blood glucose levels to where they need to be, medications, including insulin, will help. Most people eventually need to take one or more oral medications and/or insulin injections to effectively regulate blood glucose levels. It has nothing to do with willpower or personal failure, so try to let go of feeling ashamed and instead be grateful that treatments exist to help you live a longer, healthier life.

- **"If I need insulin, I must be getting sicker."** The idea that adding insulin to your treatment regimen means you are at the end of the road is completely outdated. It simply means that your pancreas is not making enough insulin and needs help. The important thing is not whether you need insulin, but whether you can control your glucose and thereby avoid the long-term complications of diabetes—to your nerves, kidneys or eyes, for example. Your goal should not be to stay away from insulin but rather to control your diabetes and prevent complications from developing.

GLUCOSE TESTING

QUESTION: I have recently been diagnosed as having diabetes and my doctor wants me to check my blood sugar on a regular basis. Would a urine test for sugar be just as good?

ANSWER: Blood glucose (sugar) testing is important in the treatment of diabetes. Starches and sugars in the diet break down into glucose. Insulin, which is released by the pancreas into the blood, helps the body use glucose for energy. If the pancreas is not able to release enough insulin for this purpose, or if the body does not efficiently utilize the insulin produced, the blood level of glucose rises. Consistently high blood glucose levels can damage the heart, blood vessels, kidneys, eyes and nerves. By carefully monitoring their blood glucose through regular testing, diabetic patients can adjust their diet, exercise and medication regimen and keep their diabetes under control. For many patients with diabetes, a target range for blood glucose is 80-160 mg/dL before meals and less than 200 mg/dL two hours after a meal. The appropriate times to monitor blood glucose depend upon the medication one is taking and the type and severity of diabetes. Type I patients, who need to take insulin, may need to check their blood glucose up to 4 times a day (before each meal and at bedtime) while Type II diabetics may need to check their blood glucose only once daily or every other day before breakfast. A doctor or diabetes health care professional should determine the appropriate times to test blood glucose levels. It should also be noted that numerous medications can affect blood glucose levels and your pharmacist can provide you with information regarding this. Urine tests for glucose are no longer recommended because they may not accurately reflect the amount of glucose in the blood at the time of the test due to differences in kidney function or urine retention caused by other conditions, such as prostate problems. In addition, various drugs or vitamins may interfere with urine glucose test results and patients who are color-blind may not be able to see the different shades of color needed to interpret the test results.

QUESTION: I have diabetes and heard about a new blood testing device that is less painful. What can you tell me about it?

ANSWER: The number of people in the United States with diabetes is growing every year. Most people with diabetes (about 90%) have type 2 diabetes, which used to be called "adult-onset" or "non-insulin dependent" diabetes. It is very important for people with diabetes to keep their blood glucose (sugar) levels at appropriate levels to prevent complications such as kidney disease, nerve disease, blindness, and cardiovascular disease. For many patients with diabetes, a target range for average blood glucose is 80-140 mg/dL before meals and 100-160 mg/dL at bedtime. Your physician can determine what target glucose levels are best, based upon your own medical situation. A doctor or diabetes healthcare professional can also help you decide the right times to test your blood glucose levels based upon the medication you are taking and the severity of the diabetes.

Recently the FDA approved a blood glucose testing device called the OneTouch FastTake Meter made by Lifescan, a Johnson & Johnson company. This new test strip meter has received FDA approval for arm testing, thereby avoiding the often painful finger stick in order to collect a blood sample for testing. Arm testing allows the patient to draw blood from almost any area of the arm, where there are less nerve endings than in their fingertips. Only a very small amount of blood is needed for this new arm testing device, which delivers test results within 15 seconds. Another new blood glucose testing device (At Last Blood Glucose System available from Amira Medical) allows patients to choose the forearm, upper arm, or thigh as a testing area. A third system (Freestyle Blood Glucose Monitoring System available from Therasense) also became available this past summer and promotes the use of the forearm as opposed to fingersticks. Although these new testing devices may not be appropriate for everyone and some individuals may have difficulty obtaining blood samples from the arm, they offer a less painful alternative for blood glucose testing.

QUESTION: I have type 2 diabetes and heard about a new over-the-counter test for blood sugar. What can you tell me about it?

ANSWER: Most people (90-95%) with diabetes have type 2 disease also referred to as "non-insulin-dependent diabetes" or "adult-onset diabetes". The incidence of type 2 diabetes increases with age and is higher in certain ethnic groups such as Blacks and Mexican Americans.

However, over the past 10 years, the prevalence of diabetes has increased by more than 30%, especially in younger age groups. For example, in people aged 30-39 years, the prevalence of diabetes has climbed by 70% in the past 10 years and is also exploding in children and teenagers. The incidence of diabetes is closely related to increasing obesity, worsening dietary habits, and sedentary lifestyles. Diabetes is a major cause of death and disability in the U.S. Complications of diabetes include heart disease, kidney disease, blindness, nerve problems, and lower-limb amputations. In view of this, monitoring and controlling blood sugar levels are extremely important.

Blood sugar (glucose) levels in the blood are usually monitored by patients and healthcare workers by utilizing devices that measure blood glucose at particular times, such as morning, before meals, or at bedtime. Another very important test for monitoring blood glucose is the "glycosylated hemoglobin" or "HbA1c" test. This test measures the average blood sugar level for the last 2 to 3 months, and provides a more complete picture of diabetes control. The American Diabetes Association (ADA) recommends that people with diabetes have this test done 2 to 4 times each year and has established a target level of less than 7%. For every 1% decrease in HbA1c levels, there is a 21% reduction in the risk for diabetes-related death, so you can see how important it is to monitor and keep this level lowered by proper diet, exercise, and medications. Now, back to your question. The FDA recently approved an over-the-counter test kit for measuring HbA1c levels. It is called A1cNow and utilizes a fingerstick blood sample providing results in about 8 minutes. No test strips are required and the test is used once and discarded. The test kit needs to be refrigerated if not used within 30 days. More information about this new product can be found at the Internet web site **www.A1cNow.com**. Be sure to seek the advice of your physician regarding the use of this test at home.

QUESTION: I heard that a new glucose monitoring system was approved for use by people with diabetes. What can you tell me about it?

ANSWER: The FDA recently approved a device that measures glucose (sugar) levels for up to 7 days in people with diabetes. It is called the STS-7 System. While a standard fingerstick test records a person's glucose level as a snapshot in time, the STS-7 Continuous Glucose Monitoring System (STS-7 System) measures glucose levels every five minutes throughout a seven-day period. This additional information can be used to detect trends and track patterns in glucose levels throughout the week that wouldn't be captured by fingerstick measurements alone. However, diabetics must still rely on the fingerstick test to decide whether additional insulin is needed. According to the FDA, the STS-7 System supplements standard fingerstick meters and test strips, providing diabetics ages 18 and older with a way to see trends and track patterns. This new system can help detect when glucose levels drop during the overnight hours, show when glucose levels rise between meals and suggest how exercise and diet might affect glucose levels. The STS-7 System, manufactured by DexCom, Inc. of San Diego, Calif., uses a disposable sensor placed just below the skin in the abdomen to measure the level of glucose in the fluid found in the body's tissues (interstitial fluid). Sensor placement causes minimal discomfort and can easily be done by patients themselves. The sensor must be replaced weekly. An alarm can be programmed to sound if a patient's glucose level reaches pre-set lows or pre-set highs. An estimated 20.8 million people in the United States—7 percent of the population—have diabetes. Most have type 2 diabetes, a condition in which the body does not properly use insulin. An estimated 5 percent to 10 percent of people with this chronic disease have type 1 diabetes, which results from the body's failure to produce insulin. People with type 1 diabetes must take insulin every day. Blood glucose (sugar) testing is important in the treatment of diabetes. Starches and sugars in the diet break down into glucose. Insulin, which is released by the pancreas into the blood, helps the body use glucose for energy. If the pancreas is not able to release enough insulin for this purpose, or if the body does not efficiently utilize the insulin produced, the blood level of glucose rises. Consistently high blood glucose levels can damage the heart, blood vessels, kidneys, eyes and nerves. By carefully monitoring their blood glucose through regular testing, diabetic patients can adjust their diet, exercise and medication regimen and keep their diabetes under control. For more information about this new glucose monitoring device, please contact DexCom, Inc., at 1-877-DEXCOM4 (1-877-339-2664).

LOW BLOOD GLUCOSE

QUESTION: My husband uses insulin each day for his diabetes. What can we do if his sugar level goes too low?

ANSWER: Low blood sugar, or hypoglycemia, can be a very serious problem in patients with diabetes. Generally, the blood glucose (sugar) level should not go below 80 mg/dL. Levels below 55 mg/dL can result in mental disturbances, coma, and possibly even death. Because of this, all patients with diabetes should carry an identification card or wear a bracelet or necklace that informs others that they are diabetic. Most cases of hypoglycemia are caused by taking too much insulin or oral anti-diabetic medication in relation to the amount of food eaten. It can also occur if a diabetic increases exercise without increasing food intake, because exercise usually causes a lowering of blood glucose (sugar). Another common cause of hypoglycemia is alcohol consumption, often after little food has been eaten for a period of time, or by combining alcohol with an oral anti-diabetic medication. Symptoms of low blood glucose include a feeling of hunger, shakiness, sweating, skipped heartbeats, and feeling faint. Even lower blood glucose can cause confusion, blurred vision, bizarre behavior, seizures, or coma. The treatment for hypoglycemia is to take glucose (sugar). Glucose tablets and liquid are available from your pharmacy for this use and it is a good idea for all diabetics to have these products readily available. If glucose products are not available, sugar-containing foods should be eaten to increase blood glucose levels rapidly. Fruit juice, sugar water, candy, sugar cubes, carbonated beverages, or milk are commonly recommended if the patient can swallow. If this doesn't help within a few minutes emergency help should be called. Some physicians will give diabetic patients a prescription for a Glucagon injection kit to treat insulin reactions, but this treatment requires patient education and training for proper use. Intravenous glucose may also be required in some situations to correct low blood glucose levels. A doctor should always be consulted to determine the cause of repeated episodes of hypoglycemia. The dose of insulin or oral anti-diabetic medications may need to be adjusted, and the diet can be changed if needed. If you have diabetes, the best way to avoid hypoglycemia is to:

- Stay on a regular schedule of eating meals, exercise, and medication.
- Check your blood glucose regularly.
- Never mix alcohol and oral anti-diabetic medications.
- If you have developed very low blood glucose in the past, it is a good idea to keep a snack containing sugar or glucose tablets with you at all times to treat early symptoms of hypoglycemia.

INSULIN PRODUCTS

QUESTION: What's the difference between the various types of insulin products?

ANSWER: Insulin is a hormone produced by the pancreas, which regulates the amount of sugar (glucose) in the blood. Its discovery in 1921 is often described as one of the major medical advances of the 20th century. The use of insulin is required for the day-to-day survival of some patients with diabetes, and it contributes to an improved quality of life and reduced complications from diabetes for many others. In the last fifteen years, several studies have shown that better control of blood glucose can significantly reduce the long-term complications of diabetes such as blindness, kidney failure, cardiovascular disease, and nerve problems. Early insulin products were made from animal sources, such as pork and beef, which had a greater potential for side effects. Today, with many advances in biotechnology, manufacturers are able to create insulin products that are almost identical to the insulin produced by the human pancreas. Normally the pancreas produces some insulin throughout the day (basal insulin) and more insulin in response to meals (postprandial insulin). Human insulin is made up of two long strings of amino acids joined together in a particular sequence. By manipulating these amino acids or adding other substances, various kinds of insulin products can be made. There are more than twenty different insulin preparations available in the U.S. They are usually differentiated by how fast they act and how long their action in the body lasts. In general, some types of insulin mimic the normal production of insulin throughout the day (basal insulin), while rapid or short acting insulins are used to counter the increase in blood glucose when a meal is eaten (postprandial). Regular insulin is short acting (5-8 hours) and has an onset of action of about 30 minutes. Two newer insulin products (insulin lispro-Humalog and insulin aspart-Novolog) have even faster actions and can be injected much closer to mealtime. Insulin preparations with intermediate durations of action (approximately 12 hours) include NPH and Lente insulin. They have a slower onset of action of about one to two hours. Two additional insulin preparations, ultralente and insulin glargine (Lantus) have an even longer duration of activity of approximately 24 hours. Finally, there are a variety of insulin mixtures available that contain both long and short acting insulins. Your physician can determine what insulin treatment regimen is best for your and your lifestyle. Every person's insulin regimen must be finely tuned to match his or her responses through careful monitoring of blood glucose levels.

QUESTION: I have type 2 diabetes and may need to go on insulin. What types of insulin are there?

ANSWER: In type 2 diabetes, either the body does not produce enough insulin or the cells of the body cannot properly use the insulin it makes (insulin resistance). Type 2 diabetes is closely associated with obesity and physical inactivity and is now being diagnosed in children and teenagers. Diet and exercise are essential components of all treatment programs for people with diabetes. When diet and exercise are not enough to control the blood sugar (glucose) levels in people with type 2 diabetes, then usually oral medications are utilized. However, many people with type 2 diabetes may also need to use insulin. This subject was recently reviewed in a Johns Hopkins Health Alert (**www. johnshopkinshealthalerts.com**, 2010).

Approximately 40% of people with type 2 diabetes eventually require some type of insulin treatment to control their blood glucose, either because their diabetes gets worse or it no longer responds to oral drugs. Many people with type 2 diabetes take insulin in combination with metformin, a thiazolidinedione, or a sulfonylurea.

Insulin was once obtained exclusively from pig or cow pancreas. Today, regular and intermediate-acting insulins are referred to as human insulins, because they are manufactured to be identical to the insulin produced by the human pancreas. Rapid—and long-acting insulins are chemically modified forms of human insulin. There are four main types of insulin:

Rapid-Acting Insulin

Insulin aspart (Novolog), insulin lispro (Humalog), and insulin glulisine (Apidra) are called insulin analogues, because their chemical structure is a modified form of human insulin that is designed to work more quickly and peak faster than regular insulin. These manufactured insulins work with time-actions that are close to the natural insulin functions in the body. Consequently, they may be effective in preventing high blood glucose (hyperglycemia) after meals and are less likely to produce hypoglycemia later on.

Regular Or Short-Acting Insulin

This type of insulin is manufactured to be the same as the insulin produced in the human body. Popular brands have an "R" (for regular) in their names, for example, Humulin R and Novolin R. Regular insulin is typically injected 30 to 60 minutes before meals and usually reaches the bloodstream within 30 minutes, in time to cover the rise in blood glucose that begins after food is eaten. Insulin action peaks two to three hours after injection and the effects generally last about three to six hours.

Intermediate-Acting Insulin

This type of human insulin called NPH insulin contains protamine, which makes the solution cloudy and slows the absorption of insulin. NPH insulins have an "N" in their names, for example, Humulin N and Novolin N. After injection, intermediate-acting insulins reach the bloodstream within two to four hours and show peak action in four to 10 hours. Duration of action is from 10 to 16 hours. Intermediate-acting insulin is often used in combination with regular or rapid-acting insulin.

Long-Acting Insulin

Both insulin glargine (Lantus) and insulin detemir (Levemir) are long-acting insulin analogues. They are often used alone in people with type 2 diabetes, or in combination with a more quick-acting insulin. Lantus is a clear solution in the vial, but it precipitates in the skin after injection, which greatly slows absorption and makes it very long acting, usually 20 to 24 hours. Levemir also is absorbed slowly, because it binds to the protein albumin in the skin. Its effects last about 14 to 18 hours.

QUESTION: I am a diabetic taking insulin shots. I keep seeing advertisements in magazines about a new type of insulin. Can you tell me more about it?

ANSWER: In 1996, the Food and Drug Administration (FDA) approved insulin lispro (tradename Humalog) for use by people with diabetes. As you know, insulin is a hormone produced by the pancreas and it regulates the amount of sugar in the blood. For many years, researchers have been trying to improve upon insulin products. Insulin was first discovered in 1921 and was a major breakthrough in the treatment of diabetes. Since that time, a number of improvements have been made in insulin including the availability of longer acting products and products of greater purity. Early insulins were also made from animal sources, such as pork and beef, and had a greater potential for side effects. Today, with advances in biotechnology, we are able to produce a "human" insulin that is identical to the insulin produced by the human pancreas and thus are no longer dependent upon animal sources. Human insulin is made up of 2 long strings of amino acids joined together in a particular sequence. With insulin lispro or Humalog, researchers found that by reversing the sequence of just two amino acids on one of the strings resulted in a type of human insulin that was absorbed faster by the body after injection and it also had a somewhat shorter duration of action compared to the regular insulin products previously on the market. These new properties allow patients with diabetes who use regular or short-acting insulin to inject their insulin lispro dose within 15 minutes of eating instead of 30-60 minutes ahead of time, like the older regular insulin injections. Because insulin lispro is a short acting insulin (like human regular insulin) it should be used in conjunction with a longer-acting insulin to regulate the blood sugar throughout the day. The side effects of this new product are the same as for human regular insulin, including the possibility of blood sugar levels that are too low (hypoglycemia). The dosage of insulin lispro is also identical to human regular insulin (1 unit of one equals 1 unit of the other).

Patients with diabetes who are switched from human regular insulin to insulin lispro and vice versa must be carefully monitored and educated about the differences in these products. Insulin lispro was approved by the FDA as a prescription only product until more experience is gained regarding its use and to allow for patient education.

QUESTION: I heard about a new type of insulin recently approved. What can you tell me about it?

ANSWER: The FDA recently approved Apidra (insulin glulisine) which is a new fast-acting insulin product. It is used to lower high blood sugar (hyperglycemia) in people with type 1 or type 2 diabetes. Human insulin is made up of 2 long strings of amino acids joined together in a particular sequence. With insulin glulisine (Apidra) researchers found that by changing the sequence of just two amino acids on one of the strings resulted in a type of human insulin that was absorbed faster by the body after injection and it also had a somewhat shorter duration of action compared to the regular insulin products previously on the market. These new properties allow patients with diabetes who use regular or short-acting insulin to inject their insulin glulisine (Apidra) dose 15 minutes before eating or within 20 minutes after starting a meal instead of 30-60 minutes ahead of time, like the older regular insulin injections. Because insulin glulisine is a short acting insulin (like human regular insulin) it normally should be used in conjunction with a longer-acting insulin to regulate the blood sugar throughout the day. The side effects of this new product are the same as for human regular insulin, including the possibility of blood sugar levels that are too low (hypoglycemia). The dosage of insulin glulisine is also identical to human regular insulin (1 unit of one equals 1 unit of the other). Patients with diabetes who are switched from human regular insulin to insulin glulisine and vice versa must be carefully monitored and educated about the differences in these products. Two other similar fast-acting insulins already on the market include insulin lispro (Humalog) and insulin aspart (Novolog).

QUESTION: Some time ago you wrote about an inhaled insulin product that may be available in the future. What about an insulin pill or patch?

ANSWER: In addition to an inhaled insulin product, an oral insulin capsule and an insulin patch are also under development. Early studies have shown that an insulin patch can provide steady blood levels of insulin throughout a 12-hour patch application. In addition, early studies also have shown that the oral administration of capsules containing insulin in combination with a special delivery agent can provide significant insulin absorption from the gastrointestinal tract. However, additional research and study will be needed before these products can be made available.

QUESTION: I have diabetes and I heard about a new type of insulin. What can you tell me about it?

ANSWER: The new insulin that you heard about is called insulin glargine with the trade name Lantus. It is somewhat different from the insulin produced by the body and is made using a biotechnology technique known as "recombinant DNA technology". Human insulin is made up of two long groups or chains of amino acids joined together in a specific sequence. The new insulin product differs from human insulin by changing three of these amino acids. This allows for the insulin to be released more slowly into the bloodstream and makes it longer acting. Several clinical studies have shown that Lantus is just as effective as another longer-acting insulin known as NPH insulin which is usually injected once or twice a day and is used in combination with regular insulin injections at mealtimes, or with oral anti-diabetic medications. Lantus only has to be injected once a day at bedtime and it is also used in combination with regular insulin or oral anti-diabetic drugs. This new insulin was approved for use in both child and adults with type 1 diabetes or in adults with type 2 diabetes. According to the World Health Organization, the incidence of diabetes is likely to more than double in the next 25 years. Over 90% of people with diabetes have type 2, which used to be called "adult-onset" or "non-insulin dependent" diabetes. When insulin cannot keep blood sugar (glucose) under control, many problems can develop such as kidney disease, cardiovascular disease, blindness, and nerve problems. Like all insulin products, the most common side effect of Lantus is low blood sugar (glucose) or hypoglycemia. It may also cause more injection-site pain than NPH insulin. In summary, Lantus is a new long-acting insulin that can be given once a day. It appears to be as effective as NPH insulin when used in combination with regular insulin at mealtimes or in conjunction with oral anti-diabetic medications.

QUESTION: I heard about a new long-acting insulin that was approved for treating diabetes. What can you tell me about it?

ANSWER: The FDA recently approved Levemir (insulin detemir) for the treatment of adults and children with type 1 diabetes and for the treatment of adults with type 2 diabetes. Type 1 diabetes results from the body's failure to produce insulin, which is a hormone needed to allow sugar (glucose) into the cells of the body and be utilized as a fuel. It is estimated that 5%-10% of people in the United States who are diagnosed with diabetes have type 1. Type 2 diabetes results from a condition in which the body cannot properly use insulin (insulin resistance), combined with a relative defficiency of insulin. Levemir is produced using a biotechnology technique known as "recombinant DNA technology" and is very similar to human insulin. It is a long-acting (basal) insulin product that is active for up to 24 hours. Depending upon the patient's condition, Levemir can be used by itself, combined with oral anti-diabetic medications, or used in combination with rapid acting insulin. Levemir is administered by subcutaneous injection in the thigh, abdominal wall, or upper arm and is given once or twice a day. Its dosage is determined based upon blood glucose levels. During clinical studies, Levemir was similar in effectiveness to NPH human insulin and Lantus (insulin glargine) in controlling blood glucose levels. This new insulin product is available in vials, and in a PenFill cartridge or prefilled syringe (FlexPen or Innolet).

AVANDIA

QUESTION: I've heard about a new oral drug for diabetes. What can you tell me about it?

ANSWER: You're probably talking about the new drug known as Avandia or rosiglitazone (rose-eh-gli-to-zone), which has recently been approved for the treatment of people with type 2 diabetes. Avandia is an oral drug that can be used together with diet control and exercise to help control blood glucose (sugar) levels in people with diabetes. It can also be used in combination with another oral medication known as Glucophage or metformin (met-for-min) together with diet and exercise. Unlike many other oral drugs that are used to treat diabetes, Avandia works by improving a person's sensitivity to insulin. This improved sensitivity is good because people with type 2 diabetes develop a resistance to the action of insulin, which controls blood glucose levels. When insulin cannot keep blood glucose under control, many problems can develop such as kidney disease, cardiovascular disease, blindness, nerve problems, etc. Clinical studies with Avandia show that about 50% to 60% of people using the drug will lower their blood glucose levels by at least 30 points (mg/dl). Avandia is in the same class of drugs as Rezulin or troglitazone (troe-gli-to-zone), which has been associated with 43 cases of acute liver failure resulting in 28 deaths and seven liver transplants. To date, however, Avandia has not caused any liver problems, which may be a big advantage of using Avandia instead of Rezulin. Side effects reported with Avandia have included weight gain due to fluid retention, headache, anemia, upper respiratory tract infection, back pain, and low blood glucose. Avandia can be taken once a day or in divided doses twice a day with or without food. Please see next question regarding new warnings for Avandia and other similar drugs.

PLEASE NOTE: The diabetes drug rosiglitazone (Avandia) and the combination drugs Avandamet and Avandaryl will no longear be available in pharmacies as of November 18, 2011. Multiple studies have linked rosiglitazone to an increased risk of heart attack. If you've successfully controlled your glucose levels with an Avandia-based medication and your doctotr feels you should continue to take it despite the known risks, he or she will need to enroll you in the FDA's Avandia-Rosiglitazone Medicine Access Program. Through the program, participants will receive Avandia by mail from FDA-certified pharmacies.

QUESTION: What can you tell me about new warnings for some diabetes drugs?

ANSWER: The FDA recently announced that it will require manufacturers of certain diabetes drugs to add a stronger warning to their labeling about the risk of heart failure. The information will be included in the form of a "Black-Box" warning and it will emphasize that the drugs may cause or worsen heart failure in certain patients and that patients should be monitored closely. Drugs that are required to have this morning include Avandia (rosiglitazone), Actos (pioglitazone), Avandaryl (rosiglitazone and glimepiride), Avandamet (rosiglitazone and metformin), and Duetact (pioglitazone and glimepiride). These medications are used in conjunction with diet and exercise to improve blood sugar control in adults with type 2 diabetes. The drugs involved are known as "glitazones" or "insulin sensitizers". Unlike other oral anti-diabetic drugs that affect insulin levels, glitazones make the body more sensitive to the action of insulin. The FDA's review of adverse event reports involving these drugs found cases of significant weight gain and edema (water retention), which may be signs of heart failure. The new strengthened warning advises healthcare professionals to observe patients carefully for signs and symptoms of heart failure, including excessive, rapid weight gain, shortness of breath, and edema after starting drug therapy. The warning also states that these drugs should not be used by people with serious are severe heart failure who have marked limits on their activity and who are comfortable only at rest or who are confined to bed or a chair. People taking these medications should contact their healthcare providers if they have any questions.

PLEASE NOTE: The diabetes drug rosiglitazone (Avandia) and the combination drugs Avandamet and Avandaryl will no longear be available in pharmacies as of November 18, 2011. Multiple studies have linked rosiglitazone to an increased risk of heart attack. If you've successfully controlled your glucose levels with an Avandia-based medication and your doctotr feels you should continue to take it despite the known risks, he or she will need to enroll you in the FDA's Avandia-Rosiglitazone Medicine Access Program. Through the program, participants will receive Avandia by mail from FDA-certified pharmacies.

QUESTION: I heard that the FDA is concerned about the safety of Avandia, which I take for diabetes. What can you tell me about this?

ANSWER: On May 21, 2007 the FDA issued a safety alert for people taking Avandia (rosiglitazone), an oral agent used to treat type 2 diabetes. While there is conflicting information available, safety data from some clinical studies have shown that there is a potentially significant increase in the risk of heart attack and heart-related deaths in patients taking Avandia. In view of this, patients who are taking Avandia, especially those who are known to have heart disease or who are at high risk of heart attack, should talk to their doctor about this new information and treatment options for their type 2 diabetes. Questions also exist regarding the safety of Actos (pioglitazone) another drug for type 2 diabetes, which is similar to Avandia. In addition, combination products containing rosiglitazone (Avandamet) and pioglitazone (ActoPlus Met, Duetact) are available. The FDA and its advisory committees will be reviewing the potential cardiovascular risks of Avandia and plan to make their results known as soon as possible.

Avandia was approved in 1999 for the treatment of type 2 diabetes. It is an oral drug that can be used together with diet control and exercise to help control blood glucose (sugar) levels in people with diabetes. It can also be used in combination with another oral medication known as Glucophage or metformin together with diet and exercise. Unlike many other oral drugs that are used to treat diabetes, Avandia works by improving a person's sensitivity to insulin. This improved sensitivity is good because people with type 2 diabetes develop a resistance to the action of insulin, which controls blood glucose levels.

PLEASE NOTE: The diabetes drug rosiglitazone (Avandia) and the combination drugs Avandamet and Avandaryl will no longear be available in pharmacies as of November 18, 2011. Multiple studies have linked rosiglitazone to an increased risk of heart attack. If you've successfully controlled your glucose levels with an Avandia-based medication and your doctotr feels you should continue to take it despite the known risks, he or she will need to enroll you in the FDA's Avandia-Rosiglitazone Medicine Access Program. Through the program, participants will receive Avandia by mail from FDA-certified pharmacies.

QUESTION: I heard that the use of Avandia is being restricted by the FDA. What can you tell me about this?

ANSWER: On September 23, 2010 the FDA announced that it will significantly restrict the use of Avandia (rosiglitazone) to patients with type 2 diabetes who cannot control their diabetes with other medications. These new restrictions are in response to data that suggest an elevated risk of cardiovascular events, such as heart attack and stroke, in patients treated with Avandia. These restrictions also apply to the diabetes medications Avandamet and Avandaryl, which contain rosiglitazone. Doctors must now document that patients have not responded adequately to other medications and cannot take Actos (pioglitazone) before they can receive a new prescription for rosiglitazone. In addition, patients will have to sign a statement indicating that they have reviewed the cardiovascular safety concerns about the drug. In Europe, the European Medicines Agency (our FDA counterpart) even took more drastic measures by recommending the suspension of all rosiglitazone-containing anti-diabetes medicines. Several FDA officials noted that Avandia and other rosiglitazone-containing products may be needed by some patients with type 2 diabetes whose disease may not be controlled on other medications or may not tolerate other medications like Actos (pioglitazone) or, in consultation with their healthcare professional, decide not to take Actos for other medical reasons. It is estimated that 600,000 Americans take Avandia, which was originally approved in 1999. Avandia, Actos, Avandaryl, Avandamet, and Duetact already contain a "Black-Box" warning about the increased risk of congestive heart failure associated with their use.

BYETTA

QUESTION: I heard about a new prescription drug that comes from the Gila Monster that is used to treat diabetes. What can you tell me about it?

ANSWER: The FDA recently approved Byetta (exenatide) for the treatment of patients with type 2 diabetes. In type 2 diabetes, either the body does not produce enough insulin or the cells of the body cannot properly use the insulin it makes (insulin resistance). Type 2 diabetes is closely associated with obesity and physical inactivity and is now being diagnosed in children and teenagers. Diet and exercise are essential components of all treatment programs for people with diabetes. When diet and exercise are not enough to control the blood sugar (glucose) levels in people with type 2 diabetes, then usually oral medications are utilized. Byetta is a new type of medication known as an "incretin memetic", meaning that it mimics the action of a hormone produced in the gut in response to food intake, which helps to lower blood glucose levels when they are too high. Strangely enough, it is a synthetically made version of a protein found in the saliva of the Gila Monster. Byetta works in a number of different ways to lower blood glucose with a variety of effects on the stomach, liver, pancreas, and brain. The FDA approved Byetta for use in patients with type 2 diabetes who are currently taking Glucophage (metformin), a sulfonylurea agent, or a combination of these two medications, but whose blood glucose levels are not adequately controlled. Sulfonylurea drugs include Diabenese (chlorpopamide), acetohexamide, Tolinase (tolazamide), Orinase (tolbutamide), Glucotrol (glipizide), Amaryl (glimapiride), and Diabeta or Glynase (glyburide). Unfortunately, Byetta must be given by subcutaneous injection twice a day. The most common side effect of Byetta is nausea, but in combination with a sulfonylurea it may increase the risk of low blood glucose (hypoglycemia) and the dosage of the sulfonylurea agent may need to be reduced.

PLEASE NOTE: Since Byetta was approved for use in 2005, the FDA has been monitoring reports of acute pancreatitis in patients receiving this medication. Patients taking Byetta who experience unexplained severe abdominal pain with or without nausea and vomiting should stop taking the drug and promptly seek medical care. Altered kidney function may also occur in patients using Byetta.

BYDUREON

QUESTION: I heard that a once-weekly treatment for type 2 diabetes was approved. What can you tell me about it?

ANSWER: The FDA recently (2012) approved Bydureon (exenatide extended-release) injection for the treatment of adults with type 2 diabetes, when used in conjunction with diet and exercise, to improve blood sugar control. Bydureon is the first once-weekly treatment of type 2 diabetes and is administered by subcutaneous injection once every 7 days. Actually, the active ingredient in Bydureon, exenatide, was originally approved in 2005 with the tradename Byetta. However, Bydureon is a long-acting, controlled-release formulation of exenatide which allows for a once-weekly injection, instead of a twice-daily injection required with Byetta. The most common side effects with Bydureon include nausea, diarrhea, headache, vomiting, constipation, itching at the injection site, a small bump at the injection site, and indigestion. Other more serious side effects can occur and it is not known if Bydureon is safe and effective in people with a history of pancreatitis or kidney problems. The manufacturer of Bydureon is being required to conduct a number of additional safety studies with this new agent, including its effects on the heart and its potential risk of thyroid cancer. It should also be noted that Bydureon should not be used together with Byetta, should not be used instead of insulin or with insulin, nor should it be used to treat type 1 diabetes. Much more information about Bydureon can be found on the Internet at **www.bydureon.com**.

CYCLOSET

QUESTION: I heard about a new oral drug for diabetes. What can you tell me about it?

ANSWER: The FDA recently approved Cycloset (bromocriptine) for the treatment of type 2 diabetes as an adjunct to diet and exercise. Bromocriptine, the active ingredient in Cycloset, has been used at a higher dose for many years to treat Parkinson's disease. It is classified as a "dopamine agonist", a drug that mimics the action of dopamine, which is in short supply in Parkinson's disease due to a lack of dopamine producing cells in the brain. Cycloset is a completely new idea for the treatment of type 2 diabetes, which represents about 90% of all cases of diabetes. The development of Cycloset for treating diabetes was based upon laboratory studies that showed brain dopamine activity to be low in metabolic disease states like diabetes. Additional studies in diabetic animals have also shown that treatment with a dopamine agonist like bromocriptine acts in the brain to "reset" the biological clock neurochemistry that improves the metabolism of glucose in people with type 2 diabetes. However, in order to do this, the bromocriptine (Cycloset) needs to be taken once daily early in the morning about 2 hours after waking up. Cycloset can be used alone or in combination with oral anti-diabetic agents. It is not as potent as other anti-diabetic agents, but works in a completely new way to lower blood glucose (sugar) levels. The most common side effects of Cycloset include nausea, dizziness, fatigue, and headache. In order to help prevent these side effects the dosage of Cycloset needs to be increased slowly over several weeks. Perhaps this novel new drug therapy for type 2 diabetes will lead to further discoveries in the future.

GLUCOVANCE

QUESTION: I heard about a new oral medication for diabetes. What can you tell me about it?

ANSWER: Actually the new medication, Glucovance, is a combination of two oral anti-diabetic drugs that have been available for quite some time. The new combination drug contains both glyburide and metformin, the two most widely prescribed oral anti-diabetic agents. Glyburide by itself is available as a generic and by the tradenames Diabeta, Micronase, and Glynase. Metformin is also available as a generic and by the tradename Glucophage. Glyburide works by increasing insulin production by the pancreas, while metformin works by blocking the production of sugar (glucose) in the liver and by increasing the patient's sensitivity to insulin. Because they work differently, this combination can be very effective in treating patients with type 2 diabetes who cannot be satisfactorily managed by diet and exercise alone. The most common side effects of Glucovance are gastrointestinal disturbances such as nausea, vomiting, and diarrhea. Less frequently, symptoms of low blood sugar (glucose) such as lightheadedness, dizziness, shakiness, or hunger may occur. In rare cases Glucovance can also cause a potentially fatal side effect known as lactic acidosis. It should be avoided in people with kidney problems, if they are over age 80 (unless they have their kidneys tested first), if they are taking medications for heart failure, if they have a history of liver disease, or if they drink alcohol excessively. This new combination drug is available in three dosage strengths and is taken orally once or twice a day with meals.

JANUMET

QUESTION: I heard a new oral drug for diabetes was approved. What can you tell me about it?

ANSWER: The FDA recently approved Janumet for the treatment of people with type 2 diabetes. It is used to help control blood glucose (sugar) in conjunction with diet and exercise. Janumet actually contains two drugs that are already on the market, sitagliptin (Januvia) and metformin (Glucophage). Sitagliptin (Januvia) was approved in 2006 but metformin (Glucophage) has been available for many years. Sitagliptin (Januvia) works to lower high blood glucose levels by blocking an enzyme in the body that leads to an increase in hormones known as incretins, which are involved in the regulation of glucose in the blood. Essentially, incretins instruct the pancreas, which makes insulin, how to react when food hits the intestinal tract. Metformin (Glucophage), on the other hand, works to lower blood glucose by decreasing its production in the liver and by making tissues more sensitive to insulin. Because they work differently, this combination can be very effective in treating patients with type 2 diabetes who cannot be satisfactorily managed by diet and exercise alone.

Janumet is taken twice a day with meals. The most common side effects of this new combination product include diarrhea, nausea/vomiting, gas, stomach discomfort, indigestion, headache, weakness, and inflammation of the nasal cavity & pharynx. In rare cases it can also cause a potentially fatal side effect known as lactic acidosis and it should be avoided by people with liver or kidney disease.

JANUVIA

<u>QUESTION</u>: I heard that a new oral drug for diabetes was approved. What can you tell me about it?

<u>ANSWER</u>: The FDA recently approved Januvia (sitagliptin) for the treatment of people with type 2 diabetes. Januvia is the first of a new class of prescription drugs called DPP-4 inhibitors. It was approved to treat type 2 diabetes when used in conjunction with a proper diet and exercise. Januvia can be given by itself or in combination with metformin (glucophage), pioglitazone (Actos), or rosiglitazone (Avandia). This new oral agent works in a very different way than other oral drugs used to treat type 2 diabetes. Januvia, which only works when the blood sugar level is elevated, blocks an enzyme in the body that leads to an increase in hormones known as incretins which are involved in the regulation of glucose (sugar) in the blood. Essentially, incretins instruct the pancreas, which makes insulin, how to react when food hits the intestinal tract. Metformin (glucophage) on the other hand works to lower blood glucose by decreasing its production in the liver and by making tissues more sensitive to insulin. Actos and Avandia also work by improving sensitivity to insulin and by blocking glucose production in the liver. When given together with Januvia, these other drugs work to complement the control of blood glucose. During clinical studies Januvia, which is taken once a day, had very few side effects. The most common side effects included stuffy or runny nose and sore throat, upper respiratory infection, and headache. Treatment with Januvia was not associated with weight gain or increased risk of hypoglycemia (low blood sugar) like other drugs used to treat type 2 diabetes. Januvia provides a new treatment option for many of these patients. A combination product containing both metformin and the active ingredient in Januvia is also being developed by the manufacturer, Merck.

<u>PLEASE NOTE</u>: The diabetes drug rosiglitazone (Avandia) and the combination drugs Avandamet and Avandaryl will no longear be available in pharmacies as of November 18, 2011. Multiple studies have linked rosiglitazone to an increased risk of heart attack. If you've successfully controlled your glucose levels with an Avandia-based medication and your doctotr feels you should continue to take it despite the known risks, he or she will need to enroll you in the FDA's Avandia-Rosiglitazone Medicine Access Program. Through the program, participants will receive Avandia by mail from FDA-certified pharmacies.

ONGLYZA

QUESTION: I heard that a new oral drug for diabetes was approved. What can you tell me about it?

ANSWER: The FDA recently approved Onglyza (saxagliptin) for the treatment of people with type 2 diabetes. Onglyza is the second of a new class of prescription drugs called DPP-4 inhibitors (the first DPP-4 inhibitor was Januvia or sitagliptin, which was approved in 2006). Onglyza was approved to treat type 2 diabetes when used in conjunction with a proper diet and exercise. Onglyza can be given by itself or in combination with metformin (Glucophage), pioglitazone (Actos) or rosiglitazone (Avandia), or glyburide (DiaBeta, Micronase, Glynase). DPP-4 inhibitors work in a very different way than other oral drugs used to treat type 2 diabetes. Onglyza, which only works when the blood sugar level is elevated, blocks an enzyme in the body that leads to an increase in hormones known as incretins which are involved in the regulation of glucose (sugar) in the blood. Essentially, incretins instruct the pancreas, which makes insulin, how to react when food hits the intestinal tract. Metformin (Glucophage) on the other hand works to lower blood glucose by decreasing its production in the liver and by making tissues more sensitive to insulin. Actos and Avandia also work by improving sensitivity to insulin and by blocking glucose production in the liver, while glyburide stimulates the secretion of insulin in the pancreas. When given together with Onglyza, these other drugs work to complement the control of blood glucose. During clinical studies, Onglyza, which is taken once a day, had very few side effects. The most common side effects included upper respiratory infection, urinary tract infection, and headache. Treatment with Onglyza was not associated with weight gain or increased risk of hypoglycemia (low blood sugar) like other drugs used to treat type 2 diabetes. Onglyza provides a new treatment option for many of these patients.

PLEASE NOTE: The diabetes drug rosiglitazone (Avandia) and the combination drugs Avandamet and Avandaryl will no longear be available in pharmacies as of November 18, 2011. Multiple studies have linked rosiglitazone to an increased risk of heart attack. If you've successfully controlled your glucose levels with an Avandia-based medication and your doctotr feels you should continue to take it despite the known risks, he or she will need to enroll you in the FDA's Avandia-Rosiglitazone Medicine Access Program. Through the program, participants will receive Avandia by mail from FDA-certified pharmacies.

PRANDIMET

QUESTION: I heard about a new oral combination medication for diabetes. What can you tell me about it?

ANSWER: The FDA recently approved Prandimet to improve control of blood glucose (sugar) in combination with diet and exercise for people with type 2 diabetes. This combination product contains two medications, repaglinide (Prandin) and metformin (Glucophage), which have been available separately for many years. Repaglinide works by increasing insulin production by the pancreas, while metformin works by blocking the production of sugar (glucose) in the liver and by increasing the patient's sensitivity to insulin. Because they work differently, this combination can be very effective in treating patients with type 2 diabetes who cannot be satisfactorily managed by diet and exercise alone. The most common side effects of Prandimet are low blood sugar (hypoglycemia), headache, diarrhea, and nausea. In rare cases, Prandimet can also cause a potentially fatal side effect known as lactic acidosis, which is caused by an accumulation of metformin in the body. The risk of lactic acidosis increases with conditions such as infection, dehydration, excessive alcohol intake, liver or kidney problems, and acute congestive heart failure. Prandimet tablets are taken 2 to 3 times daily within 15 minutes prior to meals.

PRECOSE

QUESTION: I've read about a new medication for diabetes that works differently than insulin or oral tablets. What is it and what about its side effects?

ANSWER: You're probably referring to acarbose (brand name Precose) manufactured by Bayer. This is a new drug for the treatment of patients with Type II diabetes (non-insulin dependent). Precose is the first FDA-approved medication known as an alpha-glucosidase inhibitor. The drug works by interfering with those enzymes in the small intestine that are involved in the digestion of complex carbohydrates in the diet, such as starch. This interference prevents the conversion of these carbohydrates into glucose (which is rapidly absorbed into the bloodstream), thus preventing high blood glucose levels following a meal. Unlike other oral drugs for diabetes, Acarbose does not affect insulin secretion. This drug can be used by itself or in combination with other oral hypoglycemic agents. In order to work effectively, it must be taken with meals (with the first bite), three times a day. The recommended starting dose is 25 mg (1/2 of a 50 mg tablet) orally three times daily with the dosage increased up to 300 mg per day after 4 to 8 weeks, depending upon blood glucose levels and tolerance. The most common side effects of Precose are flatulence, diarrhea and abdominal discomfort. Beginning with a low dose (25 mg) can help to minimize these side effects.

REZULIN

QUESTION: I have been taking Rezulin for my diabetes and it was taken off the market. What other similar drugs are still available?

ANSWER: Rezulin (generic name troglitazone) is an oral anti-diabetic medication that was first approved to treat patients with type 2 diabetes in January 1997. At that time, it was given a priority review by the FDA because it worked differently from other oral anti-diabetic drugs. During its clinical testing, it was found to be generally well tolerated but did affect liver function tests in some patients. After it was approved and became widely used, Rezulin was found to be associated with acute liver failure resulting in numerous deaths and liver transplants. Because of this, the FDA asked the manufacturer of Rezulin to remove the product from the market on March 21, 2000.

There are two other oral medications that were approved which work in the same way as Rezulin. These similar drugs are Avandia (generic name rosiglitazone) and Actos (generic name pioglitazone). All 3 of the drugs are known as "glitazones" or "insulin sensitizers". Unlike other oral anti-diabetic drugs which affect insulin levels, glitazones make the body more sensitive to the action of insulin. At this point in time, both Actos and Avandia appear to have a much lower risk of severe liver toxicity than Rezulin, but liver function tests should still be done periodically when taking these newer medications.

This experience with Rezulin should remind all of us that many drug side effects do not become evident until medications are used in a large number of patients. Patients using Rezulin should contact their physician about alternative treatments as soon as possible. Patients should not discontinue taking Rezulin or other treatments for diabetes until they discuss alternative therapies with their physicians. The manufacturer of Rezulin, Warner Lambert, will reimburse patients for their out-of-pocket expenses for unused supplies of Rezulin. Patients with questions regarding this process can call 1-877-798-7398 for instructions.

PLEASE NOTE: The diabetes drug rosiglitazone (Avandia) and the combination drugs Avandamet and Avandaryl will no longear be available in pharmacies as of November 18, 2011. Multiple studies have linked rosiglitazone to an increased risk of heart attack. If you've successfully controlled your glucose levels with an Avandia-based medication and your doctotr feels you should continue to take it despite the known risks, he or she will need to enroll you in the FDA's Avandia-Rosiglitazone Medicine Access Program. Through the program, participants will receive Avandia by mail from FDA-certified pharmacies.

STARLIX

QUESTION: I heard that there is a new oral medication for diabetes available. What can you tell me about it?

ANSWER: You probably are talking about Starlix (generic name nateglinide), which was approved for the treatment of patients with type 2 diabetes. Starlix is a new type of oral antidiabetic medication that works to lower blood sugar (glucose) by stimulating the pancreas to release more insulin into the blood. This new agent can be used by itself or used in combination with another oral antidiabetic drug called Glucophage (generic name metformin), when diet or exercise is not effective in controlling blood glucose. When Starlix is used together with Glucophage or metformin it can lower blood glucose levels more than when either drug is used alone because they have additive effects. When taken shortly before eating, Starlix appears to prevent "spikes" in blood glucose that occur after a meal. These "spikes" or temporary increases in blood sugar after a meal are thought to be a major cause of cardiovascular damage caused by diabetes. The recommended dose of Starlix is 120 mg three times a day, taken 1 to 30 minutes before meals. If patients taking Starlix skip a meal, they should also skip a dose. Side effects of Starlix during clinical studies have included hypoglycemia (low blood glucose), back pain, upper respiratory tract infection, flu symptoms, dizziness, joint problems, and diarrhea.

SYMLIN INJECTION

QUESTION: What can you tell me about a new type of injectable medication for diabetes?

ANSWER: The FDA recently approved Symlin (pramlintide) injection for use in combination with insulin to treat certain patients with type 1 and type 2 diabetes. It is approved for use in people with type 1 diabetes who use mealtime insulin but have failed to control their blood glucose (sugar) with insulin alone. Symlin is also approved for use in people with type 2 diabetes who use mealtime insulin with or without an oral sulfonylurea drug and/or metformin (Glucophage). Oral sulfonylurea agents include Diabenese or chlorpramide, acetohexamide, Tolinase or tolazamide, Orinase or tolbutamide, Glucotrol or glipizide, Amaryl, Diabeta, Micronase, or glyburide. The active ingredient in Symlin is similar to a hormone (amylin) that is produced in the pancreas where insulin is also made. People with diabetes do not make enough insulin or amylin. However, the hormone amylin found in Symlin works in a much different way than insulin to control (lower) glucose (sugar) levels in the blood. First of all, it slows the movement of food through the stomach, which affects how fast glucose gets into your blood after eating. It also helps to lower levels of another hormone (glucagon) that can increase glucose levels in the blood. In addition, Symlin promotes a sense of being full, which can lead to reduced food intake and potential weight loss. Clinical studies with Symlin have shown that when it is used together with insulin before meals, it can help to lower blood glucose levels and insulin doses, and promote weight reduction in people with diabetes. However it should be emphasized that Symlin is not for everyone who has diabetes and patients need to be carefully selected for this new therapy. The most worrisome concern of Symlin when used with insulin is that a person's blood glucose level will go too low (hypoglycemia). This can be very dangerous and the close monitoring of blood glucose levels and insulin dose is extremely important when using Symlin. Other medical conditions and medications can also affect blood glucose levels and patients using Symlin will need guidance and education from their physician, pharmacist, and other healthcare workers. Symlin is given by subcutaneous injection into the abdomen or thigh immediately before major meals. The dosage of Symlin and insulin used must be carefully determined by the prescribing physician. Symlin is the first of a new type of therapy for diabetes and provides a new option for many patients.

TRADJENTA

QUESTION: I heard that a new oral drug for diabetes was approved. What can you tell me about it?

ANSWER: The FDA recently (2011) approved Tradjenta (linagliptin) for the treatment of people with type 2 diabetes. Tradjenta is the third of a new class of prescription drugs called DPP-4 inhibitors (the first DPP-4 inhibitor was Januvia or sitagliptin, which was approved in 2006 and the second was Onglyza or saxagliptin approved in 2009). Tradjenta was approved to treat type 2 diabetes when used in conjunction with a proper diet and exercise. Tradjenta can be given by itself or in combination with other oral agents used to treat type 2 diaabetes such as metformin (Glucophage), pioglitazone (Actos), or glyburide (DiaBeta, Glynase).

DPP-4 inhibitors work in a very different way than other oral drugs used to treat type 2 diabetes. Tradjenta, which only works when the blood sugar level is elevated, blocks an enzyme in the body that leads to an increase in hormones known as incretins which are involved in the regulation of glucose (sugar) in the blood. Essentially, incretins instruct the pancreas, which makes insulin, how to react when food hits the intestinal tract. Metformin (Glucophage) on the other hand works to lower blood glucose by decreasing its production in the liver and by making tissues more sensitive to insulin. Actos works by improving sensitivity to insulin and by blocking glucose production in the liver, while glyburide stimulates the secretion of insulin in the pancreas.

When given together with Tradjenta, these other drugs work to complement the control of blood glucose. During clinical studies, Tradjenta, which is taken once a day, had very few side effects. The most common side effects included upper respiratory infection, stuffy or runny nose, sore throat, muscle pain, and headache. Tradjenta provides a new treatment option for many of these patients.

JENTADUETO

QUESTION: I heard that a new oral drug was approved for diabetes. What can you tell me about it?

ANSWER: The FDA recently (2012) approved Jentadueto for the treatment of adults with type 2 diabetes in conjunction with diet and exercise. Jentadueto actually contains two drugs that are already on the market, linagliptin (Trajenta) and metformin (Glucophage). Linagliptin works to lower blood glucose levels by blocking an enzyme in the body that leads to an increase in hormones known as incretins, which are involved in the regulation of glucose in the blood. Essentially, incretins instruct the pancreas, which makes insulin, how to react when food hits the intestinal tract. Metformin (Glucophage), on the other hand, works to lower blood glucose by decreasing its production in the liver and by making tissues more sensitive to insulin. Because they work differently, this combination can be very effective in treating patients with type 2 diabetes who cannot be satisfactorily managed by diet and exercise alone. Jentadueto is taken twice daily with meals. The most common side effects of this new combination product include diarrhea and inflammation of the nasal cavity and pharynx.

VICTOZA

QUESTION: I heard about a new injectable drug for diabetes. What can you tell me about it?

ANSWER: The FDA recently approved Victoza (liraglutide), a once-daily injection to treat adults with type 2 diabetes. Its use is intended to help lower blood sugar levels along with diet, exercise, and selected other diabetes medications. It is not recommended as initial therapy in patients who have not achieved adequate diabetes control on diet and exercise alone. Victoza is in a class of medicines known as glucagon-like peptide-1 GLP-1) receptor agonists that help the pancreas make more insulin after eating a meal. During clinical studies, the most common side effects of Victozta were headache, nausea, and diarrhea. However, pancreatitis (inflammation of the pancreas) can occur and Victoza should be used with caution in people with a history of pancreatitis. Because of the possibility of pancreatitis, Victoza should be stopped if there is severe abdominal pain, with or without nausea and vomiting, and should not be restarted if pancreatitis is confirmed by blood tests.

NEW INSULIN PUMP

QUESTION: What can you tell me about the new insulin pump that also monitors your blood sugar?

ANSWER: A new insulin pump that also continuously monitors blood glucose (sugar) levels was recently approved by the FDA for people who use insulin to treat their diabetes. Insulin pumps enable diabetic patients to inject insulin on both a pre-programmed and as-needed basis throughout the day and night, much like a healthy human pancreas does. This new pump (MiniMed Paradigm Real-Time Insulin Pump and Continuous Glucose Monitoring System) is the first insulin pump that actually measures a patient's blood glucose around the clock so that they can improve their glucose control. This monitoring system uses a tiny electrode sensor that is inserted under the skin using a small device and is replaced after three days of use. This sensor measures glucose levels in the fluid between body cells and this information is relayed every five minutes (288 readings per day) to the insulin pump, which displays the glucose level to the patient. It also shows a graph of glucose levels for three-hour and 24-hour periods with arrows indicating how quickly glucose is moving up or down. In addition, an alarm alerts patients when glucose levels become too high or low. This information allows patients to take immediate action to improve their glucose control after taking a confirmatory fingerstick blood glucose reading. The insulin pump/glucose monitoring system also includes a built-in calculator to help patients calculate the correct insulin dose to use. Research has shown that very good control of blood glucose levels reduces the risks of complications of diabetes such as coma, blindness, kidney failure, amputation, impotence, nerve disease, and heart disease. Diabetes is the leading cause of kidney failure and adult-onset blindness, increases the risk of heart attack deaths by 2-4 times, and leads to more than 80,000 amputations each year. Ultimately, an artificial pancreas will enable a person with diabetes to maintain normal glucose levels by providing the right amount of insulin at the right time, just as the human pancreas does in non-diabetic individuals. Until then, this newly approved insulin pump/glucose monitoring system is a big step in that direction.

INHALED INSULIN

QUESTION: What can you tell me about the new inhaled insulin product?

ANSWER: Exubera is an inhaled insulin product recently approved by the FDA for the treatment of diabetes. It is the first new insulin delivery option made available since the discovery of insulin in the 1920's. Up until now insulin, which is a large protein, needed to be given by injection. Efforts to develop noninvasive methods such as oral and nasal formulations have not been successful. The lungs, however, allow drugs to be absorbed quickly into the bloodstream. The insulin powder used with Exubera is contained in small blister packages. The blister is inserted into an inhaler device which comes with the product. The patient pumps the handle of the inhaler and then presses a button causing the blister package to be pierced. The insulin powder is then dispersed into the chamber of the device, allowing the patient to inhale the powder aerosol through the mouth into the lungs. When insulin is inhaled in this way, the drug begins to lower blood glucose (sugar) within 10 to 20 minutes, with maximum effects occurring about two hours after inhalation. The duration of glucose-lowering activity lasts for about six hours. Exubera is approved for the treatment of adults with type 1 or type 2 diabetes. In patients with type 1 diabetes, Exubera should be used along with a longer-acting injectable insulin. For people with type 2 diabetes, Exubera can be used by itself or in combination with oral anti-diabetic agents or longer-acting injectable insulins. Exubera will not totally eliminate the need for insulin injections for many patients and diabetics will have to continue prickking their fingers to check blood glucose levels. Exubera is contraindicated in patients who smoke or who have quit smoking for less than six months. It should also not be used by people with unstable or poorly controlled lung disease.

PLEASE NOTE: As of January 16, 2008, Exubera was no longer available from the manufacturer. This decision was not based on any safety or effectiveness concerns, but because too few patients were using Exubera. Further information can be obtained by calling 1-800-EXUBERA (1-800-398-2372).

DIABETES AND
NON-PRESCRIPTION MEDICATION

<u>QUESTION</u>: I have diabetes and want to know if I should be concerned about taking non-prescription medications?

<u>ANSWER</u>: Non-prescription drugs often contain ingredients that can affect your diabetes. Many include some form of sugar, which can change the level of glucose (sugar) in your blood. Some drugs also contain alcohol, which can add hidden calories to your diet. It's a good idea to avoid drugs that can affect your diabetes control, but it's not always easy to do. Choosing a non-prescription drug for relieving the symptoms of a cold or cough or even a simple headache can be a challenge. Some general guidelines for choosing non-prescription drugs are:

- Read the label carefully. Check the list of ingredients and pay close attention to any warnings or cautions.
- Avoid products containing sugar. But remember that sugar comes in many forms. Just because a product is labeled "dietetic" or "sugar-free" doesn't mean it's intended for people with diabetes. Many dietetic products have no sugar or sucrose but contain dextrose, fructose, or sorbitol, which are sugars.
- Choose products with little or no alcohol. Alcohol adds calories to your diet. The higher the alcohol content, the more calories the product contains.
- Use tablets or capsules instead of liquids. These are often a better choice because they contain no alcohol and little or no sugar.
- Avoid decongestants that are taken by mouth. These products may raise your blood glucose. Use nasal sprays or nose drops instead.
- Look for this caution statement on the label of the non-prescription drug you are thinking of buying: "Individuals with high blood pressure, heart disease, or diabetes should use only as directed by physician".

Always check with a pharmacist if you think a non-prescription drug has affected your blood glucose levels.

REUSE OF INSULIN NEEDLES

QUESTION: My wife has diabetes and needs insulin shots three times a day. The insulin needles and syringes are expensive and I wonder if I can use them more than once?

ANSWER: Many people with diabetes do not have insurance and must pay for their diabetes supplies out of their own pockets. The cost of multiple daily injections of insulin and monitoring of blood glucose levels can be costly. Before disposable needles and syringes were available, people boiled their reusable supplies to maintain sterility and prevent infections due to contamination. Today, however, the neatly packaged disposable needles and syringes are intended for one time use only. Potential problems with reusing disposable syringes and needles include dulling or bending of the needle, broken needle tips, and bacterial contamination. However, the American Diabetes Association (ADA) considers the reuse of syringes to be safe under certain conditions if precautions are undertaken. For example, the ADA considers reuse of syringes permissible as long as the syringe is properly recapped and the patient has good personal hygiene, has no open wounds, and has neither an acute illness nor weakened immune system. They also recommend discarding the syringe and needle if it becomes dull or bent or if it comes into contact with any surface other than the skin. It is probably a good idea that if single-use syringes are reused that they only be reused for one day to reduce the chance of potential problems. In addition, the needle should be recapped immediately after use and should only be used by one person and not shared with anyone else. The syringe and needle should be stored at room temperature. Wiping the needle with alcohol is not recommended because the alcohol may remove the silicon coating that makes the injection less painful. Finally, if an infection at the site of injection is suspected, a physician should be contacted immediately.

ROTATING INSULIN INJECTIONS

QUESTION: What is the best way to rotate my insulin injections each day?

ANSWER: Insulin is a hormone produced by the pancreas, which regulates the amount of sugar (glucose) in the blood. Its discovery in 1921 is often described as one of the major medical advances of the 20th century. The use of insulin is required for the day-to-day survival of some patients with diabetes, and it contributes to an improved quality of life and reduced complications from diabetes for many others. In the last fifteen years, several studies have shown that better control of blood glucose can significantly reduce the long-term complications of diabetes such as blindness, kidney failure, cardiovascular disease, and nerve problems. A Johns Hopkins Health Alert (**www.johnshopkinshealthalerts.com**, 2007) provided the following information regarding insulin injections:

- Whether you inject insulin only once a day or multiple times, it is important to change the location of the injection in a methodical and consistent pattern that also takes into account the effect of physical activity on how quickly your body absorbs the insulin. This practice, known as injection site rotation, will prevent unsightly skin changes and unwanted variations in the rate at which the insulin gets into your blood stream.
- Insulin is typically injected with a syringe or insulin pen into the layer of subcutaneous (beneath the skin) fat. Your blood vessels then absorb the insulin and ferry it to the rest of the body. Injections at the same spot too many times in a row can cause the fat to either lump up (lipohypertrophy) or waste away (lipoatrophy). These changes in the fat can impede absorption of insulin.
- **Injection tip 1—Avoid areas with relatively higher concentrations of blood vessels and nerves that might get poked accidentally.** Instead, give yourself injections in the abdomen (though not within two inches of your navel); the outsides of your upper arms, upper thighs, and hips; and the buttocks.
- **Injection tip 2—Alternate injection sites within the preferred areas rather than between them.** So, for example, if you have type

2 diabetes and take a single injection of long-acting insulin every day, you could inject on the left side of your abdomen for a while, making sure to space injections at least an inch or so apart. Then, when you complete a circuit of the left side, switch your injections to the right. By the time you return to your starting position, the tissue on the left abdomen will have had time to rest and heal.

- **Injection tip 3—Choose to use a different area for each insulin**—say, the abdomen for long-acting insulin, and the upper thighs for before-meal insulin shots. Again, switch sides for your injections to allow time for the tissue to recover.
- **Injection tip 4—Be consistent.** Due to variations in blood flow, the body absorbs insulin most rapidly in the belly area, followed by the arms, thighs, and hips or buttocks. Ideally you want your insulin to be absorbed at about the same rate each time you inject. This makes for more consistent and predictable control of blood sugar, avoiding dips and peaks. Otherwise, if you do notice an unexpected change in your blood sugar, how will you know what caused it? Was it exercise, a meal, or your medication?

Diabetes educators at the Johns Hopkins Diabetes Center encourage people to give injections in the abdomen as much as possible. It's easily accessible and absorbs insulin the quickest. But if you take multiple insulins and would like to inject in a different area, they discourage the upper arms. The outer portions of the arms are harder to reach, and arm movements can affect absorption.

TYPES OF SUGARS

QUESTION: My husband is a diabetic and I buy food that says "no sugar added", yet when I read the contents it says "alcohol sugar". What is that? Why would cookies have alcohol? Also, what is the difference between sucrose, fructose, and sorbitol?

ANSWER: I'll try to explain these confusing terms. First of all, there are many types of sugars. Sugars can come from different sources such as honey, maple syrup, molasses, corn syrup, sugar beets, sugar cane, various fruits, and many more. Regardless of the source, they are all sweet-tasting carbohydrates that are made up of the elements carbon, hydrogen, and oxygen, hence the term "carbohydrate". The way the carbohydrates are linked together determines the type of sugar. Since there are numerous chemical configurations of carbon, hydrogen, and oxygen atoms, there are numerous kinds of sugars. A saccharide is a group of carbohydrates, which includes sugars. In addition, sugars contain oxygen atoms combined to hydrogen atoms, which are called "hydroxyl" groups or "alcohol" groups. This does not mean that sugars are the same as the alcohol found in alcoholic beverages (ethanol), just that they contain the" hydroxyl" or" alcohol" chemical group (-OH).

Now that I have you all confused, let me try to explain the difference between glucose, sucrose, fructose, and sorbitol. Glucose (or dextrose) is the most important sugar (carbohydrate) in body metabolism. Without going into a lot of detail, glucose, which is formed during the digestion of more complex carbohydrates, is what humans metabolize to produce energy. It is needed by every cell and insulin enables the cells to take in glucose for energy production. Glucose is classified as a "simple sugar" or "monosaccharide" because it is not connected or linked to other carbohydrates (disaccarides, polysaccarides, etc.). Sucrose (or common white table sugar) on the other hand, is a combination of glucose and fructose. Because of this, it is classified as a disaccaride (di-meaning two, glucose and fructose). During metabolism it is broken down into both glucose and fructose. Fructose is also a "simple sugar" or "monosaccharide" found in corn syrup, honey, and fruit juices. Fructose has the same chemical composition as glucose, but the molecular arrangement is different. Finally, sorbitol is a derivative of glucose that contains the "hydroxyl" or "alcohol" group (-OH) and is found in many types of fruits and berries. It is used as a sweetening agent and does not appear to affect blood glucose levels in people with diabetes. I hope that this discussion is helpful.

ACTOS AND BLADDER CANCER

QUESTION: Can the diabetes medication Actos increase the risk of bladder cancer?

ANSWER: Yes, the use of Actos (pioglitazone) for more than one year may increase the risk of bladder cancer and the Food and Drug Administration (FDA) has issued a safety announcement regarding this risk. This safety information is based on the FDA's review of data from a planned five-year interim analysis of an ongoing, ten-year epidemiological study. The five-year results showed that although there was no overall increased risk of bladder cancer with pioglitazone use, an increased risk of bladder cancer was noted among patients with the longest exposure to pioglitazone, and in those exposed to the highest cumulative dose of pioglitazone. The FDA is also aware of a recent epidemiological study conducted in France, which suggests an increased risk of bladder cancer with pioglitazone. Based on the results of this study, France has suspended the use of pioglitazone and Germany has recommended not to start pioglitazone in new patients. The FDA will continue to evaluate data from the ongoing ten-year epidemiological study as well as conduct a comprehensive review of the results from the French study. As more information becomes available the FDA will update the public.

Additional Information for Patients
- There may be an increased chance of having bladder cancer when you take pioglitazone.
- You should not take pioglitazone if you are receiving treatment for bladder cancer.
- Tell your doctor right away if you have any of the following symptoms of bladder cancer: blood or red color in urine; urgent need to urinate or pain while urinating; pain in back or lower abdomen.
- Read the Medication Guide you get along with your pioglitazone medicine. It explains the risks associated with the use of pioglitazone.
- Talk to your healthcare professional if you have questions or concerns about pioglitazone medicines.
- Report side effects from the use of pioglitazone medicines to the FDA MedWatch program (1-800-332-1088).

FOOT CARE

QUESTION: Why is it so important for someone with diabetes to take special care of his or her feet?

ANSWER: Foot problems are the most common complication of diabetes. Patients with diabetes often develop infections that can become so severe that gangrene develops and the toe, foot or even the leg must be amputated. In fact, diabetes is the leading cause of nontraumatic amputations in America. Poor control of blood sugar (glucose) levels over a long period of time can cause damage to the tiny blood vessels and nerve endings in the feet, leading to poor circulation and less sensation in the feet. The damaged nerve supply causes the feet to lose their ability to sweat and they become dry and cracked. If the feet are not cared for every day, infections can develop in the cracked skin. Furthermore, when blood glucose is not under control, patients cannot fight infections effectively. These infections can spread deep into the tissue and then into the bone making them very difficult to treat. Patients with diabetes may not even know that they have a cut or infection because they do not feel pain because of the damage to the tiny nerve endings that signal pain.

To help avoid foot problems, proper foot care for people with diabetes should include daily inspections for cuts, sores or other problems. Patients with diabetes who can't properly examine their feet may require a mirror or magnifying glass to assist them or they may need assistance from a friend or relative. Also, there is a need for proper hydration of the feet with nonperfumed lotions or creams. Soaking of the feet is not recommended. At the first sign of redness, swelling, bruising or infection in the foot or toes, a physician or podiatrist should be consulted. Some useful foot care management tips for people with diabetes are as follows:

- Wash & inspect feet and toes daily. Use warm water and soap, and then dry thoroughly. Soaking feet is not recommended.
- Use foot creams or lubricating oils to keep the feet soft and to avoid dry, cracked skin.
- Carefully cut toenails straight across, smoothing the corners with a nail file, or have a health professional trim toenails.

- Never cut corns or calluses.
- The most common infections in a diabetic foot are infection of the tissue around the nail or between the toes, infection of the middle foot due to trauma, and infection of the sole following a puncture wound. Inspect these areas carefully each day for breaks in the skin, swelling, redness or other signs of infection.
- Wear properly fitting shoes that allow the feet plenty of room. The toes should not be rubbed or squeezed.
- Wear clean dry socks that are changed daily.
- Never walk barefooted.
- Seek medical care for all skin lesions.

REGRANEX

QUESTION: I am a diabetic with foot ulcers and I've heard about a new drug that helps heal these ulcers. Could you provide some information about this new product?

ANSWER: As I discussed in a previous column, foot problems are a common complication of diabetes. Foot ulcers or open sores that remain after the skin is damaged affect about two million diabetics in the U.S. They are more common in patients over 40 years of age and may go undetected because other complications of diabetes, such as nerve damage or eye problems, can make it difficult for patients to see or feel the ulcers as they develop. In addition, circulation problems may reduce the blood supply to the feet, resulting in slower healing and an increased risk of infection. These ulcers can lead to amputation, thus proper foot care is very important for patients with diabetes. Proper care includes trimming toenails straight across, not going barefoot, keeping the feet clean, not exposing feet to extreme heat or cold, and wearing properly fitting shoes.

The new product that you are asking about is called Regranex and is the first prescription biotechnology drug that has been approved for diabetic foot ulcers. It is known as a growth factor and works by stimulating the body to grow new tissue to heal the open wound or ulcer. It is available as a gel that is applied once a day to the wound.

Studies have shown that this gel can help to completely heal foot ulcers in up to 50% of patients when used appropriately and in conjunction with good foot care. Good foot care includes removal of dead tissue, daily dressing changes, taking pressure off the feet, and treatment of any infection. Side effects of this gel appear to be minimal with a rash occurring in about 2% of patients. Regranex comes with step-by-step instructions for its proper use, which should be followed for the best results. This new product is also being studied for the treatment of bedsores, but results are not available yet. Patients or healthcare professionals wishing more information can call 1-888-REGRANEX.

QUESTION: What can you tell me about the warning that the FDA issued about using Regranex?

ANSWER: Regranex is a topical skin preparation that is used for the treatment of leg and foot ulcers that are not healing in diabetic patients. It is known as a growth factor and works by stimulating the body to grow new tissue to heal the open wound or ulcer. It is available as a gel that is applied once a day to the wound. Studies have shown that this gel can help to completely heal foot ulcers in up to 50% of patients when used appropriately and in conjunction with good foot care. Good foot care includes removal of dead tissue, daily dressing changes, taking pressure off the feet, and treatment of any infection.

In June of 2008, the FDA announced that a "Black Box Warning" would be added to the labeling for Regranex due to a possible increased risk of cancer death in people repeatedly using this product. This warning is based upon postmarketing study data that showed there was a five-fold increased risk of cancer death in people using 3 or more tubes of Regranex. In announcing this label change, the FDA cautions health care professionals to carefully weigh the risks and benefits of treating patients with this product and also noted that Regranex is not recommended for patients with known malignancies. Growth factors like the active ingredient in Regranex, cause cells to divide more rapidly and there is concern that they will also make cancer cells grow more quickly. It should be noted that currently there is no evidence that Regranex causes new cancers, but continued patient monitoring will be needed.

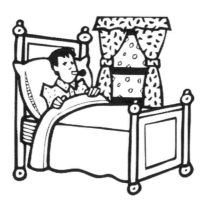

CHAPTER 9
INFECTIONS

SHINGLES

QUESTION: What can I do for shingles?

ANSWER: Shingles (also known as herpes zoster or zoster) is a viral infection caused by the varicella-zoster virus (VZV). This is the same virus that causes chickenpox in childhood and then re-emerges later in life to cause this painful condition called shingles. Following a bout of chickenpox, the virus becomes dormant and lives in the nerve tract until something "triggers" it to become active again. This may occur when a person's immune system becomes weakened by a medical condition or just due to aging. Shingles is a rare problem in young healthy adults but occurs in about 5 out of 1,000 people over age 50, and in about 10 out of 1,000 people over age 80. Some people predict that this medical problem will increase significantly in the future as baby boomers age. However, the use of a newly available vaccine to prevent chickenpox in children may lower the incidence of shingles in adults although it will take many years to determine this.

Shingles typically begins with mild aches and pains, feelings of bodily discomfort, nausea, chills, and fever. In about 90% of patients there is a sharp, stabbing pain, tenderness, and burning along the nerve tract affected. This pain can be excruciating and has been described as though you are being stabbed in the stomach with a white-hot poker. After about 3 to 5 days, lesions or a rash will appear like a belt on one side of the body or face. These lesions turn into fluid filled blisters or vesicles that later crust over in about 7-10 days. In about 90% of patients, the pain of shingles usually resolves within a month, with 97% pain free after 12 months. However, some people will still experience chronic pain for years that can be burning, shooting, aching, tearing, nagging, jabbing or lancing—sometimes called the "belt of roses from hell". This long lasting pain is called post-herpetic neuralgia (PHN). You should note that people who have never had chickenpox or with weak immune systems should stay away from people with shingles, especially when the person has the blister-like lesions.

The treatment of shingles includes bed rest, care of lesions, antiviral drugs, and pain relievers. The burning or itching from the lesions or rash may be treated with mild nonprescription products like colloidal oatmeal (Aveeno), calamine lotion, or aluminum acetate soaks (Bluboro or Domeboro). Your physician may also prescribe an antiviral medication, which can help shorten the duration and severity of pain, especially in older patients. The antiviral drugs work best when given early in the episode of shingles, so it is wise to see a doctor as soon as possible. Antiviral drugs used in this disorder include acyclovir (Zovirax), famciclovir (Famvir), and valacyclovir (Valtrex). Nonprescription pain relievers like acetaminophen (Tylenol), naproxen, or ibuprofen may be helpful, but stronger prescription pain relievers may be needed in some cases. A variety of prescription and nonprescription medications such as lidocaine patch 5% (Lidoderm) or capsaicin cream are also available to treat post-herpetic neuralgia. Fortunately, shingles rarely appears more than once during a lifetime.

QUESTION: I don't remember having chicken pox. Should I still get vaccinated for shingles?

ANSWER: Yes, according to a recent "Health After 50 Medical Letter" (The Johns Hopkins Medical Letter: Health After 50, March 2010). This Medical Letter points out that the Centers for Disease Control and Prevention (CDC) still recommends vaccination for everyone 60 and older. It is estimated that 99% of Americans over the age of 40 have actually had or come into contact with chicken pox, even if they don't remember having the virus or were never formally diagnosed with it.

The shingles vaccine, called Zostavax, is available through your primary care provider. It cuts in half your risk of developing shingles and is effective for at least six years. The vaccine can prevent a recurrence of shingles in people who have already had the disorder, but it will not reduce the severity of shingles or prevent post-herpetic neuralgia after an outbreak. However, medications are available to treat shingles.

Shingles (also known as herpes zoster or zoster) is a viral infection caused by the varicella-zoster virus. This is the same virus that causes chickenpox in childhood and then re-emerges later in life to cause this painful condition called shingles. Following a bout of chickenpox, the virus becomes dormant and lives in the nerve tract until something "triggers" it to become active again. This may occur when a person's immune system becomes weakened by a medical condition or just due to aging. Approximately one million new cases of shingles are reported each year the United States.

Shingles can be extremely painful. The virus lies dormant in nerve cells. When it reappears, it travels through nerve paths and out onto the skin, typically on one side of the body. People often describe a burning sensation; some liken shingles to the feeling of being shocked. About 25% of shingles sufferers go on to experience post-herpetic neuralgia, in which the pain lingers long after the rash has cleared up. Other possible symptoms include fever, headache, chills, and upset stomach.

The risk of developing shingles starts to rise around age 50, and the older a person is, the more severe the effects of shingles tend to be. Older people also are at the highest risk for rare but serious complications from shingles, including pneumonia, hearing problems, blindness, and encephalitis (infection of the brain).

PLEASE NOTE: Zostavax is now approved to help prevent shingles in adults 50 years of age and older.

QUESTION: What can you tell me about the new shingles vaccine?

ANSWER: Shingles (also known as herpes zoster or zoster) is a viral infection caused by the varicella-zoster virus. This is the same virus that causes chickenpox in childhood and then re-emerges later in life to cause this painful condition called shingles. Following a bout of chickenpox, the virus becomes dormant and lives in the nerve tract until something "triggers" it to become active again. This may occur when a person's immune system becomes weakened by a medical condition or just due to aging. Approximately one million new cases of shingles are reported each year the United States. Recently the FDA approved the first vaccine to prevent people over the age of 60 from getting shingles. The new vaccine will be marketed as Zostavax. Zostavax is a much more potent form of the vaccine currently used to prevent chickenpox in children. The approval of Zostavax was based upon the results of a five-year study involving about 40,000 people over the age of 60 who never had shingles. During this study, vaccination with Zostavax was shown to reduce the risk of developing shingles by 51% in all study participants. However, the vaccine was most effective in people 60 to 69 years of age who had a 64% reduction in risk. The risk reduction was lower in older people with people aged 70 to 79 having a 41% risk reduction and those 80 or older having an 18% reduction in risk. In this large study, vaccination with Zostavax was also shown to reduce the incidence of long-term nerve pain (postherpetic neuralgia) in people who developed shingles even though they received the vaccine. Zostavax is only for people who have been infected with chickenpox in the past, which represents more than 90% of adults in the United States. It is indicated for the prevention but not the treatment of shingles and people who have had shingles should not receive Zostavax.

PLEASE NOTE: Zostavax is now approved to help prevent shingles in adults 50 years of age and older.

QUESTION: I heard that the shingles vaccine has been approved for younger people. What can you tell me about this?

ANSWER: Yes, on March 24, 2011 the FDA approved the use of Zostavax, a live reduced-strength virus vaccine, for the prevention of shingles in individuals 50 to 59 years of age. Zostavax is already approved for use in individuals 60 years of age and older. In the United States shingles affects approximately 200,000 healthy people between the ages of 50 and 59, per year. It is a disease caused by the varicella-zoster virus, which is a virus

ASK THE PHARMACIST   381

in the herpes family and the same virus that causes chickenpox. After an attack of chickenpox, the virus lies dormant in certain nerves in the body. For reasons that are not fully understood, the virus can reappear in the form of shingles, more commonly in people with weakened immune systems and with aging. Shingles is characterized by a rash of blisters, which generally develop in a band on one side of the body and can cause severe pain that may last for weeks, and in some people, for months or years after the episode. The approval of Zostavax in younger people was based on a multicenter study conducted in the United States and four other countries in approximately 22,000 people who were 50-59 years of age. Half received Zostavax and half received a placebo (no active vaccine). Study participants were then monitored for at least one year to see if they developed shingles. Compared with placebo, Zostavax reduced the risk of developing shingles by approximately 70%. The most common side effects observed in the study were redness, pain and swelling at the site of injection, and headache. Zostavax was originally approved on May 26, 2006, for the prevention of shingles in individuals 60 years of age and older.

Shingles typically begins with mild aches and pains, feelings of bodily discomfort, nausea, chills, and fever. In about 90% of patients there is a sharp, stabbing pain, tenderness, and burning along the nerve tract affected. This pain can be excruciating and has been described as though you are being stabbed in the stomach with a white-hot poker. After about 3 to 5 days, lesions or a rash will appear like a belt on one side of the body or face. These lesions turn into fluid filled blisters or vesicles that later crust over in about 7-10 days. In about 90% of patients, the pain of shingles usually resolves within a month, with 97% pain free after 12 months. However, some people will still experience chronic pain for years that can be burning, shooting, aching, tearing, nagging, jabbing or lancing—sometimes called the "belt of roses from hell". This long lasting pain is called post-herpetic neuralgia (PHN). Readers should note that people who have never had chickenpox or with weak immune systems should stay away from people with shingles, especially when the person has the blister-like lesions.

QUESTION: I heard that a new prescription patch was approved to treat long-term pain after a shingles attack. What can you tell me about it?

ANSWER: The FDA recently approved Qutenza, a topical medicated patch used to relieve the pain of post-herpetic neuralgia (PNH), a serious complication that can occur after a bout with shingles. Shingles is an outbreak of rash or blisters on the skin that is caused by the same virus that causes chickenpox—the varicella-zoster virus. Anyone who once had chickenpox is at risk of shingles since the virus may become reactivated years after the initial infection. PHN is a condition affecting nerve fibers and the skin that can cause excruciating pain for weeks, months or even years. About 10 to 15 percent of patients who have shingles experience PHN and the complication is even more common in elderly patients. Qutenza contains capsaicin, a compound found in chili peppers. Although there are over-the-counter products with lower concentrations of capsaicin that are marketed for the treatment of PHN, Qutenza is the first pure, concentrated, synthetic capsaicin-containing prescription drug to undergo FDA review. Qutenza must be applied to the skin by a health care professional since placement of the patch can be quite painful, requiring use of a local topical anesthetic, as well as additional pain relief such as ice or use of opioid pain relievers. The patient must also be monitored for at least one hour since there is a risk of a significant rise in blood pressure following patch placement. The most frequently reported adverse drug reactions included pain, swelling, itching, redness, and bumps at the application site.

PERIODONTAL DISEASE

QUESTION: I heard about a new prescription product for gingivitis. What can you tell me about it?

ANSWER: The FDA recently approved Decapinol, a new prescription treatment for gingivitis, which is a common gum disease that affects most adults at some point in their lives. Gingivitis is an inflammation of the gums (gingival) generally caused by a build-up of plaque, which is a sticky matrix formed by bacteria in the mouth. Plaque forms a layer over the surface of the gums and teeth, and the bacteria release substances that cause local inflammation and damage to the gums making them bleed easily. The inhibition of and removal of this bacterial plaque can help to prevent the development of gingivitis. It is estimated that 70% to 90% of the adult population in the U.S. has some degree of gum inflammation. If left untreated, gingivitis can develop into periodontitis with inflammation, jawbone loss, and risk of tooth loss. Approximately 13% of the U.S. population may have periodontitis. Symptoms of mild gum disease include bleeding gums and bad breath. More severe disease can progress to spontaneous bleeding and loss of bone or tooth loss. In addition, bacteria may enter the bloodstream through the gums leading to systemic infections and other medical problems.

Various prescription and non-prescription antibacterial products have been used to help battle gum disease. Decapinol is an oral rinse that is effective in treating gingivitis, but it is not an antibacterial. It contains a surfactant substance (delmopinol) that acts as a physical barrier, making it harder for bacteria to stick to the teeth and gums. It also prevents bacteria from sticking to each other. This activity helps to reduce the formation of new plaque and also helps to break up existing plaque, making it easier to remove with normal tooth brushing. Because Decapinol does not actually kill bacteria in the mouth, it was approved as a medical device and not a drug. It is used as an oral rinse twice a day after normal tooth brushing and flossing. The treatment of periodontal (gum) disease may also involve dental scaling/root planing, a variety of sophisticated dental surgeries and regenerative techniques, home care, and periodic dental exams and cleaning. A dentist can determine which treatment or combination of treatments is best for their patients.

QUESTION: I've heard about some new products for gum disease. What are they?

ANSWER: Many new prescription products for periodontal (gum) disease have been approved for use during the last year. It has been estimated that three-quarters of Americans over the age of 35 suffer from periodontal disease. This chronic disorder begins as a painless infection of the gums, caused by a buildup of bacteria known as dental plaque. As the disorder progresses, the bacteria cause the gum tissue and bone around the teeth to be lost, forming pockets. If this condition is not treated, the soft tissue and bone that hold the teeth will be destroyed, resulting in tooth loosening and loss. Warning signs of periodontal disease may include bleeding gums or bad breath.

Various prescription and non-prescription antibacterial products have been available to help battle early periodontal disease. These products include rinses such as Peridex, Perioguard and some over-the-counter toothpastes. Past and current treatments of periodontal disease have also involved dental scaling/root planing, a variety of sophisticated dental surgeries and regenerative techniques, home care, and periodic dental appointments to clean and examine the teeth and gums.

Recently, three new prescription products have been made available to help treat periodontal disease. They should be used along with traditional treatment, such as scaling/root planing. PerioChip is a biodegradable chip that the dentist inserts into a periodontal pocket. It slowly releases chlorhexidine, a very potent antibacterial, over a 7 to 10 day period. Another new product is called Atridox, which is a biodegradable gel that is injected into diseased periodontal pockets by a dentist. This gel contains the antibiotic doxycycline, which is also released over a 7 to 10 day period. A third product (which also contains doxycycline) is named Periostat. It is an oral capsule that contains 20 mg of doxycycline and is taken twice a day for up to 9 months. It is thought that in this low dose (20 mg) doxycycline does not work as an antibiotic, but instead somehow prevents inflammation and bone loss around the teeth. It should be noted that any doxycycline product can make one more sensitive to light and may reduce the effectiveness of birth control tablets. Other antibacterial agents are also being tested for use in periodontal disease and should be available in the future. Periodontal disease is very treatable, so remember to brush, floss, and see your dentist regularly.

WHOOPING COUGH

QUESTION: I heard about a new whooping cough vaccine for adults. Can adults get whopping cough?

ANSWER: Yes, a person can develop whooping cough at any age. Whooping cough, or pertussis, is a highly contagious bacterial infection within the respiratory tract which results in fits of coughing that usually end in a prolonged high-pitched, deeply indrawn breath (the whoop). An infected person usually spreads the infectious organisms into the air with droplets of moisture produced by the coughing. Anyone nearby can inhale these droplets and become infected. Whooping cough typically lasts about 6 weeks with initial cold-like symptoms that are followed by severe coughing fits and gradual recovery. However, serious, sometimes fatal, complications such as pneumonia can develop. At particular risk are newborn infants who have not yet been vaccinated against this disease. Children are routinely vaccinated against whooping cough (pertussis) with a combination vaccine that also contains vaccines for both tetanus (lock jaw) and diphtheria. Immunity from these childhood vaccinations, however, wears off after about 5 to 10 years following the last childhood vaccination, leaving adults and adolescents susceptible to infection. The number of reported cases of pertussis continues to rise in the U.S. and adults are often the source of infection for infants and young children. In fact, a study conducted by the Center for Disease Control and Prevention (CDC) has reported that adults were responsible for over half of pertussis cases in infants, with parents causing the infection in 47% of cases and grandparents causing it in 8% of cases. The CDC has also reported that there were nearly 19,000 case reports of pertussis in 2004, a 63% increase over 2003 and the highest number of case reports in forty years. In view of this problem, the FDA has recently approved two new pertussis containing vaccines. The new vaccines also contain vaccines for tetanus and diphtheria. Boostrix was approved for use in adolescents aged 10 to 18 and Adacel was approved for people aged 11 through 64 years.

BIRD FLU

QUESTION: I keep reading about bird flu. What drugs are used to treat this type of flu?

ANSWER: Bird flu is an infection caused by bird (avian) flu viruses that occur naturally among birds. Wild birds worldwide carry these viruses in their intestines, but usually do not get sick from them. However, bird flu is very contagious among birds and can make some domesticated birds, including chickens, duck, and turkeys very sick and kill them. These bird flu viruses do not usually infect humans, but several cases of human infections have occurred since 1997. In June 2004 new deadly outbreaks of bird flu among poultry were reported by several countries in Asia (Cambodia, China, Indonesia, Malaysia, Thailand, and Vietnam) and it is believed that these outbreaks are ongoing. Human cases of bird flu have also been reported in some of these Asian countries with a death rate of about 70%. Most of these cases occurred from contact with infected poultry or contaminated surfaces. So far, the spread of the bird flu virus from person to person has been rare. However, public healthcare professionals are concerned that this virus may one day be able to spread more easily from one person to another and cause a worldwide outbreak of the disease (pandemic). Although there have been no reported cases of human bird flu in the U.S., it is possible that travelers returning from the affected countries in Asia could be infected. In view of this, the Center for Disease Control (CDC) advises travelers to these areas to avoid poultry farms, contact with animals in live food markets, and any surfaces that appear to be contaminated with feces from poultry or other animals. The CDC is also working with the Department of Defense and the VA to build up a stockpile of antiviral drugs to be used for treating bird flu outbreaks if needed. The two antiviral drugs that are thought to be effective for bird flu are Relenza (zanamivir) and Tamiflu (oseltamivir). The development of a bird flu vaccine is also underway. Methods to prevent the spread of bird flu are the same for regular flu and include avoiding close contact with people who area sick, staying home if sick, covering your mouth and nose with a tissue when coughing or sneezing, washing your hands frequently, and avoiding the touching of your eyes, nose, and mouth.

SWINE FLU

QUESTION: What medications are used for swine flu?

ANSWER: Swine influenza (swine flu) is a respiratory disease of pigs caused by a virus known as H1N1. Swine flu viruses do not normally infect humans, but it can occur in persons with direct exposure to pigs (e.g., people near pigs at a fair or workers in the swine industry). In addition, there have been documented cases of one person spreading swine flu to others. People may become infected by touching something with flu viruses on it and then touching their mouth or nose. The symptoms of swine flu in people are similar to the symptoms of regular human seasonal influenza (flu) and include fever, tiredness, lack of appetite, and coughing. Some people with swine flu also have reported runny nose, sore throat, nausea, vomiting, and diarrhea. The infectious period for a confirmed case of swine flu is 1 day prior to the case's illness onset to 7 days after onset.

There are four antiviral drugs available in the U.S. for the treatment of influenza: amantadine (Symmetrel), rimantadine (Flumadine), oseltamivir (Tamiflu), and zanamivir (Relenza). While most swine flu viruses have been susceptible to all 4 drugs, the current swine flu viruses isolated from humans are resistant to amantadine (Symmetrel) and rimantadine (Flumadine). At this time, the Center for Disease Control (CDC) recommends the use of oseltamivir (Tamiflu) or zanamivir (Relenza) for the treatment and/or prevention of infection with swine flu. No vaccine is available to protect humans from the swine flu. Oseltamivir (Tamiflu) is given as a capsule or oral suspension and zanamivir (Relenza) is administered by inhalation. The dosage is determined by age or body weight and the duration of treatment depends upon whether it is being used for prevention or treatment. It should be noted that there are other simple things that people can do to protect themselves from the flu, like practicing better hygiene (wash hands frequently and cover mouth and nose when sneezing) and staying away from public places or traveling if they feel sick.

BLADDER INFECTIONS

QUESTION: My daughter occasionally gets bladder infections and needs to be treated with antibiotics. What can she do to try and prevent these infections?

ANSWER: Bladder infections or cystitis is common in women, especially during the reproductive years. The reason that women get these infections more often than men is because women have a shorter urethra and the closeness of the urethra to the anus, where bacteria are commonly found. In addition, women who are sexually active, use diaphragms, or are pregnant have a greater chance of bladder infections. Sexual intercourse can cause slight injuries to the urethra and allow bacteria to get into the bladder while pregnancy can interfere with emptying of the bladder. Using a diaphragm can increase the risk of bladder infections, possibly because spermicide used with the diaphragm may suppress the normal vaginal bacteria and allow bacteria that cause cystitis to increase within the vagina. Most people with bladder infections complain of painful urination, increased frequency of urination, and/or urinary urgency. Women with this condition usually respond to a course of antibiotics. However, as with most medical problems, prevention is the key. Some steps that women can take to prevent bladder infections appear below:

- Increase daily intake of water and/or cranberry juice to at least 64 ounces because this facilitates the formation of urine and elimination of bacteria.
- Urinate often to keep the bladder as empty as possible.
- Wipe from front to back after bowel movements to prevent the spread of bacteria from the anus to the urethra.
- Avoid products such as soaps, bubble baths, and douches that are irritating to the urethra.
- Urinate after sexual intercourse to flush the urethra.
- Take showers rather than baths because this prevents the urethra from being irritated by substances in the bath water.
- Gently wash the skin around the vagina and anus daily with mild soap and water.
- Beware of spermicides because they can cause irritation.
- Beware of diaphragms because they put pressure on the urethra and can reduce urine flow; advise diaphragm users who frequently get UTIs to try a different type of contraception.

POISON IVY

QUESTION: What can I do to prevent and treat poison ivy?

ANSWER: Poison ivy rash is an allergic reaction caused by contact with a substance called urushiol (you-roo-shee-ol) found in the sap of poison ivy plants. A person may develop a rash without coming into contact with the poison ivy plant, since this sticky sap can be carried on the fur of animals, on garden tools, on sports equipment, or on any objects that have come into contact with a crushed or broken plant. Although some victims'rashes occur within a few hours or even minutes after contact with the sap, most rashes show up after 12 to 72 hours and tend to get worse over several more days. The reaction usually consists of a moist, itchy rash, often with blisters that will "weep" a clear to yellowish liquid after a few days. If untreated most skin reactions will heal within two to three weeks, but the weeping pustules can become infected if scratched or not properly cared for. Although any area of the skin can be affected by poison ivy, thinner skin unprotected by hair (such as between the toes, behind the knees, the inner side of the arm, the trunk, the face, etc.) is usually more susceptible to skin reactions.

The best treatment of poison ivy is to prevent any contact with the sap of the plant. Recognizing the poison ivy plant and staying away from it is the first rule. Poison ivy is a woody shrub or vine that grows to ten feet or more climbing trees, walls, and fences or trailing along on the ground. Although their three-leaf clusters characterize most varieties, they can also bear five and seven leaf clusters in some areas. The leaves generally have a shiny appearance due to the sap (oil), and the vines of poison ivy often look "hairy". These plants generally grow near lakes or streams in dense brush, but not always. Burning the plants vaporizes the oils, and contact with the smoke can also cause severe reactions. When contact is likely or unavoidable, protective clothing is a good idea. A nonprescription lotion named "Ivy Block" is also available and its use prior to exposure to poison ivy can decrease the chances of a reaction. It is applied to the skin and should be washed off with soap and water after the risk of exposure to poison ivy is over.

If you think you've come into contact with poison ivy, wash all exposed areas with cold running water as soon as possible. Also wash all clothing and anything else that may have come into contact with the poison ivy sap, which can remain active for months. If you do develop a rash do not scratch the blisters because this can lead to infection. Mild cases of poison ivy can be treated with cool compresses or cool showers to help relieve the itching. Calamine or Caladryl lotion can also be helpful. A lukewarm soak with Aveeno Oatmeal Bath can help relieve the itching and dry oozing blisters. Over-the-counter hydrocortisone creams or a local anesthetic spray like Dermoplast may help to reduce the itching and pain, but in severe cases of poison ivy prescription products may be needed.

TRAVELERS' DIARRHEA

QUESTION: I heard about a new drug for travelers' diarrhea. What can you tell me about it?

ANSWER: A new prescription antibiotic Xifaxan (rifaximin) was recently approved by the FDA to treat travelers' diarrhea due to Escherichia coli in people 12 years of age or older. Travelers' diarrhea is also called intestinal flu, grippe, or turista and its symptoms include diarrhea, nausea, vomiting, intestinal rumbling, and abdominal cramping. A common cause of travelers' diarrhea is the organism Escherichi coli that is found in contaminated foods or water. Travelers' diarrhea is a significant risk to U.S. citizens traveling to foreign countries, and can affect as many as 50% of travelers depending upon the countries that they visit. In order to prevent this problem, travelers should not eat food or drink beverages sold by street vendors. All food should be cooked and all fruit peeled. In addition, travelers should only drink carbonated beverages or beverages made with water that has been boiled. Ice cubes should also be made with water that has been boiled and salads containing uncooked vegetables should be avoided. In many cases of mild diarrhea, drinking plenty of fluids and eating a bland diet can be helpful and the diarrhea may go away on its own. However, more serious cases of travelers' diarrhea may require treatment with antibiotics. The main advantage of the new antibiotic Xifaxan, is that it is not absorbed into the blood stream like other antibiotics. This reduces the risk of side effects and interactions with other drugs. Xifaxan is taken orally 3 times a day for 3 days, with or without food. Common side effects of this new medication include headache, constipation, and vomiting.

WARTS

QUESTION: What causes warts and how are they treated?

ANSWER: Warts are caused by viruses known as human papillomaviruses. They are a common viral infection affecting the skin and mucous membranes, with approximately 9 million Americans contracting warts every year. It is not exactly understood how warts are transmitted, but it is assumed that warts spread by close personal contact, and that minor breaks in the skin may help to start the growth of a wart. Usually, warts appear within 3 to 4 months after exposure, although they may take up to two years to appear. Many times, warts will disappear without treatment but it is not clear why this happens. People with weak body defenses (immune systems) may have larger warts that are harder to treat.

Since there are many different types of human papillomaviruses, there are also many types of warts. Usually, warts are named according to their location. Common warts are usually found on the hands and fingers but may also occur on the face, knees or elbows. They affect 5-10% of school aged children and appear as small raised growths with a rough surface. Plantar warts are less common and are most often seen in adolescents and young adults. This wart is found on the sole of the foot and sometimes on the palm of the hand (palmar wart). Plantar warts look like calluses and they can be quite painful. Juvenile or flat warts are even less common and are mainly seen in children, often beginning where a skin break has occurred. These warts are small, slightly raised flat growths, usually pink or brown, and may occur in large numbers. Genital warts are the most serious type of warts and are known to be spread by sexual relations. They are the most common of all sexually transmitted diseases. These warts can be smooth and flat or more raised and rough.

The treatment of warts depends on the size, location and type of warts present. In many cases no treatment is necessary and warts will go away in response to natural body defenses. This is why so many folk remedies have been perceived to be helpful for the treatment of warts. Many patients have warts removed for cosmetic reasons. Warts can be treated by physicians with liquid nitrogen, electrocautery and other nondrug methods. Plantar warts may also be surgically removed by an orthopedist or podiatrist. Genital warts are often treated with a potent prescription drug known as podophyllum (po-doph-il-lum), which actually kills the wart virus. Recently, a new prescription product called Aldara became available to treat genital warts. How it works is unknown, but it appears to assist the body's defense systems. Common and plantar warts can be treated with over-the-counter preparations which usually contain salicylic acid. Salicylic acid is known as a keratolytic (ker-a-to-lit-ik) agent, which aids in the removal of dead skin. Improvement with these products should occur in 1-2 weeks and they should not be used for longer than 12 weeks. Over-the-counter products should not be used by diabetic patients or those with circulatory problems.

SKIN INFECTIONS

QUESTION: I heard that honey is being used for skin infections. Is that true?

ANSWER: Yes, honey is making a comeback, more than 4,000 years after Egyptians began applying honey to wounds. Derma Sciences, Inc., a New Jersey company that makes medicated and advanced wound care products, recently began selling the first honey-based dressing after it was approved by the FDA. Their product, named Medihoney, is made from a highly absorbent seaweed-based material, saturated with manuka honey, a particularly potent type of honey that may kill germs and speed healing. Manuka honey, which is also called Leptospermum honey, comes from hives of bees that collect nectar from manuka and jelly bushes in Australia and New Zealand. Medihoney is now being sold to hospitals, clinics, and doctors to help prevent and fight infections.

Medihoney is thought to have 3 therapeutic actions for both chronic and acute wound and skin conditions: wound protection; wound cleaning; and wound healing. It may also reduce inflammation and can eliminate the foul odor of infected wounds. In addition, Medihoney dressings may also prevent the dangerous drug-resistant staph infection known as MRSA from infecting open wounds. However, it will not work once an infection gets into the bloodstream. Some U.S. hospitals and wound care clinics are already using Medihoney dressings to treat patients with stubborn, infected wounds from injuries or surgical incisions and nonhealing pressure ulcers on the feet of people with diabetes. More information about this new product can be found at **www.medihoney.com** and **www.dermasciencesinc.com** or you can contact the company at 1-800-328-2634.

FUNGAL INFECTIONS

QUESTION: I work out at the gym on a regular basis and sometimes I get "jock itch" or "athlete's foot". What can I do for this problem?

ANSWER: "Jock itch" (Tinea cruris) and "athlete's foot" (Tinea Pedis) are common infections of the skin caused by a fungus. The fungus that causes "jock itch" likes to grow in warm, moist areas that are not exposed to light. It commonly occurs in the groin or pubic area but can also include other areas of the body that sweat a lot, such as under the arms, under the breasts, or between the buttocks. These infections are usually more frequent in men and occur most often during warm, humid weather. "Athlete's foot" is a very similar infection that causes itching and it thrives between the toes, especially when wearing shoes that prevent good ventilation. Both of these infections are highly contagious and can be easily transmitted in showers and pool areas. Some tips for avoiding these fungal infections include the following:

- Avoid going barefoot at pools and locker rooms. Wear sandals.
- Keep feet clean and dry, especially between the toes.
- Absorbent powders and astringents can help reduce moisture levels.

- Avoid sharing towels with others.
- Make sure towels, bed linens, shoes, and socks are clean and dry.
- Avoid wearing wet or damp bathing suits for long periods of time.
- Keep potentially affected areas clean and dry.
- Avoid tight clothing and synthetic fabrics.

Numerous topical non-prescription preparations are available to treat both "jock itch" and "athlete's foot". Effective ingredients in these antifungal products include clioquinol, clotrimazole, haloprogin, miconazole nitrate, providone iodine, tolnaftate, and undecylenic acid. Powders, sprays, creams, ointments, and solutions are available for over-the-counter use. In general, creams or solutions are the most efficient and effective products for getting the active ingredient into the skin. Sprays and powders are less effective because they are not rubbed into the skin. Patients should avoid spreading the infection by not scratching itchy feet, contaminating fingers or surfaces, or by sharing towels with others. To avoid reinfection, make sure to continue antifungal therapy for 10 days to 2 weeks after symptoms disappear and keep affected areas clean and dry.

QUESTION: If nystatin is a fairly safe drug, why are doctors reluctant to prescribe it?

ANSWER: Nystatin (tradename Mycostatin) is an antifungal agent that is used to treat vaginal "yeast" infections caused by a fungus named candida. These infections are also referred to as vulvovaginal candidiasis. Women aged 16 to 35 are more likely to develop this type of infection, with about 75% of women having at least one candidal vaginal infection during their child bearing years. Symptoms of a vaginal yeast infection may include itching and a white, curdy ("cottage cheese" like), or thick discharge that is mostly odorless. Other symptoms such as soreness, rash on outer lips of the vagina, and pain or burning during urination may also occur.

There are many causes of vaginal yeast infections. One cause is lowered defense against infection (immunity), which can happen when you get run down from doing too much and not getting enough rest or proper nutrition. Drugs that affect the immune system and HIV infection can also lead to these infections. Other causes include the use of antibiotics or birth control pills, pregnancy, diabetes, tight fitting clothing, menstrual periods, and sexual intercourse.

Nystatin has been available by prescription to treat vulvovaginal candidiasis for a long period of time as a topical cream or ointment, powder, or vaginal tablet. When used topically, nystatin is an effective and safe product with irritation and pain reported on rare occasions. For acute infections, vaginal tablets of nystatin are used daily for 2 weeks. If the outer skin (vulvar) area is also affected, nystatin cream or combination of cream and vaginal suppositories may be preferable. Numerous other newer oral and topical antifungal products are also available to treat this condition and can be effectively used for a shorter period of time. A convenient single-day oral tablet therapy has become very popular and many patients prefer this. I would suspect that many physicians are reluctant to prescribe nystatin because of this. It should be noted, however, that a recurrence of vaginal candidiasis is possible after any drug regimen. A special nystatin oral suspension and tablets are also used to treat candidiasis infections in the mouth.

QUESTION: I keep getting a rash under my breasts and under my arms that my doctor prescribes nystatin-triamcinolone cream for. What does this cream contain and can it be dangerous?

ANSWER: This cream is a combination of nystatin (an antifungal) and triamcinolone (a corticosteroid). Nystatin is used to treat fungal skin infections caused primarily by a fungus named Candida. The triamcinolone is helpful to reduce the inflammation, pain, and itching associated with the skin infection. Generally, when this cream is applied 2 to 3 times a day the infection will clear up in 7 to 10 days. When used topically for a limited time on small areas of the skin, the cream is usually very safe to use since only low amounts of the drugs are absorbed through the skin into the bloodstream. Once the infection is cleared up you should be able to stop the treatment and treat again only if it reoccurs. Candida infections are more common during warm, humid weather or when a person's immune system defenses are weakened. Infections with Candida can also occur when someone is taking antibiotics because the antibiotic kills the bacteria that are normally found in skin tissue, allowing the fungus to grow unchecked. Pregnant women, obese people, and people with diabetes are more prone to these infections. This fungus grows well in warm, moist conditions and that is probably why your infections are in the areas you mentioned. Therefore, you might try keeping the skin areas dry. The use of plain talcum powder or nystatin powder (by prescription only) may be helpful in preventing these infections.

QUESTION: What prescription drugs are available for treating fungal infections of the toenail?

ANSWER: Fungal infections can occur from head to toe and there are at least 50 different types of fungi that cause disease. However, the fungus called Trichophyton causes most cases of fungal nail infections. A fungal infection of the nail or nail bed is known as onychomycosis and it affects an estimated 20% of the population between the ages of 40 to 60. It is most common in men and occurs about four times more frequently in toenails compared to fingernails. Fungi that cause toenail infections thrive in moist, warm environments, like the inside of a shoe. Risk factors for developing a toenail infection include injury to the toe, long-standing athlete's foot contracted by walking barefoot around public showers, swimming pools, health clubs, hotel rooms, etc., and wearing airtight shoes for activities like hiking or biking. People with conditions such as diabetes, poor circulation, or an impaired immune system also have a higher incidence of fungal nail infections. Since toenails grow slower (9 to 18 months to grow back when removed) than fingernails (3 to 6 months to grow back), the treatment of fungal toenail infections is longer than for fingernails. Fungal toenail infections usually are not life threatening but they can cause the toenail to turn yellow-brown and can produce pain, discomfort, and psychological stress. The goals of treatment are to get rid of the fungus and to restore the toenail to its normal appearance. Current treatment options for these infections include oral (systemic) antifungal agents, surgical or chemical treatments, and the use of topical antifungal agents. The two oral (systemic) FDA approved agents considered to be first line prescription treatments are Sporanox (itraconazole) and Lamisil (terbinafine). They appear to be equally effective but require lengthy treatment due to the slow growth of toenails mentioned previously. Drug interactions may be of concern for people taking other medications, so be sure that your physician and pharmacist are aware of all the medications that you are taking (prescription and nonprescription). In addition to these oral antifungal products, a new topical solution, Penlac nail lacquer (ciclopirox), has also been approved for fungal nail infections where systemic or surgical treatment is not desired. This solution is brushed on the infected nail and is designed to remain on and penetrate the nail plate getting the active ingredient to the infected nail bed. Here again, a treatment of as long as 48 weeks may be needed. The success rate of completed cure is about 12%, but it may be an alternative for patients who refuse surgery or where drug interactions may be a major concern. It is also less expensive than the two first-line systemic antifungal treatments. Finally, when drug therapy has failed or is contraindicated, surgery and/or chemical treatment may be necessary.

QUESTION: My doctor prescribed Lamisil tablets to treat a fungus infection of my toenail. Is a generic available?

ANSWER: The FDA recently approved the first generic versions of the prescription drug Lamisil (terbinafine) used to treat fungal infections of the toenail or fingernail. Lamisil (terbinafine) is an antifungal agent that works systemically (in the bloodstream) to kill fungi that invade a fingernail or toenail or the skin underneath the nail. Effective treatment with Lamisil usually takes 6 weeks for fungal infections involving the fingernails and 12 weeks for toenails. Common side effects of Lamisil include nausea, vomiting, and headache but serious side effects involving the blood or liver can also occur. Interactions between Lamisil and other drugs are possible so be sure to make your doctor and pharmacist aware of any other medications that you take. As I noted many times before, the FDA's Office of Generic Drugs ensures that generic drugs are safe and effective through its scientific and regulatory process.

WEST NILE VIRUS

QUESTION: Is there a vaccine for the West Nile virus?

ANSWER: No, a vaccine is not available yet, but research is being undertaken to try and develop a vaccine. The West Nile virus is spread by the bite of an infected mosquito, and it can infect people, horses, birds, and other animals. It may also be transmitted from blood transfusions. People who become infected with West Nile virus may or may not have symptoms. Symptoms of infection with the virus may include mild fever, body aches, a rash, and swollen lymph glands. In more severe cases headache, high fever, neck stiffness, stupor, disorientation, coma, tremors, convulsions, muscle weakness, paralysis and, rarely, death can occur. Currently there is no specific treatment for this viral infection. In more serious cases the patient may need to be hospitalized and receive intravenous fluids and breathing support. Anti-infective medications also may be used to prevent secondary infections such as pneumonia. In addition to research for the development of a West Nile virus vaccine, a drug used to treat hepatitis C (Interferon) is also being studied to see if it is effective against the virus. In order to prevent infection with the West Nile virus, people should avoid mosquito bites by wearing long sleeves and pants and applying insect repellant when going outdoors. Repellents containing DEET are recommended but should not be used on children's hands. Eliminating standing water sources near the home may also be helpful. More information about the West Nile virus can be obtained at the Center for Disease Control (CDC) web site (**www.cdc.gov/ncidod/dvbid/westnile/index.htm**).

ANTHRAX

QUESTION: I read about the Lantana, Florida man that got anthrax and died. What drugs are used to treat anthrax?

ANSWER: The possibility of biological warfare using anthrax bacteria is a major concern, especially since the September 11 terrorist attack in New York City. Anthrax is an acute bacterial infection caused by the deadly bacterium known as Bacillus anthracis. These bacteria form spores which are difficult to destroy and can live for years in soil. People can become infected when they come into contact with infected animals or contaminated animal products, from insect bites, by inhalation, or by eating infected meat. Anthrax infection typically affects the skin, the intestinal tract, or the pulmonary tract (lungs). Pulmonary anthrax, caused by inhaling the bacteria spores, is the most serious form with a high fatality rate. The case in Lantana was Florida's first confirmed case of anthrax in 27 years and it appeared to be the pulmonary or inhalation type. Approximately 95% of human cases of anthrax are the skin type and about 5% are the inhalation type. Gastrointestinal anthrax is rare. Inhalation anthrax has an incubation period of 2 to 60 days and the first symptoms may resemble a cold or flu with fever, cough, chest discomfort, and muscle aches. This is followed by severe breathing problems and shock, usually leading to death within 24 hours. Skin anthrax often begins with a bump on the hands, arms, or head that turns into a sore. More severe symptoms may follow, including fever, swelling, and headache. The treatment of anthrax involves the use of antibiotics such as penicillin, erythromycin, a tetracycline, or a newer antibiotic called ciprofloxacin. Injectable antibiotics are required for the treatment of inhalation anthrax, while oral drugs may suffice for skin anthrax. Treatment is usually more effective when given as early as possible. Skin anthrax can usually be cured with antibiotics, but inhalation anthrax has a very high death rate.

QUESTION: It seems like Cipro is being given out like candy to people exposed to anthrax. What are its side effects?

ANSWER: Cipro or ciprofloxacin is an antiinfective drug that is classified as a fluoroquinolone antibiotic. It is prescribed for the treatment of many different types of infections and is also utilized as prophylaxis (preventative) therapy for people who have been exposed to anthrax bacteria. For postexposure prevention of anthrax, Cipro is usually given to adults in a dosage of 500 mg orally every 12 hours for 60 days. Cipro is not approved for use in children or in pregnant women. Cipro may be taken with or without food, but should not be taken together with antacids or dairy products like milk or yogurt because they interfere with its absorption from the gastrointestinal tract. Certain other prescription/non-prescription drugs and products containing iron or multivitamins containing zinc should also be avoided. Like all medications, Cipro can cause side effects, some of which can be serious. Some people may be allergic to Cipro and hypersensitivity reactions can occur. Other types of antibiotics can be used in this situation. Patients receiving Cipro should also be advised to avoid excessive sunlight or artificial ultraviolet light because it can make them more sensitive to light. The most common side effects of Cipro are nausea, diarrhea, vomiting, stomach pain or discomfort, headache, restlessness, and skin rash. However more serious side effects can occur in some people including heart attacks, convulsions, colitis, muscle damage, breathing problems, liver and kidney problems, psychotic reactions, and many other adverse effects. While most of these serious side effects are rare, they are very important if they happen to you. In addition, the overuse of Cipro (or other antibiotics) can lead to resistance to these drugs by bacteria making them ineffective. Because of the potential for side effects, Cipro is a prescription medication and must not be used without physician guidance. Like all drugs, the potential benefit of Cipro must be weighed against its potential risk. Since some anthrax infections can be deadly, Cipro or other antibiotics are useful and necessary medications for people upon confirmation of an anthrax exposure.

SARS

QUESTION: Are there any antibiotics available to treat SARS?

ANSWER: An estimated 5,000 people worldwide have been infected by a virus resulting in SARS (severe acute respiratory syndrome) and many have died. SARS is caused by a virus known as a "coronavirus". Unlike bacteria, which are much larger, a virus is a small infectious organism that needs a living cell in order to reproduce. Viruses are also harder to kill than bacteria. When viruses enter a cell they may immediately trigger a disease or may remain dormant for many years. Like bacteria, there are many different types of viruses. For example, the influenza virus causes the flu, the herpes virus produces cold sores, and the varicella virus causes chickenpox and shingles. The coronavirus that causes SARS is similar to the virus that causes the common cold and it appears to be transmitted from one person to another by droplets of fluid from coughing, sneezing, or hand contamination. Drugs that combat a viral infection are called antiviral drugs, while drugs that are used to treat infections caused by bacteria are called antibiotics.

Since antibiotics and antiviral drugs work differently from each other, antibiotics are not useful for viral infections and antiviral drugs are not useful for bacterial infections. Furthermore, available vaccines for pneumonia or the flu are also not effective for preventing SARS. Currently there are numerous antiviral drugs available to treat AIDS, herpes infections, the flu and other viruses, but none are specific for the SARS virus. These drugs and other experimental agents are being tested in the laboratory to see if they are effective against the SARS virus. Now that the genetic makeup of the virus has been determined, an attempt to make new antivirals for SARS will also be undertaken by scientists. However, this new drug development process may take several years. For now, the treatment of SARS primarily involves isolating the patients and treating their symptoms while the infection runs its course.

SMALLPOX

QUESTION: You've written a column about anthrax treatments and bioterrorism. What about smallpox?

ANSWER: Smallpox is a potentially deadly viral infection caused by the variola poxvirus. Historically, smallpox is thought to have killed more people than any other infection in human history. The last reported case of smallpox occurred in Somalia in 1977, and in 1980 the World Health Organization (WHO) declared that this disease had been eradicated throughout the globe. There currently is no evidence of smallpox transmission anywhere in the world. The WHO has recommended that all stocks of smallpox virus be destroyed, followed by the destruction of all remaining doses of smallpox vaccine. The U.S. government, however, in 1999 announced that it would not destroy its stocks of smallpox vaccine. The two known countries with existing stocks of the smallpox virus are the U.S. and Russia, but many believe that there are other stockpiles around the world. With the new threats of bioterrorism today, concern for smallpox has surfaced again. Smallpox is considered to be a potential bioweapon because it is very contagious, has a high mortality rate, and because many people are not immunized against it. Indeed, it has been noted that one of the earliest accounts of biological warfare involved the distribution of smallpox-infected blankets to the native Indians by British troops. Smallpox infection is spread through the air and produces high fever, fatigue, body aches, and a rash after an average incubation period of about 12 days. The rash generally appears first on the face, arms, and in the mouth. The rash progresses to blister and pustular lesions over 1-2 weeks and may be confused with chickenpox. The production of smallpox vaccine was discontinued in 1981. However, the Centers for Disease Control and Prevention maintain a supply to protect laboratory workers exposed to the virus. Several drug manufacturers are also now considering production of a new supply of vaccine. It appears that protection against smallpox lasts about 30 years after a 3-dose vaccination. For laboratory workers who are directly involved with the smallpox virus re-vaccination is recommended every 3 to 5 years.

Since the smallpox vaccine is currently not available for general use, scientists are now looking at the possibility of using antiviral drugs to treat smallpox. At least 20 currently available drugs have already been identified that can kill the smallpox virus in the test tube. Because potential smallpox treatments cannot be tested in infected people, researchers hope to use infected monkeys to test the antiviral drugs. Hopefully they will be successful and we will have drug treatments for smallpox available in the near future.

QUESTION: I was vaccinated for smallpox when I was young. Am I still protected now?

ANSWER: Scientists believe that childhood vaccination would not protect people against smallpox today if it were introduced into the U.S. by a terrorist group. It appears that protection (immunity) wanes after 10 to 20 years, and revaccination every 10 years is recommended for continued protection. Routine smallpox vaccination was discontinued in 1971 and has not been required for international travel since 1982. Actually the last case of smallpox in the U.S. was in 1949 and the last in the world was reported in 1977 from Somalia. In 1980 the World Health Organization officially declared that smallpox had been eliminated worldwide as a result of a global vaccination and eradication program. Today, however, the threat of smallpox has re-emerged due to the possibility of bioterrorism. In view of this, the U.S. Government has developed a smallpox vaccination program for 2003. This plan has three phases. First, members of the armed forces and emergency-room workers and those on special smallpox response teams would be vaccinated. Next up would be emergency responders, such as police, firefighters, and ambulance crews. In the final phase, the public will be offered the vaccine on a voluntary basis, probably in late spring or early summer. Due to the potential for side effects, the routine non-emergency use of the vaccine should be avoided in people allergic to the vaccine, in infants younger than 12 months (the Advisory Committee on Immunization Practices also advises against non-emergency use of the vaccine in children younger than 18 years), in people with eczema or a history of eczema or with household contacts with eczema or certain other skin conditions, anyone receiving systemic corticosteroids or immunosuppressive drugs or radiation, people with immune system deficiency, and women who are pregnant. The most frequent side effect of vaccination is the spread of infection from the vaccination site to other areas in some people. However, more serious complications such as encephalitis, infection, or severe skin lesions can occur. It has been estimated that for every one million people vaccinated approximately one or two will die from these serious complications. On the other hand, smallpox in its severe form can spread rapidly throughout a population and can be fatal in 30% or more of unvaccinated persons. There is no specific treatment or cure for smallpox, but antiviral therapy is being investigated.

VAGINAL YEAST INFECTIONS

QUESTION: What non-prescription medication can I use to treat a vaginal yeast infection?

ANSWER: Vaginal "yeast" infections are actually caused by a fungus named candida. These infections are also called candidiasis or moniliasis. Women aged 16 to 35 are more likely to develop this type of infection, with about 75% of women having at least one candidal vaginal infection during their child bearing years. Symptoms of a vaginal yeast infection may include itching and a white, curdy ("cottage cheese" like), or thick discharge that is mostly odorless. Other symptoms such as soreness, rash on outer lips of the vagina, and pain or burning during urination may also occur.

There are many causes of vaginal yeast infections. One cause is lowered defense against infection (immunity), which can happen when you get run down from doing too much and not getting enough rest or proper nutrition. Drugs that affect the immune system and HIV (AIDS) infection can also lead to these infections. Other causes include the use of antibiotics or birth control pills, pregnancy, diabetes, tight fitting clothing, menstrual periods, and sexual intercourse.

Several effective topical antifungal non-prescription medications are now available for treating vaginal yeast infections. These include clotrimazole (tradenames Gyne-Lotrimin 3, Mycelex-7, Gyne-Lotrimin 7, Mycelex-7 Combination Pack, Gyne-Lotrimin 3 Combination Pack), miconazole (tradenames Monistat-7, Femizol-M, M-Zole 3 Combination Pack, Vagistat-3 Combination Pack, M-Zole Dual Pack), tioconazole (tradenames Vagistat-1, Monistat 1), and butoconazole (tradename Mycelex-3). Use of a cream, vaginal tablet, or vaginal suppository depends upon patient preference. If the outer skin (vulvar) area is also affected, a cream or combination of a cream and vaginal suppositories or vaginal tablets is preferable for use. Side effects such as burning, itching, and irritation occur in about 7% of patients. Make sure you read the entire product labeling carefully prior to use. Symptoms usually improve within a few days, but it is important to continue using the medication for the number of days directed, even if you no longer have symptoms. Your doctor should be consulted if: you have abdominal pain, fever, skin rash, or a foul smelling discharge; there is no improvement within 3 days; or if symptoms recur within 2 months. Some tips on how to avoid vaginal yeast infections appear below:

- Wear loose, natural fiber clothing and underwear with a cotton crotch.
- Limit wearing of panty hose, tights, leggings, nylon underwear, and tight jeans.
- Don't use deodorant tampons and feminine deodorant sprays, especially if you feel an infection beginning.

- Dry off quickly and thoroughly after bathing and swimming-don't stay in a wet swimsuit for hours.

COLDS & FLU

QUESTION: What is the difference between a cold and the flu and how do you treat them?

ANSWER: The common cold and the flu are both caused by viruses—but different kinds. Most colds are caused by either "rhinovirus" or "coronarvirus" and are much less serious than the flu or influenza, which is usually caused by the influenza A or B virus. Cold symptoms usually include a runny nose, nasal congestion, sore throat, and cough. Flu symptoms on the other hand are usually more severe and can include muscle pain, high fever, chills, nausea and vomiting, dehydration, and headache. Below I have listed some of the differences between a common cold and the flu from the National Institute of Allergy and Infectious Diseases:

Common Cold
- Fever uncommon
- Headache uncommon
- Mild fatigue and weakness
- Mild general aches and pains
- Runny or stuffy nose common
- Sneezing common
- Mild-to-moderate cough
- Sore throat common
- No means of prevention

Influenza
- Fever of 102 to 104 degrees F comes on suddenly, lasts 3-4 days
- Headache prominent
- Extreme fatigue and weakness that can last 2-3 weeks
- Severe general aches and pains common
- Runny or stuffy nose sometimes occurs

- Sneezing sometimes occurs
- Cough common and can become severe
- Sore throat sometimes occurs
- Illness can be prevented with vaccination and antiviral drugs.
- Illness can be treated with pharmaceuticals within 24-48 hours after onset of symptoms.

Like most infections, prevention is the best cure. An annual flu shot often provides protection against influenza infection, but because there are so many different types of cold viruses it is unlikely that an effective vaccine will be developed for the common cold. Once someone you have contact with has a cold or the flu, some efforts will help to minimize its spread. The use and disposal of tissues, avoidance of hand-to-hand contact, periodic antiseptic spraying of shared telephones and doorknobs, using disposable eating implements, and hand washing can all be helpful. Treatment of the common cold and flu is usually a matter of treating the symptoms, but within the last year, two prescription products were approved for influenza treatment, Relenza and Tamiflu. Relenza is an inhaled antiviral while Tamiflu can be taken orally. Both of these antivirals, however, must be started within the first 2 days of flu onset and they only reduce the duration of flu by 1 to 2 days. Symptomatic treatment can include an analgesic for pain, muscle aches, and fever, but remember to avoid the use of aspirin in children with viral infections. Antihistamines and nasal decongestants can also be helpful. Cough suppressants like dextromethorphan or codeine and expectorants like guaifenesin may provide additional relief. Likewise, the use of vaporizers or humidifiers will relieve irritation of the nose and throat caused by dry air and will reduce coughs resulting from local irritation. There are far too many cold and flu products available to cover in this column. If you need advice on selecting a nonprescription product to meet your needs be sure to "Ask The Pharmacist".

QUESTION: With the flu season just around the corner, what can you tell me about the new flu drug called Relenza?

ANSWER: Relenza (generic name zanamivir) is an antiviral agent that was recently approved by the FDA for the treatment of uncomplicated flu in patients 12 years of age and older. This new agent is administered by inhalation using a Diskhaler device to deliver the medication directly to the lungs where the virus lives. The drug blocks the release of new viruses within the respiratory tract and thus reduces the spread of infection. Currently the drug is only approved for the treatment of the flu and not for preventing the flu, so annual vaccinations (flu shots) are still needed. It is interesting to note that Relenza was approved even though an FDA advisory panel of experts recommended against its approval because they thought it only provided a small benefit for flu sufferers. Studies show that this new drug will reduce the duration of flu symptoms by only 1 to 1-1/2 days, but the FDA felt that even this modest benefit is better than nothing. For Relenza to be effective, it must be used within the first 2 days of the onset of flu symptoms so only a short time is available to see a doctor and get a prescription. It also may be less effective in patients who do not have a fever or more severe symptoms (muscle aches, cough, sore throat, etc.). The recommended dose of Relenza for flu treatment is 2 inhalations twice a day (about 12 hours apart) for 5 days. Make sure you know how to use the Diskhaler before you leave the pharmacy. The most commonly reported side effects reported in studies with Relenza were sinusitis, diarrhea, and nausea, which also occurred in patients receiving a placebo (fake drug). However, the drug may cause problems in people with asthma and other lung diseases where it can pose a breathing risk. The company that makes Relenza (Glaxo Wellcome) is also investigating its use in preventing the spread of flu within a family or within institutions.

QUESTION: What can I do if I get the flu?

ANSWER: The "flu" or influenza is an infection of the lungs and airways caused by the influenza virus. It is most common during the winter months (December through March) and the best time for vaccination is October through mid-November. Symptoms of the flu develop more quickly and are more severe than a common cold. For example, colds begin with a runny nose, sneezing and may produce a cough with sputum. The flu on the other hand often causes a sudden onset of fever and a hacking dry cough. The fever usually climbs above 101 degrees, and is associated with chills, severe headache, tiredness, and body aches not often seen with a cold. Some nonprescription medications such as pain relievers, fever reducers, nasal decongestants, antihistamines, and cough remedies may help with the flu symptoms. Rest and drinking plenty of fluids also helps. However, a quick diagnosis by your physician and early treatment with a prescription antiviral medication can reduce the duration and severity of the flu symptoms. This is especially important for people at risk of serious complications such as pneumonia. People at risk of pneumonia include the very old and very young, those with a weakened immune system, or those with congestive heart failure, asthma, or chronic lung disease. Treatment with antiviral agents must be started within 2 days of the onset of flu symptoms to provide benefit; therefore, it is important to contact your physician as soon as possible. Two older oral prescription antiviral medications used to treat the flu are Symmetrel (amantadine) and Flumadine (rimantadine), but they may not be appropriate for everyone. More recently, the antivirals Relenza (zanamivir) and Tamiflu (oseltamivir) were approved to treat two types of influenza (A & B). Relenza is an inhaled product that delivers the medication directly to the lungs, and Tamiflu is given orally.

QUESTION: I heard that a new nasal flu vaccine will be available for this year's flu season. What can you tell me about it?

ANSWER: The FDA recently approved a new nasal spray flu vaccine (FluMist) for the prevention of influenza illness (flu) in healthy people 5 to 49 years of age. Since the new vaccine was only studied in people under 50 years old, it was not approved for people over 49. This is unfortunate, since people 50 and older constitute the majority of flu vaccine users. It also was not approved for children under 5 years old because during clinical trials, researchers found that this age group experienced a higher rate of asthma attacks and wheezing within 6 weeks of receiving the nasal vaccine compared to children who received a dummy drug (placebo). This new nasal vaccine will protect against the same viruses that the injected vaccine protects against during the upcoming flu season. FluMist was tested in over 20,000 healthy people prior to its approval. It was 87% effective in preventing the flu in children and significantly reduced the number of severe fever illness and upper respiratory illness with fever in adults. Common side effects of the nasal flu vaccine include runny nose, nasal congestion, cough, and sore throat. Children 5 to 8 need two doses at least 6 weeks apart the first time they get vaccinated, while people 9 to 49 need just one dose. The flu claims about 36,000 lives a year in the U.S. Children 5 to 14 have the highest infection rates, but children under 2, people over 65, and those with other medical problems are at greatest risk of developing serious complications from the flu. Limited supplies of FluMist should be available to consumers prior to the flu season, which runs from November to March.

QUESTION: I heard that it is important for flu shots to be given to young children and the elderly. Is this correct?

ANSWER: Yes. The U.S. Public Health Service Advisory Committee on Immunization Practices (ACIP) has put out a statement that encourages the use of flu shots in healthy children 6 to 23 months of age because they have been shown to be at increased risk for complications from the flu. In addition to young children, the flu vaccine should be given first to adults over 65, pregnant women who will be in their second or third trimester during the flu season, residents of nursing homes, patients with chronic disease, health care workers and household contacts of high-risk patients, and children under 9 receiving the vaccine for the first time. People receiving flu vaccine usually develop protective antibodies about 2 weeks after the shot, and are protected for about 6 months. However, in some elderly patients the antibodies fall below protective levels in 4 months or less. The best time to get a flu shot is by the end of November, but vaccination efforts can continue through December or later. Side effects from a flu shot can include soreness at the injection site, fever, muscle pain, and tiredness. The vaccine is made from inactivated virus grown in eggs and therefore allergic reactions can occur in some people. Influenza and pneumonia are a leading cause of death in the U.S., especially in older adults. The flu vaccine can prevent up to 50-60% of hospitalizations and 80% of deaths from flu-related complications among the elderly, so it is very important to get vaccinated each year.

QUESTION: I used to take Alka-Seltzer Plus Cold & Cough tablets, which contained phenylpropanolamine, and was taken off the market. What can I use now instead of this product?

ANSWER: As you probably know, last November the FDA requested that both prescription and non-prescription products that contained the decongestant phenylpropanolamine or PPA be taken off the market. The reason for this was that PPA has been associated with a number of adverse reactions including severe high blood pressure, psychiatric abnormalities (psychosis, hallucinations, delusions, manic states, suicidal behavior, etc), and stroke. It may also cause nausea, vomiting, anxiety, rapid heartbeats, tremor, and other side effects. One of the most dangerous adverse effects associated with PPA is a stroke with bleeding in the brain. This side effect may be more common in women using products containing PPA for weight control or as a nasal decongestant. Although these severe adverse reactions to PPA are uncommon, the FDA felt that many available alternative products are safer to use. Some of the best selling products for colds and weight loss contained PPA and were taken off the market or were re-formulated to contain different and potentially safer ingredients. The product you used, Alka-Seltzer Plus Cold & Cough, was one of the many products that contained PPA. In addition to the decongestant PPA, this product also contained the antihistamine chlorpheniramine, and the cough suppressant dextromethorphan. Many other non-prescription products are available containing a decongestant, antihistamine, and cough suppressant. Most of these products use pseudoephedrine as the decongestant, which is generally considered to be safer than PPA. However, products containing pseudoephedrine should not be taken by patients with heart disease, high blood pressure, thyroid disease, diabetes, or difficulty in urination due to an enlarged prostate. You may want to consider the use of topical nasal decongestants such as sprays or drops (e.g., Afrin, Neo-Synephrine). External nasal dilator strips like Breath Right may also be helpful for some people. For children under 2 years old with nasal congestion, the use of saline nasal drops can be useful. Consult with your doctor and pharmacist to determine what may be the best cold product for you to use. Also, read the product labels very carefully for its listing of ingredients, potential side effects, and precautions.

QUESTION: With flu season here again, how can we prevent its spread?

ANSWER: About 20% of Americans get the flu (influenza) each year causing more than 200,000 hospitalizations and 36,000 deaths from flu-related complications. The flu is caused by a virus and it usually spreads from one person to another by direct contact (touching, kissing, etc.), or by droplet contact from the cough or sneeze of an infected person. However, it can also spread by indirect contact when the virus is deposited on a surface such as a tabletop, desktop, doorknob, or faucet handle by an infected person. In this situation, people who touch the contaminated surface can transfer the virus to their hands and possibly to their eyes, nose, or mouth before washing their hands. Fortunately, there are some simple things that you can do to help prevent the spread of flu (and colds). The most important thing is to wash your hands frequently and properly when a family member or coworker is ill.

Proper Hand Washing

1. Wet your hands with warm, running water and apply liquid or clean bar soap. Lather well.
2. Rub your hands together vigorously and scrub all of the surfaces, including the backs of your hands, your wrists, between your fingers, and under your fingernails.
3. Continue rubbing and scrubbing for at least 10 to 15 seconds.
4. Rinse well and dry the hands with a clean or disposable towel. Use another clean towel to turn off the faucet.

It is also important to disinfect surfaces that get touched frequently. Disinfecting is different from cleaning with soap and water, which mainly removes dirt. Disinfectants have ingredients that kill viruses and other germs. A solution of household bleach (1 part bleach to 10 parts water) is an effective disinfectant, and various disinfectant wipes or sprays are also available. Some examples of surfaces and items that may need to be disinfected include doorknobs and handles, faucet handles, workplace desktops, telephones, and computer keyboards. Be sure to follow the instructions for using disinfectant products carefully, since some products need to stand for a few minutes before being wiped away. Studies have shown that the frequent use of disinfectants on commonly touched surfaces can significantly reduce the risk of infection.

QUESTION: I'm a teacher and want to protect myself from getting the flu. Can a person get sick from a flu shot?

ANSWER: With flu season just around the corner, your question is very timely. Flu season can begin as early as October and last as late as May. October and November are the best months for vaccination, but getting a flu shot in December or even later can still be beneficial. A flu shot is needed every year because different types of the influenza virus cause flu from year-to-year. The flu vaccine is made up of parts of dead influenza virus that are incapable of causing illness. These dead virus particles stimulate your body's immune system to build a defense against the influenza virus. Some people who get a flu shot develop a mild fever, fatigue, and muscle aches soon after receiving the vaccine. These symptoms are not the flu, but indicate that your body's immune system is at work producing antibodies to fight the flu virus. The flu vaccine is not 100% effective in preventing the flu, but if you catch the flu after a flu shot, the vaccine may provide you with some protection and a less severe illness. Teachers are especially vulnerable to the flu because they come into contact with so many children. The main way that the flu spreads from person-to-person is via respiratory droplets from a cough or sneeze. Sometimes the virus can also be spread when a person touches respiratory droplets from another person on a surface like a desk and then touches his or her own eyes, mouth, or nose before washing their hands. Some viruses and bacteria can live for two hours or longer on surfaces like cafeteria tables, doorknobs, and desks. To help prevent the spread of the flu, it is important to wash hands frequently, and for one to cover their mouth and nose with a disposable tissue when coughing or sneezing. If a tissue is not available, then a person's hands should be washed with soap and water every time they cough or sneeze. Hand to hand contact should also be avoided and anyone who is sick with the flu should stay at home until they recover. In addition, the use of alcohol based hand wipes, gel sanitizers, and periodic antiseptic spraying of shared items like telephones or doorknobs can be helpful. It is also important to convey this flu prevention information to the students.

STATIN DRUGS AND THE FLU

QUESTION: I heard on the news that statin drugs may reduce flu death. What do you think?

ANSWER: A recent study reported in the Journal of Infectious Diseases (2012) suggests that people taking a statin drug and are hospitalized due to the flu may have a much lower chance of dying, but more study is needed to confirm this. In this study, the medical records of over 3,000 adults with a median age of 70 years who were hospitalized during 2007-2008 due to the flu were reviewed. Researchers found that patients on statins were 41% less likely to die (3.9% among statin users and 5.5% among non-users) within 30 days, even after adjusting their data for age, the presence of heart, lung and/or kidney disease, whether they had a flu shot, or whether or not they received anti-flu medications. However, the study authors note that this was only an "observational" study and they did not know if patients taking statins were healthier than those not taking them, and more detailed studies are needed. It is not known how statins may protect people from dying from the flu, but in addition to lowering cholesterol they also have anti-inflammatory effects and infections like the flu do cause inflammation in the body. Until more information is available it is too early to make any recommendations regarding the use of statins and the flu. Currently, the best weapons against the flu are vaccinations and antiviral flu medications.

There are currently seven statin drugs available: atorvastatin (Lipitor), fluvastatin (Lescol), lovastatin (Mevacor, Altoprev), pitavastatin (Livalo), pravastatin (Pravachol), rosuvastatin (Crestor), and simvastatin (Zocor). Atorvastatin, lovastatin, pravastatin, and simvastatin are also available as generic drugs.

ANTI-VIRAL TISSUES

QUESTION: Does the new antiviral Kleenex work?

ANSWER: The new Kleenex Anti-Viral Tissue is composed of 3 layers of paper tissue with a moisture-activated middle layer that is claimed to kill 99.9% of cold and flu viruses trapped inside. This middle tissue layer is impregnated with citric acid, a common additive in detergents, and sodium lauryl sulfate, which is found in many shampoos. According to the manufacturer, these active ingredients can inactivate (kill) rhinoviruses that cause the common cold, influenza (flu) viruses, and the virus that can cause lower respiratory tract infections in children (Respiratory syncytial virus) within 15 minutes of contact. The product has not been tested against bacteria. Kleenex Anti-Viral tissue is designed to be used as a facial tissue and is not meant to be used as hand wipes or as a surface cleanser. When the tissue is used to catch a sneeze or cough, or wipe a runny nose, the moisture activates the anti-viral ingredients in that middle layer. In theory, this will help to protect your hands from nasal discharge or saliva and will help to prevent spread of the droplet containing virus to others. Viruses can remain living outsides the body for up to 48 hours or more if moisture is present. These viral-containing droplets can infect others when transferred via contact (hands, door knobs, etc.) and subsequently be absorbed through the eyes, nose, or mouth. However, to be effective the virus must be transferred into the middle tissue layer, and virus transferred from nose to tissue without passing through the treated middle layer is still infectious. Kleenex Anti-Viral tissues are a disposable tissue designed to be used once and thrown away. If these tissues are carefully disposed of after use, and combined with frequent hand washing, they may help to lower the spread of upper respiratory viral infections.

AIRBORNE FOR COLDS

QUESTION: What can you tell me about the product "Airborne" for colds?

ANSWER: According to the product's web site, Airborne was developed by an elementary school teacher who was tired of catching colds in the classroom and on airplanes. She supposedly spent 5 years developing this dietary supplement product with a team of health professionals. Airborne contains 7 herbs (lonicera, forsythia, schizonepeta, ginger, Chinese vitex, isastis root, and echinacea) along with vitamins A, C, and E, 2 amino acids (glutamine and lysine), potassium, and 4 minerals (selenium, zinc, magnesium, and manganese). Quite a "shotgun" formulation. While many of these ingredients have been purported to have viral fighting or immune stimulating effects, there is no conclusive scientific evidence that this product or any of its ingredients is effective in preventing or treating colds. Furthermore, as I've stated many times before, no health claims have been evaluated by the FDA for dietary supplements, nor has the FDA approved these products to cure or prevent any disease. Two specific concerns I have about the adult Airborne tablet is that it contains very high doses of both vitamin A (5,000 I.U.) and vitamin C (1,000 mg). Since directions for use advise taking 1 tablet at the first sign of a cold and repeating the dose very 3 hours as necessary, excessive "megadoses" of these vitamins may be ingested. Overdoses of vitamin A can cause headache, vomiting or liver damage while overdoses of vitamin C can cause diarrhea and other gastrointestinal problems or kidney stones. Airborne is also available in a children's formula (Airborne Jr) and in a lozenge form (Airborne Gummi).

QUESTION: You recently wrote about your concerns regarding the adult Airborne product for colds. What about the Airborne Gummi Lozenges?

ANSWER: In my earlier column I noted that I was concerned about the high doses of both vitamin A (5,000 IU) and vitamin C (1,000 mg) in the adult Airborne product. If these tablets are taken every 3 hours as recommended in the directions, "megadoses" of these vitamins could be ingested, which could cause side effects. As I noted, overdoses of vitamin A can cause headache, vomiting, or liver damage, while overdoses of vitamin C can cause diarrhea and other gastrointestinal problems, or even kidney stones. The Airborne Gummi Lozenges are not promoted for the treatment of colds, but for minor sore throat irritation. Each of these "cold germ" shaped lozenges contain a portion of the ingredients found in the adult Airborne product for colds. These gummi lozenges contain very small amounts of vitamin C, vitamin E, vitamin B1, riboflavin (B2), niacin (B3), vitamin B6, vitamin B12, folic acid, biotin, pantothenic acid, magnesium, and zinc. In addition, there are also very small amounts of seven herbal extracts (lonicera, forsythia, schizoepeta, ginger, Chinese vitex, isastis root, and echinacea) in each lozenge. How minute doses of these 19 different ingredients work to help a minor sore throat is questionable. Sucking on a lozenge may increase saliva formation, which can ease throat irritation, but less expensive cough lozenges can do the same thing. As I've stated many times before, for dietary supplements like Airborne products, product claims and safety have not been evaluated by the FDA. In addition, we only have the manufacturer's word that what's on the label is what is really in the product.

THE COMMON COLD & ZINC

QUESTION: Can zinc lozenges help with colds?

ANSWER: Maybe, maybe not. The common cold has been bothersome to mankind throughout history and many, many remedies or "cures" have been proposed for this ailment. Adults average 3 to 5 episodes of the common cold each year and spend over $2 billion per year on non-prescription products to get rid of their cold symptoms. All of these over-the-counter products only provide temporary, symptomatic relief but can also cause many side effects, which can make matters even worse.

In recent years, zinc has become a popular "natural" remedy for the common cold. Zinc lozenges and lollipops are now widely available and are heavily advertised to the public. Zinc has been proposed to act as an antiviral agent, but not much scientific study information is available. Other suggested ways in which zinc lozenges or lollipops may help the common cold include an antihistamine effect, stimulation of the immune system, or increased flow of saliva that helps quiet a cough and soothe an irritated throat. In available clinical studies using zinc lozenges for the common cold, about half of the studies have demonstrated a positive effect, while the other half did not. It is generally thought that zinc lozenges should be started within 24 hours of the onset of cold symptoms. The lollipops or lozenges can be sucked every 2-3 hours while awake during the cold. Side effects of using zinc lozenges or lollipops for a short period of time can include bad taste, nausea, and upset stomach. Until more information is available, pregnant and breast feeding women should avoid zinc cold remedies. Also remember that non-prescription zinc products are considered to be nutritional supplements and are not approved for safety or effectiveness by the FDA.

QUESTION: Can nasal sprays containing zinc cause a loss of smell?

ANSWER: Yes, intranasal cold remedies that contain zinc may cause the user to lose their sense of smell (anosmia) or diminish their sense of smell (hyposmia). In fact in 2009, the Food and Drug Administration (FDA) issued a public health advisory to alert consumers about the risk of permanently losing their sense of smell from zinc-containing cold remedies. Since the introduction of zinc-containing products to the market in 1999, the FDA has received more than 130 reports of anosmia associated with the use of zinc-containing intranasal products. The loss of sense of smell may be long lasting or even permanent in some people. More recently, in July 2010, researchers at the University of California San Diego described 25 cases of patients who came to a nasal dysfunction clinic complaining of anosmia after using a zinc gel nasal spray. All of these patients had intense burning "between the eyes" and perceived the loss of smell within 12 to 36 hours of using the zinc nasal spray. The researchers called for increased FDA oversight of intranasal zinc products, including homeopathic medications, in order to monitor the safety of these popular cold remedies.

Loss of the sense of smell may cause serious problems. People with anosmia may not be able to smell smoke, a gas leak, or spoiled food, for example. Anosmia is often associated with a loss of sense of taste, or ageusia. People need to be able to smell in order to taste properly. People who cannot smell are not able to appreciate flavors, could eat spoiled food, and could lose much of the pleasure of eating. Therefore, the effect of not being able to taste presents a potential danger and quality of life issue for anyone who experiences the problem of anosmia. Loss of one's sense of smell or sense of taste may also affect the work of people employed in the food industry, or other industries in which the sense of smell and taste are very important. The FDA recommends that consumers contact their healthcare provider if they experience loss of the sense of smell or taste after using any zinc-containing products that are administered into the nose. Healthcare providers and patients are urged to report adverse reactions such as loss of sense of smell or taste from the use of zinc-containing products to the FDA by phone at 1-800-FDA-TEN-88 or via the Internet at **www.fda.gov/safety/medwatch**.

USE OF ANTIBIOTICS

QUESTION: What do I need to know about my antibiotic prescription and why do I have to take if for 7 to 10 days?

ANSWER: Antibiotics are potent medications that are used to treat infections caused by bacteria. The most common bacterial infections are pneumonia, urinary tract infections, middle ear infections, some skin infections, sinusitis, and strep throat. Antibiotics are not useful for viral infections, which cause the majority of coughs, colds, and sore throats. Antibiotics work in a variety of different ways to either kill bacteria (bactericidal) or to slow down their multiplication (bacteriostatic) and allow the body's immune system to fight off the infection. Common side effects of antibiotics include diarrhea, upset stomach, increased sensitivity to sunlight, and skin rash. Most antibiotics need to be taken for at least 7 to 10 days even if you feel better after only a day or two, because you want to make sure that the bacteria have stopped multiplying. The first few doses of antibiotic kill off the weaker bacteria, but the bacteria will continue to multiply if they are not all killed causing the infection to get worse. If you do not finish the entire course of therapy, the bacteria may also become "resistant" to the antibiotic and become stronger. Infections due to "resistant" bacteria are very difficult to treat and may require hospitalization. Resistance to antibiotics occurs when they are used too often or incorrectly. You should also not use antibiotics leftover from a previous infection. Antibiotics may lose their effectiveness over time or can cause serious side effects. Outdated tetracycline for example can cause serious toxicity to the kidneys. Some newer antibiotics can be used effectively for shorter periods of time, so make sure that you pay close attention to your prescription labeling and directions. If you have any questions about your antibiotic prescription, make sure you "Ask The Pharmacist".

QUESTION: Why do antibiotics cause diarrhea?

ANSWER: Just about any antibiotic (taken orally or given by injection) can cause diarrhea. However, some antibiotics are more likely to cause diarrhea than others. This topic has been recently reviewed in a Johns Hopkins Health Alert (**www.johnshopkinshealthalerts.com**, 2011).

Antibiotics have been widely used since World War II, and they've saved countless lives since then. Bacterial illnesses such as strep throat and urinary tract infections can be easily treated, often in three to 10 days. But as with any medication, antibiotics carry the risk of digestive side effects. People taking antibiotics may develop mild diarrhea or a more serious bowel inflammation.

Many different species of bacteria live in your digestive tract. Most are helpful, others are harmful, but in healthy people the good bacteria far outnumber the bad. This balance is delicate, however, and it can be easily disrupted. When you take an antibiotic for an infection, it doesn't just target the problem bacteria. The antibiotic can kill off both good and bad bacteria in your digestive tract. Often the strongest, most treatment-resistant harmful bacteria are the ones that remain, and as they're allowed to multiply unchecked they can wreak havoc on your digestive system. Most people taking an antibiotic will be fine, but the accompanying diarrhea that affects the other 20% can range from a mild, short-lived bout of diarrhea to colitis, an inflammation of the colon. Some people may experience a more serious, perhaps even life-threatening, form of colitis caused by the bacterium Clostridium difficile (C. difficile). People over age 65 are more prone to develop antibiotic-associated diarrhea (AAD) and colitis, as are those who have recently stayed in a hospital or nursing home, have had surgery on the intestinal tract or have another illness affecting the intestines, such as inflammatory bowel disease or colon cancer. Antibiotic-associated diarrhea (AAD) involves occasional loose stools or mild diarrhea for several days. The problem typically begins five to 10 days after starting an antibiotic, however, in 25 to 40% of cases, symptoms don't appear until up to 10 weeks after treatment ends. Most cases of AAD do not require treatment and will resolve on their own within two weeks after finishing an antibiotic.

While any antibiotic, oral or injected, has the potential to cause diarrhea, the most likely candidates are stronger, broad-spectrum antibiotics, which include:

- cephalosporins like cefixime (Suprax) and cefpodoxime (Vantin)
- extended-coverage penicillins like amoxicillin
- erythromycin
- quinolones such as ciprofloxacin (Cipro) and levofloxacin (Levaquin)
- tetracyclines
- clindamycin

FLUOROQUINOLONE ANTIBIOTICS

QUESTION: I heard that some antibiotics can cause tendon rupture. What can you tell me about this?

ANSWER: The FDA recently notified manufacturers of fluoroquinolone antibiotics that a Boxed Warning in the product labeling concerning the risk of tendonitis and tendon rupture is necessary. The FDA also determined that it is necessary for manufacturers of these drugs to provide a Medication Guide to patients about possible side effects. Fluoroquinolone antibiotics are approved for the treatment or prevention of certain bacterial infections. They are not used to treat viral infections such as colds or flu. The risk of developing fluoroquinolone-associated tendonitis and tendon rupture is further increased in people older than 60, in those taking corticosteroids drugs, and in kidney, heart, and lung transplant recipients. Patients experiencing pain, swelling, inflammation of a tendon or tendon rupture should be advised to stop taking their fluoroquinolone medication and to contact their physician about changing their antibiotic. Patients should also avoid exercise and using the affected area at the first sign of tendon pain, swelling, or inflammation. Manufacturers of these products are being notified to change the labeling of their fluoroquinolone products for systemic use (e.g., tablets, capsules, and injections) but the change would not apply to fluoroquinolones for topical use such as eye or ear drops. Medications involved in this warning include: Cipro and generic ciprofloxacin, Cipro XR and Proquin XR (ciprofloxacin extended release), Factive (gemifloxacin), Levaquin (levofloxacin), Avelox (moxifloxacin), Noroxin (norfloxacin), and Floxin and generic ofloxacin.

ADULT VACCINATION CHECKLIST

QUESTION: What vaccinations should I get?

ANSWER: Recently a vaccination checklist for adults was provided in the "Johns Hopkins Health After 50 Newsletter" (November 2009). These recommendations are from the U.S. Centers for Disease Control and Prevention (CDC), and they apply to healthy older adults. You will find this checklist below and on the next page.

Vaccine
Who and How Often

- **Influenza (Flu)**
  Everyone age 50 and older; once a year at the start of the flu season (early fall, winter). The vaccine contains the strains of virus most likely to cause illness in that year.
- **Pneumococcal polysaccharide vaccine (PPSV)**
  Everyone age 65 or older or if you have a chronic respiratory condition, like asthma, or you smoke; one to two doses of the vaccine per lifetime.
- **Tetanus, diphtheria, pertussis (Td/Tdap)**
  Adults ages 19-64 should receive a dose of Tdap as a substitute for the Td shot that is given every 10 years. Those 65 and older should have a Tdap shot every 10 years. Adults who were never vaccinated for these diseases need to be given three doses of the vaccine (the first two doses four weeks apart and the last 6-12 months later).
- **Herpes zoster (Shingles)**
  A single dose for all adults 60 and older.

PLEASE NOTE: Zostavax is now approved to help prevent shingles in adults 50 years of age and older.

*   **Varicella (Chickenpox)**
    Anyone who has never had chickenpox; two doses during your lifetime.
*   **Measles, mumps, rubella (MMR)**
    For adults who have not had these childhood diseases; one to two doses per lifetime. People born before 1957 are considered to have immunity from the measles, but getting vaccinated is still a good idea.
*   **Hepatitis A**
    Travelers to regions where hepatitis A is common and anyone who wants protection; two doses per lifetime.
*   **Hepatitis B**
    Adults with multiple sex partners, partners of infected people, travelers to high-risk areas; three doses per lifetime.
*   **Meningococcal polysaccharide vaccine**
    Travelers and certain other at-risk groups; one or more doses per lifetime.

TRUVADA TO REDUCE HIV RISK

QUESTION: What can you tell me about the drug recently approved to reduce HIV risk?

ANSWER: On July 16, 2012 the FDA approved Truvada, the first drug for reducing the risk of sexually acquired human immunodeficiency virus (HIV) infection. Truvada is a two drug combination medication that was originally approved in 2004 to treat HIV-infected adults and children 12 years or older used in conjunction with other HIV medications. Truvada is now also approved to be taken once-daily and used together with safer sex practices to reduce the risk of sexually acquired HIV infection in adults who do not have HIV but are at high risk of becoming infected. In 2 large clinical studies, Truvada reduced the risk of HIV infection by 42% in about 2,500 HIV-negative gay and bisexual men and transgender women, and by 75% in approximately

4,800 heterosexual couples in which one partner was infected with HIV and the other was not. Before Truvada is prescribed, healthcare professionals need to weigh the risk versus benefit as follows:

- The person must be tested to ensure that he or she is HIV negative, and this test should be repeated every 3 months thereafter.
- Flu-like symptoms—such as fever or muscle aches—are a red flag because they could indicate the presence of early, acute HIV infection, even if test results are negative. There is a window of four to five weeks with some tests, and up to three months with others, in which the antibodies that indicate HIV infection do not appear in the blood.
- Safety concerns tied to Truvada have to do with its effect on the bones and kidneys. While effects observed in clinical trials were mild and reversible with discontinuation of the medication, people with a history of bone or kidney ailments should be regularly monitored to ensure their continued health.
- It is recommended that the person also be tested for hepatitis B because worsening of hepatitis B infections has been reported in those who have both HIV and hepatitis B when treatment with Truvada was stopped.

In addition, the FDA requires a strategy to reduce the risks of using Truvada which includes a training program for prescribers to help them counsel patients on several key points including the following:

- The drug should not become a substitute for a condom, but rather, an adjunct to condom use and other preventive measures.
- The antiretroviral must be taken daily, because its effectiveness strongly correlates to adherence. Intermittent use might spur on the development of Truvada-resistant HIV.
- Monitoring a patient's HIV status after the start of preexposure prophylaxis is crucial because if a patient subsequently becomes infected, he or she should switch from the stand-alone antiretroviral to the combination of antiretrovirals for treating (as opposed to preventing) HIV infection. Also, an HIV-positive patient who continues to take Truvada by itself risks the development of a drug-resistant virus.

About 1.2 million Americans have HIV infection with about 50,000 adults and adolescents newly diagnosed each year. The overall rate of HIV infection has remained stable at least since 2004. A key goal of anti-HIV drugs is to help stop HIV from reproducing. HIV is a virus that attacks your immune system, which is made up of millions of cells that help fight against infection and disease. Once HIV enters the body, the virus infects specialized immune system cells known as CD4 cells and multiplies (replicates) inside these cells. These new viruses are released into the blood and go on to infect other CD4 cells. As CD4 cells are attacked and destroyed by HIV, the immune system becomes less able to fight infection and disease. Anti-HIV drugs work by helping to stop or "inhibit" certain steps during the HIV replication process. When used in combination, anti-HIV therapies can help reduce the amount of HIV in the blood (viral load). Truvada works to prevent the HIV virus from establishing itself and multiplying in the body.

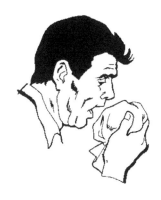

CHAPTER 10
ALLERGIES

OTC PRODUCTS

QUESTION: What non-prescription products will help my allergy symptoms?

ANSWER: Approximately one out of five Americans has allergic rhinitis, making it one of the most common chronic conditions in the country. This condition results from a hypersensitivity (allergic) reaction to foreign substances in the air, which produces inflammation of the mucosal lining in the nose. Allergy symptoms (runny nose, nasal itching, sneezing, congestion, itchy/watery eyes, and possibly itching of the throat and mouth) may occur year-round or during certain seasons of the year. Seasonal allergic rhinitis is caused by tree pollens, grasses and weeds (especially ragweed), and mold spores. Year-round (perennial) symptoms are commonly due to house dust mites, animal dander, cockroaches, or indoor mold spores. Allergic rhinitis can occur at any age, but usually develops before age 30 and heredity plays a large role. The first step in treating allergic rhinitis is identifying the foreign substance(s) (called allergens) that one is allergic to and avoiding them.

This, however, may not be easy or feasible, in which case drug therapy may be needed to control the undesirable symptoms.

Numerous non-prescription products are available to treat allergic rhinitis. The active ingredients in these products include oral antihistamines, decongestants (oral or intranasal), combinations of antihistamines and decongestants, and a relatively new type of drug called cromolyn for intranasal use. Antihistamines block the chemical histamine, which is released during an allergic reaction and causes the sneezing, itching, runny nose, and itchy/watery eyes. They do not relieve nasal congestion. Common side effects of non-prescription antihistamines include drowsiness; dry eyes, nose, and mouth; blurred vision; difficulty in urinating; and constipation. Because of these side effects, patients with glaucoma or an enlarged prostate should not use antihistamines without a physician's supervision. Intranasal decongestants cause a narrowing of nasal blood vessels, which relieves congestion. Common side effects of intranasal decongestants include local irritation, sneezing, and dryness. They should not be used more often than directed or for longer than three to five days at a time, because "rebound congestion" can occur. Oral decongestants do not cause this "rebound congestion" but can cause other side effects like nervousness, dizziness, difficulty in sleeping, increased blood pressure, difficult urination, and increased heart rate. Patients with heart disease, high blood pressure, diabetes, or an enlarged prostate should not take oral decongestants without physician supervision. Intranasal cromolyn (Nasalcrom) works differently than decongestants or antihistamines by preventing the release of inflammatory substances from mast cells, which relieves congestion, sneezing, itching and runny nose. It is relatively free of side effects, except stinging, burning or sneezing immediately after its use. Intranasal cromolyn is the non-prescription drug of choice for people who prefer intranasal therapy or who cannot take antihistamines or decongestants. A listing of some commonly used non-prescription products for treating allergic rhinitis follow:

Oral Antihistamines
Product (Active Ingredient)
- Chlor-Trimeton Allergy (Chlorpheniramine)
- Efidac 24 (Chlorpheniramine)
- Benadryl (Diphenhydramine)

Oral Decongestants
Product (Active Ingredient)
- Sudafed (Pseudoephedrine)
- Sudafed PE (Phenylephrine)

Intranasal Decongestants
Product (Active Ingredient)
- Privine (Naphazoline)
- Afrin (Oxymetazoline)
- Neo-Synephrine (Phenylephrine)
- Otrivin (Xylometazoline)

Intranasal Mast-Cell Stabilizer
Product (Active Ingredient)
- Nasalcrom (Cromolyn)

QUESTION: I take Tylenol Allergy Multi-Symptom Night Time tablets for my allergy. Is this product safe to use?

ANSWER: Tylenol Allergy Multi-Symptom Night Time tablets are a non-prescription product that contains three active ingredients: phenylephrine, diphenhydramine, and acetaminophen. This product is primarily used for the short-term treatment of symptoms associated with colds, upper respiratory infections, and allergic conditions. Like all medications, its safety depends upon using the product according to the instructions on the package and paying attention to warnings to avoid its use if you have certain other medical problems.

Phenylephrine is a decongestant that helps to reduce nasal congestion. Since this drug affects the nervous system and blood vessels it can cause side effects like nervousness, restlessness, and difficulty in sleeping. It can also increase blood pressure, speed up the heart, and produce other effects in the body. Because of this, many decongestants like phenylephrine should be avoided or used under the supervision of a physician if a person has high blood pressure, heart disease, diabetes, enlarged prostate, or an overactive thyroid.

Diphenhydramine is an antihistamine that is useful in providing relief from hay fever (allergic rhinitis) symptoms such as runny nose, sneezing, itching of the nose or throat, and itchy, watery eyes.

It also can help to reduce cough. The most common side effect of diphenhydramine is drowsiness and therefore it should not be taken when mental alertness is needed (like when driving a car), and it should not be taken with alcohol or other drugs that cause drowsiness.

Acetaminophen is a pain reliever that also reduces fever. It is a useful drug for mild to moderate types of aches and pains. An important side effect of acetaminophen is that it can cause liver damage in some people. Because of this, it should be avoided in people with liver disease or those that drink alcohol more than occasionally.

In order to reduce the possibility of side effects with any non-prescription medication, please use it only according to package instructions and be aware of any warnings noted on the package. Remember that any medicine (prescription or not) can cause side effects in some people. Many of these medicines are only intended for short-term use and they should not be taken for long periods of time. If you have any questions when purchasing a non-prescription product, make sure you "Ask The Pharmacist".

HAYFEVER

QUESTION: I heard about a new prescription nasal spray for hayfever. What can you tell me about it?

ANSWER: Hayfever or "allergic rhinitis" is a common problem, which affects almost 40% of the U.S. population. It is caused by particles in the air such as pollen, dust, animal dander, or molds which produce an allergic reaction within the airways when they are inhaled. This allergic reaction leads to the release of various chemicals including histamine and others that cause blood vessel expansion, mucus secretion, edema of the nasal mucosa, and stimulation of itch receptors. These chemicals or mediators lead to the symptoms of hayfever such as runny nose, nasal congestion, sneezing, and nasal itching. Allergies are not only bothersome, but have been linked to a variety of common and serious chronic respiratory illnesses, such as sinusitis and asthma. In addition, they may interfere with day-to-day activities or lessen the quality of life.

The FDA recently approved Patanase (olopadine) nasal spray for the relief of symptoms of seasonal allergic rhinitis or hayfever in patients 12 years of age and older. Patanase is a non-steroid histamine-blocking drug that reduces the symptoms of hayfever including nasal congestion, sneezing, itchy nose, runny nose, watery eyes and itchy eyes. It is administered as a nasal spray in a dose of 2 sprays per nostril twice a day. In short-term clinical studies, the most common side effects were a bitter taste, headache, nosebleed, nose and throat pain, post-nasal drip and cough.

QUESTION: I commonly use a nonprescription nasal decongestant for my hayfever. Are these products safe?

ANSWER: Numerous nonprescription medications are available to treat hayfever including antihistamines, cromolyn, and nasal decongestants. Nasal decongestants are available as oral products, topical nasal sprays, drops, and inhalers. Oral products usually contain pseudoephedrine, or phenylephrine while the topical nasal products contain oxymetazoline, xylometazoline, or phenylephrine. While the short-term use of decongestants can help to relieve the congestion associated with hayfever, they have little effect on the sneezing, runny nose, or nasal itching. Because of this, many combination products contain both antihistamines and nasal decongestants. Decongestants relieve nasal congestion by constricting blood vessels in the nose. However, they can also constrict blood vessels elsewhere in the body, which can increase blood pressure. Therefore, if you have high blood pressure or heart disease, you should not use nasal decongestants without your doctor's advice. These decongestants can also affect the blood sugar (glucose) and diabetic patients should not use them. In addition, nasal decongestants can cause difficulty in urination, so men with prostate problems should avoid them. Likewise, patients with thyroid disease should avoid them due to the possibility of adverse reactions.

Drug interactions with nasal decongestants can also be a problem. When taking them, you should avoid taking any additional products containing pseudoephedrine, phenylephrine, or ephedrine, which may be found in other allergy, asthma, cough-cold, or weight control products. Stimulants such as caffeine and certain drugs for depression

(MAO inhibitors) should not be used in combination with nasal decongestants. Finally, be especially cautious with herbal products or "natural" remedies that contain ma huang, ephedra, guarana, or kola nut, which can cause serious adverse reactions when taken with nasal decongestants.

Always be sure to carefully read the labeling of any nonprescription product. They should contain warnings about the potential problems with their use. If you have any doubt about the safety of a particular nasal decongestant product be sure to "Ask The Pharmacist" or consult with your doctor.

SUDAFED VERSUS SUDAFED PE

QUESTION: What is the difference between Sudafed tablets and Sudafed PE tablets?

ANSWER: Sudafed contains the nasal decongestant pseudoephedrine while Sudafed PE contains the nasal decongestant phenylephrine (PE). Under an amendment to the USA Patriot Act, as of September 30, 2006 any medication containing pseudoephedrine must be placed behind pharmacy counters or locked in cabinets to control the amounts bought by consumers and to prevent shoplifting. In addition, for customers wanting to purchase medications containing pseudoephedrine (like Sudafed) they will now have to show picture ID and sign a logbook recording where they live. The logbooks must remain on file for two years and be accessible to law enforcement authorities. The reason for these restrictions is because pseudoephedrine can be made into methamphetamine (meth) by illegal labs. Meth now leads cocaine, marijuana, and heroin as the top illegal drug problem in many states. Phenylephrine on the other hand, cannot be easily made into methamphetamine by illegal labs. Because of this, many drug manufacturers are making new versions of their oral nasal decongestant products using phenylephrine in place of pseudoephedrine (like Sudafed PE). Phenylephrine is not new to the market and has been used in nonprescription nasal sprays and other products for over 30 years. Oral phenylephrine, however, does differ from pseudoephedrine in that it must be taken more frequently and it is not absorbed into the bloodstream as well as pseudoephedrine. Some people feel that oral phenylephrine is not as effective as oral pseudoephedrine, but good studies comparing the two ingredients are not available. It should also be noted that products containing either of these ingredients should be used with caution in people with certain medical conditions including high blood pressure, glaucoma, enlarged prostate, heart trouble, diabetes, or thyroid disease. Please be sure to carefully read all package labeling and to follow dosing instructions when using any decongestant product.

INTRANASAL STEROIDS

QUESTION: I read your review of non-prescription medications for allergies and enjoyed it. I currently use a prescription product named Rhinocort for my allergies and would like some information about it.

ANSWER: As you probably know, there are numerous products available for treating allergic rhinitis, one of the most common chronic conditions in the United States. As I reviewed previously, non-prescription products for allergic rhinitis include antihistamines, decongestants, and more recently cromolyn or nasalcrom (a mast-cell stabilizer). The product that you use (Rhinocort, generic name budesonide, pronounced byoo-des-oh-nide), is another type of drug known as an intranasal steroid or corticosteroid. Intranasal steroids work differently than the non-prescription products that I discussed. They block the inflammatory response by the body to an inhaled allergen (like ragweed, tree or grass pollen, mold spores, dust mites, etc.). This inflammation blocking effect prevents or reduces nasal allergy symptoms such as sneezing, congestion, itching, and runny nose. However, eye symptoms like itching, tearing, and redness may not be helped and an oral antihistamine product (Benadryl, Chlor-trimeton, chlorpheniramine, Tavist, etc.), may also be needed. Improvement of symptoms with Rhinocort usually occurs within three days, but maximum benefits may take longer. If there is no improvement after three weeks it should be discontinued. The recommended dose is two sprays in each nostril in the morning and evening or four sprays in each nostril in the morning. After the desired effect has been obtained, the dose should be reduced to the smallest amount possible to control symptoms. The most common local side effects of intranasal steroids include nasal irritation, burning, and sneezing. Light nasal bleeding, sore throat, and headache may also occur. Rarely a yeast infection (Candida) or nasal septal perforation can occur. Other side effects such as a pounding heartbeat, nervousness, headache, and dizziness are possible. Some additional prescription intranasal steroid products include Beconase, Vancenase, Nasarel, Flonase, and Nasacort.

QUESTION: I use Flonase nasal spray for my allergies. Is a generic product available?

ANSWER: Yes, the FDA recently approved fluticasone propionate nasal spray, the first generic version of the brand name drug Flonase. Like Flonase, the generic product made by Roxane Laboratories is approved to treat the nasal symptoms of seasonal and chronic allergic and nonallergic rhinitis in both adults and children at least 4 years of age. Fluticasone is an intranasal steroid or corticosteroid that blocks the inflammatory response by the body to an inhaled allergen (like ragweed, tree or grass pollen, mold spores, dust mites, etc.). This inflammation blocking effect prevents or reduces nasal allergy symptoms such as sneezing, congestion, itching, and runny nose. Corticosteroid nasal sprays do not provide an immediate effect on allergy symptoms, but a decrease in nasal symptoms has been noted in some patients 12 hours after initial treatment. Common side effects of fluticasone nasal spray include headache, sore throat, and nose bleed. As I've noted many times before, the FDA approves all generic drugs using strict guidelines, including checking for the generic drug's chemistry by evaluating its formulation, potency, stability, and purity. The generic drug must also pass bio-equivalency testing that compares the delivery into the bloodstream of the generic drug's active ingredient to that of the brand name drug. Generic drugs are less expensive than brand-name products, and account for about 50 percent of prescriptions dispensed. The FDA approved 452 generic drug applications during 2005, the second highest total ever.

ZYRTEC-D

QUESTION: Is Zyrtec-D now available without a prescription?

ANSWER: Yes, the FDA recently approved the allergy drug, Zyrtec-D, for nonprescription use in adults and children 12 years of age and older. Zyrtec-D contains the antihistamine, cetirizine, in combination with the nasal decongestant, pseudoephedrine. Available as a prescription drug since 2001, Zyrtec-D is now approved as a nonprescription drug for the relief of symptoms due to hay fever or other upper respiratory allergies such as runny nose, sneezing, itchy, watery eyes, itching of the nose or throat, and nasal congestion. It is also useful for reducing swelling of nasal passages, for relief of sinus congestion and pressure, and for restoring free breathing through the nose. It is estimated that about 40% of the American population have an allergy problem also known as allergic rhinitis. About 60% of these people with allergies suffer from both seasonal and year-round allergies, and 30% of all allergy sufferers also have nasal congestion. The most common allergy symptoms include stuffy or runny nose, itchy and watery eyes, sneezing and congestion. Antihistamines provide relief from sneezing, runny nose, and itchy or watery eyes. Decongestants on the other hand will temporarily relieve nasal congestion and help breathing. The most common side effects of Zyrtec-D are drowsiness, tiredness, and dry mouth. This new product should not be taken by people with glaucoma, urinary retention, severe hypertension, severe coronary artery disease, or by patients taking MAO inhibitors. It should also be used with caution on patients with high blood pressure, diabetes, ischemic heart disease (like angina), increased pressure in the eye, kidney disorders, or an enlarged prostate. Sales of this new nonprescription drug are subject to the Combat Methamphetamine Epidemic Act, which places restrictions on the sale of products containing pseudoephedrine, such as limiting the amount that an individual can purchase, and imposing record keeping requirements on the retail establishments that sell the product.

ZYRTEC

QUESTION: My doctor has recommended Zyrtec 10 mg (1 tablet daily) for an allergic skin rash, which I get periodically. I've had difficulty urinating in the past when using antihistamines such as Contac. Can Zyrtec cause this problem?

ANSWER: Yes, it is also possible to have this problem with Zyrtec. Zyrtec (chemical name cetirizine) is an antihistamine that can be given once a day. Contac allergy tablets contain the antihistamine clemastine and Contac cold capsules contain the antihistamine chlorpheniramine plus a decongestant. All of these antihistamines are useful to use during allergic reactions because histamine is released during these reactions and produces symptoms such as redness, itching, and swelling. Antihistamines can, however, cause other undesirable effects such as difficult and painful urination, excessive urination, or retention of urine. They can even cause allergic reactions themselves in some people. The frequency of side effects occurring related to urination with Zyrtec is probably less than 2% of patients taking the drug. Some other newer antihistamines like Claritin may not cause problems with urination and might provide a useful alternative therapy.

CLARITIN/CLARINEX

QUESTION: I heard that Claritin will soon be sold over-the-counter. Is there any prescription drug similar to Claritin available?

ANSWER: Schering-Plough Corporation, the manufacturer of the popular allergy medication Claritin, recently announced that it plans to switch the prescription medication to an over-the-counter drug. Claritin is a once-daily antihistamine that is much less likely to cause drowsiness compared to older antihistamines like Benadryl. With Claritin coming off patent, the manufacturer has now developed a new antihistamine prescription product for treating allergy symptoms. The new product, which was recently approved by the FDA, is named

Clarinex. The active ingredient in Clarinex is actually derived from the active ingredient in Claritin and the two products are very similar.

Both Claritin and Clarinex are useful in treating the symptoms of seasonal allergic rhinitis. Approximately one out of five Americans has allergic rhinitis, making it one of the most common chronic conditions in the country. This condition results from a hypersensitivity (allergic) reaction to foreign substances in the air, which produces inflammation of the mucosal lining in the nose. Allergy symptoms (runny nose, nasal itching, sneezing, congestion, itchy/watery eyes, and possibly itching of the throat and mouth) may occur year-round or during certain seasons of the year. Seasonal allergic rhinitis is caused by tree pollens, grasses, and weeds (especially ragweed, and mold spores). Year-round (perennial) symptoms are commonly due to house dust mites, animal dander, cockroaches, or indoor mold spores. Allergic rhinitis can occur at any age, but usually develops before age 30 and heredity plays a large role. The first step in treating allergic rhinitis is identifying the foreign substance(s) (called allergens) that one is allergic to and avoiding them. This, however, may not be easy or feasible, in which case drug therapy may be needed to control the undesirable symptoms.

PLEASE NOTE: Claritin and a generic equivalent product (loratadine) are now available without a prescription. See next question.

QUESTION: Is a generic product for Claritin available?

ANSWER: Yes, the non-sedating antihistamine Claritin (generic name loratadine), which was recently switched from prescription to nonprescription status, now has a generic product available. The new generic product is made by Geneva Pharmaceuticals and it should provide a cost savings to consumers. As I've noted many times before, the FDA approves all generic drugs using strict guidelines, including checking for the generic drug's chemistry by evaluating its formulation, potency, stability, and purity. The generic drug must also pass bioequivalency testing that compares the delivery of the generic drug's active ingredient to that of the brand name drug. In addition, after a drug is approved by the FDA (brand or generic), it must maintain its approval within strict manufacturing guidelines, which require the manufacturer to provide samples to the FDA for testing from each batch made.

Loratadine is a once-daily antihistamine that is much less likely to cause drowsiness compared to older antihistamines like Benadryl. It is useful for treating the symptoms of seasonal allergic rhinitis.

ITCHY EYES

QUESTION: What nonprescription medications can I use for red, itchy eyes that I get every spring and summer?

ANSWER: Allergic conjunctivitis is a common cause of red, itchy eyes. Although allergies are best known for causing nasal symptoms, they also can be irritating to the eyes. In allergic conjunctivitis, the affected part of the eye is the conjunctiva, the thin, elastic tissue that covers the white of the eye and lines the inside of the eyelid. Conjunctivitis can be caused by either allergies or infection. In allergic conjunctivitis, the eyes become red and itchy, with a watery, stringy, or ropelike discharge. Both eyes are usually affected. In addition, people with allergic conjunctivitis often have a history of allergic rhinitis, asthma, or eczema. Infectious conjunctivitis also leads to eye redness but is more likely to produce tearing and discharge in one or both eyes. People with these symptoms may need antibiotics and should see an eye doctor. Allergic conjunctivitis can be seasonal (occurring only at specific times of the year) or perennial (occurring year-round). Seasonal allergic conjunctivitis is typically caused by outdoor allergens, such as pollen, and the perennial form is usually caused by indoor allergens, such as cockroaches, dust mites, or pet dander. Skin or blood testing by an allergist can pinpoint a patient's specific triggers.

To prevent symptoms of allergic conjunctivitis, patients should learn to avoid or limit their exposure to triggering substances. When symptoms do erupt, cold compresses on the eyes may help relieve conjunctivitis symptoms in the short term. Medications are a mainstay of treatment for allergic conjunctivitis. Some doctors recommend using artificial tears, which provide a barrier between allergens and the eye; they also help dilute and flush out the allergens that contact the eye. Other nonprescription medications used to treat allergic conjunctivitis include oral antihistamines like Benadryl (diphenhydramine), Zyrtec (cetirizine), or Claritin (loratadine); decongestant eyedrops like Visine (tetrahydrozoline), Visine LR (oxymetazoline) or Naphcon (naphazoline); and mast-cell stabilizer-antihistamine eyedrops like Alaway or Zadipor (ketotifen). In addition, combination decongestant/antihistamine eyedrops are also available over-the-counter. Various prescription medications are available to treat allergic conjunctivitis. This topic is reviewed in a recent Johns Hopkins Health Alert (**www.johnshopkinshealthalerts. com**, 2009) entitled "Remedies for Allergy Eyes".

NASAL IRRIGATION

QUESTION: Can a nasal irrigation using saltwater help with allergy and sinus problems?

ANSWER: A nasal saline (saltwater) rinse or wash if properly prepared and used may be helpful for a number of conditions such as sinusitis, rhinitis, allergies, or post-nasal drip. The nose acts to warm, moisten, and clean air before it enters the lungs. The bones of the face around the nose contain hollow spaces called paranasal sinuses, which reduce the weight of the facial bones while maintaining bone strength and shape. These air filled spaces of the nose and sinuses also humidify and warm the air, add to the sense of smell, and play a significant role in the quality of human sound. The sinuses are lined with cells that produce mucus and have tiny hairlike projections called cilia which help to remove foreign particles into the nasal cavity through small openings called ostia. The average adult produces about 1 quart of mucus in their sinuses daily, which server to keep the nose and sinuses moist and to trap inhaled irritants. As long as the mucus is thin and watery, it will flow easily along its course and eventually be swallowed. However, mucus that becomes thick can remain in the sinuses or nose leading to congestion, headache, post-nasal drip and cough. Mucus that remains stagnant also provides an opportunity for infection. Some of the causes of thickened mucus in the nose and sinuses include colds, the flu, allergies, pollution, or dry air. Nasal rinses or washes with saline solution can help to cleanse the sinuses and keep them moist. Saline rinses/washes can aid in washing away thickened mucus, allergy causing particles and irritants, such as pollens, dust particles, pollutants, and bacteria. It should be noted, however, that the mucus membranes that line the nose and sinuses are sensitive and delicate. Therefore only properly prepared saline solutions should be used for this purpose. Two nonprescription preservative free saline rinse/wash products that contain pre-measured packets of ingredients to prepare a proper saline solution are Sinus Rinse and SinuCleanse. Both of these products can be found at many pharmacies nationwide or can be obtained online (Sinus Rinse-**www.sinusrinse.com**, 1-877-477-8633; SinuCleanse-**www.sinucleanse.com**, 1-888-547-5492). Sinus Rinse uses a plastic squeeze bottle to administer the saline rinse, while SinuCleanse uses a plastic nasal washing pot known as a neti-pot. If you use these products, please make sure that you read and follow all instructions carefully. These products should not be used in certain situations, so be sure to contact your physician and pharmacist for further advice.

ALLEGRA AND JUICE

QUESTION: I read that Allegra is now available over-the-counter. Why shouldn't you take it with juice?

ANSWER: Allegra (fexofenadine) became available for purchase without a prescription (OTC) in March 2011. It is available for purchase in its original prescription strength and in various formulations. Allegra is an antihistamine that relieves symptoms due to upper respiratory allergies or hayfever, which can be caused by an allergic response to indoor or outdoor allergens. The natural body chemical histamine can react to these allergens and produce symptoms of sneezing, itching, watery eyes, and runny nose. Allegra counteracts these effects of histamine. It is recommended that Allegra be taken with water and not with fruit juice (such as apple, orange, or grapefruit). The reason for this is that these juices can significantly reduce the absorption of the active ingredient in Allegra, making it less effective. Antacids taken with Allegra can also significantly reduce its absorption and they should be avoided within 15 minutes before or after taking this medication. Please be sure to carefully read and follow all labeling and directions that come with the newly available OTC Allegra products.

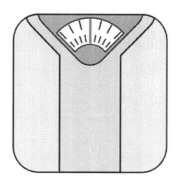

CHAPTER 11
WEIGHT CONTROL

OVER-THE-COUNTER PRODUCTS

QUESTION: What non-prescription or herbal products can I use to lose weight?

ANSWER: Excessive weight or obesity is a major public health concern that is becoming more and more common. It is estimated that about 50% of adults in the U.S. over age 20 are overweight. This compares to about 13% in 1960 and 23% in 1994. These estimates are important because obesity is a major factor in the development of serious medical problems including heart disease, high blood pressure, type 2 diabetes, sleep apnea, osteoarthritis, gallbladder disease, and some types of cancer. In simple terms, obesity is the result of an imbalance between the amount of food eaten and energy used, but its cause is not completely understood. Several metabolic, genetic, and environmental factors are involved in the development of this chronic disease. The primary treatment for obesity should include dietary changes, exercise, and behavior modification. Drug treatment alone to lose weight is of limited value.

Many non-prescription drug products for weight control that contained phenylpropanolomine were removed from the market in October 2000 because of the risk of hemorrhagic stroke. Common herbal ingredients in weight-loss products include St. John's wort, guarana, kola nut, and others. Although these products are widely promoted to the public, there is very little scientific information available to support their effectiveness or safety for weight reduction and control. Guarana and kola nut are stimulants, which can increase blood pressure and heart rate. People with heart disease, hypertension, thyroid disease, and diabetes should avoid them. St. John's wort can cause side effects including an increased sensitivity to light. In addition, many potential drug interactions can occur when using some herbal preparations together with prescription medications. Furthermore, many of these products are not standardized, and their content can vary from what is on the label. Because of these potential problems and lack of information available, I cannot recommend these products for the treatment of obesity.

HCG WEIGHT LOSS PRODUCTS

QUESTION: Why does the FDA want to remove homeopathic HCG weight loss products from the market?

ANSWER: Primarily because these over-the-counter products are unproven to help with weight loss and are potentially dangerous. In view of this, on December 6, 2011, the U.S. Food and Drug Administration and the Federal Trade Commission (FTC) issued seven Warning Letters to companies marketing over-the counter (OTC) HCG products that are labeled as "homeopathic" for weight loss. Human chorionic gonadotropin (HCG) is a hormone produced by the human placenta and found in the urine of pregnant women. HCG is FDA-approved as an injectable prescription drug for the treatment of some cases of female infertility and other medical conditions. The letters warn the companies that they are violating federal law by selling drugs that have not been approved, and by making unsupported claims for the substances. There are no FDA-approved HCG drug products for weight loss. The joint action is the first step in keeping the unproven and potentially unsafe products from being marketed online and in retail outlets as oral drops, pellets, and sprays. The labeling for the "homeopathic" HCG products states that each product should be taken in conjunction with a very low calorie diet. There is no substantial evidence HCG increases weight loss beyond that resulting from the recommended caloric restriction. Consumers on a very low calorie diet are at increased risk for side effects including gallstone formation, electrolyte imbalance, and heart arrhythmias. According to the Warning Letters, the companies have 15 days to notify the FDA of the steps they have taken to correct the violations cited. Failure to do so may result in legal action, including seizure and injunction, or criminal prosecution. Consumers and health care professionals are encouraged to report adverse events (side effects) that may be related to the use of these products to MedWatch, the FDA's voluntary reporting program, by calling 800-FDA-1088, or electronically at **www.fda.gov/medwatch/report.htm**.

EPHEDRA

QUESTION: I heard that nonprescription weight loss products containing ephedra can cause serious side effects. What are they?

ANSWER: The use of ephedra has been associated with increased heart rate and blood pressure and can lead to strokes, heart attacks, and convulsions. Additional side effects of ephedra include heart palpitations and psychiatric, gastrointestinal, or nervous system problems. In fact, ephedra along with other factors may have played a role in the recent death of a 23-year-old Baltimore Orioles pitcher. In view of these potential problems, the FDA has proposed that the following warning be added to the labels of all products containing ephedra:

WARNING: Contains ephedrine alkaloids. Heart attack, stroke, seizure, and death have been reported after consumption of ephedrine alkaloids. Not for pregnant or breast-feeding women or persons under 18. Risk of injury can increase with dose or if used during strenuous exercise or with other products containing stimulants (including caffeine). Do not use with certain medications or if you have certain health conditions. Stop use and contact a doctor if side effects occur.

When and if this warning is actually added to dietary supplements containing ephedra is not known at this time. The FDA is also trying to improve the quality of all dietary supplements by proposing requirements for good manufacturing practices to be used by makers of these products. If these requirements are approved supplement makers would need to evaluate the identity, purity, quality, strength, and composition of their products—something that is not currently required.

PLEASE NOTE: Products containing ephedra are now banned by the FDA. Please see question below.

QUESTION: What can you tell me about the ban on ephedra products?

ANSWER: The U.S. Food and Drug Administration (FDA) recently announced that it will ban dietary supplements containing ephedra, because its use has been associated with heart attacks, strokes, and convulsions. Ephedra, also known as ma huang, is included in a number of dietary supplements that are promoted for weight control, building muscle, and boosting energy. The active ingredients (alkaloids) found in ephedra are ephedrine and pseudoephedrine. These active ingredients are also contained in a large number of over-the-counter (OTC) cold and asthma remedies to relieve congestion and help breathing. Initially the FDA considered requiring a warning statement on all dietary supplements containing ephedra, but the agency now feels that a ban on ephedra supplements would be more appropriate to protect the public. The FDA has also issued a "consumer alert" urging the public to immediately stop buying and using ephedra-containing dietary supplements. Manufacturers of these supplements will have 60 days to comment on this proposed ban. It will be interesting to see how this proposal turns out, because it is the first time that the FDA has tried to ban dietary supplements that are not classified as drugs. FDA-approved drugs must show evidence of safety and effectiveness before they are marketed. However, the law requires the FDA to prove a dietary supplement poses an unreasonable risk before it can be removed from the market. Another interesting twist is that the FDA is not proposing a ban on OTC cold and asthma remedies containing pseudoephedrine or ephedrine that are used by millions of Americans.

The reasoning for this is that these products are properly labeled and are for short-term use only.

ALLI

QUESTION: I heard that a nonprescription drug for weight loss may be coming to market. What can you tell me about it?

ANSWER: An FDA advisory panel recently recommended the approval of a nonprescription weight loss medication named Alli (orlistat). Actually Alli is a lower dose (60 mg) version of the prescription drug Xenical (120 mg), which has been available since 1999. Like Xenical, Alli works mainly in the gastrointestinal tract to block the absorption of about 30% of fat that is eaten. By blocking its absorption, the fat passes through the intestine and goes out in the stool instead of into the bloodstream. During six-month clinical studies, obese people who took Alli lost a modest 5 to 6 pounds more than people who took a placebo (dummy pill). Because of the way it works, Alli can cause side effects in the gastrointestinal tract such as oily spotting from the rectum, gas, fecal urgency, increased stool frequency, and fatty/oily stools. The more fat that is eaten, the greater chance of side effects. Alli may also decrease the absorption of fat-soluble vitamins (A, D, E, K) and it is recommended that people taking Alli take multivitamins when using the medication, but not at the same time. It may also interact with some drugs such as warfarin (Coumadin) or cyclosporine (Neoral, Sandimmune, Gengraf). Alli should be used in conjunction with a diet and exercise program to assist with weight loss. If it is finally approved, Alli will be the only FDA approved weight loss drug available over-the-counter. Currently, 65% of American adults are overweight or obese, according to the National Institutes of Health. This overweight problem is associated with an increased risk of developing health problems such as high blood pressure, diabetes, heart disease, and stroke. Extra weight is also hard on the skeleton, causing lower back pain, arthritis, and joint problems.

PLEASE NOTE: Alli is now available without a prescription. Please see question on Xenical/Alli and liver injury.

QUESTION: I take Alli for weight loss and heard about counterfeit products. What can you tell me about this?

ANSWER: The U.S. Food and Drug Administration recently warned consumers about a counterfeit and potentially harmful version of Alli 60 mg capsules (120 count refill kit). Preliminary laboratory tests conducted by GlaxoSmithKline (the manufacturer of this FDA approved over-the-counter weight-loss product) revealed that the counterfeit version did not contain orlistat, the active ingredient in its product. Instead, the counterfeit product contained sibutramine, a prescription drug and controlled substance that can place people with cardiovascular disease at risk for higher blood pressure, heart attack, or stroke. Sibutramine is the active ingredient in the prescription diet drug Meridia. Sibutramine can also interact in a harmful way with other medications the person may be taking. Consumers began reporting suspected counterfeit Alli to GlaxoSmithKline in early December 2009. It has been determined that the counterfeit product has been sold over the internet, however, there is no evidence at this time that the counterfeit Alli product has been sold through other channels, such as retail stores.

The counterfeit Alli product looks similar to the authentic product, with a few notable differences. The counterfeit Alli has:

- Outer cardboard packaging missing a "Lot" code;
- Expiration date that includes the month, day, and year (e.g., 06162010); authentic Alli expiration date includes only the month and year (e.g., 05/12);
- Packaging in a plastic bottle that has a slightly taller and wider cap with coarser ribbing than the genuine product;
- Plain foil inner safety seal under the plastic cap without any printed words; the authentic product seal is printed with "SEALED for YOUR PROTECTION";
- Contains larger capsules with a white powder, instead of small white pellets.

Consumers who believe they have received counterfeit Alli should discard any fake products immediately and are asked to contact the FDA's Office of Criminal Investigations (OCI) by calling 800-551-3989 or by visiting the OCI Web site (**http://www.fda.gov/OCI**).

PRESCRIPTION PRODUCTS—XENICAL

QUESTION: I heard about a new prescription drug on TV for weight control. What can you tell me about it?

ANSWER: The new drug, approved by the FDA, is called Xenical (generic name orlistat). It was approved for the treatment of obesity to be used together with a low calorie diet.

As I noted in earlier columns, obesity (or an excess of body fat) is very common in the U.S. with at least one in three Americans being overweight (20 percent or more above what is considered normal). Being overweight is not a disgrace or a failure of willpower, but is a medical problem that needs to be treated.

If not treated, obesity can pose serious risks to your health. The heart must pump harder to support excess weight, and this can raise your blood pressure. Other risks associated with obesity can include heart attack, stroke, poor circulation, diabetes, gallstones, and some cancers. Extra weight is also hard on the skeleton, causing lower back pain, arthritis, and joint problems.

The best treatment of obesity involves a combination of reduced intake of calories, nutritional counseling, exercise, and behavior modification.

Unlike other drugs for weight loss which act on the brain to reduce a person's appetite, Xenical works mainly in the gastrointestinal tract. Here it blocks intestinal enzymes called lipases, which break down fat and help it to be absorbed by the body. By doing this, about 30% of the fat that is eaten passes through the intestine and goes out in the stool instead of into the bloodstream.

Because of the way it works, Xenical can cause side effects in the gastrointestinal tract such as oily spotting from the rectum (27% of patients), gas (24% of patients), fecal urgency (22% of patients), increased stool frequency (11% of patients), and fatty/oily stools (20% of patients). The more fat that is eaten, the more side effects. However, these side effects tend to decrease significantly after a year of taking the medication. Xenical can also decrease the absorption of some fat soluble vitamins (A, D, E, K) and supplements may be needed.

Studies have shown that Xenical together with a low calorie diet can produce a modest loss of weight. People taking Xenical lose about 7 ½ pounds more per year than dieting alone. It is taken three times a day with meals.

PLEASE NOTE: See next question on Xenical/Alli and liver injury.

XENICAL/ALLI AND LIVER INJURY

QUESTION: I've read that the FDA is reviewing reports of liver injury in people taking Xenical or Alli for weight loss. What can you tell me about this?

ANSWER: The FDA recently announced that it is reviewing adverse event reports of liver injury in patients taking the prescription weight loss drug Xenical (orlistat) and the nonprescription medication Alli (orlistat). Between 1999 and 2008, the FDA received 32 reports of serious liver injury in patients taking orlistat. Of those cases, 27 reported hospitalization and six resulted in liver failure. Thirty of the adverse events occurred outside the United States. The most commonly reported adverse events included yellowing of the skin or whites of the eyes (jaundice), weakness, and stomach pain. The FDA's analysis of these data is ongoing, and no definite association between liver injury and orlistat has been established at this time. Consumers taking Xenical should continue to take it as prescribed, and those using over-the-counter Alli should continue to use the product as directed. Consumers who have used orlistat should consult a health care professional if they experience symptoms possibly associated with development of liver injury, particularly weakness or fatigue, fever, jaundice, or brown urine. Other symptoms may include abdominal pain, nausea, vomiting, light-colored stools, itching, or loss of appetite. Consumers and healthcare professionals are also being urged to report suspected side effects from the use of Xenical or Alli to the FDA Medwatch Adverse Event Reporting program by calling 1-800-FDA-1088, or online at **www.fda.gov**.

Unlike other drugs for weight loss which act on the brain to reduce a person's appetite, Xenical and Alli work mainly in the gastrointestinal tract. Here they block intestinal enzymes called lipases, which break down fat and help it to be absorbed by the body. By doing this, about 30% of the fat that is eaten passes through the intestine and goes out in the stool instead of into the bloodstream. Because of the way they work, Xenical and Alli can cause side effects in the gastrointestinal tract such as oily spotting from the rectum (27% of patients), gas (24% of patients), fecal urgency (22% of patients), increased stool frequency (11% of patients), and fatty/oily stools (20% of patients). The more fat that is eaten, the more side effects. However, these side effects tend to decrease significantly after a year of taking the medication. These drugs can also decrease the absorption of some fat soluble vitamins (A, D, E, K) and supplements may be needed.

MERIDIA

QUESTION: My doctor prescribed Meridia to help me lose weight. What can you tell me about this medication?

ANSWER: Meridia (generic name sibutramine, pronounced sy-byu-tra-meen) is a prescription product for helping obese people to lose weight. If not treated, obesity can pose serious risks to your health. The heart must pump harder to support excess weight, and this can raise your blood pressure. Other risks associated with obesity can include heart attack, stroke, poor circulation, diabetes, gallstones, and some cancers. Excess weight is also hard on the skeleton, causing lower back pain, arthritis, and joint problems. The best treatment of obesity involves a combination of reduced caloric intake, nutritional counseling, exercise, and behavior modification. Meridia helps people lose weight by decreasing a person's appetite for food. It does this by blocking chemicals in the brain (serotonin, norepinephrine, and dopamine), which are involved in appetite control. Meridia increases the feeling of fullness, which reduces the appetite, and it may also increase metabolism in the body resulting in greater calorie use. Clinical studies have shown that people taking Meridia along with diet restrictions will lose between 5% and 10% of their initial weight within six to twelve months. Possible side effects of Meridia can include headache, dizziness, inability to sleep, dry mouth, and constipation. It can also increase the heart rate and blood pressure. Because of this, individuals with a history of heart disease, congestive heart failure, irregular heartbeat, or stroke should not take it. In addition, numerous drug interactions are possible with Meridia, so make sure your pharmacist and doctor(s) are aware of all the medicines that you take, including non-prescription products. Finally, remember that appetite control and reduced calorie intake is only one part of a successful weight reduction program as noted above.

PLEASE NOTE: Meridia was withdrawn from the market by the manufacturer on October 8, 2010 because clinical data indicated an increased risk of heart attack and stroke. Physicians are advised to stop prescribing Meridia and patients should stop taking this medication. Patients should talk to their health care provider about alternative weight loss and weight loss maintenance programs. Please see next question.

QUESTION: Why was the weight loss drug Meridia taken off the market?

ANSWER: The manufacturer (Abbott Laboratories) voluntarily withdrew its anti-obesity medication, Meridia (sibutramine) from the U.S. market on October 8, 2010 after coming under pressure from health regulators who said that the drug increases the risk of heart attack and stroke. Food and Drug Administration scientists said that they requested the withdrawal because Meridia's risks were not outweighed by the very modest weight loss that people achieve on this medication. Physicians are advised to stop prescribing Meridia and patients should stop taking this medication. Patients should talk to their healthcare provider about alternative weight loss and weight loss maintenance programs. Meridia was approved by the FDA in 1997 for weight loss and maintenance of weight loss in obese people, as well as in certain overweight people with other risks for heart disease. The approval was based on clinical study data showing that more people taking Meridia lost at least 5% of their body weight than people taking a dummy pill (placebo) who relied on diet and exercise alone. The FDA requested the market withdrawal of Meridia based upon a clinical study that showed a 16% increase in the risk of serious heart events, including non-fatal heart attack, non-fatal stroke, the need to be resuscitated once the heart stopped, and death in a group of patients taking Meridia compared to a placebo.

FEN-PHEN

QUESTION: I used to take "fen-phen" pills to lose weight. I've heard that they were taken off the market because of heart side effects and I'm worried. What should I do?

ANSWER: "Fen-phen" refers to the use of dexfenfluramine (Redux) or fenfluramine (Pondimin) and phentermine (Ionamin) in combination for weight control. Both fenfluramine and dexfenfluramine were voluntarily removed from the market in September 1997 because numerous reports of valvular heart disease were associated with their use. Since the withdrawal of these medications, several medical organizations have developed guidelines for people who took these diet drugs. A major concern is that patients who develop heart valve disease may be at risk of developing heart infections known as bacterial endocarditis after some medical and dental procedures. Because of this, the following recommendations have been issued for patients who took "fen-phen" drugs for any length of time:

• Patients should see a physician for a medical history and cardiovascular examination to determine whether there are signs or symptoms of heart or lung disease.
• Patients who have signs or symptoms of heart or lung disease, such as a new heart murmur or shortness of breath, should have an echocardiogram performed.

- An echocardiogram should be strongly considered for all patients, with or without symptoms, before any procedure for which the American Heart Association recommends the use of antibiotics to prevent heart infection (bacterial endocarditis). An echocardiogram will help to determine if there are heart valve problems for which antibiotics may be needed to prevent heart infections.

Some procedures for which antibiotics should be given to prevent heart infections in people with heart valve problems include dental procedures where bleeding may occur, surgery for the removal of adenoids or tonsils, or surgery involving the respiratory tract, gastrointestinal tract, or genitourinary tract. These guidelines will be updated as more information becomes available. Furthermore, the public should be aware that "herbal fen-phen" preparations are not approved for weight control and that side effects are also possible when using these products. Any drugs for weight control should be used in conjunction with a sound long-term program of diet, behavior modification and exercise.

BELVIQ

QUESTION: I heard that a new weight-loss drug was approved. What can you tell me about it?

ANSWER: On June 27, 2012 the FDA approved Belviq (lorcaserin) for chronic weight management in obese and overweight adults who have at least one weight-related medical complication such as diabetes, high-blood pressure, or high cholesterol. This new weight-loss prescription drug is to be used in conjunction with a healthy reduced-calorie diet and exercise. Belviq is the first new prescription weight-loss medication to be approved by the FDA in 13 years and provides a new treatment option. It works by activating a receptor in the brain, which may help a person eat less and feel full after eating smaller amounts of food. During clinical studies involving nearly 8,000 obese and overweight people with and without diabetes, Belviq treatment for up to one year was associated with an average weight loss of about

3-4% of body weight. While this loss was modest, the drug appeared safe enough for approval. Belviq is taken as a 10 mg tablet twice daily and should be discontinued if a 5% weight loss is not achieved by the end of 3 months. The most common side effects of Belviq in non-diabetic patients are headache, dizziness, fatigue, nausea, dry mouth, and constipation. In people with diabetes, the most common side effects are low blood sugar (hypoglycemia), headache, back pain, cough, and fatigue. A number of drug interactions are also possible with Belviq, so be sure that your doctor and pharmacist are aware of all other medications that you take (prescription and nonprescription). After the drug is marketed the drug manufacturer will conduct studies to determine if it is also effective in obese pediatric patients, and to determine if its long-term use is associated with major adverse cardiac events such as heart attack or stroke. The FDA has also concluded that Belviq may have some abuse potential and has asked the U.S. Drug Enforcement Administration (DEA) to determine what schedule it should be placed into. In view of this, Belviq is not expected to be available until early 2013.

QSYMIA

QUESTION: I heard that a new weight-loss drug was approved. What can you tell me about it?

ANSWER: In July 2012, the FDA approved the second new drug for weight-loss within the last 2 months, after a 13-year-long drought in the diet drug pipeline (Belviq was approved in June 2012). The new medication, Qsymia, actually contains two very different drugs that have been available for quite some time. Qsymia contains the appetite suppressant phentermine along with the anticonvulsant topiramate in a controlled-release capsule. Exactly how this drug combination works to produce weight-loss is poorly understood, but each of the ingredients have multiple and different effects in the brain and other parts of the body. Qsymia was approved for use in combination with a reduced-calorie diet and exercise for weight management in obese adults and overweight adults who have at least one weight-related condition such as high blood pressure, type 2 diabetes, or high cholesterol. During clinical studies, patients who took Qsymia once-daily in the morning had an average weight loss of about 7-9% after one year compared to those taking a "dumy pill", and approximately 60-70% of patients lost at least 5% of their body weight compared to 20% of patients treated with a "dummy pill". The most common side effects of Qsymia include tingling of the hands and feet, dizziness, altered taste sensation, insomnia, constipation, and dry mouth. However, other more serious adverse effects can occur and Qsymia must not be taken by patients who are pregnant, have glaucoma, or have hyperthyroidism. In addition, Qsymia will only be dispensed through specially certified pharmacies. Much more information about this weight-loss drug can be found online at **www.Qsymia.com**.

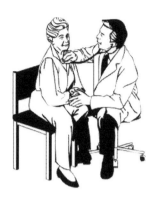

CHAPTER 12
ARTHRITIS AND PAIN

RHEUMATOID ARTHRITIS

QUESTION: I have rheumatoid arthritis, which causes pain and swelling in my hands. What treatments are available to help me?

ANSWER: Rheumatoid arthritis is a chronic disease that affects five to eight million Americans. It occurs much more commonly in women and some people have an inherited likelihood to get the disease. Although the cause of rheumatoid arthritis is not entirely understood, the disease results when a person's immune system, which normally helps the body to get rid of infections or tumors, begins to attack joint tissues causing inflammation and pain. The usual signs and symptoms of rheumatoid arthritis include morning stiffness in and around the joints, swelling of the finger or wrist joints, swelling of three or more joints, and lumps that appear just under the skin. Other symptoms include feelings of tiredness, weakness, and poor appetite. The joints usually affected are those in the hands, wrists, and feet but swelling and pain may occur in the elbows, shoulders, hips, knees, and ankles. The treatment of rheumatoid arthritis may involve rest, physical therapy, surgery when appropriate, and medications to ease the pain and reduce the inflammation or swelling. Rest helps to avoid aggravating the inflamed joints while physical therapy helps to keep the joints and muscles limber. Medications are usually selected based upon the severity of the disease. For mild cases, anti-inflammatory drugs such as aspirin or ibuprofen may be used. If they do not work, other drugs such as Ridaura, Solganal, Aurolate, or Myochrysine (gold compounds), Cuprimine or Depen (a chelating or binding agent), or Plaquenil (an antimalarial drug) may be added to the anti-inflammatory drug. In some people a steroid drug may also be useful for a short time while waiting for the stronger drugs to work. The strongest drugs used to treat rheumatoid arthritis are called immunosuppressive agents because they block the person's immune system from attacking the joint tissues. Examples of these drugs include Imuran, Rheumatrex, Methotrexate, or Cytoxan. This latter group of drugs is saved for patients who do not respond to any other treatment. Agents used to treat rheumatoid arthritis may have potentially serious side effects and should only be taken exactly as directed. Also, because of the possibility of drug interactions, make sure that your doctor(s) and pharmacist is kept informed of all the medications that you are taking.

QUESTION: I have rheumatoid arthritis and I heard about some new medications for this problem. What can you tell me about them?

ANSWER: Rheumatoid arthritis (RA) is one of the most severe forms of arthritis and it affects 5 to 8 million people in the U.S. It occurs about 3 times more often in women than men. The exact cause of RA is not known, but the immune system of the body is involved. Instead of protecting the body from disease, the immune system attacks the joints, causing inflammation, pain, and joint damage. RA is a chronic disorder that typically comes and goes. Symptoms include swelling, pain, tenderness, redness, or warmth in one or more joints. Many people also have joint stiffness, especially upon awakening. In some people, this disease can be severely painful and can cause joint deformation or permanent damage to joints and can even affect other organs of the body. In other people RA is a more mild disease causing little disability.

The treatment of RA involves a combination of medication, rest, special exercises, and joint protection. Anti-inflammatory drugs are usually prescribed initially. Drugs such as aspirin, non-steroidal anti-inflammatory drugs (NSAIDs) like ibuprofen (Motrin), or acetaminophen (Tylenol) can be very effective in reducing the pain and inflammation. If these medications are not effective, more potent drugs can be tried like corticosteroids, gold salts, penicillamine, and drugs to suppress the immune system like methotrexate. These more potent drugs, however, also have the potential for more serious side effects and may not be effective in some people.

The newer drugs approved for RA include Enbrel, Remicade, and most recently Humira. They are all biotechnology drugs that block a substance in the body known as tumor necrosis factor or TNF. The amount of this substance (TNF) found in the joints of people with RA is much higher than in people without RA and it is believed to be a major cause of joint inflammation and destruction. All 3 of these drugs must be given by injection. Remicade is given intravenously while Enbrel and Humira are given subcutaneously (just below the skin). Humira is administered every other week and has been shown to not only improve the painful symptoms of RA, but also to actually prevent it from getting worse. It may be used to treat RA by itself or can be used in combination with other drugs for RA like methotrexate. Patients can obtain information about Humira by calling 1-800-4-HUMIRA (448-6472) or at **www.humira.com**.

PLEASE NOTE: The FDA has recently warned that patients taking Cimzia, Enbrel, Humira, or Remicade (also known as tumor necrosis factor (TNF) blockers) should be aware that they are more susceptible to serious fungal infections. Patients taking these drugs who develop a persistent fever, cough, shortness of breath, and fatigue should promptly seek medical attention.

QUESTION: I receive Humira injections for rheumatoid arthritis. Can this increase my risk of getting shingles?

ANSWER: Yes it may, according to a recent study reported in the "Journal of the American Medical Association". Humira and other similar drugs such as Embrel and Remicade are known as tumor necrosis factor (TNF) inhibitors, which are used to treat a variety of inflammatory conditions including rheumatoid arthritis, plaque psoriasis, Crohns disease, and others. All TNF inhibitors affect a person's immune system and because of this patients are at increased risk for infections, some of which can be very serious such as tuberculosis or blood infections. This new study looked at the incidence of herpes zoster infection (shingles) in patients with rheumatoid arthritis who were receiving a TNF inhibitor and it found that the risk getting shingles may be higher in people receiving these drugs. Based upon the results of this study it is recommended that patients treated with TNF inhibitors be carefully monitored for early signs and symptoms of shingles. The researchers, however, did note that more study is needed. Anyone who is receiving treatment with these agents should discuss the risk of infections or shingles with their physician.

Shingles (also known as herpes zoster or zoster) is a viral infection caused by the varicella-zoster virus (VZV). This is the same virus that causes chickenpox in childhood and then re-emerges later in life to cause this painful condition called shingles. Following a bout of chickenpox, the virus becomes dormant and lives in the nerve tract until something "triggers" it to become active again. This may occur when a person's immune system becomes weakened by a medical condition or just due to aging. Shingles is a rare problem in young healthy adults but occurs in about 5 out of 1,000 people over age 50, and in about 10 out of 1,000 people over age 80. Some people predict that this medical problem will increase significantly in the future as baby boomers age.

QUESTION: I heard about a new type of drug for rheumatoid arthritis. What can you tell me about it?

ANSWER: The FDA recently approved Actemra (tocilizumab), a new type of injectable product used to treat adults with rheumatoid arthritis who have not adequately responded to or cannot tolerate other rheumatoid arthritis medications. In numerous clinical studies, patients treated with Actemra experienced greater improvement in their tender or swollen joints than patients treated with a "dummy pill" (placebo). Actemra works by blocking the effect of certain protein (interleukin-6) that is overabundant in people with rheumatoid arthritis and is associated with inflammation. The most common side effects of Actemra during clinical studies were upper respiratory tract infections, headache, inflammation of the nose or nasal passage, high blood pressure, and impaired liver function tests. However, since Actemra can suppress the body's immune system, it can also have some serious side effects, including infections, liver abnormalities, and damage to digestive organs. Actemra is administered by intravenous infusion every 4 weeks in their doctor's office.

QUESTION: I have rheumatoid arthritis (RA) and I heard about a new medication for this problem. What can you tell me about it?

ANSWER: The new drug approved by the FDA to help people with RA is named Arava or leflunomide (chemical name). During clinical testing, Arava reduced the signs and symptoms of RA in over 40% of the people who took it. It also was shown to slow the damage to joints. How the drug works is not completely understood, but it does affect the immune system and is called an immunomodulatory drug. The most common side effects with Arava are diarrhea, rash, hair loss, and possible abnormal liver function tests.

PLEASE NOTE: Arava labeling now has a Boxed Warning to highlight the risk of severe liver injury in patients using this drug and how this risk may be reduced. The FDA previously required a Boxed Warning stating that Arava was contraindicated in pregnant women, or women of childbearing potential who were not using reliable contraception.

VACCINES TO BE AVOIDED BY PEOPLE WITH RHEUMATOID ARTHRITIS

QUESTION: Should I avoid certain vaccines if I have rheumatoid arthritis?

ANSWER: Although the cause of rheumatoid arthritis (RA) is not entirely understood, the disease results when a person's immune system, which normally helps the body to get rid of infections or tumors, begins to attack joint tissues causing inflammation and pain. Because the immune system is affected in people with RA, they are about twice as likely to get infections compared to others. In addition, many of the medications used to treat RA work by suppressing the immune system. In view of this, vaccines play a very important role in protecting people with RA from getting infections. However, some vaccines are not appropriate for people with RA, because they contain live organisms. This topic has been recently reviewed in a Johns Hopkins Health Alert (**www.johnshopkinshealthalerts.com**, 2011) which provides the following advice regarding vaccine safety for people with RA:

Must-Have Vaccines

- Influenza vaccine—Even if you are taking one or more RA medications, you can expect to get good protection against the flu virus.
- Pneumococcal vaccine—This vaccine protects against common types of pneumonia, bacteremia (blood infection), and meningitis. All adults should get the pneumococcal vaccine at least once.
- Tetanus-diphtheria-pertussis—Everyone needs protection from diphtheria and tetanus, and if you're under 65 years old, you should get the vaccination for pertussis as well.

Vaccines To Avoid

Most vaccines are safe and fairly effective in people with RA, but there are some that you should avoid, because they use live viruses or bacteria. Also avoid attenuated vaccines, which use a weakened—but not dead—organism.

- FluMist—This inhaled nasal flu spray vaccine is made from attenuated virus and should not be used by people with RA.
- MMR—Typically given to people born in 1957 or later, the MMR, or German measles, vaccine should not be given to people taking certain immunosuppressive medications used to treat RA.
- Herpes zoster—As with the MMR vaccine, the herpes zoster vaccine may be inappropriate in people taking certain immunosuppressive medications, such as steroids or other drugs used to treat RA.
- Bacillus Calmette-Guérin (BCG)—This vaccine is sometimes administered to prevent tuberculosis, but it should not be given to a person with RA because it is made from an attenuated strain of bacterium that causes tuberculosis.

- Varicella (chickenpox)—Varicella vaccination is not usually required for anyone born in the United States before 1980 and should not be administered to anyone taking immunosuppressive drugs.
- Smallpox—This vaccine, which is made from a live virus that is related to (but milder than) smallpox, is rarely administered in the United States. However, in the event of a public emergency, it would be made available to anyone exposed to the smallpox virus.
- Yellow fever—This is a live oral vaccine. Consult with your rheumatologist and an infectious disease specialist about what to do if you must go to a country where yellow fever is endemic. But don't be surprised if they won't administer it.

OSTEOARTHRITIS

QUESTION: I have osteoarthritis and would like to know what medications can help this problem?

ANSWER: Osteoarthritis is one of the oldest and most common diseases of man. It probably affects almost everyone over the age of 60 to some extent, but only some have it bad enough to cause painful joints. It is different than rheumatoid arthritis, which usually begins at an earlier age and has a different cause. Osteoarthritis is commonly called "wear-and tear" arthritis and is caused by the breakdown of joint cartilage—the cushion between the bones that works like a shock absorber. As the cartilage breaks down, the bones begin to rub together, causing pain and loss of movement. It usually affects the hands and weight-bearing joints, such as the knees, hips, feet and back. A good treatment program for osteoarthritis can help reduce joint pain and stiffness, and improve joint movement and function. A treatment program may include joint protection, exercise, heat and cold treatment, weight reduction, surgery when necessary, and various medications. Acetaminophen (Tylenol) is frequently used initially for the pain associated with osteoarthritis. Anti-inflammatory drugs such as aspirin or ibuprofen in addition to numerous other anti-inflammatory prescription products are also effective in reducing joint pain, stiffness, and swelling. However, these anti-inflammatory drugs can cause injury to the stomach lining, especially in the elderly. Using "coated" aspirin products and taking these medications with meals can help to avoid these stomach problems. Topically applied anti-inflammatory drugs with fewer side effects are being researched and in the future may become available for use. Topical capsaicin, which is the irritant found in chili pepper and red pepper, may also be helpful in relieving the pain of osteoarthritis of the hands, knees, and feet of some patients. In addition to these medications, the use of two dietary supplements, glucosamine and chondroitin sulfate have been promoted for people with osteoarthritis. Glucosamine, which occurs naturally in the human body, is said to play an important role in the body's maintenance and repair of cartilage. Chondroitin is said to prevent certain chemicals from breaking down cartilage in joints. The use of these so-called "chondroprotective" agents together represents an attempt to actually stop the breakdown of cartilage and rebuild it. However, these effects have not been proven yet in clinical studies. Another potential treatment of osteoarthritis involves the injection of a solution of sodium hyaluronate into the joint. This fluid is similar to synovial fluid, a natural joint liquid, which helps joints move smoothly and easily. Two products containing sodium hyaluronate have been approved for patients with osteoarthritis of the knee. These products (Hyalgan and Synvisc) may be helpful when pain relievers such as acetaminophen, physical therapy, and exercise have not been successful. They work like synovial fluid to lubricate the knee joints and act as a shock absorber to provide pain relief. For more information about arthritis of all types, write to the Arthritis Foundation at P.O. Box 19000, Atlanta, GA 30326 or call toll-free at 1-800-283-7800.

QUESTION: What nonprescription drugs are available to treat osteoarthritis?

ANSWER: Osteoarthritis is the most common type of arthritis, affecting some 21 million people in the U.S. Osteoarthritis, also called "wear and tear" arthritis, is a joint disease that mainly affects the cartilage or slippery tissue that covers the ends of bones in a joint. Fluid inside the joint (synovial fluid) lubricates the joint and keeps the cartilage smooth. Healthy cartilage allows bones in the joint to glide over one another, and it absorbs energy from the shock of physical movement, like walking. In osteoarthritis, cartilage breaks down and wears away. This allows the bones in a joint to rub together, causing pain and swelling. Over time, the joint may even lose its normal shape. Osteoarthritis usually affects middle-aged and older people and is the most common cause of limited activity after the age of 70. With increasing age, our ability to rejuvenate our bone tissues and lubricating fluids gradually diminishes, exposing the cartilage to damage that is repaired more slowly than normal.

The treatment of osteoarthritis usually involves the use of medications and non-drug measures. Non-drug treatment may include exercises that avoid impact on the affected joints, weight reduction to reduce stress on joints, application of hot packs or cold packs to relieve joint pain and stiffness, and the use of assistive devices like a cane or walker. There are several nonprescription medications that are used to treat the pain and inflammation associated with osteoarthritis. Acetaminophen (Tylenol) is a good initial choice for pain relief and it does not irritate the stomach like other medications. However, alcohol use should be limited or avoided when taking acetaminophen because of potential liver problems. Nonsteroidal anti-inflammatory drugs (NSAIDs) may be useful if acetaminophen does not relieve the pain. Unlike acetaminophen, nonprescription NSAIDs reduce both pain and inflammation but can also irritate the stomach and should be taken with food. NSAIDs may also cause fluid retention and should be avoided by patients with congestive heart failure (CHF), especially if they are elderly. Over the counter NSAIDs include salicylates, aspirin, ibuprofen (Motrin, Advil), naproxen (Aleve), and ketoprofen (Orudis KS, Actron). The topical application of camphorated or mentholated rubs or capsaicin cream—a natural component of hot peppers, may also be useful in some people, but they should never be used with a heating pad. The use of dietary supplements containing glucosamine and chondroitin also appear to be somewhat beneficial, but the FDA has not evaluated their safety or efficacy and more study is needed. You should consult your physician and pharmacist to determine the best treatment options for you.

ANTI-INFLAMMATORY DRUGS

QUESTION: What's the difference between aspirin, Tylenol, ibuprofen, and the new anti-inflammatory drugs that I'm hearing so much about?

ANSWER: As you may know, aspirin is a very useful drug for the treatment of a variety of conditions. It has the ability to reduce fever (antipyretic), control pain (analgesic), reduce inflammation (anti-inflammatory), and to prevent blood from forming clots (anti-coagulant). In fact, if aspirin was introduced as a new drug today it would be considered a remarkable product. However, aspirin use is not without side effects and can cause gastrointestinal irritation and bleeding. Tylenol (acetaminophen) is also an effective drug for the treatment of fever and pain like aspirin, but it does not reduce inflammation or prevent the blood from clotting like aspirin does. An advantage of using acetaminophen over aspirin for pain or fever is that it is less irritating to the gastrointestinal tract and may be useful in patients where this is a concern. On the other hand, a potential problem with using acetaminophen is that it can cause damage to the liver and should not be used by people with liver disease or those who drink alcohol more than occasionally. Ibuprofen is one of many prescription and non-prescription drugs known as non-steroidal anti-inflammatory drugs (NSAID's). NSAID's can also reduce fever, control pain, and reduce inflammation. Ibuprofen does not produce the same anti-coagulant effects as aspirin, but it can also increase bleeding time at higher doses. The most common side effect with ibuprofen is gastrointestinal irritation, but it is less likely to cause gastrointestinal bleeding than aspirin. A less common but more serious side effect of ibuprofen is damage to the kidneys. Regarding the treatment of pain, it should be noted that some types of pain respond better to aspirin or acetaminophen or a particular NSAID and that there can be differences in response to pain from one person to another. In addition, interactions with other medications and side effects will vary between all of these different drugs. The new anti-inflammatory drugs that you are hearing about are known as COX-2 inhibitors. They are a new type of NSAID that may not significantly irritate the gastrointestinal tract, cause damage to the kidneys, or increase bleeding time. The new

COX-2 inhibitors work exactly the same way as the currently available NSAID's to stop inflammation. They both affect an enzyme in the body called cyclooxygenase or COX for short. However, there are two types of COX: COX-1, which acts to protect the kidneys and the lining of the gastrointestinal tract and COX-2, which is largely responsible for causing inflammation and pain. The problem with available NSAID's is that they interfere with both COX-1 and COX-2. The new COX-2 inhibitors only block COX-2 and therefore reduce inflammation with a lower risk of hurting the stomach or kidneys.

CELEBREX, VIOXX, AND BEXTRA

QUESTION: I've heard about new drugs for arthritis. What can you tell me about them?

ANSWER: Celebrex, Vioxx, and Bextra are new non-steroidal anti-inflammatory (NSAID) drugs used to treat pain and inflammation. They are known as COX-2 inhibitors. The proposed advantage of these new drugs is that they may not irritate and cause damage to the gastrointestinal tract like the older NSAID products (e.g., ibuprofen (Motrin, Advil), naproxen (Anaprox, Naprosyn, Aleve), ketoprofen (Orudis, Actron), sulindac (Clinoril), tolmetin (Tolectin), diclofenac (Voltaren, Cataflam), and many others). All of these drugs (new and old) relieve pain and inflammation by interfering with an enzyme called cyclooxygenase (COX). This interference prevents the production of hormone like chemicals called prostaglandins, which cause pain and inflammation. However, there are two types of COX enzymes, COX-1, which helps protect the gastrointestinal tract, and COX-2, which is largely responsible for the pain and inflammation. Therefore COX-2 inhibitors are more specific for pain relief and leave COX-1 enzymes alone to protect the gastrointestinal tract. I know this seems somewhat complicated, but the bottom line is that these new COX-2 inhibitors are not more effective than the older drugs like ibuprofen, but they may have fewer gastrointestinal side effects. Only time will tell if these newer and more expensive products are significantly safer. They are used for the treatment of acute pain in adults and for the relief of the signs and symptoms of osteoarthritis. Osteoarthritis is the most common form of arthritis and it affects mostly older people (about half are age 65 or older). In osteoarthritis, also called "wear and tear" arthritis, cartilage in between bone joints breaks down and the bones rub together causing pain. Remember that none of these NSAID drugs (old or new) can "cure" osteoarthritis but only provide relief of symptoms. COX-2 inhibitors may be a good choice to use for individuals who may be at risk for gastrointestinal problems (i.e., history of peptic ulcer disease, etc.), but patients still need to remain alert for possible ulceration and bleeding (i.e., abdominal discomfort; dark, tarry stools; etc.) and notify their doctor as soon as possible if this occurs.

PLEASE NOTE: Vioxx was withdrawn from the market on September 30, 2004 due to its increased risk for causing heart attacks and strokes. The use of Vioxx has also been associated with an increased risk of kidney problems and heart arrhythmia events. Please see the next question. Bextra was withdrawn from the market in April, 2005 due to cardiovascular risks and a risk of serious, sometimes fatal, skin reactions in patients using this medication. Celebrex remains on the market, but with a black-box warning in its labeling about an increased risk of serious and potentially life-threatening gastrointestinal and cardiovascular events associated with use of the drug.

VIOXX WITHDRAWN FROM MARKET

QUESTION: I've heard that Vioxx was withdrawn from the market because it may cause heart attacks and strokes. How can a painkiller have these side effects?

ANSWER: At this point in time we really don't know exactly how Vioxx can lead to heart attacks or stroke and can only speculate. Vioxx was voluntarily withdrawn from the worldwide market on September 30, 2004, because a recent study showed that people taking Vioxx for more than 18 months had a much higher risk of serious cardiovascular problems, such as heart attacks and strokes, compared to people not taking the drug. Interestingly, this study was trying to determine if Vioxx was also effective in preventing the recurrence of polyps in people with a history of colorectal cancer so that even more people could use the drug. The study was supposed to go on for 3 years, but was stopped after 18 months because of the cardiovascular risks identified. An earlier study in 2000 also indicated that Vioxx might cause heart problems, but still other studies did not. How a drug like Vioxx that is used for pain and inflammation can also cause effects on the heart points out how complex drug therapy can be. Even "simple" drugs like aspirin can have many effects and the study of how drugs work or "pharmacology" can be very complicated. One of the theories behind why Vioxx could cause heart problems is that it may adversely affect blood clotting activities. Another is that it may cause the body to retain fluid or increase blood pressure leading to cardiovascular problems. Still another theory involves a decrease in protection of the heart by Vioxx due to its effect on certain enzymes in the body. The removal of Vioxx from the market has opened the door for many additional questions to be answered. For example, is the FDA too close to the drug manufacturers? Should these highly potent drugs be mass-marketed to the consumer in advertisements and on television? Should we slow down the drug approval process in order to get more safety information before a new drug is approved? What's the next blockbuster killer drug, wrapped in a heavy dose of fancy advertising, and possibly lurking in your medicine cabinet? Only time will tell.

CELEBREX AND CARDIOVASACULAR RISK

QUESTION: I take Celebrex for osteoarthritis. Can it cause heart problems like Vioxx?

ANSWER: The short answer to your question is we don't know for sure at this point in time. Vioxx, Celebrex, and Bextra (valdecoxib) are all non-steroidal anti-inflammatory drugs (NSAIDs) that were approved to treat pain and inflammation. They were developed in an attempt to make them less likely to irritate or damage the gastrointestinal tract like other older NSAIDs such as ibuprofen (Motrin, Advil), naproxen (Anaprox, Naprosyn, Aleve), and many other products. These older NSAIDs work by blocking an enzyme called cyclooxygenase or COX for short. This enzyme blocking activity prevents the production of hormone like chemicals called prostaglandins, which cause pain and inflammation. However, there are two types of COX enzymes—COX-1 which helps protect the gastrointestinal tract and affects blood clotting and COX-2 which is largely responsible for the pain and inflammation. The newer NSAIDs (Vioxx, Celebrex, and Bextra) were designed to only block or inhibit COX-2 in order to reduce the pain and inflammation, but not hurt the gastrointestinal tract. Because of this they are known as COX-2 inhibitors. However, not all three of these NSAIDs inhibit COX-2 in the same way and they are all different chemicals. Vioxx has the greatest COX-2 activity, followed closely by Bextra. But Celebrex has much less COX-2 activity and might even have some COX-1 activity. Because of this, it has been suggested that perhaps Celebrex may not increase the risk of cardiovascular problems, such as heart attacks and strokes in the same way as Vioxx. In fact, several studies in arthritis patients lasting about 6 months have not found a significant difference in cardiovascular side effects for people taking Celebrex. On the other hand, a recent report from Canada has linked Celebrex to 14 deaths and numerous heart-related side effects over the past 5 years. Longer-term studies using Celebrex in patients at risk of cardiovascular disease are now needed to definitely find out if this drug is associated with a greater risk of heart attacks and strokes. In view of this, the manufacturer of Celebrex, Pfizer, has announced that it will conduct a large study in patients with osteoarthritis and a recent heart attack to determine if their drug can cause cardiovascular problems. The FDA has also asked the manufacturer of Celebrex to add a boxed warning to the Celebrex Prescribing Information that calls attention to cardiovascular and gastrointestinal risks associated with use of the drug.

HEATWRAPS FOR PAIN

QUESTION: I heard about using heatwraps to relieve pain. What can you tell me about them?

ANSWER: ThermaCare Therapeutic HeatWraps are a nonprescription product that provides a low-level of heat therapy to help relieve various types of pain. They appear to be effective for the temporary relief of minor muscular and joint aches and pain due to overexertion, strains, sprains, and arthritis. They may also be useful for the temporary relief of minor menstrual cramping and associated backache. These disposable wraps are air-activated self-heating devices with a thin, flexible design that allows them to be worn comfortably and discreetly beneath clothing for up to 8 hours a day. They come in several different shapes depending upon the area needing heat therapy. There are back-wraps, neck-to-arm wraps, and menstrual wraps that are worn inside of panties. Because these HeatWraps are activated when exposed to air, they should only be opened when someone is ready to use the wrap. The wrap may take up to 30 minutes to heat completely and it is usually worn for 8 hours each day of treatment but should not be used for more than 7 days in a row (4 days for menstrual cramps and backache). HeatWraps may cause skin redness or irritation in some people and they should not be used with medicated lotions, creams, or ointments, and should not cover any medicated skin patches such as estrogen or nicotine patches. This product appears to be a convenient and portable form of heat therapy to help relieve pain, decrease muscle stiffness, increase flexibility, and reduce disability in patients with acute muscular low back pain. They also appear to be useful in reducing muscle tension in patients with neck and shoulder muscle pain and to reduce the pain associated with osteoarthritis, sprains, strains, and menstruation. Nonprescription pain relievers like ibuprofen (Motrin, etc.) or acetaminophen (Tylenol) can help provide additional pain relief when used with these wraps. More information about the HeatWraps can be obtained from the manufacturer at 1-800-323-3383 or at **www. thermacare.com**.

SALONPAS PATCH

QUESTION: I saw a TV ad about a nonprescription pain-relieving product called Salonpas Patch. What can you tell me about it?

ANSWER: The Salonpas Pain Relief Patch is an over-the-counter pain-relieving patch that has been approved by the FDA for the temporary relief of mild to moderate aches and pains of muscles and joints associated with arthritis, sprains, strains, bruises, and simple backache. Each soft, thin, stretchable patch contains menthol 3% (a topical pain reliever) and methyl salicylate 10% (a topical non-steroidal anti-inflammatory drug or NSAID). Both of these ingredients are also known as "counterirritants" and have been used for musculoskeletal pain over many decades. Methyl salicylate appears to provide pain relief and anti-inflammatory effects, while also increasing blood flow and creating a feeling of warmth. In addition, menthol produces a cooling sensation when applied to the skin. The FDA approved the Salonpas Pain Relief Patch based upon numerous clinical and non-clinical studies that showed it was safe and effective for temporary pain relief over an 8 to 12 hour period. The onset of significant pain relief with the patch usually occurs within 1 hour of application. Because the patch is applied to the skin at the site of pain, there is less chance of systemic side effects seen with oral pain-relieving medications. However, since some of the active ingredients are absorbed through the skin, the potential for NSAID side effects such as stomach bleeding may occur and users of this product are advised to carefully read all product information and labeling. The Salonpas Pain Relief Patch should be applied to a clean and dry affected area and left in place for up to 8 to 12 hours. Only one patch should be applied at a time and no more than 2 patches per day should be used. The patches should not be used by children under age 18 or by pregnant or breast-feeding women without their doctor's OK. The patches should also not be used on the face or on rashes, on wounds or damaged skin, with a heating pad, if allergic to aspirin or NSAIDs, when sweating, or right before or after heart surgery (please see product labeling for all precautions regarding its use). Salonpas is the trade name for other marketed nonprescription pain products including ointments, gels, and sprays. Readers can request a free sample of Salonpas Pain Relief Patch at **www.salonpas.us/try-now**.

DARVON
(PROPOXYPHENE) WARNING

QUESTION: I heard that the FDA is "going after" Darvon medications. What can you tell me about this?

ANSWER: Darvon (propoxyphene) and Darvocet (propoxyphene plus acetaminophen) are opioid medications that have been marketed since 1957 to relieve mild to moderate pain. Recently, the FDA has announced that it is taking several actions to reduce the risk of overdose in patients using medications containing propoxyphene because of information linking this drug to fatal overdoses. The agency is requiring manufacturers of propoxyphene containing products to strengthen the label, including the boxed warning, emphasizing the potential for overdose when using these products. These manufacturers will also be required to provide a medication guide to patients stressing the importance of using the drugs as directed. In addition, the FDA is requiring a new safety study assessing unanswered questions about the effects of propoxyphene on the heart at higher than recommended doses. Findings from this study, as well as other data, could lead to additional regulatory action. The most frequent side effects of propoxyphene include lightheadedness, dizziness, sedation, nausea, and vomiting. Pain is one of people's most common medical complaints. In addition to propoxyphene containing products, pain can be treated with other narcotic based drugs (e.g., oxycodone and codeine) aspirin, acetaminophen, ibuprofen, and other drugs. All pain medicines have side effects. Aspirin can cause bleeding of the stomach and intestines and other serious problems. Acetaminophen, the main ingredient in Tylenol and other drugs, can cause liver damage. Codeine, one of the most widely used opioids, can cause severe constipation. It is important that healthcare professionals and consumers be aware of all the risks associated with pain medications, including propoxyphene, when making decisions on how to treat pain. As with all prescription and non-prescription drugs and supplements, you should consult with your physician when choosing a pain medication.

PLEASE NOTE: On November 19, 2010, the U.S. Food and Drug Administration (FDA) recommended against continued prescribing and use of the pain reliever propoxyphene because new data show that the drug can cause serious toxicity to the heart, even when used at therapeutic doses. The FDA has requested that companies voluntarily withdraw propoxyphene from the United States market.

VOLTAREN (DICLOFENAC SODIUM) WARNING

QUESTION: I heard that Voltaren (diclofenac sodium) might be linked to liver failure and death. What can you tell me about this?

ANSWER: The FDA recently announced that treatment with all products containing diclofenac sodium might increase liver dysfunction, resulting in severe liver reactions and liver transplantation or death. Diclofenac sodium is a nonsteroidal anti-inflammatory drug (NSAID) that is used to relieve the pain of rheumatoid arthritis, osteoarthritis, ankylosing spondylitis, in addition to other conditions. Products that contain diclofenac sodium include Voltaren, Voltaren XR, Voltaren topical gel, Voltaren ophthalmic solution, Pennsaid topical solution, Solaraze topical gel, Arthrotec, and generic products. Cases of drug-induced liver toxicity with diclofenac sodium have been reported within the first month of treatment, but can occur at any time during treatment. The FDA has advised physicians to monitor liver function tests in patients receiving long term therapy with diclofenac sodium. If patients have abnormal or worsening of liver test results, physicians are advised to discontinue diclofenac sodium treatment immediately if liver disease symptoms develop. It is also recommended that physicians advise their patients receiving diclofenac sodium of the signs and symptoms of liver toxicity, including nausea, fatigue, lethargy, diarrhea, itching, jaundice, right upper abdominal pain or tenderness, dark urine, rash, or flu-like symptoms and what to do if these signs and symptoms occur. In order to reduce the risk for liver toxicity in patients receiving diclofenac sodium, the lowest effective dose should be used for the shortest time possible. In addition, caution should be exercised in prescribing diclofenac sodium with other drugs that can cause liver toxicity.

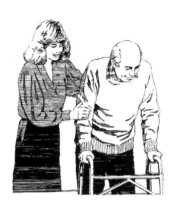

CHAPTER 13
PARKINSON'S DISEASE

DRUGS FOR PARKINSON'S DISEASE

QUESTION: What drugs are used to treat Parkinson's disease?

ANSWER: Parkinson's disease (PD) is a slowly progressive brain disorder in which various cells (neurons) within the brain die or become impaired, causing a wide variety of symptoms. Movement problems are common in people with PD, including shaking or tremor, muscle stiffness and rigidity, slow movement, and walking or postural changes. Other movement or muscle related symptoms can include small, cramped handwriting, stiff facial expression, muffled speech, swallowing problems, lack of arm swing, and diminished manual dexterity. In the past, these movement problems received the most attention and numerous medications have been developed to treat them. More recently, however, PD has been redefined to include a number of other non-movement disorders that can occur, such as pain, sleep disturbances, constipation, depression, anxiety and panic disorder, psychosis, and dementia. In fact, symptoms such as constipation, loss of smell, or sleep disorders may actually occur years before the movement problems begin. One interesting thing about PD is that no two patients' symptoms are exactly the same. For example, some patients may have tremor or shaking, while others do not. While it is beyond the scope of this column to discuss the treatment of all the potential problems associated with PD, I will briefly review the drugs used to treat the movement disorders part of the disease. Movement problems in PD are primarily due to the loss of a chemical in the brain known as dopamine. About 60-80% of the brain cells that make dopamine need to be lost or damaged before movement problems start. Drugs to replace dopamine, such as levodopa/carbidopa (Sinemet), are often used. In addition, drugs that prevent the breakdown (metabolism) of levodopa in order to increase brain concentrations of dopamine may be used, such as rasagiline (Azilect), selegiline (Zydis), tolcapone (Tasmar), or Entacapone (Comtan). Two other popular medications, ropinirole (Requip) or pramipexole (Mirapex), which "mimic" the action of dopamine in the brain may also be used. Amantadine is another unique medication that may be helpful for many patients with PD. Furthermore, older drugs known as anticholinergics (benztropine or trihexyphenidyl) may be beneficial for some younger patients with tremor. Neuroprotective medications to stop or low the progression of PD are also being studied with hopes that PD can be better treated in the future. In summary, PD is now considered a multi-system brain disorder with many movement and non-movement symptoms. Numerous medications are available to treat these problems, but much more research is needed to better understand and hopefully cure or slow down this terrible disease process.

MIRAPEX

QUESTION: What can you tell me about Mirapex?

ANSWER: Mirapex (generic name pramipexole) is known as a dopamine receptor agonist and is used to treat Parkinson's disease. Parkinson's disease is an illness that causes a reduction in the amount of a chemical known as dopamine produced in the brain. This chemical helps the body to function normally, and the loss of dopamine causes physical symptoms such as rigidity, tremors, slowed movement, a shuffled walk and postural instability. Mirapex is believed to work by going to dopamine receptors in the brain and stimulating them to work, causing an improvement in symptoms. Patients taking the drug can function better in their daily living activities and also show improvements in their movements. Mirapex can be used by itself or in combination with other drugs to treat early Parkinson's disease. It is also useful in treating patients with advanced Parkinson's disease who are also taking levodopa, a commonly used anti-Parkinson's drug. Some patients with advanced disease may also be able to reduce their dose of levodopa when taking Mirapex. The most common side effects reported by patients taking Mirapex during clinical trials were nausea, dizziness, drowsiness, inability to sleep, a decrease in blood pressure when rising up, movement disorders, constipation, weakness, and hallucinations. The decrease in blood pressure (fainting) when rising up is known as postural hypotension and this may occur more frequently during the initial treatment period with Mirapex. Please note that when Mirapex therapy is initiated for treating Parkinson's disease, the dosage must be gradually increased over a number of weeks to avoid side effects. If you have any questions about your dosage schedule, please talk to your doctor and/or pharmacist.

PLEASE NOTE: A generic version of Mirapex (pramipexole) and a once-daily tablet (Mirapex ER) were approved in 2010.

QUESTION: I heard that Mirapex, which I take for Parkinson's, can cause someone to gamble a lot. What can you tell me about this?

ANSWER: There have been several reports in the medical literature of patients who developed a compulsive gambling disorder after taking Mirapex for Parkinson's disease. The most recent report appeared in the medical journal Archives of Neurology, which described 11 patients with Parkinson's disease who became pathological gamblers while taking their medication. Nine of these patients were taking Mirapex and two were taking Requip. While gambling is common in our society, it becomes pathological when a person cannot resist gambling impulses despite severe personal, family, or work consequences. Both Mirapex and Requip are known as dopamine agonists drugs which work by increasing the amount of a chemical known as dopamine in the brain. Parkinson's disease is an illness that causes a reduction in brain dopamine and leads to physical symptoms such as rigidity, tremors, slowed movement, a shuffled walk, and postural instability. Most of the patients in this recent report had either no gambling history or occasional gambling history before starting on their medication, but developed uncontrollable gambling behaviors with some losing in the hundred's of thousands of dollars. In addition to the pathological gambling, some of these patients also developed a compulsive eating disorder, increased alcohol consumption, increased spending habits, and an obsession with sex. These compulsive behaviors resolved when the dosage of medication was lowered or discontinued in most cases. The incidence of pathological gambling with Mirapex appears to be more frequent than with Requip, but more information is needed. It has been estimated that this side effect occurs in approximately 1.5% of patients receiving Mirapex, but again more study is needed. Why these side effects can occur with Mirapex or Requip is not entirely understood, but it is known that there are dopamine receptors in the brain associated with emotions that include pleasure and reward-seeking. It should also be noted that Requip and Mirapex are also approved for the treatment of restless leg syndrome.

APOKYN

QUESTION: I heard about a drug for people with advanced Parkinson's disease. What can you tell me about it?

ANSWER: The FDA approved Apokyn (apomorphine), which is an injectable drug to treat people with advanced Parkinson's disease. This drug is used to treat episodes of "hypomobility" or so-called "off" periods in which the patient becomes immobile or unable to perform activities of daily living. An estimated 1.5 million Americans have Parkinson's disease, which results in tremors, rigidity, postural instability, slowness, and difficulty moving. Within 3 to 5 years of treatment with standard drug treatments such as levodopa, many patients experience episodes of "hypomobility" when they cannot get up from a chair, or have trouble walking or even speaking. Apokyn may be beneficial in these patients during episodes of "hypomobility" and it is the first therapy approved for this use. How this new drug works in Parkinson's disease is not clearly understood, but it is believed to stimulate certain chemical receptors in the brain. Apokyn is given by subcutaneous injection and it must be taken together with an antiemetic drug because it causes severe nausea and vomiting. It can also cause serious low blood pressure and fainting in some people. The most common side effects of Apokyn include yawning, abnormal movements, nausea and vomiting, sedation or sleepiness, dizziness, runny nose, hallucinations, edema, chest pain, increased sweating, flushing, and pallor. Some serious drug interactions can also occur when Apokyn is taken with some other medications

AZILECT

QUESTION: I heard about a new once-daily treatment for Parkinson's disease. What can you tell me about it?

ANSWER: The FDA recently approved Azilect (rasagiline) tablets as the first once-daily oral treatment for PD. It can be used by itself to treat early PD or can be given in combination with levodopa to treat moderate to advanced disease. Clinical studies with Azilect have shown that it improves activities of daily living and symptoms of movement disorders. Once-daily Azilect works in a similar way to Eldepryl (selegiline), another drug used to treat PD. Both of these drugs block an enzyme in the brain that is responsible for the breakdown (metabolism) of the chemical dopamine. This blocking activity helps the brain to conserve the depleted supply of this chemical. Azilect can interact with numerous other drugs, so it is important that the patient's physician and pharmacist are made aware of all other prescription and nonprescription products being taken. Also, in order to prevent a dangerous increase in blood pressure, patients taking Azilect should avoid tyramine-rich foods and beverages such as aged cheeses, air-dried meats, pickled herring, yeast extract, aged red wines, tap/draft beers, sauerkraut, and soy sauce.

PLEASE NOTE: In December 2009 the FDA eased restrictions regarding the use of Azilect (rasagiline) with many over-the-counter cough/cold medications. However, the use of cough/cold products containing dextromethorphan (DM) is still contraindicated. In addition, patients taking Azilect no longer need to follow a general dietary restriction of ordinary levels of tyramine, which is found in certain foods and beverages, such as air-dried and fermented meats, aged cheeses, red wine, tap/draft beer, herring, sauerkraut, and most soybean products. But, due to potential mild increased sensitivity in some patients, ingestion of very high levels of tyramine (more than 150 mg) should be avoided to prevent a dangerous increase in blood pressure. If patients eat foods very rich in tyramine and do not feel well soon after eating, they should contact their healthcare provider. Please consult with your physician and/or pharmacist if you have any questions about Azilect.

QUESTION: What medications should I avoid when taking Azilect?

ANSWER: Azilect (rasagiline) is approved for the treatment of the signs and symptoms of Parkinson's disease and can be used by itself or in combination with Sinemet (levodopa/carbidopa). Azilect is known as a MAO-B inhibitor and primarily works to prevent the breakdown (metabolism) of dopamine, a brain chemical in short supply in Parkinson's disease and needed for proper movement. By preventing its breakdown, Azilect increases the amount of dopamine in the brain and helps people with Parkinson's disease move better. There are a number of drugs that can interact with Azilect and should be avoided when taking this medication. These "contraindicated" medications include:

- Pain relievers: meperidine (Demerol); tramadol (Ultram); methadone (Dolophine, Methadose, Diskets); or propoxyphene (Darvon, Darvon-N)
- Muscle relaxant: cyclobenzaprine (Flexeril, Fexmid, Amrix).
- Cough suppressant: dextromethorphan (many cough and cold preparations contain dextromethrophan or DM).
- Supplement: St. John's wort
- Antidepressant MAO inhibitors: phenelzine (Nardil), tranylcypromine (Parnate), or isocarboxazid (Marplan)
- MAO-B inhibitor: selegiline (Zelapar, Eldepryl, Emsam).

- Likewise, some other antidepressants and some products for colds or weight loss can pose a problem in people taking Azilect and should be used with caution. In addition, the antibiotic ciprofloxacin (Cipro) can increase blood levels of Azilect and no more than 0.5 mg per day of Azilect should be taken when receiving ciprofloxacin. In view of these potential drug interactions, people taking Azilect should inform their physician(s) and pharmacist(s) about all the medications (prescription and non-prescription) and supplements that they are taking.

It should also be noted that in December 2009 the FDA eased restrictions regarding the use of Azilect with many over-the-counter cough/cold medications. The restriction against the use of Azilect with amine-containing products, such as pseudoephedrine, phenylephrine, phenylpropanolamine, and ephedrine, has been removed. However, the use of cough/cold products containing dextromethorphan (DM) is still contraindicated. Furthermore, there is no longer a contraindication for use of Azilect with general or local anesthetics. In addition, patients taking Azilect no longer need to follow a general dietary restriction of ordinary levels of tyramine, which is found in certain foods and beverages, such as air-dried and fermented meats, aged cheeses, red wine, tap/draft beer, herring, sauerkraut, and most soybean products. But, due to potential mild increased sensitivity in some patients, ingestion of very high levels of tyramine (more than 150 mg) should be avoided to prevent a dangerous increase in blood pressure. If patients eat foods very rich in tyramine and do not feel well soon after eating, they should contact their healthcare provider. Please consult with your physician and/or pharmacist if you have any additional questions about Azilect.

TASMAR

QUESTION: What can you tell me about Tasmar?

ANSWER: Tasmar (generic name tolcapone) is used to treat Parkinson's disease in patients taking levodopa/carbidopa (Sinemet), but are not responding satisfactorily to it. Tasmar is a new type of medication known as a COMT inhibitor or blocker. COMT stands for catechol-o-methyltransferase (cata-col-o-methil-trans-fir-ace), a real tongue twister. COMT is an enzyme needed by the body to metabolize or inactivate dopamine and levodopa, which forms dopamine. By blocking the breakdown of levodopa and dopamine, Tasmar increases the amount of dopamine in the brain, thus improving a patient's symptoms. Studies show that Tasmar can produce a 20% to 30% reduction in a patient's "off time" and a similar increase in "on time". "Off time" is when Parkinsons patients are having symptoms and "on time" is a period of normal function. Patients taking Tasmar may also be able to reduce their dosage of levodopa.

Tasmar is taken 3 times daily. Side effects of Tasmar can include movement disorders, nausea, diarrhea, sleep disorders, dizziness, loss of appetite, lightheadedness when rising up, and sleepiness. However, Tasmar can also cause potentially fatal liver failure in some people and frequent monitoring of liver function is required.

COMTAN

QUESTION: What can you tell me about Comtan for Parkinson's disease?

ANSWER: The new drug that recently became available to treat Parkinson's disease is Comtan (generic name entacapone). It is similar to the drug Tasmar, which I wrote about in a previous column, but it does not have a warning about potentially fatal liver failure like Tasmar. Comtan is useful in patients with Parkinson's disease who are already receiving levodopa in combination with another drug called carbidopa (trade name Sinemet). Many of the patients who take this combination find that it becomes less effective—the so-called "wearing off" effect. Comtan works by blocking the metabolism of levodopa in the body. It blocks an enzyme abbreviated COMT and is known as a COMT inhibitor. By blocking its metabolism, Comtan increases the amount of levodopa available to get into the brain where it can be converted to dopamine and correct its deficiency. Studies show that the use of Comtan in conjunction with Sinemet (levodopa/carbidopa) increases the amount of time that a patient has relatively good function (called "on" time). Most patients can also reduce their dose of Sinemet (levodopa/carbidopa) when they take Comtan. Side effects of Comtan can include nausea, diarrhea, abdominal pain, discoloration of the urine, movement disorders, insomnia, hallucinations, and low blood pressure when arising. Comtan is taken orally with each dose of Sinemet (levodopa/carbidopa).

NEUPRO

QUESTION: I heard about a skin patch for Parkinson's disease. What can you tell me about it?

ANSWER: The FDA approved Neupro transdermal system for the treatment of early Parkinson's disease. It is the first skin patch approved for the treatment of symptoms of this disorder. Neupro contains the drug rotigotine, which works by mimicking the effects of dopamine in the body. The patch is designed to continuously deliver rotigotine through the skin into the bloodstream over a 24-hour period. It is applied once a day to healthy skin on the front of the abdomen, thigh, hip, flank, shoulder, or upper arm. The most common side effects of Neupro include skin reactions at the patch site, dizziness, nausea, vomiting, drowsiness, and insomnia. Other potential safety concerns include sudden onset of sleep while engaged in routine activities such as driving or operating machinery (sleep attacks), hallucinations, and decreased blood pressure on standing up. This new drug is also being tested for its potential use in patients with Restless Legs Syndrome.

PLEASE NOTE: Neupro patches were withdrawn from the market by the manufacturer in April, 2008. The reason for this recall was that some of the patches had snowflake-like crystals on the patch, which may reduce its clinical performance. However, in 2012 the U.S. Food and Drug Administration (FDA) re-approved Neupro for the treatment of the signs and symptoms of advanced stage idiopathic Parkinson's disease (PD) and as a treatment for moderate-to-severe primary Restless Legs Syndrome (RLS).

REQUIP XL

QUESTION: I heard about a new once-daily medication for Parkinson's disease. What can you tell me about it?

ANSWER: The FDA recently approved Requip XL (ropinirole extended-release) tablets for treatment of the signs and symptoms of Parkinson's disease (PD). This once-daily extended-release tablet has been shown to reduce the amount of "off" time while awake by approximately 2 hours per day. Patients with Parkinson's disease may experience what is commonly known as "off" time when their medication wears off and their symptoms return. Requip immediate-release tablets have been available for treating Parkinson's disease since 1997, but it needs to be taken 3 times a day. Recently, a generic version of Requip immediate-release tablets (ropinirole) was also approved by the FDA. PD is an illness that causes a reduction in the amount of a brain chemical known as dopamine. This chemical helps the body to function normally, and a loss of dopamine causes physical symptoms such as rigidity, tremors, slowed movement, a shuffled walk, and postural instability. Ropinirole is thought to work by stimulating dopamine receptors in the brain. The most common side effects of Requip XL are sudden uncontrolled movements, nausea, dizziness, hallucination, drowsiness or sleepiness, stomach pain/discomfort, and low blood pressure when arising.

PARKINSONISM

QUESTION: Can some drugs cause symptoms like Parkinson's disease?

ANSWER: Yes, there are a number of drugs that can produce a condition known as "parkinsonism", which causes some of the same neurologic symptoms that people with Parkinson's disease have. The symptoms may include tremor, stiffness, slow movements, unstable balance, or any combination of these effects. It has been estimated that about 7% of people with parkinsonism have developed their symptoms following treatment with particular medications, which can lead to an incorrect diagnosis for Parkinson's disease. In addition, people with Parkinson's disease may also develop worsening symptoms if treated with these medications inadvertently. Medications that can cause drug-induced parkinsonism decrease or block the action of the brain chemical known as dopamine, which is needed for proper movement. People with actual Parkinson's disease develop their symptoms due to a progressive loss of dopamine-producing cells in the brain. However, their symptoms do not become apparent until 70 to 80% of the dopamine-producing cells are depleted. The incidence of drug-induced parkinsonism increases with age and is more common in women than men. When patients present with symptoms consistent with Parkinson's disease and they are taking a drug known to produce parkinsonism, the drug should be discontinued whenever possible, but no drug should be withdrawn without first discussing the situation with your doctor. Drug-induced parkinsonism is usually reversible, but it may take weeks to months or longer before the symptoms disappear completely, especially if patients have been taking the medication for a long time. Some of the types of medications that can cause drug-induced parkinsonism include antipsychotic drugs, drugs for nausea and vomiting, antihypertensive drugs, and others. While not a complete listing, some of the drugs implicated in causing parkinsonism-like symptoms include the following:

- Amiodarone (Cordarone, Pacerone)
- Chlorpromazine (Thorazine)
- Fluphenazine
- Haloperidol (Haldol)
- Lithium (Lithobid)
- Methydopa
- Metoclopramide (Reglan)
- Olanzapine (Zyprexa)
- Perphenazine
- Pimozide (Orap)
- Prochlorperazine (Compazine)
- Promethazine (Phenergan)
- Quetiapine (Seroquel)
- Reserpine
- Resperidone (Risperdal)

- Thioridazine
- Tranylcypromine (Parnate)
- Trifluoperazine
- Valproic acid (Depakene, Depakote)

NEUROPROTECTION

QUESTION: Are there any supplements that can slow the progression of Parkinson's disease?

ANSWER: Parkinson's disease (PD) is a progressive neurodegenerative disease that affects more than 1.5 million people in the United States. The incidence of PD increases after the age of 60, and it affects both women and men equally. Dr. James Parkinson first described the symptoms of PD 1817 and he called it "Shaking Palsy". PD is an illness that causes a reduction in the amount of a brain chemical known as dopamine. This chemical helps the body to function normally, and a loss of dopamine causes physical symptoms such as rigidity, tremors, slowed movement, a shuffled walk, and postural instability. By the time PD has progressed enough to cause symptoms, approximately 60% to 80% of the brain cells that produce dopamine have already been lost. That is why it is so important to try to preserve and protect the remaining 20% to 40% of these brain cells (neurons). While the cause(s) of PD are unknown at this time, it is thought that the environment and genetics play a role. With few exceptions, most cases of PD are associated with an accumulation of an abnormal protein in the brain known as "Lewy bodies". In addition, mechanisms that may contribute to neuron cell death include stress from chemicals created during normal metabolic processes (oxidative and nitrative stress), excessive excitation of the neurons by chemicals, inflammation in the neurons, and the inability of mitochondria (the principal energy source of neurons) to function. The goal of "neuroprotective" therapy is to try and stop these processes that lead to neuron cell death. Unfortunately, at this time, no supplements have been proven scientifically to have "neuroprotective" ability in humans. However, many supplements have the potential for "neuroprotection" based upon animal and laboratory studies. Some of these supplements include coenzyme Q10 (CoQ10), creatine, caffeine, nicotine, anti-inflammatory agents, alpha lipoic acid, Vitamins C, D, and E, folic acid, selenium, curcumin/tumeric, taurine, fish oil, B-vitamins, acetyl-L-carnitine, N-acetyl-cysteine, and others. Anyone considering taking a supplement for PD should consult with his or her physician for advice.

QUESTION: I heard on TV that a drug might slow down the progression of Parkinson's disease. What can you tell me about this?

ANSWER: Recently, the New England Journal of Medicine published the results of a study called ADAGIO which looked at whether the drug Azilect (rasagiline) would slow down the progression of Parkinson's disease. This 18-month study involved almost 1,200 patients with early stage Parkinson's disease and was conducted in 129 research centers around the world. Half of the patients in the study took daily doses of 1 milligram or 2 milligrams of Azilect for 36 weeks, while the other half took a placebo (dummy pill). After that, all study participants taking a placebo were then switched to Azilect (1 or 2 milligrams daily) for the next 36 weeks. At the 18-month point, the patient's symptoms were measured and were compared to their symptoms at the beginning of the study. What the results showed is that patients taking Azilect 1 milligram daily for the entire 18-months had less worsening of their symptoms than patients only taking Azilect 1 milligram daily for just the last 9-months. In other words, it appeared that Azilect 1 milligram daily "protected" the patients from their disease progression. However, the clinical improvements in these patients were relatively small. In addition, patients taking Azilect 2 milligrams daily did not show any significant Improvements in symptoms. Why the Azilect 1 milligram daily dose was effective in slowing functional decline but the 2 milligram daily dose was not cannot be explained at this point. In view of these results, some neurologists may support the use of Azilect for slowing down the disease progression and some may not. More research and longer-term study of these patients may be needed to better determine if Azilect will indeed modify the outcome of this disease. It should also be noted that Azilect is already approved for the treatment for Parkinson's disease. It is classified as a MAO-B inhibitor, which blocks the breakdown of the chemical dopamine in the brain, making it work longer and better to improve movement problems associated with Parkinson's disease. Brain levels of dopamine are in short supply in Parkinson's disease due to the progressive death of brain cells (neurons) that produce it. The potential "neuroprotective" effects of Azilect, however, appear to be unrelated to its effects on dopamine.

QUESTION: I heard that some types of blood pressure medication might help prevent Parkinson's disease. What can you tell me about this?

ANSWER: A study recently published in the journal "Annals of Neurology" suggests the possibility that a certain type of blood pressure medication may help to prevent or slow down the progression of Parkinson's disease. These medications have been used for many years to treat high blood pressure and are known as L-type calcium channel blockers of the dihydropyridine class. Drugs in this class include felodipine (Plendil), isradipine (Dynacirc), nicardipine (Cardene), and nifedipine (Procardia). Amlodipine (Norvasc) also falls into this class, but it did not show a beneficial effect in this study, probably because it has a more difficult time getting into the brain compared to the other agents. In this Danish study involving more than 11,000 patients, researchers found that people taking one of these medications had a 26-30% risk reduction in developing Parkinson's disease. Other antihypertensive medications, including amlodipine, did not show this risk reduction. Exactly how these specific blood pressure medications may work to prevent or slow down Parkinson's disease is not well understood. Brain cells (neurons) rely on calcium to function, and it has been suggested that this may make them more susceptible to aging and oxidative stress. This could decrease the neuron's capability to create energy and function properly, leading to brain cell death (neurodegeneration). It should be noted that this is only one retrospective study and much more research is needed to determine, if indeed, these drugs may be neuroprotective. In addition, since many people with Parkinson's disease have low blood pressure problems (orthostatic hypotension), additional blood pressure lowering could be problematic.

Parkinson's disease is a slowly progressive brain disorder in which various cells (neurons) within the brain die or become impaired, causing a wide variety of symptoms. Movement problems are common in people with Parkinson's disease, including shaking or tremor, muscle stiffness and rigidity, slow movement, and walking or postural changes. Other movement or muscle related symptoms can include small, cramped handwriting, stiff facial expression, muffled speech, swallowing problems, lack of arm swing, and diminished manual dexterity. In the past, these movement problems received the most attention and numerous medications have been developed to treat them. More recently, however, Parkinson's disease has been redefined to include a number of other non-movement disorders that can occur, such as pain, sleep disturbances, constipation, depression, anxiety and panic disorder, psychosis, and dementia. In fact, symptoms such as constipation, loss of smell, or sleep disorders may actually occur years before the movement problems begin.

QUESTION: Can ibuprofen lower the risk of Parkinson's disease?

ANSWER: A study recently reported at the 2010 annual meeting of the American Academy of Neurology suggests that the commonly used non-steroidal anti-inflammatory drug (NSAID) ibuprofen, may reduce the risk of getting Parkinson's disease. This study included more than 136,000 men and women who did not have Parkinson's disease at the start of the study. The study participants were followed over a six-year period and approximately 300 were diagnosed with the disease during that time span. Patients in the study reported on their use of NSAIDs using a questionnaire. Results from the study showed that people who took three or more tablets of ibuprofen tablets a week showed a 40% lower risk of getting Parkinson's disease compared to those who did not take ibuprofen. In contrast, the risk of Parkinson's disease was not lower for people who regularly used acetaminophen (Tylenol), aspirin, or other NSAIDs. Exactly how ibuprofen may work to protect against Parkinson's disease is not known, but its ability to reduce inflammation may be involved. It should be noted that the study's results do not establish a direct cause and effect relationship between ibuprofen and Parkinson's disease and more study is needed. In addition, ibuprofen use can cause gastrointestinal bleeding and affect the kidneys.

CLINICAL RESEARCH STUDIES

QUESTION: I have Parkinson's disease and would like to find out about research studies. Can you give me any information?

ANSWER: April is a good time to talk about Parkinson's disease (PD), since it is the month Dr. James Parkinson was born and is designated as Parkinson's Awareness Month each year. If you have access to the Internet, two good web sites to find information about research studies are **www.clinicaltrials.gov** and **www.pdtrials.org**. If you don't have access to the Internet another good starting point is the Parkinson's Disease Foundation (1-800-457-6676; **www.pdf.org**). This organization has numerous free resources regarding PD, including a booklet entitled "Getting Involved in Parkinson's Research". Clinical research trials (studies) are very important and participants in these trials can play a more active role in their own health care, gain access to new research treatments before they become available, and can help others by contributing to medical research. If you are considering whether to take part in a clinical trial, the National Institutes of Health (NIH) suggests asking the following questions before signing on:

- What is the purpose of the study?
- Who is going to be in the study?
- Why do researchers believe the experimental treatment being tested may be effective? Has it been tested before?
- What kinds of tests and experimental treatments are involved?
- How do the possible risks, side effects, and benefits in the study compare with my current treatment?
- How might this trial affect my daily life?
- How long will the trial last?
- Will hospitalization be required?
- Who will pay for the experimental treatment?
- Will I be reimbursed for other expenses?
- What type of long-term follow up care is part of this study?
- How will I know that the experimental treatment is working? Will results of the trials be provided to me?
- Who will be in charge of my care?

ER

You should also know that every clinical trial in the U.S. must be approved and monitored by an Institutional Review Board (IRB) to make sure the risks of the study are as low as possible and are worth any potential benefits. In addition, you will learn the key facts about a clinical trial (Informed Consent) before deciding whether or not to participate and you may withdraw from the study at any time.

QUESTION: You recently wrote a column about Parkinson's disease and research studies. I heard that the Michael J. Fox Foundation has a good web site for research pertaining to Parkinson's.

ANSWER: Yes, the Michael J. Fox Foundation for Parkinson's Research recently (2012) launched the Fox Trial Finder web site at **www.foxtrialfinder.org**. This Internet site is a new clinical trial matching tool that matches volunteers to clinical research trials (studies) that are underway and for which they may be qualified for. It also lets people know by e-mail alert when new clinical trials are being launched that they may be interested in joining. Using the Fox Trial finder is easy and straightforward. A person with Parkinson's disease, their care partner, or anyone without this disease can use the web site. Once on the web site, the potential study volunteer completes a profile by answering some basic questions (gender, age, race, diagnosis, symptoms, medications, geographic location, etc). Possible research study matches are then instantly identified. For each study listed, the volunteer can indicate if they are interested in making contact with the clinical study team to get more information. All of this is done anonymously and without any obligation on the volunteer's part. The Fox Trial Finder also provides details about each trial that a volunteer may be a match for, including its purpose, description, and location. Remember your privacy is assured and a clinical trial team member will never see your personal information unless you provide it. If a potential study volunteer does not have access to the Internet, your local public library should be able to help. Clearly, participation in clinical trials is extremely important as nearly 80% of all clinical trials finish late or may not even be completed due to low participation rates. This means it will take much longer to bring new treatments to patients with disease.

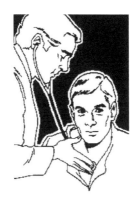

CHAPTER 14
OTHER MEDICAL PROBLEMS

FIBROMYALGIA

QUESTION: What drugs are used to treat fibromyalgia?

ANSWER: Fibromyalgia is a soft-tissue syndrome characterized by widespread chronic musculoskeletal pain, morning stiffness, poor sleep, and fatigue. Other symptoms can include anxiety, depression, headache, numbness or tingling, and irritable bowel syndrome. In the past, fibromyalgia has also been called rheumatism, fibrositis, and fibromyositis. Fibromyalgia is thought to affect about 2% of the U.S. population or about 3.7 million people. It is more common in women especially those over the age of 50. The prevalence of fibromyalgia also increases with age, rising to 7.4% of women aged 70-79 years of age. The diagnosis of fibromyalgia is made based upon the patient's symptoms. Although its cause is unknown, fibromyalgia may be triggered by physical or mental stress, inadequate sleep, an injury, exposure to dampness or cold, certain infections, and occasionally by rheumatoid arthritis or related disorders.

There is no known cure for fibromyalgia and no drugs have been specifically developed for its treatment. However, a few existing drug treatments can produce improvement in 30-50% of patients with this disorder. Goals of treatment include pain relief along with improved sleep, depression, and energy levels. Medications commonly used for this condition include antidepressants, cyclobenzaprine (a muscle relaxant), ondansetron (an anti-nausea drug), corticosteroids like prednisone, sedatives to help sleep, pain relievers such as acetaminophen (Tylenol), NSAIDs (like ibruprofen and others), or tramadol (Ultram), and injections with lidocaine, an anesthetic agent. Herbal treatments that may be helpful include SAMe, capsaicin, or malic acid. In addition, non-drug treatments like cardiovascular fitness training, biofeedback training, and behavioral therapy may be beneficial in some patients with fibromyalgia.

QUESTION: I heard that a new drug was approved for fibromyalgia. What can you tell me about it?

ANSWER: The FDA recently approved Savella (milnacipran) for the treatment of fibromyalgia. It is not known exactly how Savella works to improve the symptoms of fibromyalgia (such as pain and decreased physical functioning), but some researchers believe that abnormalities in certain brain chemicals (neurotransmitters) may be involved in fibromyalgia. Savella primarily affects the brain chemicals norepinephrine and serotonin, which are thought to play a role in fibromyalgia. This activity is different from Lyrica (pregabalin), the only other drug approved for the treatment of fibromyalgia, which seems to work by reducing the number of electrical pain signals that the brain cells send to each other. Savella is taken orally twice a day. Its most common side effects are nausea, headache, constipation, insomnia, and hot flushes, but other more serious adverse effects can occur. Milnacipran has also been marketed in Europe and Japan as an antidepressant for many years.

MIGRAINE HEADACHES

QUESTION: What medications can I use for migraine headaches?

ANSWER: Approximately 23-million Americans have migraine headaches which can be debilitating or disabling. These headaches occur more frequently on one side of the head, are pulsating or throbbing and are accompanied by nausea or vomiting in most people. Migraines may also be associated with sensitivity to light or sound and can be aggravated by routine physical activity, such as climbing stairs. Certain foods and beverages may also bring on or "trigger" a migraine attack in certain people. Some of these dietary triggers are:

- Alcoholic drinks
- Coffee, tea, cola
- Aged cheese
- Chocolate
- Monosodium glutamate (MSG)
- Smoked fish
- Nuts
- Pickled foods

The exact cause of migraine headaches is not known, but research shows that a chemical known as serotonin (sar-o-ton-in) is the main culprit. This chemical, which is found in the brain, can cause blood vessels to narrow or constrict and stimulate pain receptors. Levels of serotonin are unusually high just before a migraine and unusually low during the migraine attack. Many people who suffer from migraine have a family history of this problem and it is three times more common in women than in men. Migraine usually begins when a person is in their late teens or early adulthood and attacks can increase or decrease during menstruation, pregnancy and menopause. Some people can even feel when a migraine is coming. If untreated, most migraine headaches can last at least four hours and up to 72 hours.

Fortunately, there are numerous medications available to treat and prevent migraine headaches. Non-drug measures can also help, such as avoiding dietary "triggers", stress management, application of ice and/or heat, and getting enough sleep. An effective non-prescription product is Excedrin Migraine, which is a combination of acetaminophen, aspirin, and caffeine. Other over-the-counter agents, which can benefit some migraine sufferers, include ibuprofen or similar products and sinus medications containing pseudoephedrine. The list of prescription products for the treatment of migraine is too lengthy to go into detail for this column, but many new drugs known as "triptans" are now available.

"Triptans" act like serotonin mentioned earlier, which is reduced during a migraine attack. These products include naratriptan (trade name Amerge), sumatriptan (trade name Imitrex), and zolmitriptan (trade name Zomig). Other useful prescription medications include ergot products (e.g., Ergomar, Cafergot, Migranal, etc.), some antidepressants or anticonvulsants, Midrin, Fioricet, beta-blockers (e.g., Inderal, Tenormin, etc.) and a number of other types of drugs. If non-prescription products are not effective, your physician can help select the best prescription drug or drugs for you. As always, make sure that your physician and pharmacist know all the medications that you take (prescription and non-prescription) to avoid dangerous drug interactions or side effects.

QUESTION: I heard about a new combination prescription drug for migraine headache. What can you tell me about it?

ANSWER: The new combination prescription drug for treating migraine headaches is Treximet. Treximet tablets contain sumatriptan (85 mg) in combination with naproxen (500 mg). Sumatriptan is a "triptan" drug that acts like the brain chemical serotonin, which is in low amounts during a migraine attack. It works by causing blood vessels in the brain to narrow or constrict, which helps to relieve the migraine headache. Sumatriptan alone has been available for quite some time as the prescription drug Imitrex. Naproxen is an anti-inflammatory drug that has pain-relieving properties. Together, sumatriptan and naproxen help to relieve the pain of migraine headaches more effectively by working in different ways. Its dosage is one tablet with no more than 2 tablets in 24 hours. During clinical study the most common side effects of Treximet were dizziness; nausea; sleepiness; chest discomfort and chest pain; neck, throat and jaw pain; tightness and pressure; numbness/tingling; upset stomach; and dry mouth. However, serious side effects can occur in some people and patients taking Treximet need to be monitored closely by their physician.

QUESTION: I get migraine headaches and heard about a new drug treatment being approved. What can you tell me about it?

ANSWER: Some of the commonly used prescription medications used to treat migraine headache are known as "triptans". They work by reducing the swelling of blood vessels surrounding the brain during a migraine headache. The new drug you are talking about is Relpax (eletriptan) and it is a "triptan" drug. It is taken orally and has been shown to provide headache relief in about 55-70% of people within about 2 hours or less. There are now 7 different "triptan" drugs available by prescription to treat migraine. "Triptans" can cause serious side effects in some people and patients taking them need to be monitored by their physician. More information about Relpax can be obtained by calling 1-866-4RELPAX (1-866-473-5729) or at **www.relpax.com**.

QUESTION: I heard that there is a new prescription nasal spray for migraine headaches. What can you tell me about it?

ANSWER: The new prescription medication you heard about is Zomig (zolmitriptan) Nasal Spray. Previously, it was only available in tablet form. Zomig is a "triptan" drug that acts like the chemical serotonin referred to earlier. The advantage of the nasal spray is that it is fast acting and can relieve some migraine headaches within 15 minutes after using it. In clinical studies, approximately 90% of people using Zomig Nasal Spray had headache relief within 2 hours. The most common side effects of Zomig Nasal Spray are taste disturbance, abnormal touch sensation, increased sensitivity to touch, sleepiness, and dizziness. However, numerous other adverse reactions are possible in some people. Another prescription "triptan" nasal spray, Imitrex (sumatriptan) is also available for treating migraine headaches.

QUESTION: Can riboflavin help to prevent migraine headaches?

ANSWER: It may. Riboflavin or vitamin B-2 is an essential water-soluble vitamin that is commonly found in multiple vitamin preparations to treat or prevent riboflavin deficiency. This vitamin enables the body to break down sugar and fat and is key to converting the vitamin niacin into its active form. It is also the vitamin that may turn your urine bright yellow. Milk and dairy products are rich sources of riboflavin. Other sources include fortified bread, cereals, beef liver, and eggs. The recommended dietary allowance (RDA) of riboflavin is 1.3 mg per day for men and 1.1 mg per day for women, but much higher daily doses (400 mg) may be needed for migraine prevention. Migraine headaches are a debilitating neurovascular disorder that now affects about 28 million Americans. Adult females are at greater risk for this disorder, which affects nearly 18% of women and 6% of men in the U.S. It is not known exactly how riboflavin may help to prevent migraine headache, but its beneficial effects may be due to an increased energy production in the cells of cerebral blood vessels. It has been shown that patients with migraine have reduced energy production within their cells in between attacks and this may be a factor in migraine headache development. The use of high-dose riboflavin for the prevention of migraine has been studied in a small number of clinical trials. Results from these studies have shown that riboflavin may be effective in decreasing the number and severity of migraine attacks. It also appears to be safe with relatively few side effects. However, larger and longer-term studies are needed to substantiate these beneficial effects. It should also be noted that riboflavin is not FDA-approved for the prevention of migraine headache.

QUESTION: I heard about a new liquid medication for migraine headaches. What can you tell me about it?

ANSWER: The FDA recently approved Cambia (diclofenac) for the treatment of migraine headache attacks with or without aura in adults. About 25% of people with migraine attacks experience an aura, which involves temporary, reversible disturbances in vision, sensation, balance, movement, or speech. Commonly, people see jagged, shimmering, or flashing lights or develop a blind spot with flickering edges. Less commonly, people experience tingling sensations, loss of balance, weakness in an arm or leg, or difficulty talking. The aura occurs within the hour before the migraine and ends as the migraine begins. Actually Cambia is not a new drug, but a new dosage form. Cambia contains the active ingredient diclofenac, a non-steroidal anti-inflammatory drug (NSAID) that has been available for many years. Cambia comes in a powder-containing packet, which is emptied into a cup and mixed with 1-2 ounces of water for drinking immediately when the migraine attack occurs. This liquid formulation may provide for significant pain relief within 15 to 30 minutes after a single dose. The safety and effectiveness of a second dose has not been established. The most common side effects of Cambia during clinical studies were nausea and dizziness.

GOUT

QUESTION: What can I do for gout?

ANSWER: Gout, or gouty arthritis, was first described by Hippocrates in the fifth century BC. It results from excessive uric acid production, which causes sodium urate crystals to accumulate in the joints leading to attacks of painful joint inflammation. This painful inflammation of joints was once considered a "disease of kings" because the foods that contribute to high uric acid levels were only available to the wealthy in early times. Gout affects more than 3 million Americans and is more common in men than in women. It often runs in families and most often affects the joints in the feet, particularly at the base of the big toe. However it also can affect other joints including the ankle, knee, wrist, and elbow. Gout attacks can be caused by many factors such as dehydration, trauma, fever, heavy alcohol consumption, certain drugs, and a diet high in purines, which are converted to uric acid in the body. Foods high in purines include anchovies, bacon, beer, game meats, herring, organ meats, sardines, scallops, turkey, asparagus, mushrooms, and sweetbreads. Some medical conditions can also contribute to gout such as obesity, high blood pressure, hypothyroidism, abnormal kidney function, certain cancers and blood disorders, and radiation treatment. People who suffer from gout should avoid foods that contain large amounts of purines and limit their alcohol consumption. It is also important for them to exercise regularly, maintain optimal weight, drink plenty of water to help their kidneys flush out excess uric acid, and avoid crash diets because rapid weight loss can increase uric acid levels. While there is no cure for gout, drugs are available to prevent or treat acute attacks. Medications that lower uric acid levels such as allopurinol and probenecid can be prescribed to prevent attacks of gout. These products are usually recommended for people who have experienced multiple gout attacks and over time will help to slowly dissolve deposits of uric acid in the joints. The anti-gout drug, colchicine, can also be prescribed for the prevention and treatment of gout attacks. Acute gout attacks are most commonly treated with anti-inflammatory drugs such as ibuprofen or naproxen. These medications are usually taken (with food or milk) at the first sign of an acute gout attack since it usually takes these drugs 12-24 hours to relieve symptoms. Left untreated, gout can destroy cartilage and bone leading to deformed joints and limiting movement. In addition, chronically elevated uric acid levels can lead to kidney disease and failure. Your physician will be able to determine if you have gout and recommend appropriate treatment.

QUESTION: I heard about a new injectable drug for treating gout. What can you tell me about it?

ANSWER: The FDA recently approved Krystexxa (pegloticase injection) for the treatment of adults with chronic gout who are not helped by existing drugs used to treat gout. About 3% of the three million adults who suffer from gout are not helped by conventional oral therapy. Gout occurs due to an excess of the bodily waste uric acid, which is eventually deposited as needle-like crystals in the joints or in soft tissue. These crystals can cause intermittent swelling, redness, heat, pain, and stiffness in the joints. Krystexxa is an enzyme that lowers uric acid levels by metabolizing it into a harmless chemical that is excreted in the urine. During two 6-month studies involving 212 patients with chronic gout who did not respond to an oral conventional drug therapy for gout (allopurinol), Krystexxa was able to lower uric acid levels in the blood and to reduce deposits of uric acid crystals in joints and soft tissue. Krystexxa is given by intravenous injection every 2 weeks. Its most common side effects include gout attacks (flares), injection site bruising, nausea, irritation of the nasal passages, constipation, chest pain, allergic reactions, and vomiting.

QUESTION: I heard that a new drug was approved to treat gout. What can you tell me about it?

ANSWER: The FDA recently approved Uloric (febuxostat), the first new treatment for gout in more than 40 years. It was approved to treat (reduce) high levels of uric acid in patients with gout. Uloric works like allopurinol (Zyloprim), which has been available to treat gout for many years. Both of these drugs block an enzyme in the body (xanthine oxidase), which is needed to make uric acid. People with gout have high levels of uric acid in their blood because they either produce too much of it, don't get rid of it effectively, or a combination of both. During clinical studies involving more than 3,000 people with gout, Uloric was found to be more effective than allopurinol in reducing uric acid levels. The most common side effects of Uloric during these studies were nausea, joint pain, rash, and abnormalities in liver function tests. Uloric is taken in a dose of 40 mg or 80 mg orally once a day.

ALCOHOL DEPENDENCE

QUESTION: I heard about a new drug to help treat people who are dependent on alcohol. What can you tell me about it?

ANSWER: The FDA recently approved a new drug to treat alcohol dependent people who want to remain alcohol-free after they have stopped drinking. The new prescription drug is called Campral (generic name acamprostate) and is available as a delayed-release tablet that is taken 3 times a day. It is the first new mediation in nine years to be approved in the U.S. for the treatment of alcohol dependence. Treatment with Campral should be part of a comprehensive management program that includes psychosocial support. It is not known exactly how the new medication works to help keep people alcohol free. It works differently from other currently available medications that either blocks the "high" associated with alcohol use or that induce vomiting if alcohol is ingested. Campral appears to interact with certain neurotransmitter systems in the brain that are involved with alcohol-induced behavior to restore a normal balance. It does not affect blood alcohol levels or diminish withdrawal symptoms and does not appear to cause aversion to alcohol. Campral may not be effective in people who are actively drinking at the start of treatment, or in people who abuse other substances in addition to alcohol. The most common side effects of Campral reported during clinical studies have been diarrhea, headache, intestinal gas, and nausea. Alcohol dependence is a chronic disease that accounts for approximately 100,000 deaths per year. Nearly 14 million Americans have a problem associated with alcohol.

QUESTION: I heard about a new drug that is injected once a month for alcohol dependence. What do you tell me about it?

ANSWER: The FDA recently approved Vivitrol injection for the treatment of alcohol dependence. The active ingredient in Vivitrol is naltrexone, which has been available for quite some time as an oral tablet that is used for the same indication. Vivitrol is an extended-release form of naltrexone that is injected once-a-month for the treatment of alcohol dependence in patients who are able to abstain from drinking and who also are receiving psychosocial support, such as counseling or group therapy. It is not known exactly how this drug works to reduce alcohol consumption, but it does interact with receptors (opioid) in the brain that are known to be involved with alcohol craving. During clinical study, the use of Vivitrol injection was shown to reduce the number of heavy drinking days and allowed some patients with alcohol dependence to maintain complete abstinence without relapse. The most common side effects of Vivitrol include nausea, vomiting, headache, dizziness, fatigue, and reactions at the site of injection. However, it can also cause injury to the liver when given in excessive doses. Alcohol dependence is a chronic disease with underlying neurological and genetic factors. The four most common symptoms of this disease are cravings, loss of control over drinking, withdrawal symptoms (including sweating, nausea, shakiness, and anxiety) and an increased tolerance for alcohol. About 18 million people in the United States are dependent on or abuse alcohol, and half of them are considered alcohol dependent. Approximately 75% of people treated for alcohol problems relapse back to drinking within the first year, and it is important that psychosocial support, such as counseling, is used in conjunction with any medication treatment.

PLEASE NOTE: In October 2010, Vivitrol was also approved to treat and prevent relapse after patients with opioid dependence have undergone detoxification treatment.

SENSITIVE TEETH

QUESTION: How do certain toothpastes help sensitive teeth?

ANSWER: Tooth (dentinal) hypersensitivity affects more than 40 million people in the U.S. each year and up to 30% of adults have this problem at some time during their lifetime. People with sensitive teeth experience pain from hot/cold and sweet/sour solutions as well as when hot/cold air touches the teeth. The pain can vary from mild to sharp and excruciating. In healthy teeth, porous tissue called dentin is protected by your gums and by your teeth's hard enamel shell. Dentin contains microscopic holes (tubules) that connect to tooth nerves and trigger pain when dentin is exposed and irritated. Dentin can be exposed by receding gums caused by improper brushing or gum disease, fractured or chipped teeth, clenching or grinding your teeth, or erosion due to aging. Excessive flossing or toothpick use can also cause dentin exposure. Pain from sensitive teeth is not always constant and can come and go. Constant pain could be a sign of a more serious problem, so it is important to discuss your symptoms with your dentist to determine the cause and proper treatment. The use of a soft-bristle toothbrush and desensitizing toothpastes may be helpful for some people with sensitive teeth. Active ingredients commonly used in these toothpastes are potassium nitrate and/or stannous fluoride. Potassium nitrate works by interrupting the signals between the nerve cells in the tooth. By blocking these signals, nerve excitement and pain are prevented. Stannous fluoride on the other hand works by closing off (occluding) the dentin tubules. This prevents fluid flow in the tubules, which leads to nerve excitation and pain. For optimum effectiveness, users should apply at least a 1-inch strip of the desensitizing toothpaste to a soft-bristle toothbrush and brush thoroughly for at least 1 minute twice daily. The onset of effect with these products is not immediate and may take from several days to 5 weeks. The desensitizing toothpaste should be used until the sensitivity subsides or as long as a dentist recommends its use. Some desensitizing toothpastes include Aquafresh Sensitive, Biotene Sensitive, Colgate Sensitive Maximum Strength, Crest Sensitivity Protection, Crest Pro-Health, Oragel Sensitive Pain-Relieving Toothpaste for adults, Oragel Gold Sensitive Teeth Gel,

Pepsodent Sensitive, Rembrandt Whitening Toothpaste for Sensitive Teeth, and Sensodyne Exra Whitening.

HYPERSALIVATION

QUESTION: Can some drugs cause you to salivate more?

ANSWER: Yes, there are some drugs that can cause excessive salvation or "hypersalivation". Saliva is the liquid that keeps the mouth moist. It lubricates the teeth, gums, and tongue and helps to wash debris from the mouth. Saliva also helps people taste, digest, and swallow foods. Normally, over 16 ounces of saliva is produced daily by the salivary glands in the mouth. Saliva contains a number of ingredients such as electrolytes, immunoglobulins, anti-infective compounds, along with digestive and other proteins. Dryness of the mouth is a fairly common complaint, especially in the elderly, and many drugs can cause this condition, known as xerostomia. However, hypersalivation can also be a side effect of medications. Listed below are some medications that can cause hypersalivation in certain individuals.

Some Medications That Can Cause Hypersalivation
Trade Name (Generic Name)

- Akarpine (pilocarpine)
- Clozaril (clozapine)
- Exelon (rivastigmine)
- Geodon (ziprasidone)
- Haldol (haloperidol)
- Isopto-atropine (atropine)
- Isopto-carpine (pilocarpine)
- Klonopin (clonazepam)
- Mestinon (pyridostigmine)
- Orap (pimozide)
- Prozac (fluoxetine)
- Requip (ropinirole)
- Resperdal (risperidone)
- Salagen (pilocarpine)

- Soriatane (acitretin)
- Symbyax (olanzapine and fluoxetine)
- Topamax (topiramate)
- Trecator-SC (ethionamide)
- Urecholine (bethanechol)
- Xanax (alprazolam)
- Xyrem (sodium oxybate)
- Zyprexa (olanzapine)

SINUSITIS

QUESTION: What nonprescription products are helpful for sinusitis?

ANSWER: Sinusitis, or inflammation of the sinuses, is a very common medical problem that affects about 30% of the population at some point in their life. This inflammation may last for a short period of time (acute sinusitis) or may persist for 3 months or longer (chronic sinusitis). Sinusitis is usually categorized as infectious or allergic. Infectious sinusitis can be caused by a virus, a fungus, or by bacteria. Allergic sinusitis is caused by an allergic reaction to dust, mold, pollen, or some other substance in the environment. Acute sinusitis commonly occurs in conjunction with a cold where nasal congestion blocks the sinuses and prevents drainage of mucus into the nose and mouth. The sinus mucus builds up and thickens, which can lead to infection in the sinuses. Sinusitis causes nasal and sinus congestion, runny nose, sinus pain or pressure, headache, and sometimes pain or tingling in the upper teeth. It can also cause impaired taste and sense of smell, or bad breath.

The treatment of sinusitis is based upon its cause. Sinusitis caused by bacteria requires treatment with antibiotics and a physician should be consulted to diagnose the problem. There are numerous nonprescription products that are available to help relieve the symptoms of sinusitis. These include oral decongestants such as pseudoephedrine (Sudafed, Drixoral, others), or nasal decongestants (Afrin, Dristan, Privine, Otrivin, others). Decongestants are indicated for the temporary relief of nasal congestion and nasal decongestants should not be used for more than 3 to 5 days to avoid "rebound" or worsening congestion. Guaifenesin (Mucinex) may be a useful agent to help thin and loosen mucus, allowing sinus drainage. Drinking fluids (a minimum of 8 glasses of water per day), which keeps secretions thin, is also encouraged. The anti-inflammatory drug cromolyn (Nasalcrom nasal solution) may be useful in some people. Using nasal saline sprays (Ocean, Afrin saline, Salinex, others) can be helpful to improve drainage of thick mucus. In addition, mechanical devices which help to keep the nose open such as Breathe-Right and the use of a vaporizer can be useful. Antihistamines can be used, but only for allergic sinusitis because they tend to be drying to the mucus, which thickens it and hinders sinus drainage. Many other prescription and nonprescription products are available to treat sinusitis, so your pharmacist and physician should be consulted for more information. Also, be sure to read product labeling carefully to prevent side effects and drug interaction problems.

HEMORRHOIDS

QUESTION: I heard about a new nonprescription device used to treat hemorrhoids. What you tell me about it?

ANSWER: More than 10 million people in the U.S. complain of hemorrhoidal symptoms and about half of the population has hemorrhoids by the age of 50. Hemorrhoids are swollen (dilated) veins around the anus and rectal areas. They are similar to the twisted and swollen varicose veins, which develop on the legs of some people. Hemorrhoidal veins usually become swollen due to aging, obesity, sitting or standing for a long time, straining during bowel movements, heavy lifting with straining, or pregnancy. Hemorrhoids that occur in the anal canal are called internal hemorrhoids while those that form near the anal opening are called external hemorrhoids. Both internal and external hemorrhoids may stay in the anus or protrude outside the anus. Symptoms of hemorrhoids include itching, pain, burning, and bright red blood on the toilet paper or in a bowel movement. Since other conditions can produce these symptoms, including serious conditions such as colorectal or anal cancer, people who experience these symptoms should consult a doctor who can confirm the diagnosis of hemorrhoids and recommend appropriate treatment.

Medications that are commonly used to treat hemorrhoids include anti-inflammatory, local anesthetic or vasoconstrictor creams, ointments, or suppositories. These preparations can help shrink inflamed tissue and relieve pain or itching. Taking stools softeners or a laxative like psyllium can relieve straining with bowel movements. In addition, moist towelettes containing witch hazel or other ingredients can soothe swollen tissues when used after a bowel movement. Your pharmacist can help you select one of the numerous nonprescription products that are available.

Many nondrug measures can also be used to prevent or treat hemorrhoids. These include increasing fluid intake, regular exercise, and a high fiber diet to prevent constipation and straining. People with hemorrhoids should be encouraged to avoid sitting on the toilet longer than five minutes, to reduce straining and decrease pressure on the hemorrhoidal vessels. In addition, taking warm sitz baths can promote good hygiene and relieve symptoms, especially after bowel movements. Recently, the FDA approved a new type of nonprescription device to treat hemorrhoids that is sold under the brand name Hemor-Rite Cryotherapy. The Hemor-Rite device is a small anatomically designed device that contains coolant materials and is kept frozen in the freezer until it is used. After applying a glycerin lubricant, the neck of the device is inserted into the anal canal and is left in place for six to eight minutes, or until it reaches body temperature for a maximum of 10 minutes. This direct application of cold to the swollen hemorrhoidal veins by the neck and base of the device provides prompt relief of itching, pain, and swelling due to its vasoconstriction and numbing effects. It is recommended that the device be used for a minimum of four times a day for the first week and then twice a day until symptoms disappear. The manufacturer also recommends its use every two days as a form of hemorrhoid prevention. The device is reusable for a six-month period. In between uses, the Hemor-Rite device should be cleaned, placed in its storage case, and stored in the freezer for least two hours before it is used again. This new device comes with a storage case, a bottle of glycerin lubricant, and complete instructions for use. Please read the full instructions carefully before use. Currently the

Hemor-Rite Cryotherapy device is only available on the Internet at **www.hemorrite.com** or by calling 1-866-HEMORITE (436-6748). If both drug and nondrug measures to treat hemorrhoids are not effective, other procedures may be needed including surgery. Your doctor will be able to determine what treatment option is best for you.

QUESTION: What nonprescription products are useful for hemorrhoids?

ANSWER: Nonprescription medications that are commonly used to treat hemorrhoids include anti-inflammatory, local anesthetic or vasoconstrictor creams, ointments, or suppositories. These preparations can help shrink inflamed tissue and relieve pain or itching. Active ingredients found in these nonprescription products include the following:

Local Anesthetics
Benzocaine, benzyl alcohol, dibucaine, lidocaine, or pramoxine

Vasoconstrictors
Ephedrine, epinephrine, phenylephrine

Anti-Inflammatories
Hydrocortisone

Taking stool softeners or a laxative like psyllium can relieve straining with bowel movements. In addition, moist towelettes containing witch hazel or other ingredients can soothe swollen tissues when used after a bowel movement. Your pharmacist can help you select one of the numerous nonprescription products that are available.

Many nondrug measures can also be used to prevent or treat hemorrhoids. These include increasing fluid intake, regular exercise, and a high fiber diet to prevent constipation and straining. People with hemorrhoids should be encouraged to avoid sitting on the toilet longer than five minutes, to reduce straining and decrease pressure on the hemorrhoidal vessels. In addition, taking warm sitz baths can promote good hygiene and relieve symptoms, especially after bowel movements.

ANAL FISSURE

QUESTION: What can you tell me about a new prescription medication for anal fissure?

ANSWER: The FDA recently approved Rectiv (nitroglycerin) intra-anal ointment for the treatment of moderate to severe pain associated with chronic anal fissure. Approximately 700,000 people in the United States receive a diagnosis of or treatment for an episode of anal fissures each year. An anal fissure is a small tear in the skin that lines the anus, and it can occur in many ways, such as passing large or hard stools, straining during a bowel movement, or following an episode of diarrhea. When an anal fissure occurs, it typically causes severe pain and bleeding with bowel movements. Chronic anal fissure has been shown to significantly affect patients' quality of life. An episode can take 6 to 8 weeks to heal, and if healing does not occur surgery may be required. Rectiv ointment is a prescription medicine that reduces pressure in the anal canal and improves blood flow in this area. In clinical studies it has been shown to significantly reduce the pain associated with chronic anal fissure. Rectiv is applied intra-anally every 12 hours for up to 3 weeks. The most common side effects of Rectiv are headache and dizziness. Rectiv should not be used by people taking medications for erectile dysfunction (such as Viagra, Cialis or Levitra), people with severe anemia (low n umbers of red blood cells), people with high pressure in their skull (for example following head trauma or bleeding in the brain), or those allergic to the ingredients in the ointment. Rectiv is the only FDA approved prescription product for patients with chronic anal fissure pain.

DUPUYTREN'S CONTRACTURE

QUESTION: Can Mederma Gel help someone with Dupuytren's contracture?

ANSWER: Dupuytren's (doo-pa-trens) contracture is a benign condition, which causes a tightening of the flesh beneath the skin of the palm, and can result in permanently bent fingers that are drawn inward towards the palm and wrist. It is a fairly common hereditary disorder that is caused by a progressive thickening and shrinking of the bands of fibrous tissue (fascia), which reinforces the skin of the palm. Fascia looks like a cloth, having fine threads that run lengthwise from the palm to the fingers, and as these threads shorten they produce a curling of the affected fingers that can result in a clawlike hand. Trying to straighten the fingers pulls the shortened the bands taut, and they feel like a wire under the skin, called a cord. This disease is named after Guillaume Dupuytren who was Napoleon's surgeon and lectured on this condition, which has also been referred to as a Viking or Celtic disease. Interestingly, the author of "Peter Pan" was thought to have this disorder, which may have been the idea for Captain Hook's hook, and the Papal Benediction sign, with bent ring and small fingers, may have started with a pope having this condition. Dupuytren's contracture is estimated to affect 3 to 5% of the United States population and is six times more common in men than women. What actually causes this condition is unknown, but numerous enzymes, growth factors, and other body chemicals are involved in this very complex disease process. The treatment of Dupuytren's contracture is dependent upon the extent of the disease and many nonoperative and surgical therapies have been tried. Surgery is usually needed when the hand cannot be placed flat on a table or when the fingers curl so much that hand function is limited. Surgery to remove the diseased fascia is difficult, because it surrounds nerves, blood vessels, and tendons. A minimally invasive treatment known as needle aponeurotomy is also available. Dupuytren's contracture may recur spontaneously, even after surgery. Mederma is a topically applied greaseless gel that is available without prescription to help scars appear softer and smoother. It contains an onion (allium cepa) extract that has been shown to have a variety of medicinal properties and chemical effects in the body. Massage therapy to the affected areas with this onion extract gel product several times a day has been suggested for the treatment of Dupuytren's contracture. However, very little information is available on this subject and Mederma is not approved by the FDA for this use. Onion extract theoretically has some clinical effects that may be beneficial, but I could find no solid scientific clinical information on its use for this disorder. People with Dupuytren's contracture should consult with their physician or a hand specialist to determine what treatment is best for them.

QUESTION: What can you tell me about a new drug for the disease that causes bent fingers?

ANSWER: The FDA recently approved Xiaflex (collagenase) injection to treat Dupuytren's (dū-pwē-trans) contracture, a disorder caused by the buildup of an abnormal amount of collagen in the hands. The collagen builds nodules in the palms of the hand, which eventually causes an internal ropelike cord to form and grow into the fingers, causing them to be bent inward towards the wrist and unable to extend. Prior to Xiaflex, surgery was the only effective treatment of this disorder. The incidence of Dupuytren's contracture disease is highest in Caucasians, particularly those of Northern European descent. Most cases of Dupuytren's contracture occur in patients older than 50 years. The most frequently affected parts of the hand associated with Dupuytren's contracture are the joints called the metacarpophalangeal joint, or MP joint, which is the joint closest to the palm of the hand and the proximal interphalangeal joint, or the PIP joint, which is the middle joint in the finger. The little finger and ring finger are most frequently involved. Xiaflex is injected directly into the collagen cord of the hand and should be administered only by a health care professional experienced with injections of the hand, as tendon ruptures may occur. In one 66 patient study, 44% of those injected with Xiaflex were treated succcssfully, compared to 5% for patients who received a placebo. In another 306 patient study, 64% of patients given Xiaflex were treated successfully, compared to only 7% of patients receiving the placebo. The most common adverse reactions in patients treated with Xiaflex were fluid build up, swelling, bleeding, and pain in the injected area. Although no serious allergic reactions have been observed, such a response would not be unexpected because this foreign protein could prompt an immune system reaction. For information and questions on Xiaflex, patients and physicians can contact the manufacturer (Auxilium Pharmaceuticals) at 1-877-XIAFLEX.

NEURONTIN (GABAPENTIN)

QUESTION: I had a pain prescription filled for the drug Neurontin, but the information that came with it said it was for convulsions. I'm confused—what can you tell me about this medication?

ANSWER: Neurontin (generic name gabapentin) is currently approved to treat two conditions: epilepsy and postherpetic neuralgia. It has a long been used in combination with other drugs to treat various types of seizures in people with epilepsy. In 2002 it was also approved to treat pain following shingles (herpes zoster) in adults, which can be very difficult to treat in many people. How Neurontin works in the treatment of these disorders is not known. Gabapentin is an amino acid that is similar to a brain chemical known as gamma-aminobutyric acid or GABA that is involved in the conduction of nerve impulses within the central nervous system. It has been found to have many effects in the body and has been used in a number of conditions including multiple sclerosis, nerve-related pain (neuropathic pain), bipolar disorder, prevention of migraine headaches, dementia-related behavior problems, Parkinson's disease, hot flashes, panic disorder, ALS (Lou Gehrig disease) and many others. Since the treatment of these disorders is not approved by the FDA, they are known as "off-label" uses of Neurontin (gabapentin). There is some clinical study documentation that Neurontin may be effective in several of these conditions, and in others there may be very little documentation. It is up to the prescribing physician to decide if Neurontin may be useful in each individual patient situation. However, when you get your prescription filled, only information regarding FDA approved indications for Neurontin will be provided by your pharmacy in most situations.

NEUROPATHIC PAIN

QUESTION: I heard about a new drug for nerve pain in people with diabetes or shingles. What can you tell me about it?

ANSWER: The FDA recently approved Lyrica (pregabalin) for the treatment of nerve (neuropathic) pain that is caused by diabetes or herpes zoster (shingles). It was also approved for treating certain types of epilepsy in combination with other anti-epileptic drugs. Neuropathic pain is cause d by damage to sensory nerves that results from underlying conditions such as diabetes or shingles and the pain can be severe. Nearly one-half of Americans with diabetes will develop some form of this painful disorder over the course of their disease. The pain from this condition, known as diabetic neuropathy, is different from arthritis or muscle pain and is often described as burning, tingling, sharp stabbing, or pins and needles in the feet, legs, hands or arm. Herpes zoster or shingles produces painful skin lesions and is caused by the reactivation of the chickenpox virus later in life. Pain due to shingles is known as postherpetic neuralgia and is often described as constant stabbing, burning, or electric shock-like sensations. It is the most common complication of shingles, and an estimated 150,000 Americans develop this problem each year. How Lyrica works to relieve pain in these disorders is not exactly known, but it appears to block nerve conduction in over-excited nerve cells.

The most common side effects of Lyrica include dizziness, sleepiness, dry mouth, edema, blurred vision, weight gain, and difficulty with concentration or attention. People taking this medication need to be cautioned against operating machinery or driving due to these side effects. Lyrica is very similar to another medication, Neurontin (gabapentin), which is also used for treating some of these same disorders. Lyrica is taken orally 2 or 3 times a day depending upon the condition, and its dose needs to be adjusted in people with impaired kidney function.

DENGUE FEVER

QUESTION: I recently returned from a trip to the Dominican Republic with Dengue fever. What can I do to treat this?

ANSWER: Dengue (den-gay) fever is a common problem worldwide in tropical and sub-tropical areas including Caribbean regions like the Dominican Republic and Puerto Rico. It is caused by a virus that is transmitted by mosquitoes. After an incubation period of about 2 to 7 days, the typical patient experiences a sudden onset of high fever, chills, headache, and severe generalized body, joint, and muscle aches. These aches are often so painful that the disease has been called "break-bone fever". In addition, a body rash similar to measles can develop in about one-half of people afflicted with Dengue fever. Other symptoms may occur including loss of appetite, nausea, vomiting, and skin sensitivity. Children with this illness may have a more mild illness with low fever, fatigue, runny nose, and cough. Dengue fever usually lasts about one week and is nonfatal. However a more severe form of this illness, which involves bleeding, is possible in some people and can be fatal. Prevention is the best therapy for this disorder, including the use of insect repellants containing 20-30% DEET and avoidance of mosquitoes during peak periods of the day (dawn and dusk). While no specific treatment is available for Dengue fever, acetaminophen (Tylenol, etc.) preparations may be helpful for pain and fever. Aspirin and non-steroidal anti-inflammatory medications should be avoided because of the potential for bleeding or the development of Reye's syndrome in children. Antihistamines like diphenhydramine (Benadryl) may be useful for itching if a rash develops. Patients should rest, drink plenty of fluids, and consult a physician. Ask your physician and pharmacist about what nonprescription or prescription medications may be helpful in your specific situation. Also, be sure to read all package labeling carefully and follow their instructions accordingly.

RESTLESS LEG SYNDROME

QUESTION: I heard about a new drug for restless leg syndrome. What can you tell me about it?

ANSWER: The FDA recently approved Requip (ropinirole) for the treatment of restless legs syndrome. It is the first and only medication that has been approved for this disorder. Requip has been available since 1997 to treat Parkinson's disease, but the treatment of restless leg syndrome is a new indication for this medication. Restless leg syndrome is a relatively common problem that affects up to 10% of American adults and is more common in women and people over the age of 50. About one-third or more of people with this syndrome also have family members with this problem. Individuals with this disorder have a compelling urge to move their legs when sitting still or when lying in bed before going to sleep. During sleep, the legs may move spontaneously and uncontrollably, which can cause the person to wake-up. In addition, people with restless leg syndrome may have uncomfortable or sometimes painful sensations in the legs often described as creeping-crawling, tingling, pulling, or tightening. Walking or moving the legs can temporarily relieve these symptoms, but they can significantly disrupt a patient's sleep and daily activities. The cause of this neurological disorder is unknown, but researchers believe that it may be related to a chemical known as dopamine, that carries the signals between nerve cells that control body movement. Requip is thought to work by stimulating dopamine receptors in the brain. During clinical studies, the most common side effects of Requip were nausea, sleepiness, vomiting, dizziness, and fatigue.

QUESTION: I take Requip for restless legs syndrome. Is there a generic available?

ANSWER: Yes, the FDA recently approved the first generic versions of Requip (ropinirole) tablets for the treatment of restless legs syndrome. The labeling of the generic versions of ropinirole hydrochloride may differ from that of Requip because some uses of the drug are protected by patents. In addition to treating restless legs syndrome, Requip is also FDA-approved to treat symptoms of Parkinson's disease. The generic products are not approved for treatment of Parkinson's disease because this indication is protected by patent. Manufacturers of the generic drugs may seek approval for that use once the patent for the Parkinson's disease indication expires later this year. The generic ropinirole hydrochloride tablets will have the same safety warnings as Requip, cautioning about patient reports of falling asleep while engaged in activities of daily living, including while driving. Although many of these patients reported sleepiness while on the drug, some patients perceived that they had no warning signs and believed that they were alert immediately prior to falling asleep. Some of these events have been reported as late as one year after the start of treatment.

As I've noted many times before, the FDA approves all generic drugs using strict guidelines, including checking for the generic drug's chemistry by evaluating its formulation, potency, stability, and purity. The generic drug must also pass bio-equivalency testing that compares the delivery into the bloodstream of the generic drug's active ingredient to that of the brand name drug. Generic drugs are less expensive than brand-name products, and account for about 56% of prescriptions dispensed.

QUESTION: What drugs are used to treat the restless legs syndrome?

ANSWER: Non-drug therapy of the restless legs syndrome includes a reduction or elimination of caffeine and alcohol use, in addition to smoking cessation. Massaging or raising the legs, using a vibrator, leg movement exercises, and walking around can also be helpful in some people with this problem. If these measures do not help, prescription drug therapy can be initiated. The type of drug utilized is based upon the severity of the symptoms with more potent medications used for severe cases. Patients with mild restless legs syndrome may benefit from drugs known as benzodiazepines (e.g. Klonapin, Valium, Restoril, or Halcion) or opiods (e.g. codeine). People with moderate to severe symptoms and disruptive sleep may have the anti-Parkinson's drug ropinirole (Requip) or pramipexole (Mirapex) prescribed. If these agents are not effective, other drugs might prove helpful including some anticonvulsant medications or a drug called clonidine (Catapres). In addition, some patients may respond better to combination therapy. Your physician can determine what therapy is best for you.

QUESTION: I have restless leg syndrome. Can the Prilosec that I take for heartburn make my restless leg syndrome worse?

ANSWER: Although more research is needed, it may be possible that drugs like Prilosec (omeprazole) could make the symptoms of your restless leg syndrome (RLS) worse. Prilosec (omeprazole) is one of a group of drugs known as proton pump inhibitors or PPIs. These drugs are very effective in treating "heartburn" or gastroesophageal reflux

5

disease (GERD) because they block the production of stomach acid. However in doing so, PPIs may also reduce the amount of iron absorbed from the foods that we eat and from supplements that we take. To be properly absorbed in our gastrointestinal tract, iron has to be broken down by the acid in our stomach and some studies indicate that RLS may be associated with iron deficiency in certain people. While the exact cause of RLS is unknown, it may be related to a chemical in the body known as dopamine that is important in controlling body movement. Iron is essential for the production of dopamine, and it has been suggested that iron deficiency may play a role in RLS. Therefore, there may be an association between PPI use, low iron stores in the body, and RLS, but more study needed. In addition to Prilosec (omeprazole), other PPI medications include AcipHex (rabeprazole); Kapidex (dexlansoprazole); Nexium (esomeprazole); Prevacid (Lansoprazole); Protonix (pantoprazole); and Zegerid (omeprazole/ sodium bicarbonate).

QUESTION: I heard that a new drug was approved for the treatment of restless legs syndrome. What can you tell me about it?

ANSWER: The FDA recently approved Horizant (gabapentin enacarbil) for the treatment of adults with restless legs syndrome (RLS). Horizant is an extended-release tablet formulation that is taken orally once a day with food at about 5 PM. Horizant is converted into gabapentin, an anti-seizure drug, after it is absorbed by the body. Exactly how Horizant helps in the treatment of RLS is not known. The most common side effects of Horizant include sleepiness/ sedation and dizziness. Because of this, Horizant can impair one's ability to operate complex machinery and cause significant driving impairment. Patients being treated with this medication should not drive until they have gained sufficient experience to assess whether it impairs their ability to drive. In addition, like other drugs used to treat seizures in people with epilepsy, Horizant's labeling contains a warning that it may cause suicidal thoughts and actions in a small number of people.

AGE-RELATED MACULAR DEGENERATION (AMD)

QUESTION: I heard about a new drug to treat age-related macular degeneration. What can you tell me about it?

ANSWER: The FDA recently approved a new drug therapy to help slow vision loss in people with the eye disease known as neovascular (wet) age-related macular degeneration or AMD. AMD occurs when the central part of the eye's retina, known as the macula, is damaged. This can lead to severe, irreversible loss of vision and is the leading cause of severe vision loss in people over the age of 50. There are two types of AMD, wet and dry. Dry AMD is the most common form, representing about 90% of all cases of AMD. However, dry AMD accounts for only 10% of the severe vision loss associated with this disease. There is no generally accepted treatment for dry AMD, although vitamins, antioxidants, and zinc supplements may slow its progression. Over time, dry AMD cases often develop into wet AMD. Wet AMD occurs when abnormal blood vessels start to grow under the center of your retina. These new blood vessels may be very fragile and often leak blood and fluid, which can damage your macula or create a scar on your retina, causing vision problems. The vision loss may be permanent, because abnormal blood vessels and scar tissue actually replace normal retina tissue. An early symptom of wet AMD is vision change, when straight lines appear wavy. Wet AMD can lead to a rapid loss of central vision that impairs activities such as recognizing faces, reading, driving a car, crossing streets, or basic tasks. An estimated 2 million people in the U.S. currently have wet AMD, with an increase of 200,000 new cases each year. This number is expected to increase as the baby boomer generation ages.

The new drug that was approved for the treatment of wet AMD is named Macugen (pegaptanib). It is the first in a new class of ophthalmic drugs that acts to block the abnormal blood vessel growth and leakage of blood and fluids within the eye. Mucugen is given by intravitreal injection once every 6 weeks. Studies have shown that patients treated with Macugen show a significant decrease in vision loss when receiving the drug for 1 year. However, the drug appears to be less effective during the second year of treatment and its effectiveness beyond 2 years has not been shown.

QUESTION: I heard about a new drug that improves vision in people with age-related macular degeneration (AMD). What can you tell me about it?

ANSWER: The FDA recently approved Lucentis (ranibizumab) for the treatment of neovascular (wet) age-related macular degeneration, the leading cause of blindness in people over the age of 55. It is the first drug shown to actually help improve the vision of people with AMD. Lucentis works in a similar way to Macugen (pegatanib), which has been available since 2005 to treat wet AMD. Both of these drugs inhibit the growth of blood vessels when injected into the eye. During clinical studies, both Lucentis and Macugen have demonstrated that they can slow the progression of vision loss in people with wet AMD. However, clinical studies with Lucentis have also shown that 34-40% of patients receiving this drug experienced a significant improvement in vision during 12 months of treatment. Lucentis is given by intravitreal injection once a month.

QUESTION: I heard that a new drug was approved for age-related macular degeneration. What can you tell me about it?

ANSWER: The new drug that was approved for the treatment of wet AMD is named Eylea (aflibercept). It belongs to a new class of ophthalmic drugs that act in a complex way to block abnormal blood vessel growth and leakage of blood and fluids within the eye. Other similar drugs include Macugen and Lucentis. Studies have shown that patients treated with Eylea had a significant improvement in visual acuity when treated over a 52-week period. Eylea is given by intravitreal injection once a month for the first 3 months and then once every 2 months after that.

MULTIPLE SCLEROSIS

QUESTION: I heard about a new drug for multiple sclerosis. What can you tell me about it?

ANSWER: The FDA recently approved Tysabri (natalizumab), which is a new type of treatment for multiple sclerosis (MS). About 400,000 people in the U.S. are afflicted with this disorder, which most commonly affects young adults between the ages of 20 and 40 and is twice as common in females compared to males. The term "multiple sclerosis" refers to the many areas of scarring (sclerosis) that results when nerves in the eyes, brain, and spinal cord are damaged or destroyed by this disease. Most people with MS have periods of relatively good health, which alternates with debilitating flare-ups or relapses and the disorder often worsens over time. The cause of MS is not known, but it may be due to a virus (or something else) that triggers a reaction against the body's own tissues early in life. This reaction, which is called an autoimmune reaction, results in inflammation and damage or destruction of nerves. Heredity may also play a role and about 5% of people with MS have a brother or sister who is affected and another 15% have a close relative with this disorder. A person's environment during their first 15 years of life also appears to play a role, with many more people developing MS who grew up in a temperate climate compared to a tropical climate. Symptoms of MS may include vision problems, loss of balance, numbness, difficulty walking, paralysis, psychological problems, and many other adverse effects. The treatment of MS can include corticosteroids, interferon injections, and other immunosuppressive drugs to try and prevent the body's immune system from attacking nerves. Many other drugs are used to control symptoms of this disease. The newly approved drug Tysabri works in a different way. It appears to prevent inflamed immune cells from escaping from the bloodstream into the brain where they cause damage to nerve fibers and their insulation (Myelin). During clinical studies, Tysabri reduced the number of patient relapses with MS by 54-66%. The drug is given intravenously every 4 weeks and seems to be more effective than many other treatments. Tysabri is also being studied for its potential use in Crohns disease, ulcerative colitis, and rheumatoid arthritis. (**Please see next column**).

QUESTION: Why was the new drug for multiple sclerosis that you wrote about a few weeks ago taken off the market?

ANSWER: The makers of Tysabri, a new drug to treat multiple sclerosis (MS) announced that they were voluntarily suspending sales of the drug as of Monday, February 23, 2005. This decision was made after one patient died and another patient developed a serious disease of the central nervous system known as progressive multifocal leukoencephalopathy or PML for short. PML is a rare and frequently fatal disease that primarily affects people with weakened immune systems. It is believed to be caused by activation of a virus that resides in a dormant state in up to 80% of healthy adults. How the virus is activated is not known. Both of these patients had been taking Tysabri for more than 2 years in combination with Avonex (interferon), another drug used to treat MS. Tysabri was also being studied for use in the treatment of Crohns disease, ulcerative colitis, and rheumatoid arthritis. Its use in these clinical studies was also suspended. The manufacturers of Tysabri are convening an expert panel to try and better understand the potential risk of PMI in patients receiving Tysabri, with hopes that they can resume marketing of this new drug in the future. The withdrawal of this drug within a month after its approval by the FDA points out the difficulty in identifying rare side effects during initial clinical studies. Tysabri was used in about 3,000 patients in clinical trials of MS, Crohns disease, and rheumatoid arthritis. However, reports of PML did not show up until the drug was approved and made available for use in many more patients and for longer periods of time.

PLEASE NOTE: In June 2006, the FDA allowed Tysarbi to be made available in a restricted-distribution system called TOUCH (Tysarbi Outreach: Unified Commitment to Health). The drug manufacturers Biogen and Elan developed this system. Doctors, patients, and pharmacies must register with TOUCH and agree to abide by the program's provisions before Tysarbi can be prescribed and administered at authorized infusion centers. In February 2010, the FDA warned the public that the risk of developing progressive multifocal leukoencephalopathy (PML), a rare but serious brain infection associated with the use of Tysabri (natalizumab), increases with the number of Tysabri infusions received. This new safety information, based on reports of 31 confirmed cases of PML received by the FDA as of January 21, 2010, will now be included in the Tysabri drug label and patient Medication Guide.

QUESTION: What can you tell me about the new drug for multiple sclerosis?

ANSWER: The FDA recently approved Ampyra (dalfampridine) to improve walking in people with multiple sclerosis (MS). Ampyra is known as a potassium channel blocker that improves nerve conduction and function. It is taken orally as a 10 mg extended-release tablet twice a day, approximately 12 hours apart. In clinical studies, Ampyra was shown to significantly improve the walking ability (both distance and speed) of MS patients compared to a "dummy" pill (placebo). The most common adverse events reported in clinical trials were urinary tract infection, insomnia, dizziness, headache, nausea, weakness, back pain, balance disorder, swelling in the nose or throat, constipation, diarrhea, indigestion, throat pain, and burning, tingling, or itching of skin. However, given at doses greater than recommended, Ampyra can cause seizures. Multiple sclerosis is a chronic, usually progressive disease in which the immune system attacks and degrades the function of nerve fibers in the brain and spinal cord. More than 400,000 Americans have MS. Most people living with MS are diagnosed between the ages of 20 and 50, and women are affected two to three times more often than men. Worldwide, MS may affect an estimated 2.5 million people. Research indicates 64%-85% of people with MS have difficulty walking, and 70% of people with MS who have difficulty walking report it to be the most challenging aspect of their MS. Within 15 years of an MS diagnosis, 50% of people with MS often require assistance walking and, in later stages, up to a one third are unable to walk. Ampyra will be sold through a network of specialty pharmacies coordinated by the manufacturer (Acorda Therapeutics). If you have additional questions about this product please call Ampyra Support services at 1-888-881-1918.

QUESTION: I heard that a new oral drug for multiple sclerosis might be approved soon. What can you tell me about this?

ANSWER: In June 2010, an FDA advisory committee voted to recommend approval of Gilenya (fingolimod) as a first-line treatment for relapsing multiple sclerosis (MS). Gilenya is the first in its class of oral MS drugs recommended for approval and a final decision regarding its approval is expected by the end of 2010. While not fully understood, Gilenya is thought to work in a complex way on the body's immune system. The availability of oral agents to treat relapsing MS in anxiously anticipated, especially for those patients with a fear of injections or for those who have not responded to, or who are unable to tolerate current therapies. In clinical studies, MS patients treated with oral Gilenya had significantly lower relapse rates, a longer time to first relapse, were more likely to be relapse-free for a 24-month period, and had fewer new or enlarged brain lesions compared to MS patients receiving a dummy pill (placebo). In addition, when compared with interferon injection (a widely used drug for MS), MS patients treated with Gilenya had a lower relapse rate, prolonged time to disability progression, and fewer new or enlarged brain lesions after 12 months of treatment. The most common side effects of Gilenya in clinical studies were fatigue, infections, back pain, diarrhea, cough, abnormal liver function, and hyperpigmentation of the skin. Additional oral agents for the treatment of MS are also being studied.

MS affects about 400,000 people in the United States. There are four basic presentations of MS, the most common being the relapsing form. The exact cause of MS is unknown, but what is known is that the myelin sheath, an insulating cover surrounding nerve axons, is damaged by an immune action leading to damage to the brain and spinal cord. This damage, which can be seen on MRI scans as a lesion, leads to visual disturbances, muscle weakness, coordination difficulties, and memory and cognition problems. It most commonly occurs in people ages 20-40, and affects women 2 to 3 times more often than men. Common complaints include weakness, fatigue, pain, bladder and bowel problems, as well as balance, visual, and other sensory disturbances. There is no cure for MS. The strategies for treating MS include: reducing the number of attacks, reducing the number of lesions observed in MRI scans, slowing the progression of disability, and improving the speed of recovery.

PLEASE NOTE: Gilenya was approved for the treatment of multiple sclerosis by the FDA in September 2010. After a safety review by the FDA in May 2012, Gilenya is now contraindicated in patients with certain pre-existing or recent heart conditions or stroke, or who are taking certain antiarrhythmic medications. Patients taking Gilenya should contact their healthcare professional and seek immediate care if they develop dizziness, tiredness, irregular heartbeat, or palpitations which are signs of a slowing heart rate.

CARPAL TUNNEL SYNDROME

QUESTION: I have been diagnosed with carpal tunnel syndrome. Are there any treatments for this problem other than surgery?

ANSWER: Carpal tunnel syndrome is a painful condition that is caused by compression of the median nerve, which is located on the palm side of the wrist (this area is referred to as the carpal tunnel). The compression of the nerve is due to swelling and bands of fibrous tissue that occur due to a variety of reasons. This disorder is more common in women and may affect one or both hands. People at risk for this problem include those who do not position their computer keyboard properly and those whose work requires repeated forceful movements with the wrist extended. Prolonged exposure to vibrations from certain power tools has also been implicated. Some drugs have also been associated with the development of carpal tunnel syndrome, including beta blockers (Inderal, propranolol, Lopressor, metoprolol, others) and Valium (diazepam), but their relationship to this disorder is unclear. In addition, pregnant women and people who have diabetes, an under-active thyroid gland, gout, or rheumatoid arthritis are at increased risk for this syndrome. Symptoms of carpal tunnel syndrome include odd sensations, numbness, tingling, and pain in the first three fingers on the thumb side of the hand, or the arm and shoulder. The pain may be worse at night because of the way the hand is positioned.

The best treatment of carpal tunnel syndrome is to avoid activities and positions that overextend the wrist or put pressure on the median nerve. The use of wrist splints (especially at night) and adjusting the angle of the computer keyboard can be very helpful. Anti-inflammatory drugs like aspirin, ibuprofen (Motrin, Advil), or naproxen (Aleve) may be beneficial for some patients. Injections of corticosteroids into the carpal tunnel can bring long-lasting relief to others with this disorder. If these measures do not help, surgery in which fibrous tissue is removed may be the best way to relieve pressure in the affected nerve and provide pain relief. Your doctor can advise you on the best way to treat your carpal tunnel symptoms.

PULMONARY ARTERIAL HYPERTENSION

QUESTION: I've heard that the medicine in Viagra is now used to treat another medical problem. What can you tell me about this?

ANSWER: The FDA recently approved a new medication named Revatio to treat a rare medical problem known as pulmonary arterial hypertension or PAH. The active ingredient in Revatio is sildenafil, which is also the active ingredient in the erectile dysfunction drug Viagra. Pulmonary arterial hypertension is a rare, aggressive and life-shortening vascular disease. It is caused by dangerously high pressure in the blood vessels that go from the heart to the lungs. Symptoms of PAH include difficulty breathing, dizziness, and fatigue. If this condition is left untreated, patients have an average survival time of less than 3 years from the time of diagnosis. It is estimated that PAH affects approximately 100,000 people in the world. This new treatment is the first oral treatment for PAH to be approved for patients with an early stage of the disease. Studies have shown that it reduces arterial hypertension, improves heart function, and increases the exercise capability of patients. Revatio works in the same way as Viagra does to relax and expand blood vessels. However, its smooth muscle relaxing effects for treating PAH are more important in the pulmonary blood vessels as opposed to the blood vessels in the penis, which is important for Viagra's effectiveness in erectile dysfunction. Revatio is taken in a dosage of 20 mg three times a day for the treatment of PAH. The

Revatio 20 mg tablet is white and round to distinguish it from Viagra's blue diamond-shaped tablet for erectile dysfunction.

SPORTS INJURIES

QUESTION: I like to play softball. What can I do for minor injuries?

ANSWER: More than 10 million people are treated for sports injuries each year in the U.S. The most common types of sports injuries are bruises, sprains, and strains. Sprains are caused by the stretching or tearing of the ligaments that connect bones to each other, while strains are caused by the stretching or tearing of muscles or tendons. The initial treatment of acute sports injuries is aimed at reducing pain and swelling and preventing further damage to the injured area. The most common recommended treatment is known as PRICE therapy, which stands for Protection, Rest, Ice, Compression, and Elevation. This therapy works best if started as soon as possible after the injury, preferably within 10 to 15 minutes. The injured area should be protected against further injury. Devices like slings, splints, canes, or crutches may be helpful depending upon the injured area. The injured part should also be rested to prevent further injury and allow for healing. Ice helps to stop swelling. A simple way to apply ice to the injured area is to wrap the ice in a damp towel or cloth and place it on the injured area. In general, ice should not be applied for more than 15-30 minutes at a time to prevent tissue damage and this can be repeated every 2 hours while you are awake. You can also use a bag of frozen vegetables wrapped in a damp towel. Compression decreases swelling and supports the injured area. The most common way to apply compression to the injured part is to use an elastic bandage or wrap, such as an Ace bandage. The compression wrapping should be snug, but not so tight that it cuts off circulation. The injured part should also be elevated as far above the heart as possible, as soon as possible and kept elevated as much as possible for the first 72 hours following injury. In addition, nonprescription pain relievers can be helpful. For many years, experts have recommended the use of nonsteroidal anti-inflammatory drugs (NSAIDs) like ibuprofen. However, now more and more experts recommend using acetaminophen (Tylenol) instead. Be sure to read package labels for these products carefully for proper dose, possible side effects, and potential for drug interactions. Aspirin is usually not recommended because it can increase the risk of bleeding. Medical attention is needed for head injuries, more severe sports injuries, when symptoms persist for more than 2 weeks despite PRICE therapy and medications, if symptoms get worse, if you think you might have broken a bone, if you cannot move or put weight on an injured joint, or if you are unsure about the seriousness of the injury or how to care for it.

QUESTION: I heard that a prescription patch was approved to treat sports injuries. What can you tell me about it?

ANSWER: The FDA recently approved Flector Patch for the topical treatment of acute pain due to minor strains, sprains, and contusions. It is the first prescription patch approved in the U.S. for this type of topical treatment. The Flector Patch contains diclofenac, a non-steroidal anti-inflammatory drug (NSAID) that reduces pain and inflammation due to an injury when applied directly to intact skin. Since diclofenac is released from the patch directly to the injured area, less of the drug is absorbed into the bloodstream, which reduces its potential for side effects. One patch is applied to the most painful area twice daily. It should not be applied to damaged or non-intact skin and should not be worn when bathing or showering. During clinical studies, the most common side effects of Flector Patch were application site conditions such as itching, rash, burning, etc. and gastrointestinal problems such as nausea. However, other side effects can occur so be sure to read the information supplied with your prescription.

Soft tissue injuries, such as sprains, strains, and contusions, are a common occurrence associated with sports activities. Sprains are a traumatic stretching of ligament possibly with a partial or total tear, whereas strains involve the fibrous membrane that covers and supports muscles or muscle tendons. Contusions (bruises) are caused by a sudden forceful blow to body tissue. When soft tissue is acutely injured, an inflammatory reaction occurs, resulting in swelling and pain. NSAIDs are commonly used short-term to treat this pain and inflammation.

TINNITUS (EAR NOISES)

<u>QUESTION</u>: Is there anything available to treat constant tinnitus?

<u>ANSWER</u>: Tinnitus, or abnormal ear noise, is usually described as sounding like steam escaping from a small pipe, ringing, roaring, pulsating, chirping (crickets), whistling, blowing, or humming in the ear. Some people learn to cope with this problem, while others suffer all the time. Sleepiness, chronic fatigue, depression, and personality changes are commonly reported in people who cannot tolerate their ear noises. The exact cause of tinnitus can be very difficult to determine, but it is usually associated with a hearing loss. Some of the causes of tinnitus include exposure to high noise levels; infections of the ear, head, neck, and teeth; various ear or nerve disorders; a variety of foods; and certain drugs. Some of the foods associated with tinnitus are coffee, wine, tea, cheese, chocolate, and grain based spirits. Drugs that can cause this problem include certain antibiotics known as aminoglycosides (e.g., gentamicin, tobramycin), some diuretics (e.g., Lasix or furosemide), salicylates like aspirin, quinidine for heart rhythm problems, quinine for leg cramps, NSAIDs like ibuprofen or naproxen, and others.

The treatment of tinnitus depends upon the cause. If it is due to an infection, then the infection must be treated. If it is caused by a drug or food that can be identified, then these need to be eliminated if possible. Sometimes relief of tinnitus may be obtained by "masking" it with background music or other sounds that are more pleasant to listen to than the tinnitus. Hearing aids or biofeedback techniques may also be helpful. Other treatments that have been tried with varying success include the use of gingko biloba, injections of local anesthetic drugs like lidocaine, anticonvulsant drugs, antihistamines, sedatives, and vitamin B-12. Non-prescription eardrops are not effective and are not recommended for the treatment of tinnitus. Unfortunately, sometimes nothing will help. You need to get a thorough medical examination and evaluation to determine the cause of your constant tinnitus and its appropriate treatment.

<u>QUESTION</u>: Can some medications cause ringing in the ears?

<u>ANSWER</u>: Yes, there are several medications that can cause ringing in the ears, or tinnitus. It has been estimated that some 36 million Americans suffer from tinnitus, many of whom with symptoms severe enough to disrupt concentration, interrupt sleep, or even cause depression or anxiety. Tinnitus, or abnormal ear noise, may be described as ringing, chirping, humming, or buzzing by those who suffer from this problem. Two well-known causes of tinnitus are age-related hearing loss and damage to specialized cells, called hair cells, which line the inner ear and detect sound waves. Certain medical conditions and unhealthy habits such as smoking, too much caffeine or alcohol can also cause tinnitus. Some of the more common types of medications that can cause tinnitus are listed on the next page:

Drug Type
Example (Generic Name, Trade Name)
- **Antibiotics**
  Gentamicin (Garamycin)
  Neomycin
  Tobramycin (Nebcin)
  Streptomycin
- **Antidepressants**
  Amitriptyline (Pamelor, Aventyl)
  Nortriptyline
- **ACE inhibitors**
  Captopril (Capoten)
  Ramipril (Altace)
- **Diuretics**
  Bumetanide (Bumex)
  Furosemide (Lasix)
- **Anti-cancer drugs**
  Cisplatin (Platinol-AQ)
  Paclitaxel (Taxol, Onxol)
- **Heart medications**
  Nifedipine (Procardia, Adalat, others)
  Quinidine
  Propranolol (Inderal)
  Verapamil (Calan, Isoptin, Verelan, others)

- **Anti-Parkinson's drugs**
  Levodopa (Larodopa, Sinemet)
- **Pain relievers**
  Aspirin
  Ibuprofen (Motrin, Advil, others)
  Naproxen (Naprosyn, Anaprox, Aleve, others)
- **Vitamin**
  Vitamin A

HEEL SPURS

QUESTION: What can I do for a heel spur?

ANSWER: Heel spurs (plantar fascitis) are growths of extra bone at the heel and can be caused by excessive pulling on the heel bone by tendons or connective tissue attached to the bone. People with "flatfeet" (abnormal flatness of the sole and arch of the feet) have an increased risk of heel spurs. Heel spurs can be very painful when they are developing, especially when walking. Sometimes the area around the heel spur can become inflamed causing a throbbing pain. Sports activities can also aggravate a heel spur. In some cases the foot can adapt to the spur and the pain can actually decrease as the spur gets larger. A physician or podiatrist can usually diagnose heel spurs during a physical examination and x-rays can confirm diagnosis. The treatment of heel spurs is aimed at relieving the pain and inflammation. Rest, ice, and nonpresecription anti-inflammatory pain relievers such as ibuprofen (Motrin, Advil) or naproxen (Aleve) may be helpful. Periodic stretching of the calf muscles can also be useful. In addition, wrapping the arch with padding and using comfortable shoe inserts or orthotics can provide relief. In some cases injections of corticosteroids and local anesthetic agents into the painful area of the heel may be needed. Surgery may be an option in severe cases, but most painful heel spurs resolve without surgery. Your podiatrist or physician can help determine which treatment is best for you.

BIPOLAR DISORDER

QUESTION: I heard about a new drug for bipolar disorder. What can you tell me about it?

ANSWER: The FDA has approved the drug Equetro for the treatment of acute manic episodes associated with bipolar disorder. Equetro is an extended-release capsule that contains carbamazepine, which has been used since 1997 for the treatment of epilepsy and trigeminal neuralgia. Bipolar disorder is one of the six leading mental health disorders worldwide. It is estimated that each year more than 2 million American adults, or about 1% of the population aged 18 years and older, are afflicted with bipolar disorder, also known as manic depression. This disorder is characterized by episodes of mania and depression, with periods of normal mood in between. It can have devastating effects on an individual's life, although proper diagnosis and early treatment can usually alter the course of the illness. It is not known exactly how Equetro works in the treatment of bipolar disorder, but it does alter nerve transmission and various chemical activities in the brain. Common side effects of Equetro include dizziness, sleepiness, nausea, vomiting, and lack of coordination. However, serious blood disorders can rarely occur and it can cause fetal harm in pregnant women. In addition, numerous troublesome drug interactions are possible. Equetro is given twice daily in adults with acute manic episodes of bipolar disorder. Some other drugs used for this disorder include lithium (Eskalith), the anticonvulsant valproic acid (Depakote, Depakene), olanzapine (Zyprexa), quetiapine (Seroquel), and risperidone (Risperdal)

QUESTION: I heard about a new combination drug for bipolar depression. What can you tell me about it?

ANSWER: A new combination prescription drug was recently approved by the FDA for the treatment of depressive episodes associated with bipolar disorder. The product is called Symbyax and it contains two drugs that alter chemicals in the brain. The two drugs in Symbyax have been available for some time, olanzapine (Zyprexa) and fluoxetine (Prozac). How they work in combination to reduce depression in people with bipolar disorder is not known, but several brain chemicals are affected including serotonin, norepinephrine, and dopamine. Symbyax is taken as a single capsule once daily in the evening.

Bipolar disorder, which used to be called manic-depressive illness, is a complicated mental illness in which patients have debilitating mood swings that range from deep depression and feelings of extreme guilt, sadness, anxiety, and sometimes suicidal thoughts to episodes of mania with abnormal euphoria, elation, and irritability. In between these mood swings everything can be normal. Patients with bipolar disorder spend about three times longer in the depressive state than in the manic phase and it takes longer to recover from it. The depressive state is associated with a higher mortality rate. It is estimated that one in four people with bipolar depression will attempt suicide at least once and the risk of suicide is 35 times greater than for patients in the manic phase. It has been estimated that almost 10 million Americans have bipolar disorder. Symbyax is the first FDA-approved medication to treat bipolar depression, which is very difficult to treat.

NASAL POLYPS

QUESTION: What medications are used to treat nasal polyps?

ANSWER: Nasal polyps are inflamed fleshy outgrowths of the mucous membrane of the nose that usually develop in the area where the sinuses open into the nasal cavity. A polyp is shaped like a tear drop when it's developing and looks like a peeled, seedless grape when it's mature. Sinuses are hollow cavities in the bones around the nose. When polyps develop in this "paranasal" area they may block drainage from the sinuses and cause nasal congestion and/or sinus infections. Large polyps can prevent nasal breathing and force someone to breath through their mouth. They can also cause headaches, facial pain, and a reduced sense of smell. The exact cause of nasal polyps is not known and there are many theories about polyp formation. Some people believe that they result from allergies or chronic sinus infections. The medical treatment of nasal polyps usually involves the use of nasal spray or drops containing corticosteroids, which can help to reduce inflammation and shrink the polyps to relieve nasal obstruction. Some examples of nasal corticosteroids include Flonase (fluticasone), Nasonex (mometasone), and Rhinocort (budesonide). Oral corticosteroids like prednisone can also be used, but they are associated with more side effects. Unfortunately, in some cases the effects of corticosteroids is short lasting and polyps frequently re-grow. Antibiotics are used when a sinus infection is present. In many cases, the most effective treatment for nasal blockage due to polyps is surgical removal and an ear, nose, and throat (ENT) doctor must be consulted.

IRON DEFICIENCY ANEMIA

QUESTION: Will iron tablets help me if I'm anemic?

ANSWER: If your anemia is due to a deficiency of iron, oral iron supplements can be an effective treatment. There are many types of anemia, but iron deficiency anemia is the most common form of anemia. Anemia is a condition in which the number of red blood cells or amount of hemoglobin in them is below normal. Red blood cells contain hemoglobin, which enables them to carry oxygen from the lungs and deliver it to all parts of the body. Iron deficiency anemia results from a lack of iron in the body, which is needed to make hemoglobin. Normally we obtain iron from our diet, and it is absorbed and stored for future use. If there is not enough iron in our body due to a poor diet, poor absorption of iron, or a loss of iron because of bleeding, iron stores can become low causing anemia. The anemia will eventually lead to symptoms such as fatigue, shortness of breath, pale skin, irritability, dizziness, fast heart rate, an inability to exercise, and other symptoms. The diagnosis of iron deficiency anemia is made by measuring the amount of hemoglobin and red blood cells in the blood. Blood tests that measure levels of iron can also be used to diagnose iron deficiency anemia. In addition, tests for blood in the stool or urine may be performed to check for bleeding. Pregnant women are at risk for iron deficiency anemia because more iron is needed to support the growth of their baby. Menstruating women are also at greater risk due to increased iron loss through bleeding. Children and teenagers also need increased iron during periods of rapid growth. In men and postmenopausal women, iron deficiency anemia is more likely due to gastrointestinal bleeding. Because excessive bleeding is the most common cause of iron deficiency anemia, the first step in treatment is to locate the source of bleeding and stop it. Many patients with iron deficiency anemia can be treated with oral iron supplements such as ferrous sulfate, ferrous fumarate, or ferrous gluconate. However, iron supplements should never be used without first confirming that the patient is iron deficient and anemic. The standard adult dose of ferrous sulfate is one 300 mg tablet three times a day. Iron tablets should be kept out of reach of children, who can be fatally poisoned from taking only a few tablets. Side effects of iron supplements include nausea, stomach complaints, constipation, and dark stools. Iron is absorbed best on an empty stomach, but food may help to avoid stomach upset. Milk or antacids may interfere with iron absorption and should not be taken within 2 hours of taking iron supplements. Correcting iron deficiency anemia with iron supplements usually takes 1-2 months, even after the bleeding has stopped. In addition, iron supplements should be continued for 6-12 months to replenish the body's reserves. Iron rich foods include meats, fish, poultry, egg whites, beans, whole grain breads and cereals, and green leafy vegetables.

CHRONIC OBSTRUCTIVE PULMONARY DISEASE (COPD)

QUESTION: I heard about a new inhaled medication for treating chronic bronchitis and emphysema. What can you tell me about it?

ANSWER: Chronic bronchitis and emphysema are also known as chronic obstructive pulmonary disease or COPD. People with chronic bronchitis have a persistent cough that produces sputum and is caused by inflammation in the airways. There is also scarring and swelling of the airways along with smooth muscle contraction or bronchospasm. Emphysema is an enlargement of the tiny air sacs in the lungs and the destruction of their walls. Both of these conditions produce obstruction to airflow and difficulty breathing. Symptoms of COPD include cough, sputum production, and shortness of breath. These symptoms may worsen if the person develops a respiratory tract infection. An estimated 24 million Americans suffer from COPD, with over 50% under the age of 65. However, over 95% of all deaths from COPD occur in people over age 55. It is the fourth leading cause of death in the U.S. and is projected to become the third leading fatal illness by 2020. Smoking is a major cause of COPD and about 10 to 15% of smokers develop this condition.

The newly FDA-approved treatment for patients with COPD is called Spiriva and contains the drug tiotropium. Spiriva capsules contain a dry powder form of tiotropium that is inhaled using a special deice called a HandiHaler which comes with the product. When inhaled into the lungs, Spiriva helps to expand the airways (bronchodilation) and reduce the production of mucous (sputum). This improves the ability to breathe and quality of life for patients with COPD. Spiriva is given by inhalation once a day and its most common side effect is dry mouth, which occurs in about 10-15% of patients.

QUESTION: I heard about a new inhaler for chronic bronchitis or emphysema. What can you tell about it?

ANSWER: The FDA recently approved Arcapta Neohaler (indacaterol) for the long term, once-daily maintenance treatment of airflow obstruction in patients with chronic obstructive pulmonary disease (COPD), including chronic bronchitis and/or emphysema. When inhaled, the active ingredient in Arcapta Neohaler works locally in the lungs to open or expand the bronchial breathing tubes. Arcapta Neohaler is a long-acting agent and is the first once-daily product of this type to be approved in the U.S. for COPD. The most common side effects of Arcada Neohaler include throat pain, inflammation of the nose/throat, headache, and nausea. It is contraindicated in patients with asthma without the use of a long-term asthma control medication. This new product will be dispensed with a Medication Guide that includes instructions for use and information about risks of taking the drug.

Chronic Obstructive Pulmonary Disease or COPD is a chronic, progressive lung disease that is commonly caused by tobacco smoking, air pollution or occupational exposure, and results in airflow obstruction and debilitating bouts of breathlessness. More than 12 million people in the US are affected, while another estimated 12 million people are believed to have the disease but remain undiagnosed. COPD ranks as the third leading cause of death in the US and a major cause of serious long-term disability.

QUESTION: I heard about a new drug approved to treat COPD. What can you tell me about it?

ANSWER: The FDA recently (2012) approved Tudorza Pressair (aclidinium bromide inhaler) for the long-term maintenance treatment of bronchospasm (narrowing of the airways in the lung) associated with chronic obstructive pulmonary disease (COPD), including bronchitis and emphysema. Tudorza Pressair is a long-acting anticholinergic (antimuscarinic) drug that when inhaled works by helping to open the airways in the lungs, assisting people with COPD to breathe. It is used by inhalation twice a day, but is not indicated for acute use as a rescue medication to treat sudden breathing problems and is not recommended for people younger than 18 years of age. The most common side effects of Tudorza Pressair include headache, inflammation of the nasal passage, and cough.

INSOMNIA

QUESTION: What nonprescription products can I use to help me sleep?

ANSWER: Insomnia or the inability to obtain sleep of sufficient quality or quantity to feel refreshed the following morning is a very common complaint. It is estimated that approximately 50% of adults are periodically affected by insomnia and about 90% have insomnia sometime during their life. There are numerous causes of insomnia, which can be transient (lasting less than 7 days), short-term (lasting from 7 days to 3 weeks), or long-term (lasting over 3 weeks). Causes of transient insomnia may include acute stress in one's life, time-zone changes, or environmental disturbances like excess noise or light and temperature changes. Eating a large meal or drinking alcohol before bedtime can also cause transient insomnia. Short-term insomnia is usually caused by more severe stress such as loss of a job or a death in the family. Long-term insomnia, on the other hand, may be caused by underlying medical or psychiatric problems such as depression, restless leg syndrome, sleep apnea, pain, congestive heart failure, thyroid disease, need to urinate, or various drugs. In order to improve sleep, the underlying cause of insomnia should be corrected, if possible, and principles of good sleep hygiene should be followed. These principles include:

- Establish a routine time for bedtime and awakening
- Avoid daytime naps
- Avoid alcohol, caffeine, and other central nervous system stimulants (e.g., decongestants)
- Administer medications associated with insomnia in the morning (e.g., diuretics)
- Reduce lighting at least 1 hour prior to bedtime
- Exercise regularly, but avoid exercising just prior to bedtime
- Mask noises or use soft earplugs, if necessary
- Use the bedroom only for sleeping, reading, or sexual activity
- Avoid engaging in stressful activities or unpleasant tasks near bedtime
- Limit fluid intake close to bedtime
- Avoid eating large meals immediately prior to bedtime

Nonprescription sleep aids include the antihistamine diphenhydramine found in such products as Benadryl, Compoz, Nytol, Sominex, and doxylamine found in Unisom. Combination products containing the pain reliever acetaminophen and diphenhydromine are also available without a prescription in products like Extra Strength Tylenol PM or Exedrin PM. It should be noted that these antihistamines can cause dizziness, sedation, confusion, dry mouth, constipation, urinary retention, and next-day "hangover" sedation may occur in some patients. People using antihistamines should also avoid alcohol and it is not advisable for patients to drive or operate machinery when taking these medications. In addition, doxylamine should not be used by women who are pregnant or breastfeeding. Always read the package labeling for more complete information. Other nonprescription sleep aids include the herbs Valerian, Kava or Chamomile and the hormone melatonin. Patients should not take any nonprescription sleep aid for more than 10 consecutive days, and if the insomnia persists a physician should be consulted.

QUESTION: I have trouble going to sleep and I heard about a new prescription drug that can help. What can you tell me about it?

ANSWER: Insomnia or difficulty in sleeping or in falling asleep is reported to occur in 13-45% of the adult population. It is more commonly a problem in females and in the elderly. Short tern insomnia lasting from 1 to 3 weeks can be caused by stress such as the loss of a job, starting a new job, illness, death of a friend or family member, and upcoming marriage or divorce, moving, or financial difficulties. Insomnia lasting more than 3 weeks may be caused by underlying medical or psychiatric/psychologic problems, or the abuse of certain drugs or alcohol. The new drug that you heard about is named Sonata (generic name zaleplon), which was approved for the short-term (2-3 weeks) treatment of insomnia in adults. Studies in both young and elderly adults have shown that Sonata can shorten the time it takes to fall asleep in most people with insomnia. Therefore, it may be of particular benefit for people who have trouble falling asleep within 30 minutes after lying down. The drug is very short acting, however, and it does not increase the duration of sleep or reduce the number of awakenings during the night. In addition, because of its short action, Sonata does not appear to cause sedative effects, memory loss, or difficulty concentrating the next day like many other sleep medications. The most common side effects of this new drug include headache, weakness, lightheadedness, difficulty with coordination, drowsiness, and dizziness. Some interactions with other drugs are also possible so be sure that your doctor and pharmacist are aware of all other medications that you take, both prescription and nonprescription. The use of alcohol should also be avoided while on this medication. Sonata should be taken immediately before bedtime or as soon as possible after having difficulty in falling asleep. Like other drugs for insomnia, its use should be limited to 7 to 10 days and re-evaluation by a doctor is recommended if it needs to be taken for a longer period of time.

QUESTION: I heard about a new drug for insomnia. What can you tell me about it?

ANSWER: The FDA recently approved Lunesta (eszopiclone) for the treatment of insomnia. It is indicated for the treatment of adult and elderly people who have difficulty in falling asleep as well as those who are unable to sleep through the night. An estimated 100 million adult Americans suffer from either chronic or occasional insomnia, which left untreated, may become progressively worse and in turn potentially affect a person's emotional, mental, and physical health. The dose of Lunesta ranges from 1 to 3 mg given immediately before bedtime. However, doses of Lunesta should be individualized and based upon the person's primary complaint, age, liver function, and other medications being taken. Also, because sleep problems often may be associated with underlying physical or psychiatric causes, it is recommended that each person should be fully evaluated before receiving Lunesta. If sleep has not improved after 7 to 10 days of medication use, further assessment is recommended. Lunesta has a rapid onset of hypnotic and sedative effects. In order to minimize the risks for falls, excessive sedation, and daytime drowsiness, Lunesta should be taken only when people are able to sleep for at least 8 hours. Alcohol should be avoided with Lunesta, and this sleep aid should be used with caution in people with depression, those who are pregnant or breastfeeding, and in patients with poor respiratory function. The most common side effects of Lunesta include headache, dry mouth, dizziness, drowsiness, and unpleasant taste. Patients using Lunesta should use extreme caution when driving or operating machinery until they know how the drug will affect them. Unlike other sedative/hypnotic medications that are generally indicated for short-term use, Lunesta has been approved for longer-term treatment if needed.

QUESTION: I heard about a new drug to help you go to sleep. What can you tell me about it?

ANSWER: The FDA recently approved the prescription drug Rozerem for the treatment of insomnia. Insomnia is characterized by difficulty falling asleep, difficulty staying asleep, or poor quality sleep, which can lead to serious daytime consequences including tiredness, low motivation, disturbances of judgment, and reduced coordination. Insomnia, which affects about one-third of American adults, has also been linked to a variety of health problems, including obesity, diabetes, high blood pressure, heart disease, and depression. Rozerem is the first and only prescription medication that has shown no evidence of abuse and dependence and, as a result, has not been designated as a controlled substance by the U.S. Drug Enforcement Administration (DEA). This new sleep medication works differently than other hypnotic drugs. Rozerem is chemically related to the natural hormone melatonin, which helps regulate the body's "master clock" or sleep-wake cycle, and is thought to work by stimulating certain melatonin receptors in the brain. It is a new treatment option for adults who have difficulty falling asleep, and it may work for some people in ways that other sleep medications do not. In clinical studies, Rozerem was shown to reduce the time for falling asleep and it did not appear to impair a person's learning ability, memory, ability to concentrate, or level of alertness. The most common side effects of Rozerem during clinical studies were headache, drowsiness, fatigue, dizziness, and nausea. Several drug interactions may also occur when Rozerem is used with other medications and should be avoided by people engaging in hazardous activities that require concentration (such as operating a motor vehicle or heavy machinery). Rozerem is usually taken within 30 minutes of going to bed.

QUESTION: I heard about a new drug to help you sleep. What can you tell me about it?

ANSWER: The FDA recently approved Silenor (doxepin tablets) for the treatment of insomnia that is characterized by difficulty with sleep maintenance. It is approved for both short term and long term insomnia in adults and the elderly. Sleep maintenance difficulty is defined as waking frequently during the night and/or waking too early and being unable to return to sleep. During clinical studies, Silenor demonstrated maintenance of sleep into the 7th and 8th hours of the night without causing meaningful residual effects the next day. Silenor does not appear to have abuse potential and has not been classified as a controlled substance. As with other hypnotics, doxepin may cause unpredictable sleep-driving and other complex behaviors while sleeping, as well as amnesia, anxiety, and other neuropsychiatric events. Doxepin may also exacerbate depression symptoms and suicidal thoughts in patients with depression. The drug has depressant side effects, and patients should avoid driving, operating heavy machinery, or drinking after taking doxepin and should take caution on mornings following treatment. Additional adverse effects include sedation, upper respiratory tract infection, nausea, and hypertension. Exactly how Silenor works to help sleep maintenance is not known, but it does block the effects of histamine and may also have an effect on melatonin, both of which are involved in the sleep-wake cycle. Actually, doxepin, the active ingredient in Silenor has been used extensively to treat depression and anxiety disorders for about 30 years under the tradename Sinequan. However, the dosage of doxepin in Silenor is much lower (3-6 mg) than dosage used to treat depression and anxiety. It is estimated that approximately 70 million American adults suffer from insomnia, characterized by difficulty falling asleep, waking frequently during the night, waking too early and not being able to return to sleep, or waking up not feeling refreshed.

QUESTION: I take Ambien to help me get to sleep. How does it work and what are its side effects?

ANSWER: Ambien or zolipidem (generic name) is classified as a sedative-hypnotic drug and is used for the short-term treatment of insomnia. It is not chemically related to barbiturates like phenobarbital or the benzodiazepine drugs used for sleep like Dalmane (flurazepam), Restoril (temazepam), or Halcion (triazolam). Exactly how Ambien induces sleep is not exactly known, but it appears to interact (bind) with certain receptors in the brain believed to be responsible for sedation and sleep. Ambien has been shown to reduce the time to fall asleep, decrease the number of awakenings, and to increase total sleep time. The sleep induced by Ambien seems to be more natural and causes less sedation the next day compared to some of the other drugs mentioned above. The most common side effects of Ambien during short-term treatment (up to 10 nights) were drowsiness, dizziness, and diarrhea. During longer-term treatment (28 to 35 nights), the most commonly observed side effects were dizziness and drugged feelings. However, numerous other side effects can occur. Because it can cause drowsiness, patients taking Ambien need to be cautioned about performing tasks requiring alertness, coordination, or physical dexterity. Alcohol and other CNS depressants should also be avoided when taking Ambien. An extended-release formulation of zolpidem (Ambien CR) was also recently approved for the treatment of insomnia characterized by difficulty in falling asleep and/or maintenance of sleep. These tablets consist of a two-layer dosage form with one layer releasing the drug contents immediately and another layer that allows a slower release of additional content. It should be noted that both of these Ambien products are Schedule IV controlled substances and can cause dependence.

QUESTION: You recently wrote about Ambien. How does it compare to other prescription drugs used for insomnia?

ANSWER: As I've noted before, approximately one in three American adults complain of some type of insomnia and 20 million Americans suffer from chronic insomnia. Insomnia is characterized by difficulty in falling asleep, difficulty staying asleep, or poor quality of sleep leading to impairment of next-day functioning. It has also been linked to a variety of health care problems including obesity, diabetes, hypertension, heart disease, and depression.

For many years, tranquilizers known as benzodiazepines have been prescribed for insomnia. This group of drugs would include Valium (diazepam), Halcion (triazolam), Xanax (alprazolam), Restoril (temazepam) and others. However, because of their long-lasting effects, they may leave you groggy and/or disoriented the next-day. The newer agents such as Ambien (zolpidem), Sonata (zaleplon), Lunesta (ezopiclone), and Rozerem (ramelteon) are classified as non-benzodiazepine sleep-aids. They more precisely target chemical receptors in the brain involved with sleep and in general have fewer side effects than the benzodiazepines. They are expensive and are not available as generic drugs yet. Ambien induces sleep quickly, but may cause grogginess if you sleep less than eight hours. A recent report has described bizarre behavior in several motorists who exceeded a safe dose of Ambien or who took the drug and did not go to bed. Some of these people crashed their cars with no memory of it. Sonata appears to be effective for people who have trouble staying asleep. Lunesta on the other hand appears to help people fall asleep quickly, but should only be used when you expect to get eight hours of sleep, or it may result in temporary memory loss. Rozerem helps with sleep-onset problems but it is not recommended for restarting sleep if you wake up during the night. Your physician can evaluate your sleep situation and determine if medication is needed and if so, the right drug for you. People taking sleeping aids should keep in touch with their doctor for regular reevaluation of progress as well as side effects.

QUESTION: I take Ambien to help me sleep. Is there a generic available?

ANSWER: Yes, the FDA has recently approved generic versions of Ambien (zolipidem). Ambien was the 13th highest-selling brand name drug in the U.S. during 2006, with yearly sales of approximately $2.2 billion. Ambien or zolipidem (generic name) is classified as a sedative-hypnotic drug and is used for the short-term treatment of insomnia. It is not chemically related to barbiturates like phenobarbital or the benzodiazepine drugs used for sleep like Dalmane (flurazepam), Restoril (temazepam), or Halcion (triazolam). Exactly how Ambien induces sleep is not exactly known, but it appears to interact (bind) with certain receptors in the brain believed to be responsible for sedation and sleep. Ambien has been shown to reduce the time to fall asleep, decrease the number of awakenings, and to increase total sleep time. The sleep induced by Ambien seems to be more natural and causes less sedation the next day compared to some of the other drugs mentioned above. The most common side effects of Ambien during short-term treatment (up to 10 nights) were drowsiness, dizziness, and diarrhea. During longer-term treatment (28 to 35 nights), the most commonly observed side effects were dizziness and drugged feelings. However, numerous other side effects can occur. Because it can cause drowsiness, patients taking Ambien need to be cautioned about performing tasks requiring alertness, coordination, or physical dexterity. Alcohol and other CNS depressants should also be avoided when taking Ambien. In March of 2007, the FDA also called for all companies that produce sedative-hypnotic drugs such as Ambien to revise their product labeling to include stronger warnings about potential adverse effects, such as severe allergic reactions and complex sleep-related behavior, such as "sleep-driving". As I've noted many times before, the FDA approves all generic drugs using strict guidelines, including checking for the generic drug's chemistry by evaluating its formulation, potency, stability, and purity. The generic drug must also pass bio-equivalency testing that compares the delivery into the bloodstream of the generic drug's active ingredient to that of the brand name drug. Generic drugs are less expensive than brand-name products, and account for about 56% of prescriptions dispensed.

QUESTION: I heard that an oral spray was approved to treat insomnia. What can you tell me about it?

ANSWER: The FDA recently approved Zolpimist oral spray for the short-term treatment of insomnia characterized by difficulties in falling asleep. Zolpimist contains the active ingredient zolpidem, which has been available as an oral tablet for many years in products like Ambien or Ambien CR and is also available as a generic product. Zolpimist oral spray is administered as 2 sprays (10 mg) directly into the mouth over the tongue once daily immediately before bedtime. A lower dose of 1 spray (5 mg) is recommended in elderly or debilitated patients or in patients with liver impairment or those taking central nervous system depressants. This new oral spray provides for rapid absorption from the oral mucosa and gastrointestinal tract.

Zolpidem is classified as a sedative-hypnotic drug and is used for the short-term treatment of insomnia. It is not chemically related to barbiturates like phenobarbital or the benzodiazepine drugs used for sleep like Dalmane (flurazepam), Restoril (temazepam), or Halcion (triazolam). Exactly how zolpidem induces sleep is not exactly known, but it appears to interact (bind) with certain receptors in the brain believed to be responsible for sedation and sleep. Zolpidem has been shown to reduce the time to fall asleep, decrease the number of awakenings, and to increase total sleep time. The sleep induced by zolpidem seems to be more natural and causes less sedation the next day compared to some of the other drugs mentioned above. The most common side effects of zolpidem during short-term treatment (up to 10 nights) were drowsiness, dizziness, and diarrhea. During longer-term treatment (28 to 35 nights), the most commonly observed side effects were dizziness and drugged feelings. However, numerous other side effects can occur. Because it can cause drowsiness, patients taking zolpidem need to be cautioned about performing tasks requiring alertness, coordination, or physical dexterity. Alcohol and other CNS depressants should also be avoided when taking zolpidem.

QUESTION: I heard that a new under the tongue medication was approved for insomnia. What can you tell me about it?

ANSWER: The FDA recently approved Edular sublingual (under the tongue) tablets for the short-term treatment of insomnia characterized by difficulties in falling asleep. Edular contains the active ingredient zolpidem, which has been available as an oral tablet for many years in products like Ambien or Ambien CR and is also available as a generic product. In addition Zolpimist, an oral spray product that contains zolpidem, is available. The usual adult dose of Edular is a 10 mg tablet placed under the tongue once a day immediately before bedtime. The tablet should not be swallowed or taken with water and should not be taken with or immediately after a meal. A lower 5 mg dose is recommended for elderly or debilitated patients and in patients with liver function problems or those taking central nervous system depressants. This new sublingual tablet provides for fast and effective absorption from the oral mucosa where the tablet disintegrates.

Zolpidem is classified as a sedative-hypnotic drug and is used for the short-term treatment of insomnia. It is not chemically related to barbiturates like phenobarbital or the benzodiazepine drugs used for sleep like Dalmane (flurazepam), Restoril (temazepam), or Halcion (triazolam). Exactly how zolpidem induces sleep is not exactly known, but it appears to interact (bind) with certain receptors in the brain believed to be responsible for sedation and sleep. Zolpidem has been shown to reduce the time to fall asleep, decrease the number of awakenings, and to increase total sleep time. The sleep induced by zolpidem seems to be more natural and causes less sedation the next day compared to some of the other drugs mentioned above. The most common side effects of zolpidem during short-term treatment (up to 10 nights) were drowsiness, dizziness, and diarrhea. During longer-term treatment (28 to 35 nights), the most commonly observed side effects were dizziness and drugged feelings. However, numerous other side effects can occur. Because it can cause drowsiness, patients taking zolpidem need to be cautioned about performing tasks requiring alertness, coordination, or physical dexterity. Alcohol and other CNS depressants should also be avoided when taking zolpidem.

QUESTION: I heard about a new drug for early wakening at night. What can you tell me about it?

ANSWER: The FDA recently approved Intermezzo (zolpidem) to treat insomnia characterized by middle-of-the-night waking followed by difficulty returning to sleep. The active ingredient of Intermezzo (zolpidem) was actually first approved for insomnia in 1992 under the trade name Ambien, but Intermezzo is formulated as a sublingual (under the tongue) tablet in a lower dose (1.75 mg or 3.5 mg). Intermezzo is not indicated for the treatment of middle-of-the-night insomnia when the patient has fewer than 4 hours of bedtime remaining before the planned time of waking. The recommended dose of Intermezzo is 1.75 mg for women and 3.5 mg for men, taken only once per night as needed for a middle-of-the-night awakening. The dose is lower in women because they clear the drug from the body at a lower rate than men. The 1.75 mg dose is also recommended for people over the age of 65. The most common side effects of Intermezzo are headache, nausea, and fatigue. Insomnia is a common condition in which a person has trouble falling or staying asleep. It can range from mild to severe, depending on how often it occurs and for how long. Insomnia can cause excessive daytime sleepiness and lack of energy. It also can make a person feel anxious, depressed, or irritable. People with insomnia may have trouble focusing on tasks, paying attention, learning, and remembering. Middle-of-the-night awakening with difficulty falling back to sleep is a form of insomnia that is estimated to affect millions of adults in the United States. Intermezzo is the first and only prescription sleep aid indicated for dosing in the middle of the night to treat this form of insomnia.

ANTIDEPRESSANTS AND SUICIDE

QUESTION: I've read that some antidepressant drugs may lead to suicide. Is this true?

ANSWER: There have been reports of suicide attempts by both children and adults who have been treated with some antidepressants.

However, it is not really clear at this point if certain antidepressant drugs actually cause some people to commit suicide or whether the underlying mental illness being treated is to blame. Until this question is answered, the FDA has recently requested that doctors who prescribe certain antidepressants to closely monitor their patients for warning signs of suicide, especially when therapy is initiated or when the dosage is changed. These antidepressants work by altering the brain's level of serotonin, which is a chemical that helps nerve cells communicate. The brand and generic names of some of these drugs are listed below:

- Prozac or Sarafem (fluoxetine)
- Zoloft (sertraline)
- Paxil (paroxetine)
- Luvox (fluvoxamine)
- Celexa (citalopram)
- Lexapro (escitalopram)
- Wellbutrin (bupropion)
- Effexor (venlafaxine)
- Serzone (nefaxodone)
- Remeron (mirtazapine)

The FDA has also asked the manufacturers of these drugs to add or strengthen suicide-related warnings on their products' labeling. In addition, they have asked a Columbia University team to review information from numerous studies to try and determine if there is any link between the drugs and suicide attempts and thoughts in children.

CATAPLEXY/NARCOLEPSY

QUESTION: I heard that the "date-rape" drug has been approved to treat narcolepsy. Is this true?

ANSWER: The FDA has recently approved Xyrem (sodium oxybate), also known as GHB or the "date-rape" drug for treating people with a condition known as cataplexy. Cataplexy is a dangerous complication of the sleep disorder known as narcolepsy. People with narcolepsy have recurring episodes during which they suddenly fall asleep for a few seconds or up to an hour. Because of this, they have trouble working, driving, or enjoying social activities because they may fall asleep. Some people with narcolepsy also have cataplexy, a condition in which they lose all control of muscles and collapse. Cataplexy is usually triggered by strong emotions such as laughter, anger, or surprise. It is estimated that about 140,000 Americans have narcolepsy, which usually begins with excessive daytime sleepiness and sleep attacks during the second and third decades of life. Its cause is unknown but may involve various chemicals in the brain.

The notorious "date-rape" drug (GHB) marketed as Xyrem will only be made available to patients under a very restricted distribution program called the Xyrem Success Program, which involves prescriber and patient education along with the use of a single centralized pharmacy. GHB has been abused as a party drug to get high, and when mixed with alcohol it can knock a person out, which is why it has also gained a reputation as the "date-rape" drug. The drug is odorless and colorless and when slipped into drinks, victims often have no memory of what happened. GHB also used to be sold as a dietary supplement in health food stores, but by the mid 1990's the government declared its use illegal and in 2000 toughened penalties were enacted for abusers. How the drug works in patients with narcolepsy is unknown, but it may help to improve sleep and allow better daytime performance. It is taken at night and is commonly used in conjunction with daytime prescription stimulants. Patients with narcolepsy who would like more information can call toll free at 1-877-679-9736.

ORAL RINSES

QUESTION: My dentist suggested that I start using an oral rinse called Periomed. What can you tell me about this product?

ANSWER: Periomed oral rinse is a prescription product that is used to help reduce gum inflammation and bleeding (gingivitis), reduce tooth sensitivity, and prevent plaque accumulation and dental caries (cavities). It contains 0.63% stannous fluoride concentrate as the active ingredient. The use of fluoride preparations like Periomed is thought to decrease gingivitis and dental carries in 3 ways. First they make the dental enamel more resistant to acids; secondly, they interfere with the growth and function of dental plaque bacteria; and thirdly they help to replace minerals in dental enamel. Fluoride rinses work together with the fluoridation of water and toothpastes containing fluoride to reduce the incidence of dental carries and gingivitis. As many as 85% of all people over the age of 40 have gum disease and at least 90% of geriatric patients suffer from inflammation or degeneration around their teeth. In addition, stannous ("tin containing") fluoride, as found in Periomed, also has been shown to reduce sensitivity in people with sensitive teeth. It has been reported that about 25% of patients treated in a dental practice have one or more teeth that are sensitive to cold, heat, touch, sweet, or sour substances. It appears that the "tin" in stannous fluoride forms a deposit on small tubes of tooth dentine and blocks sensitivity sensations. Stannous fluoride is retained in the mouth for a prolonged period of time after oral use. Periomed oral rinse is normally used once daily after brushing with a fluoride toothpaste. One tablespoonful of a diluted solution of the concentrated oral rinse is swished in the mouth and between the teeth for one minute and then spit out. This is then repeated one more time. The rinse should not be swallowed. It is also a good idea not to eat or drink for 30 minutes after the treatment. Periomed, which is available in mint, tropical fruit, and cinnamon flavors, may cause temporary surface staining of the teeth, which is not permanent and may be removed by adequate brushing.

CANKER SORES

QUESTION: What can I do for canker sores?

ANSWER: Canker sores are a common problem affecting 20% to 55% of all Americans at one time or another. They are small, painful sores that occur inside the mouth. A canker sore appears as a round white spot with a red border and they almost always form on soft loose tissues that are not attached to bone, like inside the lip or cheek or on the tongue. The cause of these sores is not known, but stress and/or genetics may play a role. Other possible factors that may contribute to canker sores include food allergies, bacteria in the mouth, hormonal changes, nutritional deficiency, other diseases, and injury such as biting the inside of the cheek or lip. Many people report a strange sensation in the affected area, such as burning, prickling, or tightness just before the sore appears. Sometimes the sore can be so painful that you are unable to eat, drink, talk, whistle, or sing. However, most canker sores are not serious and heal on their own within 7-10 days.

The main goal in treating canker sores is to control the discomfort and pain in addition to protecting the sores from irritation. The application of topical local anesthetic gels or pastes can help provide temporary pain relief. Sample anesthetic products include Orabase-B, Benzodent cream, Anbesol, Tanac, and Oragel Mouth-Aid. Coating the ulcer sores with topical protectants such as Orabase, denture adhesives, or benzoin tincture can also be effective in providing symptomatic relief. In addition, the use of orthodontic waxes to cover sharp appliances, such as braces, can be helpful. Finally, the use of cleansing products that are swished and spit out can be useful in the treatment of canker sores. Some examples of these products, which should not be used for more than 7 days, are Amosan Oral Wound Cleanser, Cank-Aid, Gly-Oxide, Oragel Perioseptic Spot Treatment Oral Cleanser, Peroxyl Antiseptic Dental Rinse, and Proxigel. A Sodium bicarbonate mouth swish (one-half to 1 teaspoonful in 4 ounces of water) used up to four times a day can also be appropriate for people over 2 years of age. Other helpful measures include the avoidance of irritating foods (potato chips, crackers, spicy foods, pineapple, citrus fruits, and chocolate) and sipping acidic juices and soft drinks through a straw to lessen contact with the canker sore to avoid pain. It should also be noted that sores in the mouth can be a sign of more serious problems such as oral cancer and if a person experiences rash or fever with the sores, or if irritation, pain, or redness persists, he or she should see a doctor or dentist.

QUESTION: I heard that licorice root extract can help heal canker sores. What can you tell me about this?

ANSWER: Canker sores are a common problem. Most are not serious and heal on their own within 7-10 days. It should also be noted that sores in the mouth can be a sign of more serious problems such as oral cancer and if a person experiences rash or fever with the sores, or if irritation, pain, or redness persists, he or she should see a doctor or dentist.

Recently it was reported in the journal "General Dentistry" that canker sores (also known as recurrent aphthous ulcers) can be treated with a licorice root herbal extract. The authors of this study examined the effects of using a medicated adhesive patch (with extract from the licorice root) for treating canker sores compared to no treatment. After 7 days of treatment, the ulcer size in the group of people who received the adhesive patch with licorice extract was significantly smaller, while the ulcer size in the no-treatment group increased by 13%. The study authors note that in its original form licorice root extract has a very strong taste. However, when it is combined with a self-adhering, time-release, dissolving oral patch, the taste is mild and pleasant. While the exact mode of action for licorice root extract as an anti-ulcerogenic agent is unknown, the therapeutic use of licorice dates back to the Roman Empire.

COLD SORES

QUESTION: Can lysine help get rid of cold sores?

ANSWER: A "cold sore" or "fever blister" is an infection that usually occurs on the lips or occasionally inside the nose or mouth. They are caused by the herpes simplex virus type 1 (HSV-1) and are known medically as herpes simplex labialis or herpes labialis. It is a common problem in younger people with at least 70% of children getting this infection by age 14. Once an individual is infected, attacks can potentially occur throughout life, but the incidence drops after the age of 35. Many people experience symptoms that a cold sore is coming before the blisters actually form. This is known as a "prodrome" and may include a numbness, soreness, burning, or swelling. A variety of things can trigger a cold sore including sunlight, tanning booths, stress or excitement, fatigue, windburn, fever, the menstrual cycle, or dental work. The blisters formed by this infection can rupture and the skin can crack causing pain during eating, drinking, or talking. Eventually scabs will form, and complete healing occurs in about 10 to 14 days without scarring. Infected individuals can pass the infection to others and therefore direct contact and sharing of glasses should be avoided. People with cold sores should also avoid touching the lesions, since they may transfer the virus to other people, or to objects that others may touch.

Many health-food stores and magazines have promoted the use of lysine for cold sores or fever blisters. Lysine is an essential amino acid that is required for proper human nutrition. Good dietary sources of lysine are meat, cheese, yogurt, poultry, sardines, nuts, eggs, wheat germ, and soybeans. The use of lysine has been advertised to decrease the frequency, severity, and duration of cold sores. The basis for this is that lysine has been shown to prevent the reproduction of the herpes simplex virus in some laboratory studies. However, the results from several studies in humans have been mixed. Most of these studies show that lysine may be effective in reducing the frequency of outbreaks of cold sores, but only a few studies have actually found that lysine decreases the severity or duration of the infection. In addition, the FDA has not approved lysine for its use in the treatment of cold sores or fever blisters. The adult dose of lysine used in the clinical studies has ranged from one to four grams daily. Oral lysine appears to be fairly safe and well tolerated, but people with kidney or liver disease should not use it.

QUESTION: A few weeks ago you talked about the use of lysine for cold sores. I heard about a new nonprescription cream that also helps. What can you tell me about it?

ANSWER: The newly approved nonprescription product for treating cold sores is marketed as Abreva cream (generic name docosanol). It is the first topical nonprescription antiviral agent approved for the treatment of cold sores. Abreva cream does not actually kill the cold sore virus, but prevents it from spreading. Studies have shown that it can shorten healing time as well as the duration of symptoms such as tingling, pain, burning, and itching. This new topical cream is most effective when treatment is started as soon as possible after the first sign of the tingle, redness, bump, or itch that can signal the onset of a cold sore. Abreva cream should be rubbed in gently but completely, and applied five times a day until the lesion is healed. The cream should not be applied directly inside the mouth, or in or near the eyes. Abreva appears to be well tolerated with few side effects. Cosmetics, such as lipstick, may be applied over the cream, but the use of a separate applicator like a cotton swab is recommended to prevent the spread of infection.

QUESTION: What nonprescription products are useful for cold sores?

ANSWER: There are numerous nonprescription (OTC) products available to treat cold sores. Currently, Abreva is the only OTC product approved by the FDA to shorten healing time as well as both the severity and the duration of the symptoms associated with cold sores. In addition, a number of topical OTC products are available to provide relief of symptoms such as pain and itching, but not for reducing the duration of symptoms. Some of these products include Ambesol Cold Sore Therapy, Blistex Medicated, Campho-phenique, Carmex, Chapstick Medicated, Herpecin-L, and Zilactin. People with cold sores may also benefit from the use of a cool, wet compress or ice on the affected area, keeping the lesions clean by cleansing the affected area with a mild soap solution, and using skin protectants to keep lesions moist.

DRY MOUTH

QUESTION: My mouth always seems to be dry and it is difficult to chew my food. What can I do about this?

ANSWER: Dryness of the mouth or xerostomia is a fairly common complaint, especially in the elderly. More than 50% of the elderly population has occasional oral dryness, while 10% to 25% experience it constantly. Although xerostomia is usually not a serious condition, it may cause considerable discomfort and difficulty in eating. It may also be associated with medical disorders such as rheumatoid disease, diabetes, hypertension, or depression and therefore its cause needs to be determined. Additional causes of xerostomia include irradiation of the head and neck, numerous types of medications, and various other medical conditions. A listing of some of the most common types of medication that can cause dryness of the mouth can be found in the table at the end of this column. Like tears, saliva serves a number of important functions including anti-infective action, protection of the mucosa, lubrication, and assisting with the digestion of food. A sufficient amount of saliva is necessary for the maintenance of good oral health, and normally over 16 ounces of saliva is produced each day by the salivary glands. Saliva contains a large number of ingredients such as electrolytes, immunoglobulins and other anti-infective compounds, along with digestive and other proteins. Besides difficulty in tasting or eating food and swallowing, a lack of saliva can also lead to dental cavities and sores within the mouth. The treatment of xerostomia is dependent upon its cause. If the dry mouth is due to a medication it should be discontinued if possible or switched to one without the drying effects if there is an alternative available. Tobacco, alcohol, caffeine containing beverages, and mouthwashes containing alcohol should be avoided. Spicy or acidic foods should also be avoided since they may burn the mucosa or lead to damaged teeth. Patients with xerostomia should try to sip water after every bite of solid food to help cope with dry mouth. In addition, the use of sugar-free gum and hard candy to help stimulate saliva flow can be helpful. Non-prescription mouth moisteners or artificial saliva are also available. The idea behind using saliva substitutes is that they provide a long lasting coating of the oral mucosa. They usually contain carboxymethylcellulose and/or mucins for lubrication. Some representative saliva substitute products are MouthKote, Salivart, and Oral Balance. Some patients may benefit from using olive oil as a mucosal lubricant. Finally, a number of prescription medications and other treatments are available to treat xerostomia.

Some Types Of Medications That
Can Cause Dry Mouth (Xeristomia)

- Antihypertensives
- Appetite Suppressants
- Anticholinergics
- Antihistamines
- Anticonvulsants
- Antiparkinson agents

- Bronchodilators
- Antipsychotics
- Antidepressants
- Tranquilizers
- Diuretics

DRY EYES

QUESTION: I heard about a new prescription eyedrop to treat dry eyes. What can you tell me about it?

ANSWER: People often complain of having dry eyes. Chronic dry eye disease, also known as keratoconjunctivitis sicca, is a painful and irritating condition due to a lack of tear production caused by inflammation in the eye. Tears are a salty fluid that continuously bathes the surface of the eye to keep it moist and flush away foreign particles. Tears also contain antibodies that help protect the eye from infection. Tears are produced by the lacrimal (tear) glands, located near the outer corner of the eye. If the tear glands do not produce enough tears, the eye can become painfully dry and can be damaged. Dry eye disease is very common and the incidence increases with age, after menopause, and in people with certain medical problems such as rheumatoid arthritis, diabetes, lupus, or a condition known as Sjogren's syndrome. It has been estimated that up to 25% of patients visiting eye clinics report dry eye symptoms. People with dry eye disease typically complain of eye discomfort, including a dry, gritty feeling, or feeling like something is in their eye. This dryness can lead to inflammation and eye damage and may increase the risk of eye infections. The treatment of dry eye disease usually involves the use of non-prescription tear-replacement products, commonly known as artificial tears. The new drug that you heard about is a prescription eyedrop named Restasis (cyclosporine ophthalmic emulsion). Restasis has anti-inflammatory effects in the eye and it significantly increases tear production in people with chronic dry eye disease, or keratoconjunctivitis sicca. One drop is placed in each eye twice a day and it can be used together with artificial tears. It should not be used while wearing contact lenses. The most common side effect of Restasis is a burning sensation in the eye. More information about this new treatment can be found on the Internet at **www.Restasis.com**.

GLAUCOMA

QUESTION: My mother has glaucoma and I heard about a new type of drug treatment being tested. What can you tell me about it?

ANSWER: Glaucoma is a common eye disorder that is caused by an increased pressure within the eyeball. This increased pressure results from an inability of eye fluid (aqueous humor) to properly drain from the eye, which eventually damages the optic nerve. It is the second leading cause of irreversible blindness in the United States, right behind diabetes. Approximately 3 million Americans over the age of 40 have glaucoma, but only about half of these cases are diagnosed. That is because most people with glaucoma do not have symptoms in the early stages of the disease and do not seek medical attention until the glaucoma is advanced and eye damage has already occurred. Risk factors for developing glaucoma include aging, a family history of glaucoma, diabetes, African-American descent, and very nearsightedness.

Although there is no cure for glaucoma, various drugs and laser surgery can be used to lower the pressure in the eye in order to try and prevent loss of vision. Most of the currently available drugs to treat glaucoma either work by helping to increase the drainage of fluid (aqueous humor) from the eye or they decrease the production of this fluid.

Numerous types of eyedrops and a few oral medications are available for the treatment of glaucoma. It is very important to use these eyedrops correctly to prevent side effects and to make sure that the drops are absorbed into the eye. In addition, when more than one eyedrop medication is used, the various eyedrops should be used at least 10 to 15 minutes apart or they will simply wash each other out of the eye.

The experimental drug treatment for glaucoma that you heard about recently will probably not be available for several years. These drugs are known as nitric oxide blocking agents. Researchers have found that there are increased levels of nitric oxide in the eyes of patients with glaucoma, which can be toxic to eye tissue. These nitric oxide blocking drugs may reduce the harmful effects on the eye and provide a new approach to the treatment of glaucoma in the future. Several other drugs are also currently being tested and researched.

QUESTION: My father has glaucoma and I heard about two new drugs recently approved for this condition. What are they?

ANSWER: The FDA recently approved two new eyedrops for the treatment of glaucoma, Travatan Z and Lumigan. Both work by helping to increase the outflow of aqueous humor from the eye. They are synthetic drugs that are similar to naturally occurring substances in the eyes known as prostaglandins that help to regulate the pressure in the eyes. These new eyedrops are administered once a day in the evening and some studies have shown that they may be more effective in reducing the pressure in the eye than currently available drugs. Side effects that can occur with these new medications include a gradual darkening of the eye color and eyelid skin, and an increased thickness, number, and darkness of eyelashes. Itching and redness of the eyes and eyelids can also occur. Both Travatan Z and Lumigan appear to be similar in effectiveness for glaucoma but more study is needed.

QUESTION: I heard about a new type of eyedrop medication for glaucoma. What can you tell me about it?

ANSWER: Numerous types of eyedrops and a few oral medications are available for the treatment of glaucoma. It is very important to use these eyedrops correctly to prevent side effects and to make sure that the drops are absorbed into the eye. In addition, when more than one eye drop medication is used, the various eyedrops should be used at least 10 to 15 minutes apart or they will simply wash each other out of the eye.

The new type of ophthalmic medication to treat glaucoma that was recently approved by the FDA is named Rescula (generic name undprostone). Rescula belongs to a new class of glaucoma drugs known as docosanoids, which are derived from a compound that is vital to the development and function of the retina of the eye. It appears to lower intraocular pressure by boosting the outflow of fluid (aqueous humor) from the eye. It will probably be used for patients who do not respond to other medications or who cannot tolerate other medications. The Rescula eyedrops are used twice a day either alone or in combination with other drugs. Contact lenses should be removed prior to using this eye drop, but may be reinserted 15 minutes later. The most common side effects of Rescula are burning, stinging, dry eyes, itching, and redness which occur in about 10 to 25% of patients. Long-term use may also affect the length of eyelashes and eye color.

ALZHEIMER'S DISEASE (AD)

QUESTION: I have a friend with Alzheimer's disease (AD). What drugs are available or being tested to treat this disease?

ANSWER: Alzheimer's disease is a devastating degenerative brain disorder in which patients develop brain lesions known as amyloid plaques and tangled proteins within the nerves of the brain. These "plaques and tangles" result in a decrease in mental function and an increase in behavioral problems. This disease is named after a German physician, Alois Alzheimer, who first described this disorder in 1906. Alzheimer's disease is not a normal part of aging and approximately 6% of people over 65 years of age and 35% of those over 85 years of age may be afflicted with this brain disorder. Some early onset types of Alzheimer's disease can occur as early as age 40. The first symptom of this disease is usually short-term memory loss, such as forgetting appointments, losing keys, getting lost traveling in familiar surroundings, and having difficulty handling money. As the disease progresses, the patient typically has difficulty performing routine tasks at home or work. Speech also becomes difficult and the patient may try to compensate by using evasive speech and confabulations. Later, the patient becomes unable to do routine chores and may neglect personal hygiene and appearance. Judgment and reasoning can become severely impaired, and supervision is required to protect the patient from accidental injury to self or others. In the final stages, the patient may become vegetative, unable to recognize family members, and unable to communicate. Mood disturbances, disruptive behavior, and psychosis can present problems for caregivers. Repetitive asking of questions, rummaging through drawers, perpetual humming or grunting, and fingernail clicking are common. Once a patient is diagnosed, life expectancy is approximately 10-11 years. The exact cause of Alzheimer's disease is not known, but the "plaques and tangles" in the brain lead to a decrease in the production of a brain chemical known as acetycholine, which is needed for brain cells to function. At the present time, there is no cure for this disease and the goal of therapy is to increase the quality of life for the patient.

Information Resource: Alzheimer's Association, 919 N. Michigan Avenue, Suite 1100, Chicago, IL 60611-1676 (800)272-3900.

QUESTION: I have a friend with Alzheimer's disease (AD). What drugs are available or being tested to treat this disease?

ANSWER: In continuation of last week's column, I will now review the drugs that are being used to treat Alzheimer's disease or are being studied for their effectiveness in this disorder. As I noted last week, the "plaques and tangles" in the brain of patients with Alzheimer's disease lead to a decrease in the production of the brain chemical known as acetylcholine which is needed for proper brain cell function. In view of this, several drugs have been developed or are being developed that increase the levels of this chemical in the brain. They do this by preventing the breakdown of acetylcholine or by causing a release of this chemical. Other drugs that act on brain receptors and work to protect brain cells or neurons are also being studied. In addition, antioxidants have been used in an attempt to reduce oxidative stress in the brain that may be a factor in the development of Alzheimer's disease. Anti-inflammatory agents may prove to be useful in some patients to reduce or prevent inflammation within the brain. Likewise, estrogen replacement therapy is being studied for use in postmenopausal women. Estrogen therapy is thought to improve cerebral blood flow and help to repair brain cells. Furthermore, a group of drugs known as neuronal growth promoters that stimulate nerve growth and protect brain cells are being studied. Please note that many of these drug studies are in their early stages and much more information concerning their effectiveness and safety will be needed. Finally, a host of other agents are being used to treat the behavioral problems seen in patients with Alzheimer's disease (AD). These include antipsychotics, tranquilizers or sedatives, anticonvulsants, mood stabilizers, and antidepressants. Below I have listed many of the drugs used for the treatment of Alzheimer's disease or that are undergoing study for this use. Please note that I have not included medications used to treat behavioral problems in these patients.

Drugs That Increase Acetylcholine In The Brain

- Tacrine (Cognex)
- Donezepil (Aricept)
- Rivastigmine (Exelon)
- Metrifonate
- Galanthamine
- Eptastigmine
- Huperzine A
- Linopiridine

Possible Neuroprotective Drugs

- AF-102B
- AIT-082
- Anti-Inflammatory Drugs
- Antioxidants
- Bapineuzumab
- Cerebrolysin
- Egb-761 (ginkgo biloba extract)
- Estrogen Replacement Therapy
- Neuronal Growth Promoters
- Nonsteroidal anti-inflammatory drugs (NSAIDs)
- Propentofylline
- Selegiline
- Solanezumab
- Vitamin E
- Xanomeline

A good information resource for Alzheimer's disease is: Alzheimer's Association, 919 N. Michigan Avenue, Suite 1100, Chicago, IL 60611-1676 phone (800)272-3900 **http://wwww.alz.org**

QUESTION: I heard about a new drug for Alzheimer's disease. What can you tell me about it?

ANSWER: The exact cause of Alzheimer's disease is not known, but the "plaques and tangles" in the brain interfere with chemicals that are needed for proper functioning. There is no known cure for this disease. Currently, there are four drugs approved for the treatment of mild-to-moderate Alzheimer's disease (Aricept, Razadyne, Exelon, and Cognex). They work by raising levels of a chemical known as acetylcholine, which is needed for brain cells to function. Recently, a new type of drug was recommended for approval for patients with more severe forms of the disease. It is called memantine (Namenda) and has been used in Germany to treat dementia since 1982. Memantine works by blocking a brain chemical known as glutamate that can damage or destroy nerve cells. It is not a miracle drug, but appears to provide modest improvement in performance for patients with moderate-to-severe Alzheimer's disease. There is no evidence that memantine has any effect in early stages of Alzheimer's or that it alters the course of the disease. Side effects of memantine include dizziness, headache, constipation, and confusion.

QUESTION: I heard about a new prescription medication for Alzheimer's disease (AD). What can you tell me about it?

ANSWER: The latest approved prescription drugs for Alzheimer's disease are named Exelon (generic name rivastigmine) and Razadyne (generic name galantamine).

   Although the cause of Alzheimer's disease is not known, it is associated with a loss of neurons (nerve cells) in the brain and a reduced amount of the neurotransmitter chemical known as acetylcholine. Several drugs have been developed that increase the amount of acetylcholine in the brain and improve mental functioning. They are known as acetylcholinesterase inhibitors. The newly approved products, Exelon and Razadyne, fall into this class of drugs, which increase the concentration of acetylcholine in the brain and work to improve memory, attention, and other cognitive abilities. Clinical studies have shown that Exelon can improve mental function in about 25% of patients with Alzheimer's disease, but the improvements are modest. The most common side effects associated with the use of Exelon are nausea, vomiting, loss of appetite, and dizziness. Likewise, Razadyne was approved for the treatment of mild to moderate Alzheimer's disease. It is derived from daffodil bulbs and has been shown to improve or stabilize mental function during clinical studies. The most frequent side effects of Razadyne are nausea, vomiting, loss of appetite, diarrhea, and weight loss. Unfortunately, like the other available drugs in this class (Cognex and Aricept), Exelon and Razadyne do not alter the progression of the disease.

QUESTION: What can you tell me about the new skin patch to treat Alzheimer's disease (AD)?

ANSWER: The FDA recently approved Exelon Patch, the first and only skin patch for the treatment of Alzheimer's disease. The once-daily patch was approved to treat patients with mild to moderate Alzheimer's disease and was also approved to treat patients with mild to moderate Parkinson's disease (PD) dementia. Alzheimer's disease, which afflicts about 5 million Americans, is a progressive, degenerative disease that alters the brain, causing impaired memory, thinking, and behavior. It is estimated that by 2030, the number of people in the U.S. over the age of 65 with Alzheimer's disease will reach almost 8 million. Parkinson's disease is a chronic and progressive neurological condition that affects approximately 1.5 million Americans. About 2 out of 5 people with Parkinson's disease have dementia characterized by impairments in memory and attention. Exelon, which contains the active ingredient rivastigmine, has been available as an oral capsule for many years to treat Alzheimer's disease. Rivastigmine is not a cure for this disease, but acts by blocking the breakdown of a chemical in the brain called acetycholine, which is needed for brain cells to function. The new once-daily Exelon Patch appears to be similar in effectiveness to Exelon Capsules, which are taken twice a day for the treatment of Alzheimer's disease. The Exelon Patch delivers rivastigmine through the skin into the bloodstream over a 24 hour period, which provides a convenient dosage form. In addition, since the drug enters the bloodstream directly, it reduces some of the gastrointestinal side effects seen with the capsule form such as nausea and vomiting.

QUESTION: Are there any generic drugs available to treat Alzheimer's disease?

ANSWER: Yes, the FDA recently gave its nod to two generic drugs for treating dementia related to Alzheimer's disease. In December 2009 a generic form of Aricept (donepezil) orally disintegrating tablets was approved and in January 2010 the FDA gave tentative approval to a generic version of Namenda (memantine). The generic donepezil product should be available soon, but generic memantine needs to get final FDA approval, which will depend upon a determination of patent expiration for Namenda. Donepezil works by raising levels of a chemical known as acetylcholine, which is needed for brain cells to function. On the other hand, memantine works by blocking a brain chemical known as glutamate that can damage or destroy nerve cells. Donepezil is approved for the treatment of dementia in patients with mild to moderate or severe Alzheimer's disease. Memantine, however, is only approved for moderate to severe Alzheimer's disease. Neither of these agents is a miracle drug, but do appear to provide modest improvement.

QUESTION: What can you tell me about the new medical food for Alzheimer's disease?

ANSWER: The use of "medical foods" goes back to the early 1970's, when infant formulas were developed for patients with rare inherited metabolic disorders. In the past 20 years, commercially prepared "medical foods" have been marketed for various medical conditions. Recently Axona, a "medical food" containing a formulation of medium-chain triglycerides, was marketed for the clinical dietary management of the metabolic processes associated with mild to moderate Alzheimer's disease (AD). The rationale for using Axona is that researchers have found a reduction in glucose utilization in the brain in patients with Alzheimer's disease and in younger people at risk for AD. Medium-chain triglycerides are metabolized in the liver into compounds (ketone bodies) that are transported into the brain, which provide an alternative fuel source in the brain in place of glucose. Some clinical studies have shown that the use of Axona results in improvements in the Alzheimer's Disease Assessment Scale. Although medium-chain triglycerides are generally considered safe, in clinical studies with Axona, about 25% of patients developed diarrhea, and a few patients showed significant increases in blood triglyceride levels. In addition, Axona contains milk and soy products, so it is not recommended in people who are allergic to these ingredients. It should also be noted that "medical foods" are exempt from labeling requirements for health claims and nutrient content, and are not reviewed or approved by the FDA. The manufacturer of Axona recommends taking one packet of its product dissolved in 4-8 ounces of water with breakfast each day. However, the evidence for use of medium-chain triglycerides to prevent or treat AD is limited and the long-term effects of taking this "medical food" are unknown. Alzheimer's disease is the most common neurodegenerative disease, affecting approximately 5.2 million Americans. As with all prescription and non-prescription drugs and supplements, you should consult with your physician before taking any "medical food". More information about Axona can be found at **www.about-axona.com.**

QUESTION: Can statin drugs reduce the risk of Alzheimer's disease?

ANSWER: Numerous studies have looked at this question and the results have been mixed. Some studies show that Alzheimer's disease is rarer in people who take statins, but other studies show the opposite. In the most recent and largest study to date it was concluded that the use of statins, but not of non-statin cholesterol-lowering drugs, was associated with a lower risk of Alzheimer's disease. The results of this study (The Rotterdam study) were reported in the January 2009 issue of the Journal of Neurology, Neurosurgery and Psychiatry. The Rotterdam study involved almost 7,000 participants over the age of 55 who were followed for an average of 9 years. During this time, 582 subjects were diagnosed with Alzheimer's. When compared with the non-statin user, people taking statins had a significant 43% reduced risk of Alzheimer's disease. This protective effect was similar for various types of statin drugs. On the other hand, the use of other cholesterol-lowering drugs such as fibrates or nicotinic acid did not show a similar protection benefit. It is not clearly understood how statins may prevent Alzheimer's disease but their effects on cholesterol may lead to a decrease in the production of dangerous proteins found in the brains of people with this disease. Statins may also work by reducing inflammation in the brain or by improving circulation in the brain. Clearly, much more study in this area is needed, but the results reported in this recent study are very interesting. There are currently seven statin drugs available: atorvastatin (Lipitor), fluvastatin (Lescol), lovastatin (Mevacor, Altoprev), pitavastatin (Livalo), pravastatin (Pravachol), rosuvastatin (Crestor), and simvastatin (Zocor). Aorvastatin, lovastatin, pravastatin, and simvastatin are also available as generic drugs.

QUESTION: I heard on TV that insulin nasal spray may help slow Alzheimer's disease. What can you tell me about this?

ANSWER: Results of a pilot study recently reported in the medical journal Archives of Neurology suggests that intranasal insulin may improve memory and activities of daily living in patients with Alzheimer's disease (AD). Patients in this study received either intranasal insulin using a special device to help get it into the brain, or a placebo (dummy medication) for a 4-month period and were then given tests to see if their memory improved. The study involved 104 men and women with AD, with an average age of about 72. Study results showed that treatment with intranasal insulin improved delayed memory using story recall testing and also preserved caregiver-rated activities of daily living. It is not known exactly how insulin may help in AD, but insulin is critical for normal brain function and progressive reductions in glucose (sugar) metabolism in the brain have been well documented in AD. It should be emphasized, however, that this was a small pilot study of short duration and much larger and longer studies will be needed to support the use of intranasal insulin therapy for patients with AD. People should not try to treat themselves with insulin, which can be deadly if misused.

QUESTION: What can you tell me about curcumin and Alzheimer's disease?

ANSWER: Curcumin has been used as a traditional Indian (Ayruvedic) and Chinese medicine for thousands of years. It is derived from tumeric, a plant found in southern Asia that is widely used as a yellow food color and spice, including an ingredient in curry powder. Curcumin is known as a "polyphenolic" or "curcuminoid" compound that has many effects including antioxidant and anti-inflammatory properties. It has also been reported that curcumin may boost the immune system to help remove amyloid plaques from the brain. All of these effects may help people with Alzheimer's disease and perhaps other neurodegenerative disorders. However, naturally occurring curcumin is not readily absorbed from the gastrointestinal tract and man-made (synthetic) curcumin products have been developed to try and overcome this problem. At this point in time, no dosage of curcumin can be recommended for medicinal use and more research is needed. Currently, studies of curcumin used alone and in combination with other agents such as vitamin D are underway to determine the therapeutic effects, dosage, and safety of curcumin in Alzheimer's and other diseases.

STATINS AND COLON CANCER

QUESTION: Can statin drugs reduce the risk of colon cancer?

ANSWER: While statin drugs have a number of effects in addition to lowering high cholesterol levels and reducing the risk of heart disease and stroke, they do not appear to be useful in curbing the risk of colorectal cancer. A recent study involving more than 400,000 Canadians suggests that there is no significant reduction in the risk of colon cancer in people who regularly take statin medications. In this study, statin users were followed up for 3 to 7 years and the incidence of colorectal cancer was similar to that for people who never used statins. Colon cancer is the third leading cancer and the second leading cause of cancer deaths in the U.S. It has been estimated that over 145,000 new cases of colon cancer will be diagnosed in the U.S. this year, and ninety percent of people who get this disease are over the age of 50. Colonoscopy is considered the gold standard for finding, removing, and possibly preventing colorectal cancer. It can detect up to 95% of colon cancers and can be used to remove precancerous polyps before they develop into cancer. Current guidelines recommend that colonoscopy screening begin at age 50 for individuals at average risk for getting colorectal cancer. There are currently seven statin drugs available: atorvastatin (Lipitor), fluvastatin (Lescol), lovastatin (Mevacor, Altoprev), pitavastatin (Livalo), pravastatin (Pravachol), rosuvastatin (Crestor), and simvastatin (Zocor). Atorvastatin, lovastatin, pravastatin, and simvastatin are also available as generic drugs.

OVERACTIVE BLADDER

QUESTION: What can be done for an overactive bladder?

ANSWER: An overactive bladder (also called urge incontinence) is the most common cause of urinary incontinence in the elderly. The incidence of this disorder increases with age, primarily as a result of age-related problems or events. The aging process is associated with a decrease in bladder capacity and its ability to empty completely, involuntary bladder muscle contractions, and sex-specific changes. Elderly women may experience bladder problems due to estrogen deficiency, while elderly men commonly may have bladder problems due to prostate gland enlargement. A number of other medical problems such as Alzheimer's disease, stroke, Parkinson's disease, urinary tract infection, and diabetes can also cause bladder problems.

The symptoms of an overactive bladder are described as urgency and frequency, with patients reporting symptoms throughout the day and several times each night. The urgency to urinate can be great and may result in a sudden leakage of urine. In addition, many patients often experience a sensation that they have not emptied their bladder completely.

The treatment of an overactive bladder can involve both medications and non-drug measures. Non-drug therapies include behavioral bladder training, pelvic floor exercises, biofeedback, and in serious cases, surgery. Drug therapy to reduce bladder muscle contractions and promote the storage of urine are often needed. The normal process of urination is complicated and involves many nerves and bladder muscles that contract or relax. Drugs used to treat an overactive bladder work on these nerves and muscles and help to reduce the urge to urinate and the frequency of urination. The most commonly used medications are known as anticholinergic drugs. The two agents used most in clinical practice are Ditropan (oxybutynin) and Detrol (tolterodine). Other similar drugs include Urispas (flavoxate), Bentyl (diclyclomine), and Levsin (hyoscyamine). These drugs can also cause sedation and should not be used in people with glaucoma, myasthenia gravis, or gastrointestinal obstruction disorders. In addition, they should be used with caution in people with a history of heart disease. Other side effects of these medications include dry mouth, blurred vision, and constipation. Another drug used for overactive bladder is Tofranil (imipramine), which is an antidepressant, but also has a number of other effects, which may benefit some patients. Your doctor can help decide what therapy is best for you.

QUESTION: I heard about a new prescription product for overactive bladder. What can you tell me about it?

ANSWER: The new product you heard about is named Sanctura and contains the anticholinergic drug trospium. It is given orally twice a day and its most common side effects are dry mouth, constipation, and headache. Sanctura should not be used in people with urinary retention, gastric retention, or glaucoma. Other commonly used anticholinergic drugs for overactive bladder include Ditropan (oxybutynin) and Detrol (tolterodine).

QUESTION: I heard about a new patch for overactive bladder. What can you tell me about it?

ANSWER: The new patch you heard about is named Oxytrol and contains the anticholinergic drug, oxybutynin. The Oxytrol transdermal system or patch slowly releases the drug, which is absorbed through the skin over a 4-day period. A new patch is applied to the abdomen, hip, or buttock twice a week, providing a convenient way to help control overactive bladder. Oxytrol has been shown to reduce the number of incontinence episodes, reduce urinary frequency, and increase the amount of urine voided. The most common side effects of this patch include irritation and itching where the patch is applied, dry mouth, constipation, diarrhea, vision problems, and pain when urinating.

QUESTION: I've heard about a new drug for overactive bladder. What can you tell me about it?

ANSWER: Actually the FDA recently approved 2 new drugs for the treatment of overactive bladder, VESIcare (solifenacin) and Enablex (darifenacin). An overactive bladder (also called urge incontinence) is the most common cause of urinary incontinence in the elderly and I've written several columns on this topic. Overactive bladder is a medical condition that causes the bladder muscle (called the detrusor muscle) to contract while the bladder is filling with urine, instead of when the bladder is full. People with this problem feel the urge to urinate more often and many times without warning. An important concern for people with overactive bladder is the fear of having an accident in public. Because of this, they gradually develop coping behaviors such as restricting fluid intake, carrying extra clothing, "mapping" bathroom locations, or even choosing not to leave the friendly confines of their home. Numerous medications are available to treat this disorder including Ditropan (oxybutynin), Detrol (tolterodine), Urispas (flavoxate), Bentyl (dicyclomine), and Levsin (hyocyamine). Now you can add to this list VESIcare and Enablex, which have been shown to reduce the symptoms of overactive bladder such as urinary frequency, urgency, and incontinence episodes. They also have been shown to increase the volume of urine voided per urination. Like many of the other drugs used to treat this disorder, VESIcare and Enablex work by blocking the nerve impulse (anticholinergic) that causes the bladder muscle to contract. They may also cause fewer side effects (such as dry throat) than some other drugs used to treat overactive bladder, but more comparison studies are needed. Both VESIcare and Enablex are given orally once daily. Their most common side effects are dry mouth and constipation.

QUESTION: I heard about a new prescription product for overactive bladder. What can you tell me about it?

ANSWER: The new product you heard about is named Toviaz and contains the anticholinergic drug fesoterodine. It is given once a day and its most common side effects are dry mouth and constipation. Toviaz should not be used in patients with urinary retention, gastric retention, or uncontrolled narrow-angle glaucoma. Other commonly used anticholinergic drugs for overactive bladder include Enablex (darifenacin), Urispas (flavoxate), Oxytrol (oxybutrin), Detrol (tolterodine), Vesicare (solifenacin), and Sanctura (trospium).

QUESTION: I heard about a topical gel that was approved to treat overactive bladder. What can you tell me about it?

ANSWER: The new topical gel that you head about is named Gelnique and contains the anticholinergic drug, oxybutynin. The gel is applied once a day to the abdomen, upper arms/shoulders or thighs. During a clinical study involving almost 800 patients with overactive bladder, Gelnique was effective in reducing the number of incontinence episodes and urinary frequency, and produces an increase in urine volume per void. The most frequently reported treatment related side effects of Gelnique in this study included dry mouth and application-site reactions (itching, rash, redness). Like other anticholinergic drugs, Gelnique should not be used by people who have urinary retention, gastric retention, or narrow-angle glaucoma.

QUESTION: I heard about a new prescription product for overactive bladder that comes in a pump. What can you tell me about it?

ANSWER: The FDA recently approved Anturol (oxybutynin) 3% topical gel for the treatment of overactive bladder (OAB) in patients with symptoms of urge urinary incontinence, urgency, and frequency. The active ingredient in Anturol, oxybutynin, has been available in different dosage forms for a long time, but this new product comes with a pump delivery system to help apply a proper dose of gel topically once daily to the thigh, abdomen, upper arm, or shoulder. After being applied to the skin, the oxybutynin is absorbed into the bloodstream over a 24-hour period where it blocks the nerve impulses that cause the bladder muscle to contract, which reduces bladder spasms and delays the desire to urinate in people with OAB. Since Anturol gel is applied topically, it can help to reduce some of the side effects seen with oxybutynin given orally. During clinical study, Anturol was shown to reduce the number of incontinence episodes and to improve urinary frequency and volume of urine per urination. The most common side effects of Anaturol gel are dry mouth, and skin reactions where it is applied.

OAB is characterized by a sudden, uncomfortable need to urinate with or without urge incontinence (urine leakage), and usually includes more frequent urination and nocturia (waking up at least once during the night to urinate). It affects as many as 33 million adults in the U.S., which is more common than diabetes or asthma. More than an "inconvenience", OAB is disabling and associated with a marked decrease in health-related quality of life as well as higher rates of depression. The disease affects both men and women, however, women experience more severe symptoms earlier in life.

QUESTION: I heard that a new drug was approved to treat adults with an overactive bladder. What can you tell me about it?

ANSWER: In June 2012, the FDA approved Myrbetriq (mirabegron) for the treatment of overactive bladder (OAB). Symptoms of OAB include the need to urinate too often (urinary frequency), the need to urinate immediately (urinary urgency), and the involuntary leakage of urine as a result of the need to urinate (urge urinary incontinence). Myrbetriq is an extended-release tablet that is taken once a day. It is a new type of medication that relaxes the bladder's smooth muscle (detrusor) while it is filling and increases the bladder's capacity to hold urine. Other agents used to treat OAB work by inhibiting involuntary bladder contractions. During clinical studies, once-daily Myrbetriq was shown to help patients with OAB reduce the number of times they urinate each day and reduce the number of times they had a wetting incident. In addition, patients with OAB were able to expel more urine when they urinated, demonstrating the drug's effectiveness in improving the storage capacity of the bladder. The most common side effects observed during clinical studies with Myrbetriq were increased blood pressure, common cold-like symptoms, urinary tract infection, constipation, fatigue, elevated heart rate, and abdominal pain. This new drug is not recommended for use in people with severe uncontrolled high blood pressure, end stage kidney disease, or severe liver problems.

EARWAX

QUESTION: What can I do for excessive earwax?

ANSWER: Earwax or cerumen is a yellowish substance secreted by glands in the outer portion of the ear canal (the tube that leads to the eardrum). Actually, cerumen serves as a protective coating and along with hairs that line the outer half of the ear canal, helps to protect the ear from injury and infection. Earwax contains antibodies against bacteria and is slightly acidic, which discourages the growth of bacteria and fungi. People with abnormally narrow ear canals and/or excessive hair growth in the canal are predisposed to impacted cerumen because the normal flow of cerumen to the opening of the ear is disrupted. Earwax impaction is also a common problem for people who use hearing aids, which may push earwax inward when they are placed in the ears. In fact, some people think they are having difficulty hearing because their hearing aid is not working or needs a new battery when earwax is actually causing their hearing problem. In addition, older people may experience impacted earwax due to the formation of a drier cerumen, which is more difficult to expel from the ear. Improper use of cotton swabs to clean the ear canal can also lead to impaction of earwax. Symptoms of impacted earwax include ear discomfort, a feeling of fullness, and difficulty hearing.

Proper, routine cleaning can help to prevent earwax buildup. Cotton swabs can be used around the outer part of the ear and the opening of the ear canal and cotton balls can be used to clean and dry the outer ears after bathing. However, cotton swabs or any other object should never be inserted into the ear canal, because you can puncture the eardrum or cause an infection. Mildly impacted earwax can often by dislodged with an over-the-counter (OTC) earwax softener such as Debrox, Murine Ear Drops, AuroEar Drops, and others. Make sure that you follow the package directions closely for proper use. Other agents such as a drop or two of warm (not hot) mineral oil, or olive oil (sweet oil) twice a day have also been used as home remedies, but you should consult your doctor or pharmacist before using these agents. After the cerumen is softened, the ear should be gently irrigated, using an ear bulb syringe filled with warm water. The ear should be flushed with warm water, holding your head upright and then turning it sideways so that the water drains. Earwax problems that persist require help from a doctor. Be sure to consult a doctor if you have pain, swelling, tenderness, persistent hearing loss, or a milky discharge. These may be signs of an ear infection. Also, never put any solution in our ears if you have signs of a perforated eardrum, such as earache or sudden pain in the ear, partial hearing loss, slight bleeding, or discharge. If you think that you have impacted earwax please consult your doctor or pharmacist for more information.

DEPRESSION

QUESTION: I am a 69 year old male and have had insomnia and frequent periods of depression most of my adult life. I've tried numerous drugs over the years to help, but nothing seems to work. Do you have any advice for me?

ANSWER: Depression is a very common illness, which affects the whole body. During their lives, about 5.8% of the population will suffer from depression. It is more common than heart disease or cancer. Depression is twice as common in women as in men and depressive symptoms may occur in approximately 15% of people over the age of 65. Symptoms of depression include feelings of hopelessness, sadness, worthlessness, and changes in appetite and sleep behavior. The cause of depression is not clearly known, but patients with depression have symptoms that suggest that the illness may be due to a disorder affecting the chemicals in the brain that are used to conduct nerve impulses. Numerous antidepressant medications are available to treat depression and you have taken many of these as noted in your letter. They all work a little differently on the brain chemicals and have different side effects. These drugs are not addicting, but work to return a person's moods to normal. All antidepressants take several weeks to reach their full effect and it is important to continue the medication for the full course of therapy to prevent symptoms from coming back. In many cases the side effects of antidepressants will decrease over time. Your pharmacist and doctor should be made aware of all your medications, because antidepressants can interact with many drugs and alcohol. Some newer antidepressant medications include Remeron (generic name, mirtazapine), Effexor (generic name, venlafaxine), and Serzone (generic name, nefazodone). Your doctor can help to determine which antidepressant might be best for you.

Chronic or long-term insomnia (difficulty in sleeping) is a very common symptom of depression. Therefore, it is important to get appropriate treatment for depression first and not just rely on drugs that help you sleep. Some helpful principles for good sleep are as follows:

Principles Of Good Sleep Hygiene

- Follow a regular sleep pattern: go to bed and arise at about the same time daily.
- Make the bedroom comfortable for sleeping. Avoid temperature extremes, noise, and lights.
- Make sure the bed is comfortable.
- Engage in relaxing activities prior to bedtime.
- Exercise regularly but not late in the evening.
- Use the bedroom only for sleep and sexual activities, and not as an office, game room, etc.
- If tense, practice relaxation exercises.
- If hungry, eat a light snack, but avoid eating meals or large snacks immediately prior to bedtime.
- Eliminate daytime naps.
- Avoid caffeine use after noon.
- Avoid alcohol or nicotine use later in the evening.
- If unable to fall asleep, do not become anxious; leave the bedroom and participate in relaxing activities until tired.

QUESTION: I heard about a new antidepressant being approved. What can you tell me about it?

ANSWER: The new antidepressant is called Lexapro (escitalopram). It is the first new antidepressant approved by the FDA in the last 4 years. Lexapro is manufactured by Forest Pharmaceuticals and is very similar to another antidepressant, Celexa, from the same company. Lexapro is known as a selective serotonin reuptake inhibitor or SSRI. It works by altering the amount of a brain chemical called serotonin, which is believed to be involved in depression. During clinical studies, Lexapro was found to be similar in effectiveness compared to other SSRI drugs. It may be somewhat faster acting than some other antidepressants, but more studies and experience with using this new drug will be necessary to determine this. Lexapro is taken once daily. Side effects include nausea, diarrhea, dry mouth, difficulty in sleeping, increased sweating, fatigue, and an ejaculation disorder in men. Patients on the drug should not use alcohol or be taking MAO inhibitors (monoamine oxidase inhibitors).

QUESTION: I heard about a new type of antidepressant recently approved. What can you tell me about it?

ANSWER: The FDA recently approved a new type of antidepressant called Cymbalta (generic name duloxetine). Cymbalta belongs to a new class of antidepressant drugs that work on two different brain and spinal cord chemicals are involved in depression, serotonin and norepinephrine. These brain chemicals are believed to help regulate a person's emotions and sensitivity to pain. Because Cymbalta helps to restore balance between two different brain chemicals it is known as a dual-reuptake inhibitor. By working on both of these chemicals, Cymbalta treats the emotional and physical symptoms of depression, which can have a tremendous impact on a person's quality of life. Emotional symptoms can include feelings of sadness or crying, lost interest in favorite activities, feeling overwhelmed or stressed, feeling suicidal or like life isn't worth living, and difficulty concentrating. Physical symptoms of depression can include sleep changes, vague aches and pains, headaches, changes in appetite and weight, tiredness, and problems with digestion. Nearly 19 million Americans suffer from depression each year and it is a leading cause of disability. During clinical testing, many people taking Cymbalta began to see an improvement in symptoms within one to four weeks. However, not everyone responds to treatment and results will vary from person to person. In addition, people taking certain other medications such as MAO inhibitors or thioridazine should not use Cymbalta. It should also be avoided by people with uncontrolled narrow-angle glaucoma, people with liver disease, or by people with substantial alcohol use. Some of the common side effects of Cymbalta are nausea, dry mouth, constipation, decreased appetite, fatigue, sleepiness, and increased sweating. Cymbalta can be taken once daily.

QUESTION: I take Paxil for depression. Is a generic product available?

ANSWER: Yes, there are now generic paroxetine (Paxil) products available. They come in 10 mg, 20 mg, 30 mg, and 40 mg dosages. As I've noted before, the FDA approves all generic drugs using strict guidelines, including checking for the generic drug's chemistry by evaluating its formulation, potency, stability and purity. The generic drug must also pass bio-equivalency testing that compares the delivery into the bloodstream of the generic drug's active ingredient to that of the brand name drug. The use of generic drugs has grown substantially in the past 15 years, rising from 25% of all new prescriptions in 1987 to 40% in 2002. Generic drugs are less expensive because generic manufacturers don't have all the investment costs of the developer of a new drug. Also, once generic drugs are approved, there is greater competition, which helps to keep the price down. Generic drugs do not look the same as brand-name drugs because trademark laws do not allow a generic drug to look exactly like the brand-name drug. However, the active ingredient in the generic product must be identical to the brand-name product. Paroxetine (generic name for Paxil) is an effective antidepressant medication that is also used to treat panic disorder, obsessive-compulsive disorder, social anxiety disorder, posttraumatic stress disorder, and other conditions. It is known as a "selective serotonin reuptake inhibitor" or SSRI and works by altering the levels of certain chemicals within the brain.

QUESTION: I recently heard that generic Prozac became available. Are there other new generics coming soon?

ANSWER: After a number of legal battles, generic Prozac or fluoxetine is now available. Two other popular medications, Mevacor (lovastatin) and Buspar (buspirone) also recently became available as generic drugs. As I've noted many times before, the FDA approves all generic drugs using strict guidelines, including checking for the generic drug's chemistry by evaluating its formulation, potency, stability, and purity.

The generic drug must also pass bio-cquivalency testing that compares the delivery into the bloodstream of the generic drug's active ingredient to that of the brand name drug. Generic drugs are less expensive than brand-name products, and account for about 40 percent of prescriptions dispensed.

QUESTION: How long will I have to take my antidepressant medication?

ANSWER: This question was recently addressed in a Johns Hopkins Health Alert (**www.johnshopkinshealthalerts.com**, 2010). Today, experts recognize that major depression and anxiety are long term, often recurrent illnesses. But it isn't necessarily permanent, and many people with mood disorders can eventually stop taking antidepressant medication. Although antidepressant medications aren't addictive and, when discontinued, don't cause the same type of withdrawal reaction as medications like opiates for pain, your body may still experience withdrawal-like symptoms. If you quit antidepressant medication cold turkey, you could experience physical discomfort or a relapse of your condition. Some people can be tapered off antidepressant medication after an extended period of stability, but these changes need to be timed carefully. Antidepressant medications usually produce a significant improvement in four to six weeks, although it may take 12 weeks or longer on a therapeutic dose to see the full benefit. This is known as the acute phase. If your condition has improved after this time, you move on to a continuation phase with the goal of preventing a relapse (the return of the same depressive episode). Continuation treatment lasts anywhere from four months to a year, and you will continue to take the same dosage of the antidepressant medication that worked in the acute phase. If you remain symptom free at the end of the continuation phase, you are recovered, and many people require no further treatment. Your doctor may prescribe slightly lower doses of your antidepressant medication in the maintenance phase than during the acute or continuation phases. Maintenance treatment may be especially important for older adults, for whom research indicates high rates of recurrence: 50-90% over a two—to three-year period, as cited by a study in "The New England Journal of Medicine". Despite these guidelines, there is no "one size fits all" when it comes to treatment length. However, recent evidence shows that many people require a year or more of antidepressant therapy to treat a major episode of depression or anxiety adequately. You should consult with your doctor to determine how long you will need to take your antidepressant medication.

QUESTION: I heard that a new drug was approved to treat depression. What can you tell me about it?

ANSWER: The FDA recently approved Viibryd (vilazodone) to treat major depressive disorder. Major depressive disorder, also called major depression, is characterized by symptoms that interfere with a person's ability to work, sleep, study, eat, and enjoy once-pleasurable activities. Episodes of major depression often recur throughout a person's lifetime, although some may experience only a single occurrence. Signs and symptoms of major depression include: depressed mood, loss of interest in usual activities, significant change in weight or appetite, insomnia or excessive sleeping (hypersomnia), restlessness/pacing (psychomotor agitation), increased fatigue, feelings of guilt or worthlessness, slowed thinking or impaired concentration, and suicide attempts or thoughts of suicide. All people with major depression do not experience the same symptoms. Exactly how Viibryd works to treat depression is not fully understood, but it has a dual mechanism of action in the brain and enhances the activity of the brain chemical known as serotonin. During clinical study, Viibryd was able to significantly improve the symptoms of patients with major depression compared to a dummy pill (placebo). The most frequent side effects reported by patients taking Viibryd in clinical trials included diarrhea, nausea, vomiting, and insomnia. Viibryd did not appear to cause significant weight gain or negatively impact sexual desire or function seen with many other antidepressants. However, like all other antidepressant drugs, Viibryd labeling has a boxed warning and a patient medication guide describing the increased risk of suicidal thinking and behavior in children, adolescents, and young adults aged 18 to 24 during initial treatment.

EXCESSSIVE SWEATING

QUESTION: I seem to sweat a lot more than other people. Can Zocor cause this?

ANSWER: Zocor is a "statin" drug that is used to lower high cholesterol levels. While some drugs in this class ("statins") can cause sweating, Zorcor does not appear to be one of them. Sweat is made by the sweat glands in the skin and is carried to the skin's surface by ducts. Sweating helps to cool the body by evaporation. Thus, people usually sweat more when it's warm. The evaporation of water from the skin can also occur without the production of visible sweat and is known as "insensible" sweat. Excessive sweating (also know as hyperhidrosis) may affect the entire surface of the skin, but often it's limited to the palms, soles, armpits, or groin. It can be caused by various medical conditions such as infections, nervous disorders, migraine, or thyroid problems. Abnormal sweating may also be associated with certain foods, hot drinks, or with hot flashes during menopause. If the excessive sweating is due to a medical problem, appropriate therapy for that condition needs to be addressed. Heavy sweating of the palms, soles, or armpits can be controlled to some degree with a nighttime application of aluminum chloride solution (Drysol), which requires a prescription. When using this product, the sweaty area must be completely dried prior to its application. For maximum effect the area can be covered with plastic wrap after application of the solution. The plastic wrap is removed in the morning and the area is then washed. In some people excessive sweating may stop after 2 or more treatments. There are several other types of treatments for hyperhidrosis that may also be effective. You should discuss this problem with your doctor so that the most appropriate therapy can be selected for your situation.

OSTEOPOROSIS

QUESTION: What drugs are used to treat osteoporosis?

ANSWER: Osteoporosis is a bone disorder that can lead to fractures affecting about 10 million Americans, about 80% of whom are women. Another 18 million people have a condition known as low bone mass, which puts them at high risk for osteoporosis. As the population ages, osteoporosis will become much more common. This disease produces a loss of bone mass throughout the skeleton, making the bones more fragile which increases the risk of fractures, particularly in the hip, spine, and wrist. Osteoporosis is caused by an imbalance between the formation of new bone and bone breakdown due to hormone deficiencies, aging, medication, or other causes. Some of the risk factors for osteoporosis and fractures include the following:

- Advanced age
- Dementia
- Being female
- Personal or family history of fracture
- White or Asian race
- Alcoholism
- Cigarette smoking
- Estrogen or testosterone deficiency
- Inadequate calcium, vitamin D, and vitamin K in diet
- Physical inactivity
- Low body weight or small body build

Osteoporosis, like high blood pressure, is often called a "silent disease" because bone loss occurs without symptoms, and may go undetected until a fracture occurs. Preventative measures for people of all ages are very important and should include adequate intake of calcium and vitamin D, along with regular weight-bearing exercise, smoking cessation, and moderation in alcohol intake. But even with enough dietary calcium intake and a healthy lifestyle, many postmenopausal women and others at risk of osteoporosis can continue to lose bone. The most commonly used tool to diagnose osteoporosis and predict fracture risk is a test for bone mineral density (BMD).

There are 3 types of prescription medications available to prevent and treat osteoporosis: hormone replacement therapy (HRT); selective estrogen receptor modifiers (SERMS); and bisphosphonates. A fourth type of medication, calcitonin, is used for treatment only. HRT is useful for osteoporosis prevention and treatment in postmenopausal women because one-third to one-half of bone loss in older women is due to estrogen deficiency. SERMs like Evista act similar to estrogen to increase bone mineral density in postmenopausal women, but have a lower risk of causing breast cancer than HRT. Bisphosphonates like Fosfamax or Actonel reduce bone loss and are probably the best agents for actually building up bone density in the spine and hip. Finally, the hormone calcitonin works by inhibiting bone loss but may not be as effective as the other drugs. It does, however, have analgesic activity and may be useful in patients with significant pain. Many other new treatments are also being tested for the prevention and treatment of osteoporosis.

QUESTION: What can you tell me about a new warning for osteoporosis medications?

ANSWER: In October 2010, the FDA issued a warning about the increased risk of thigh bone (femur) fracture in patients using bisphosphonates long-term for osteoporosis. This warning applies to oral bisphosphonates including Fosamax (alendronate), Fosamax Plus D, Actonel (risedronate), Actonel with Calcium, Boniva (ibandronate), Atelvia (risedronate), and their generic products, as well as injectable bisphosphonates such as Reclast (zoledronic acid), and Boniva (ibandronate). While it is not clear whether bisphosphonates are the cause, atypical thigh bone (femur) fractures, a rare but serious type of femur fracture, have been predominantly reported in patients taking these drugs. The optimal duration of bisphosphonate use for osteoporosis is unknown, and the FDA is highlighting this uncertainty because these fractures may be related to use of these medications for longer than 5 years. The labeling of these bisphosphonate products will now include a warning about this risk. Patients taking bisphosphonates for osteoporosis should not stop using their medication unless told to do so by their physician. Patients should also report any new thigh or groin pain to their healthcare provider and be evaluated for a possible thigh bone fracture. Healthcare professionals should also be aware of the possible risk of thigh bone fracture in patients taking these drugs and consider periodic re-evaluation of the need for continued bisphosphonate therapy in patients who have been on these drugs for longer than 5 years.

QUESTION: How long should someone take osteoporosis drugs?

ANSWER: This a good question, but there is no clear-cut answer at this point in time. Recently (2012), the FDA provided a Consumer Update regarding this question, which provides useful information about this subject.

If you're one of the 44 million Americans at risk for osteoporosis—a disease in which bones become weak and are more likely to break—you may be taking bisphosphonates. This class of drugs has been successfully used since 1995 to slow or inhibit the loss of bone mass. Doctors commonly prescribe such brand-name drugs as Actonel, Atelvia, Boniva, and Fosamax (as well as a number of generic products) for osteoporosis. In fact, more than 150 million prescriptions were dispensed to patients between 2005 and 2009. Bones go through a continual process of remodeling, in the form of bone resorption (disintegration) and bone formation. Bone loss related to osteoporosis occurs when resorption is greater than formation. Bisphosphonates decrease bone resorption, thereby slowing bone loss. During treatment, bisphosphonates become part of the newly formed bone and can stay there for years, through many cycles of resorption and formation. Patients continue to be exposed to the effects of the drug even long after they've stopped taking it. Bisphosphonate labels have carried a safety warning about severe jaw bone decay (osteonecrosis of the jaw) since 2002. In October 2010, the FDA warned patients and health care professionals about the increased risk of unusual thigh bone fractures and directed manufacturers to include the warning in the safety labels and medication guides that come with prescription medications. The FDA continues to evaluate the possible association of bisphosphonates with esophageal cancer. These associations would suggest that health care professionals may want to reconsider how long patients should continue taking the drugs.

Researchers at the FDA have taken a close look at the long-term benefit of bisphosphonates to treat osteoporosis. Their review of clinical studies measuring the effectiveness of long-term bisphosphonates use shows that some patients may be able to stop using bisphosphonates after three to five years and still continue to benefit from their use. According to the review, further investigation is needed on the long-term risks and benefits of these drugs.

In view of the above information, decisions to continue treatment must be based on individual assessments of risks and benefits and on patient preference. If you are taking bisphosphonates:

- Talk to your physician about whether or not you should continue this therapy. Re-evaluate the decision on a periodic basis.
- Don't stop taking these (or any) prescribed drugs without talking to your physician first. If you do make the decision to discontinue use, talk to your physician before stopping therapy.
- Tell your health care professional if you develop new hip or thigh pain (commonly described as dull or aching pain), or have any concerns with your medications.
- Report unusual side effects of your bisphosphonate medication to the FDA's MedWatch program.

QUESTION: My wife takes Fosamax for osteoporosis and was told by her doctor not to drink any coffee in the morning. Why is that?

ANSWER: Fosamax (generic name alendronate) is a type of drug known as a "bisphosphonate". Bisphosphonates are used to treat osteoporosis because they work to prevent the breakdown of bone (bone resorption) by the osteoclast bone cells. This helps to bring the maintenance of bone by the body back into balance. Bisphosphonates like Fosamax are useful drugs for osteoporosis but their activity can be affected by other drugs and foods or drinks. For example, Zantac (ranitidine), which is used for heartburn, may increase the activity of Fosamax while calcium supplements or antacids can interfere with the absorption of Fosamax when taken together. The use of Fosamax can also increase the risk of gastrointestinal problems when taken with aspirin. In addition food, coffee, or orange juice can significantly reduce the absorption and clinical effects of Fosamax. In view of these interactions, Fosamax tablets should be taken with a full glass of plain water first thing in the morning and at least 30 minutes before any other beverage or food. Patients taking Fosamax should also avoid lying down for at least 30 minutes after taking this medication to reduce the chance of irritation to the swallowing tube (esophagus). If supplemental calcium and vitamin D are also being utilized with Fosamax, they should not be taken within 30 minutes of Fosamax so that they don't interfere with its absorption from the stomach.

QUESTION: Can Fosamax cause muscle pain?

ANSWER: Yes, and the FDA recently informed healthcare professionals and patients about the possibility of severe and sometimes incapacitating bone, joint, and/or muscle pain in patients taking bisphosphonate drugs. Bisphosphonates include alendronate (Fosamax), etidronate (Didronel), ibandronate (Boniva), pamidronate (Aredia), risedronate (Actonel), tiludronate (Skelid), and zoledronic acid (Zometa, Reclast). Although severe musculoskeletal pain is listed as a side effect in the prescribing information for bisphosphonates, the association between bisphosphonates and severe musculoskeletal pain may be overlooked by healthcare professionals, which may delay diagnosis, prolong pain and/or impairment, and necessitate the use of pain relievers. The severe musculoskeletal pain may occur within days, months, or years after starting to take a bisphosphonate drug. Some patients have reported complete relief of symptoms after discontinuing the bisphosphonate, whereas others have reported slow or incomplete resolution of the problem. Patients who develop severe musculoskeletal pain while taking a bisphosphonate drug should discuss the various treatment options with their physician, which may include temporary or permanent discontinuation of the drug.

QUESTION: Can Fosamax cause jaw disease?

ANSWER: Fosamax or alendronate is a popular medication used for the treatment and prevention of osteoporosis. It belongs to a class of drugs known as bisphosphonates, which are used to treat osteoporosis because they prevent the breakdown of bone (bone resorption). Recently, a study reported in the Journal of the American Dental Association suggests that use of alendronate (or other bisphosphonates) may be linked to a dangerous condition known as osteonecrosis of the jaw (ONJ). ONJ, sometimes called jawbone death, occurs when bone in the jaw fails to heal after trauma, such as a tooth extraction. The exact cause of ONJ is unclear. Researchers in this recent study looked at the dental records of 208 patients with a history of alendronate use and found that 9 of 66 patients who had teeth extracted developed ONJ. This rate of ONJ occurrence is much higher than previously thought. In fact, recently an expert panel for the American Dental Association concluded the risk of ONJ apparently remains low for people taking bisphosphonates. Other reported risk factors for developing OJ include cancer chemotherapy, use of corticosteroids, and poor oral hygiene. The risk for ONJ also appears to be higher in people receiving bisphosphonates by injection. Patients receiving bisphosphonates who need dental work should discuss the potential risk of ONJ with their dentist, especially if they have any other risk factors noted above. In addition to Fosamax (alendronate), other bisphosphonates include Didronel (etidronate), Skelid (tiludronate), Actonel (risedronate), Reclast, Zometa (zoledronic acid), Boniva (ibandronate), and Aredia (pamidronate).

QUESTION: Is a generic Fosamax available?

ANSWER: Yes, the FDA recently approved the first generic versions of Fosamax, which is used to treat osteoporosis. Fosamax (generic name alendronate) is a type of drug known as a "bisphosphonate". Bisphosphonates are used to treat osteoporosis because they work to prevent the breakdown of bone (bone resorption) by the osteoclast bone cells. This helps to bring the maintenance of bone by the body back into balance. Bisphosphonates like Fosamax are useful drugs for osteoporosis but their activity can be affected by other drugs and foods or drinks. For example, Zantac (ranitidine), which is used for heartburn, may increase the activity of Fosamax while calcium supplements or antacids can interfere with the absorption of Fosamax when taken together. The use of Fosamax can also increase the risk of gastrointestinal problems when taken with aspirin. In addition food, coffee, or orange juice can significantly reduce the absorption and clinical effects of Fosamax. In view of these interactions, Fosamax tablets should be taken with a full glass of plain water first thing in the morning and at least 30 minutes before any other beverage or food. Patients taking Fosamax should also avoid lying down for at least 30 minutes after taking this medication to reduce the chance of irritation to the swallowing tube (esophagus). If supplemental calcium and vitamin D are also being utilized with

Fosamax, they should not be taken within 30 minutes of Fosamax so that they don't interfere with its absorption from the stomach.

QUESTION: What can you tell me about taking Fosamax for osteoporosis?

ANSWER: Fosamax (generic name alendronate) is a type of drug known as a "bisphosphonate". Other bisphosphonates include Actonel (risedronate), Boniva (ibandronate), and Reclast (zoledronic acid). Bisphosphonates are used to treat osteoporosis because they work to prevent the breakdown of bone (bone resorption) by the osteoclast bone cells. This helps to bring the maintenance of bone by the body back into balance. Bisphosphonates like Fosamax are useful drugs for osteoporosis but their activity can be affected by other drugs and foods or drinks. For example, Zantac (ranitidine), which is used for heartburn, may increase the activity of Fosamax while calcium supplements or antacids can interfere with the absorption of Fosamax when taken together. The use of Fosamax can also increase the risk of gastrointestinal problems when taken with aspirin. In addition food, coffee, or orange juice can significantly reduce the absorption and clinical effects of Fosamax. In view of these interactions, Fosamax tablets should be taken with a full glass of plain water first thing in the morning and at least 30 minutes before any other beverage or food. Patients taking Fosamax should also avoid lying down for at least 30 minutes after taking this medication to reduce the chance of irritation to the swallowing tube (esophagus). If supplemental calcium and vitamin D are also being utilized with Fosamax, they should not be taken within 30 minutes of Fosamax so that they don't interfere with its absorption from the stomach.

A recent Johns Hopkins Health Alert (**www.johnshopkinshealthalerts.com**, 2011) also offers the following strategies that have proven successful at increasing adherence to bisphosphonate medications:

• Minimize the risk of side effects. To reduce the risk of gastrointestinal side effects with an oral bisphosphonate be sure that you take the bisphosphonate in the morning on an empty stomach with a 12-oz glass of water while standing or sitting in an upright position. For

30 minutes afterward, do not lie down or eat or drink anything other than water.

- Reduce the dosing frequency. Dosing regimens that are less frequent can help with the inconvenience of once-a-day oral bisphosphonates. Once-weekly regimens of Fosamax or Actonel appear to be just as effective and may minimize the risk of gastrointestinal side effects. Actonel and Boniva are available in a tablet that can be taken once a month.

- Switch to another formulation. If you still cannot tolerate oral forms of bisphosphonates because of the side effects, two intravenous (I.V.) forms are available: I.V. Boniva, which is given every three months, and I.V. Reclast, which is given once a year or once every two years.

- Lower your costs. If cost is a factor, there is an inexpensive, generic form of Fosamax known as alendronate. It is available in the weekly dose.

QUESTION: You've written about osteoporosis in women. What about osteoporosis in men?

ANSWER: Osteoporosis is commonly thought of as a women's health problem and it is much more common in women, especially postmenopausal women. However, osteoporosis can also occur in men, and about 20% of all people with osteoporosis are men. While there are other causes, most cases of osteoporosis in men are age-related and tend to occur in men over the age of 70. Men are at lower risk of developing osteoporosis because they have larger bones, better bone quality, are less likely to fall than women, and they do not have the accelerated bone loss that women do during menopause. Other risk factors for developing osteoporosis such as genetics, adequate nutritional intake (calcium, vitamin D, and protein), lack of exercise, adverse lifestyle practices (such as smoking or alcoholism), sex hormone levels (estrogen or testosterone), certain diseases and medications, are similar between men and women. Like women, the management of osteoporosis in men includes regular exercise, prevention of falls, adequate calcium and vitamin D intake, stopping smoking, reducing alcohol intake, and various prescription drug treatments. Drug therapy for men with osteoporosis is somewhat limited compared to women.

There are, however, a few drugs available that help to prevent bone loss and to increase new bone formation for men. In summary, while the incidence of osteoporosis in men is much lower than in women, its consequences such as increased bone fractures can be just as devastating. The diagnosis of osteoporosis in both men and women can be made by your physician based upon a special test that measures bone mineral density (BMD).

QUESTION: I heard about a new skin patch to prevent osteoporosis. What can you tell me about it?

ANSWER: The FDA recently approved a low-dose estrogen skin patch for the prevention of postmenopausal osteoporosis in women who are at significant risk for this disorder. The new, clear, dime-sized, patch is called Menostar and is applied to the lower abdomen once a week. It contains the estrogen, estradiol, and is the lowest dose estrogen therapy currently available for prevention of postmenopausal osteoporosis. The decline in estrogen production that occurs during menopause results in an acceleration of bone loss and bone resorption (bone removal). Osteoporosis continues to be under-recognized and under-treated in postmenopausal women. According to the National Osteoporosis Foundation, as many as 8 million women suffer from osteoporosis and another 22 million women have bone density deficiency, putting them at risk for bone fracture and its complications. In fact, 24% of women over 50 years old who suffer a hip fracture die within a year of the fracture. Risk factors for osteoporosis include low bone mineral density (BMD), low estrogen levels, family history of osteoporosis, previous fracture, small frame, light skin color, smoking, and alcohol intake. Women with extremely low or unstable estrogen levels are at a 2 1/2 times greater risk for osteoporosis and debilitating bone and hip fractures compared to other postmenopausal women. Estrogen therapy decreases bone loss and helps to restore the balance between bone loss and bone formation. The approval of Menostar was based upon a clinical study involving more than 400 postmenopausal women that showed significant increases in bone mineral density (BMD) after two years in postmenopausal women receiving the patch therapy. These studies also showed that Menostar did not cause significant endometrial problems and therefore the patch does not require a daily or monthly progestin drug to protect against endometrial cancer in women with a uterus. The most frequently reported site effects of Menostar during clinical study were skin irritation at the application site, joint pain, and a white or yellow vaginal discharge.

QUESTION: I heard about a new drug for osteoporosis that you only take once a month. What can you tell me about it?

ANSWER: The FDA recently approved Boniva (ibandronate) for the treatment and prevention of osteoporosis in postmenopausal women. Boniva is a bisphosphonate drug that works by preventing the breakdown of bone and bring the maintenance of bone by the body back into balance. In clinical studies, it has been shown to significantly increase bone mineral density (BMD) in postmenopausal women. It is the first available treatment option for osteoporosis that only needs to be taken once a month. The most common reported side effects with Boniva in clinical studies were stomach pain, high blood pressure, upset stomach, joint pain, nausea, and diarrhea. Other similar drugs include Fosamax and Actonel.

QUESTION: I heard about a new drug for osteoporosis. What can you tell me about it?

ANSWER: The FDA recently approved Atelvia (risedronate) delayed-release tablets for the treatment of postmenopausal osteoporosis. Atelvia is a bisphosphonate drug that works to prevent the breakdown of bone (bone resorption). This helps to bring the maintenance of bone by the body back into balance. Actually, Atelvia is a new version of an older medication, Actonel (risedronate), which has been used for many years to treat postmenopausal osteoporosis and other conditions. The main difference between Atelvia and Actonel is that it can be taken with food, whereas patients taking Actonel are instructed to take it on an empty stomach. Dosing instructions for Atelvia call for patients to take it immediately after breakfast with 4 ounces of water. In contrast, Actonel's label indicates that it should be taken with 6-8 ounces of water at least 30 minutes before the first food or drink of the day, other than water. In addition, there are several dosing schedules for Actonel—5 mg daily, 35 mg weekly, 150 mg once a month, or 75 mg taken on two consecutive days a month. Atelvia on the other hand, is taken as a 35 mg delayed-release tablet once a week. Patients taking either Actonel or Atelvia should not lie down for 30 minutes after taking the medication to avoid irritation of the upper gastrointestinal tract. Side effects and cautions for Atelvia are similar to those for Actonel.

The decline in estrogen production that occurs during menopause results in an acceleration of bone loss and bone resorption (bone removal). Osteoporosis continues to be under-recognized and under-treated in postmenopausal women. According to the National Osteoporosis Foundation, as many as 8 million women suffer from osteoporosis and another 22 million women have bone density deficiency, putting them at risk for bone fracture and its complications. In fact, 24% of women over 50 years old who suffer a hip fracture die within a year of the fracture. Risk factors for osteoporosis include low bone mineral density (BMD), low estrogen levels, family history of osteoporosis, previous fracture, small frame, light skin color, smoking, and alcohol intake.

MUSCLE SPRAINS

QUESTION: I bike ride a lot. What is good for muscle sprains?

ANSWER: Sprains occur when a person's ligaments (tissues that surround joints and connect one bone to another) have been overstretched by some type of trauma. Mild sprains can produce pain, tenderness, edema, and reduced function, while more severe sprains can actually cause tearing and bleeding with complete loss of muscle function. Acute injuries to muscles, ligaments, and tendons are best treated with a combination approach known as PRICE-protection, rest, ice, compression, and elevation. Ice or other forms of cold is beneficial when applied soon after the injury and for up to 48-72 hours. After this time application of heat is probably better. Treatment can also include topical (external) pain relievers (analgesics) or oral pain relievers. Most nonprescription topical analgesic products contain menthol, methyl salicylate, camphor, or capsaicin. These ingredients are known as counterirritants that produce reversible, transient inflammation or irritation of the skin. It is not known exactly how they work but they are thought to produce itching, burning, warmth, or cooling sensations that mask the deeper pain from the injury. They don't cure the pain, but simply make the underlying pain more bearable. Products with counterirritants should not be applied to wounds or damaged skin and not covered with a bandage or used more than 3-4 times a day. Nonprescription oral analgesics that may provide relief from sprain injuries include acetaminophen (Tylenol), aspirin, and non-steroidal antiinflammatory drugs (NSAIDs) such as ibuprofen (Motrin, Advil), naproxen (Aleve), or ketoprofen (Orudis KT).

SMOKING CESSATION

QUESTION: I really want to quit smoking. What medications are available to me, without a prescription to help me quit?

ANSWER: Both nicotine gum (Nicorette) and nicotine patches (Nicoderm, Nicotrol) which used to require prescriptions, are now available over-the-counter (OTC). They are considered to be nicotine replacement therapies and are useful in preventing or lessening the severity of withdrawal symptoms (anxiety, inadequate sleep, craving tobacco, hunger, gastrointestinal problems, headaches, drowsiness), which occur when you quit smoking. These withdrawal symptoms are produced because the nicotine in cigarette smoke is addictive. The nicotine containing medications make it easier to abstain from tobacco by replacing the nicotine formerly obtained from cigarette smoking. Cigarettes contain 6-11 milligrams of nicotine and the typical pack-a-day smoker absorbs 20-40 milligrams of nicotine each day. Nicotine gum (Nicorette or Nicorette DS) is available in a 2 or 4-milligram form. The 4-milligram gum enables people trying to quit smoking to absorb more nicotine with less chewing effort. Chewing nicotine gum (10-12 doses/day) provides one-third to one-half the usual daily nicotine intake of smoking 30 cigarettes per day. The usual duration of nicotine gum usage is about 12 weeks. The gum should be chewed slowly for 30 minutes for slow and even absorption. Only one piece of gum should be chewed whenever the urge to smoke occurs and you should not drink liquids while chewing. The nicotine (transdermal-thru the skin) patches come in two basic systems. The Nicoderm patch comes in three strengths, and uses a tapering approach over a 10-week period. Nicotrol is available in a 15-milligram/day patch only and is used over a six-week period. Only one patch at a time should be used and after use they should be folded in half and disposed of in a child-and-pet-proof container. Nicotine side effects from both the gum and patch can occur. This can include increased heart rate, heart arrhythmias, increased blood pressure, increased blood sugar, increased breathing, and a reduced appetite. Chewing the gum can also cause oral sores and tired jaw muscles, while the patches can produce a skin rash in some people. People using any of these medications should not smoke, because they can get nicotine toxicity. These nicotine preparations have been proven successful in large numbers of people with proper education and support. Recently, a nicotine lozenge (Commit) has also become available which contains 2 or 4 milligrams of nicotine per lozenge. Help for successful smoking cessation can be obtained from several organizations, including the American Cancer Society (1-800-227-2345), the American Lung Association (1-800-586-4872) and the American Heart Association (1-800-242-8721). The short and long-term benefits of quitting smoking are many and include a lower risk for heart disease, emphysema and various cancers.

QUESTION: I've heard about a new, nonprescription lozenge to help you quit smoking. What can you tell me about it?

ANSWER: Up until now, several nonprescription products containing nicotine have been available to help people stop smoking. These include nicotine gum (Nicorette or generic forms), and nicotine patches (Nicotrol, Habitrol, Nicoderm CQ, or generic forms). Recently, a new nicotine lozenge product was approved by the FDA to help people quit smoking. The new lozenge product is named Commit and is available in two strengths (2 mg and 4 mg) for either heavy or light smokers. The lozenge should be moved around the mouth to gradually release the nicotine. All of these products are considered to be nicotine replacement therapies and are useful in preventing or lessening the severity of withdrawal symptoms (anxiety, inadequate sleep, craving tobacco, hunger, gastrointestinal problems, headaches, drowsiness), which occur when you quit smoking. These withdrawal symptoms are produced because the nicotine in cigarette smoke is addictive. These nicotine-containing medications make it easier to abstain from tobacco by replacing the nicotine formerly obtained from cigarette smoking. Cigarettes contain 6-11 milligrams of nicotine and the typical pack-a-day smoker absorbs 20-40 milligrams of nicotine each day. You should follow the dosage instructions carefully for all of these nicotine products since side effects can occur. Side effects can include increased heart rate, heart arrhythmias, increased blood pressure, increased blood sugar, increased breathing, and a reduced appetite. People using any of these nicotine products should not smoke, because they can get nicotine toxicity. These nicotine preparations have been shown to be effective when used with proper education and a support program. Help for successful smoking cessation can be obtained from several organizations, including the American Cancer Society (1-800-227-2345), the American Lung Association (1-800-586-4872), and the American Heart Association (1-800-242-8721). The short and long-term benefits of quitting smoking are many and include a lower risk for heart disease, emphysema, and various cancers.

QUESTION: I heard that a new drug was approved to help you quit smoking. What can he tell me about it?

ANSWER: The FDA recently approved Chantix (varenicline) as an aid to smoking cessation treatment. Chantix is the second nicotine-free smoking cessation drug available for use since Zyban (bupropion) was approved in 1997. Most other drugs to stop smoking are nicotine-replacement therapies sold by prescription and over-the-counter in gum, patch, lozenge, nasal spray, or inhaler dosage forms. Chantix works in two ways to help people stop smoking. First of all it reduces the pleasure of smoking and secondly it lessens the withdrawal symptoms that lead smokers to light up again and again. It does this by interacting with the same receptors in the brain that nicotine binds to when inhaled in cigarette smoke. This interaction with nicotine receptors affects the release of a chemical known as dopamine in the pleasure centers of the brain, which reduces the pleasure of smoking and the craving to smoke that occurs when the effect of nicotine wears off. Chantix tablets are taken twice a day for 12 weeks with an additional course of 12 weeks recommended for people who have successfully stopped smoking at the end of the first 12 weeks of treatment. All patients who are prescribed Chantix will also have the opportunity to enroll in a free behavioral support program sponsored by the manufacturer. During clinical studies, about 40-50% of people taking Chantix were able to quit smoking by the end of 12 weeks of treatment. However, the number dropped to about 20% during the 40-week period following treatment. The most common side effects of Chantix during these studies were nausea, sleep disturbance, constipation, gas, and vomiting. One in five American adults, or nearly 45 million people, smoke cigarettes. It is the single most preventable cause of death in the United States and is responsible for a growing list of cancers, as well as chronic diseases including those of the lung and heart. **Please see the next column regarding Chantix's safety.**

QUESTION: Why is the FDA investigating the safety of Chantix, the stop smoking medication?

ANSWER: The FDA has received numerous reports of suicidal thoughts, aggressive and erratic behavior, and drowsiness in patients who have taken Chantix (varenicline), a prescription medicine to help adults stop smoking. A preliminary FDA assessment of the reports involving suicidal thoughts revealed that many of the cases involved new-onset of depressed mood, suicidal ideation, and changes in emotion and behavior within days to weeks of starting Chantix treatment. The FDA is also aware of a case of erratic behavior leading to the death of a patient using Chantix and several reports of patients who experienced drowsiness that affected their ability to drive or operate machinery while taking Chantix. When the FDA completes its investigation of Chantix it will communicate its findings to the public. In the meantime, it recommends the following steps be taken:

• Health care professionals should monitor patients taking Chantix for behavior and mood changes.
• Patients taking Chantix should contact their doctors if they experience behavior or mood changes.

• Patients should use caution when driving or operating machinery until they know how quitting smoking with Chantix may affect them.

Chantix is the second nicotine-free smoking cessation drug available for use since Zyban (bupropion) was approved in 1997. Most other drugs to stop smoking are nicotine-replacement therapies sold by prescription and over-the-counter in gum, patch, lozenge, nasal spray, or inhaler dosage forms. Chantix works in two ways to help people stop smoking. First of all it reduces the pleasure of smoking and secondly it lessens the withdrawal symptoms that lead smokers to light up again and again. It does this by interacting with the same receptors in the brain that nicotine binds to when inhaled in cigarette smoke. This interaction with nicotine receptors affects the release of a chemical known as dopamine in the pleasure centers of the brain, which reduces the pleasure of smoking and the craving to smoke that occurs when the effect of nicotine wears off.

QUESTION: I heard that the FDA now requires warnings on Chantix and Zyban. What are the warnings about?

ANSWER: The FDA recently announced that it is requiring the manufacturers of the smoking-cessation drugs Chantix (varenicline) and Zyban (bupropion) to put a "Boxed Warning" in the prescribing information for these products. The warning will highlight the risk of serious mental health events that may occur when taking these drugs including changes in behavior, depressed mood, hostility, and suicidal thoughts. Similar warnings will also be required for bupropion marketed as the antidepressant Wellbutrin and for generic versions of bupropion. In addition to the "Boxed Warning", the FDA is requesting more information in the Warnings section of the prescribing information and updated information in the Medication Guide for patients that further discusses the risk of mental health events when using these products. The manufacturers are also required to do an additional study on Chantix and Zyban to determine the extent of the side effects. Since its approval in 2006, Chantix has been associated with 98 completed suicides and 188 attempts. Bupropion, approved for smoking cessation in 1997, has been associated with 14 completed suicides and 17 attempts. Although both drugs are associated with serious adverse events, they are effective at helping people quit smoking and the risk of these adverse events must be weighed against the significant health benefits of quitting smoking. Patients should immediately contact their health care professional if they experience any of the mental health events noted. In addition, any adverse event associated with these products should be communicated to the FDA's MedWatch reporting program by telephone at 1-800-FDA-1088, by fax at 1-800-FDA-0178, online at **www.fda.gov/medwatch**, or by mail to 5600 Fishers Lane, Rockville, Maryland 20852-9787.

QUESTION: I want to quit smoking. What are my options?

ANSWER: I've written about many smoking cessation products in previous columns, but let me provide a review of your options based upon a Johns Hopkins Health Alert (**www.johnshopkinshealthalerts. com**, 2008). Despite a steady decline in the number of smokers, tobacco continues to cause twice as many deaths per year as AIDS, alcohol abuse, motor vehicle collisions, illicit drug use, and suicides combined. Understandably, knowledge of the dangers of smoking or the benefits of quitting smoking is typically not enough to motivate people to quit. Nicotine is highly addictive, and the habitual act of smoking adds a further psychological obstacle to becoming cigarette free.

The large majority of would-be quitters don't succeed on their first attempt. Research suggests that people who get help with quitting tend to be more successful. The American Heart Association recommends:

- **Smoking Cessation Strategy 1**—Nicotine replacement therapy (NRT): The nicotine patch, inhaler, gum, or lozenges are available over-the-counter (OTC).

- **Smoking Cessation Strategy 2**—Zyban (bupropion): A prescription antidepressant that replaces the "high" of nicotine by increasing the brain's supply of dopamine.

- **Smoking Cessation Strategy 3**—Chantix (varenicline): A prescription drug that blocks nicotine receptors in the brain.

- **Smoking Cessation Strategy 4**—Smoking cessation counseling: Individual therapy and support groups.

In addition, although many studies show that NRT products can help you quit smoking, you shouldn't rule out going cold turkey—quitting smoking all at once, rather than tapering your nicotine use. Cold turkey may be a cheaper, quicker, and more effective option, particularly for lighter smokers. A survey of over 6,000 California smokers, published in the Journal of the American Medical Association, found that moderate to heavy smokers (those who smoked 15 or more cigarettes per day) benefited the most from NRT. But NRT didn't increase the chances of quitting for those who smoked less than 15 cigarettes per day.

The bottom line: No matter how you approach quitting, you will need a genuine desire to quit and a lot of willpower. The good news is that 20 minutes after quitting your heart rate will improve. After a few weeks, blood circulation improves, cilia—the tiny hairlike fibers in the lungs that remove mucus—grow back, and your risk of pancreatic and esophageal cancer drops. A year later, your risk of heart disease is cut in half, and if you stay smoke free for 10 years, the same can be said for your risk of lung cancer.

Help for successful smoking cessation can be obtained from several organizations, including the American Cancer Society (1-800-227-2345), the American Lung Association (1-800-586-4872) and the American Heart Association (1-800-242-8721). The short and long-term benefits of quitting smoking are many and include a lower risk for heart disease, emphysema and various cancers.

QUESTION: What can you tell me about E-cigarettes?

ANSWER: E-cigarettes (or "electronic cigarettes") are being promoted as a healthier and cleaner alternative to cigarettes. They are battery-operated, stainless steel devices that look like real cigarettes and contain a nicotine solution of various strengths and flavors, but no tobacco. When you suck on the device, the liquid heats up and produces a fine mist (not smoke) that you inhale. They were developed in China and are sold on the Internet and in shopping malls in the United States under various brand names. Some people use them to try and quit smoking or to get around smoking bans. While their tips glow to simulate real cigarettes, there is no secondhand smoke, but there is no evidence that they actually help people quit smoking or that they are safe. E-cigarettes deliver a vapor of nicotine to the lungs, which may have harmful effects such as increased blood pressure and heart rate, and they may still be addicting. The World Health Organization, the American Cancer Society, the American Lung Association, and the FDA do not support use of these products. In fact, the FDA recently announced that E-cigarettes contain carcinogens and toxic chemicals such as diethylene glycol, an ingredient used in antifreeze. Because these products have not been submitted to the FDA for evaluation or approval, they have no way of knowing if they are safe or effective. Until more information about E-cigarettes is available, it is recommended that smokers try other forms of nicotine replacement products, such as gums, lozenges, and patches first.

QUESTION: What can you tell me about cytisine and smoking cessation?

ANSWER: Cytisine is an extract derived from the seeds of the Golden Rain acacia plant. This extract has properties and effects very similar to nicotine and it has been used in tablet form for over 40 years in Eastern Europe as a smoking cessation agent. Although cytisine has not been clinically studied in the U.S. and is not approved as a smoking cessation product here, several European studies have shown that it is a relatively inexpensive and effective drug to kick the smoking habit (addiction). Recently, the results of a study using cytisine for smoking cessation were reported in the New England Journal of Medicine (2011). This study involved 740 adult half-a-pack daily smokers in Poland who received either cytisine tablets or a placebo (dummy tablet) for 25 days. All study participants also received a minimal amount of counseling during the study. The patients were judged to have stayed off cigarettes if they reported that they had smoked fewer than 5 cigarettes per month during the year after they stopped taking the tablets. Results from the study sh owed that at the one-year mark the sustained abstinence rate was three and a half times higher for the smokers getting cytisine tablets compared to a placebo (8.4% vs. 2.4%). The risks of death, hospitalization, and other serious side effects were small and comparable in both groups, but gastrointestinal side effects such as up set stomach, dry mouth, and nausea were more common in the cytisine groups. As noted earlier, cytisine products have not been approved for use in the U.S. and it is unclear if they will ever be marketed here.

One in five American adults, or nearly 45 million people, smoke cigarettes. It is the single most preventable cause of death in the United States and is responsible for a growing list of cancers, as well as chronic diseases including those of the lung and heart. Help for successful smoking cessation can be obtained from several organizations, including the American Cancer Society (1-800-227-2345), the American Lung Association (1-800-586-4872) and the American Heart Association (1-800-242-8721). The short and long-term benefits of quitting smoking are many and include a lower risk for heart disease, emphysema and various cancers. In addition, you can save a lot of money.

ZYBAN

QUESTION: I've heard that there is an oral drug product available that you can take to help you stop smoking. What is it?

ANSWER: You're probably thinking of Zyban, recently approved as an aid to stop smoking. Zyban (generic name bupropion) is a prescription medication available in tablet form, manufactured by Glaxo Wellcome. Actually bupropion (Bu-pro-pee-on) has been available for quite some time for the treatment of depression and is marketed under the tradename Wellbutrin. Unlike other smoking cessation products available such as nicotine gum (Nicorette) and nicotine patches (Nicoderm, Nicotrol), Zyban is a non-nicotine product.

As I reviewed in a previous column, nicotine products prevent or lessen the severity of withdrawal symptoms such as anxiety, inadequate sleep, craving tobacco, hunger, gastrointestinal problems, etc., which occur when you quit smoking. Zyban, on the other hand, is thought to actually work in the brain to reduce the urge to smoke and to help reduce nicotine withdrawal symptoms. Some studies have shown that Zyban may be more effective than nicotine patches but more information is needed.

In contrast to nicotine replacement therapy, Zyban therapy should begin 1 to 2 weeks before a targeted "quit day" to allow time for the drug to work in the brain. The initial dosage is a 150 mg tablet daily for the first 3 days and then 150 mg twice a day for 7 to 12 weeks. Zyban use should also be part of a comprehensive smoking cessation program, which includes counseling to increase its chance of success.

The most common side effects of Zyban therapy are dry mouth and difficulty in sleeping. However, more serious side effects such as seizures can occur and a dose over 300 mg per day should not be used. Zyban should not be used for people with a seizure disorder, bulimia, or anorexia nervosa. In addition, since Wellbutrin contains the same active ingredient, Zyban should not be used in people taking this medication or any other medication containing bupropion. Like all medications, you should consult your doctor and pharmacist to prevent any possible drug interactions.

Help for successful smoking cessation can also be obtained from several organizations, including the American Cancer Society (1-800-227-2345), the American Lung Association (1-800-586-4872) and the American Heart Association (1-800-242-8721). The short and long-term benefits of quitting smoking are many and include a lower risk for heart disease, emphysema and various cancers.

QUESTION: I heard that the FDA now requires warnings on Chantix and Zyban. What are the warnings about?

ANSWER: The FDA recently announced that it is requiring the manufacturers of the smoking-cessation drugs Chantix (varenicline) and Zyban (bupropion) to put a "Boxed Warning" in the prescribing information for these products. The warning will highlight the risk of serious mental health events that may occur when taking these drugs including changes in behavior, depressed mood, hostility, and suicidal thoughts. Similar warnings will also be required for bupropion marketed as the antidepressant Wellbutrin and for generic versions of bupropion. In addition to the "Boxed Warning", the FDA is requesting more information in the Warnings section of the prescribing information and updated information in the Medication Guide for patients that further discusses the risk of mental health events when using these products. The manufacturers are also required to do an additional study on Chantix and Zyban to determine the extent of the side effects. Since its approval in 2006, Chantix has been associated with 98 completed suicides and 188 attempts. Bupropion, approved for smoking cessation in 1997, has been associated with 14 completed suicides and 17 attempts. Although both drugs are associated with serious adverse events, they are effective at helping people quit smoking and the risk of these adverse events must be weighed against the significant health benefits of quitting smoking. Patients should immediately contact their health care professional if they experience any of the mental health events noted. In addition, any adverse event associated with these products should be communicated to the FDA's MedWatch reporting program by telephone at 1-800-FDA-1088, by fax at 1-800-FDA-0178, online at **www.fda.gov/medwatch**, or by mail to 5600 Fishers Lane, Rockville, Maryland 20852-9787.

DRUGS AND VISION PROBLEMS

QUESTION: Can some prescription medications cause vision problems?

ANSWER: Yes, numerous prescription medications can cause either temporary or permanent vision disorders. For example, some medications can cause side effects like blurred vision, double vision, dry eyes, puffy eyelids, increased sensitivity to light, excessive tearing, etc. These problems are usually only short-term and disappear over time or when the medication causing the problem is discontinued. However, according to a Johns Hopkins Vision Health Alert (**www. johnshopkinshealthalerts.com**, 2007) the long-term use of some prescription medications can result in more serious or permanent vision disorders. For example, some drugs used to treat irregular heartbeats such as Cordarone (amiodarone) and Lanoxin (digoxin) can cause blurred vision, yellow vision, or blue-green halos around objects. In addition, some antimalarial drugs such as Aralen (chloroquine) and Plaquenil (hydroxychloroquine) (which also may be used to treat rheumatoid arthritis and lupus) can cause visual disturbances like blurred vision, but long-term therapy may lead to a permanent disease of the retina (retinopathy). Likewise, corticosteroids taken orally or by inhalation can lead to glaucoma or cataracts. Erectile dysfunction drugs like Viagra, Cialis, and Levitra can also produce blurred vision, increased sensitivity to light, or temporarily cause objects to have a blue tinge. Furthermore, some medications used to treat mental disorders like Thorazine (chlorpromazine) and Mellaril (thioridazine) may lead to blurred vision, changes in color vision, and difficulty seeing at night. Finally, (Nolvadex (tamoxifen), which is used to reduce the risk of breast cancer, may cause blurred vision, changes to the retina and cornea, and cataracts. Please note that these are only a few common examples of prescription medications that can cause vision problems. If you develop any visual problems while receiving drug therapy for any medical condition, be sure to let your physician or ophthalmologist know so that they can properly monitor these effects.

ASPIRIN AND CANCER

QUESTION: I recently heard that aspirin might be used to treat a rare type of cancer. What can you tell me about aspirin?

ANSWER: Hardly a month goes by without some new use being proposed for aspirin. I've said before that if aspirin were a new drug today, it would be considered a real medical wonder drug and probably would require a prescription. British and Greek scientists have now suggested that aspirin may help to treat a rare cancer known as turban tumour syndrome, in which huge mushroom-shaped tumors grow out of the scalp and other hairy parts of the body. It is thought that this cancer is caused when the body's inflammatory response becomes overactive and that aspirin may be an effective treatment. The history of aspirin is interesting and goes all the way back to 400 BC when Hippocrates used willow-leaf tea to relieve pain. In 1763, dried willow leaves were also used for rheumatic fever. By 1823, the active ingredient in willow was extracted and named salicin. Later it was found that salicin is changed to salicylic acid in the body, which irritates the stomach. Then, in 1893 German scientists found that they could reduce its irritant effects by changing salicyclic acid to acetyl salicylic acid or aspirin. In 1897, Bayer's scientist Felix Hoffman (no relation) patented aspirin and clinical studies were started. By the 1930's, the patent ran out and aspirin became a generic drug. In 1974, evidence of the beneficial effects of aspirin for cardiovascular disease began to appear and during 1982 a Nobel Prize was awarded for the discovery of the role of aspirin in preventing blood clots. By 1989 it was suggested that aspirin may prevent dementia, and in 1995 that it may protect against bowel cancer. Finally, in the last few years, studies have suggested that aspirin may reduce the risk of various cancers and Alzheimer's disease. However, not all news about aspirin has been good. For instance it can cause serious gastrointestinal bleeding and increase the risk of Reye's syndrome in young people that can lead to seizures, coma, and death. Aspirin can also cause severe hypersensitivity reactions in some people, and should not be used by women who are pregnant or breastfeeding. In addition, aspirin can interact with other drugs and you should consult with your doctor and pharmacist before its use.

QUESTION: Can a daily "baby" aspirin help prevent colon cancer?

ANSWER: It may, according to the results of a study recently published in the medical journal "Gut". Results from this epidemiolgic study showed that the regular daily use of low-dose (75 mg) aspirin for at least 5 years may reduce the risk of colorectal cancer by 37%. After just one-year of daily low-dose aspirin (75 mg), the risk of colorectal cancer was reduced by 13%. This Scottish case-control study recruited over 5,000 men and women aged 16 to 79 years old. Approximately 2,000 of the study participants had colorectal cancer and approximately 3,000 did not. The study participants filled out a detailed questionnaire about their lifestyle, medications used, and cancer history. Analysis of the study questionnaire data showed that the risk of colorectal cancer was lower in people who used aspirin or nonsteroidal anti-inflammatory drugs (NSAIDs) on a regular basis. NSAIDs include such drugs as ibuprofen (Motrin, Advil, etc.), naproxen (Aleve, etc.), and many others. Some studies have shown similar benefits with NSAIDs or higher dose aspirin (325 mg), but a key finding of this Scottish study was that even a much lower daily dose of aspirin (75 mg) was associated with a lower incidence of colorectal cancer.

The authors of this study note that more, well designed studies are needed to confirm their findings. It should also be noted that aspirin and NSAIDs can cause serious gastrointestinal bleeding in some people and this risk must be weighed against its potential beneficial effects in cancer prevention and cardiovascular protection. People need to consult with their physician to determine if daily aspirin therapy is appropriate for them and what dosage should be used.

QUESTION: Can daily aspirin use prevent cancer?

ANSWER: According to the results of a large clinical study funded by the American Cancer Society and reported in the Journal of the National Cancer Institute, the use of adult-strength (325 mg or more) aspirin taken daily for 5 years or more was associated with a 15% reduced overall cancer incidence. The investigators in this study looked at the association between long-term daily use of adult-strength aspirin and the overall incidence of 10 types of cancer in 69,810 men and 76,303 women who participated in a cancer prevention study. Although the statistical methods in this observational study are somewhat complicated, results indicated that long-term daily adult-strength daily aspirin use was linked to a reduced incidence of colorectal cancer among men and women combined (30% decrease) and a reduced incidence of prostate cancer (20% decrease) in men. In addition, there was a reduction in breast cancer (15% decrease) among women, but this was not statistically significant. There was no association between long-term aspirin use and the risk for lung cancer or other individual cancers such as bladder, kidney, and pancreatic. The authors of this study note that more, well designed studies are needed to confirm their findings. It should also be noted that aspirin can cause serious gastrointestinal bleeding in some people and this risk must be weighed against its potential beneficial effects in cancer prevention and cardiovascular protection. People need to consult with their physician to determine if daily aspirin therapy is appropriate for them and what dosage should be used.

QUESTION: Can aspirin be helpful for women with breast cancer?

ANSWER: The results of a recent study reported in the Journal of Clinical oncology found that women with breast cancer who take aspirin on a regular basis at least 2 days a week may have a lower risk of dying from breast cancer or having their breast cancer spread to other parts of the body (metastasis). This observational study involved 4,164 female registered nurses who were diagnosed with breast cancer between 1976 and 2002 and were followed until they died or until June 2006, whichever came first. The study results showed that breast cancer survivors taking aspirin at least 2 days a week had a nearly 50% lower risk of breast cancer death and risk of distant metastasis compared to those who did not take aspirin. The study did not look at the dose of aspirin used, but most regular use was likely for heart disease prevention at the 81 mg/day level, the researchers suggested. Results from this study, however, did not find an association between aspirin use and the incidence of breast cancer. It is not known how aspirin may affect cancer growth, but aspirin does have anti-inflammatory effects and also blocks an enzyme known as cyclooxygenase, which could play a role in blocking breast cancer growth by decreasing the amount of estrogen produced. It should be noted that in spite of the positive findings from this study, more research is needed to confirm any benefits. Experts point out that this was an observational study and was limited by the use of self-reporting by patients. The study's authors caution women who are undergoing breast cancer treatment to talk to their doctors before taking aspirin because it can cause serious gastrointestinal bleeding and can interact with other medications.

QUESTION: What's the latest information about daily aspirin use?

ANSWER: I've written several columns in the past about the use of daily aspirin to prevent cardiovascular problems and/or cancer. Aspirin has numerous effects in the body including the prevention of blood clotting and anti-inflammatory properties. The anti-clotting effect of aspirin is a two-edged sword—it may help prevent heart attacks and strokes, but can also lead to serious gastrointestinal bleeding. Therefore, any potential benefits of regular daily aspirin use must be weighed against its potential risks. Recently (2012), researchers reviewed and analyzed 9 studies of aspirin use in the United States, Europe, and Japan that included over 100,000 participants who had never had a heart attack or stroke. Results from this retrospective analysis reported in the journal Archives of Internal Medicine showed that regular aspirin users were 10% less likely to have any type of heart attack and 20% less likely to have a nonfatal heart attack compared to non-aspirin users. However, aspirin users were also about 30% more likely to have a serious gastrointestinal bleeding event. The overall risk of dying during the study was the same for aspirin users and non-aspirin users as was the risk of dying from cancer. The study researchers concluded that the regular use of aspirin in people without prior cardiovascular disease might be more harmful than it is beneficial, but that treatment decisions need to be considered on a case-by-case basis depending on the individual's risk factors and family history. Risk factors for heart disease include high blood pressure, obesity, lack of exercise, smoking, diabetes, or high cholesterol levels. Risk factors for gastrointestinal bleeding can include a history of gastrointestinal bleeding, alcohol use, smoking, or the use of medications such as NSAIDs, corticosteroids, or blood thinners in addition to aspirin. Anyone regularly using aspirin or planning to start regular aspirin use should discuss this therapy with their physician.

PHENYLKETONURIA

QUESTION: I received a trial package of Listerine Pocket Paks in the mail. On the container it says phenylketonurics: contains "phenylalanine". Are these safe to use?

ANSWER: Some people are born without an enzyme that is needed to convert the amino acid phenylalanine into another amino acid tyrosine, which is then eliminated from the body. Without this enzyme, toxic levels of phenylalanine build up in the blood causing brain damage and mental retardation. In the United States, approximately one in 16,000 babies are born with this problem known as penylketonuria or PKU. In the U.S., newborns are screened for this disorder. Phenylketonuria occurs in most geographic groups and in both sexes, but it is rare in Jews of Eastern European ancestry and in blacks. The symptoms of PKU are usually absent in newborns. Symptoms in children who have undiagnosed or untreated PKU include seizures, nausea and vomiting, aggressive or self-injurious behavior, hyperactivity, and sometimes psychiatric symptoms. Affected children often give off a "mousy" body odor caused by a by-product of phenylalanine in their urine and sweat. The treatment of PKU consists of limiting the intake of phenylalanine. Phenylalanine intake must be restricted beginning in the first few weeks of life to prevent mental retardation. A restricted diet, started early and well maintained, makes normal development possible and prevents brain damage. However, if very strict control of diet is not maintained, affected children may have difficulties in school. Most doctors now believe that a phenylalanine-restricted diet should continue for life. Now back to your question. Yes this Listerine product is safe to use, unless you have PKU, which is usually diagnosed early in life.

LEPROSY

QUESTION: I read in the paper that leprosy is spreading in the U.S. What drugs are used to treat leprosy?

ANSWER: Yes, it has been reported that leprosy, also know as Hansen's disease, is on the rise in the United States. Leprosy has usually been regarded as a plague of the past that occurred in biblical times or was confined to poor and distant countries. It has been estimated, however, that there are now more than 7,000 people in the U.S. affected with leprosy. Most of the people with leprosy in this country are immigrants from other countries, but some people have also contracted leprosy here. Leprosy is a nonfatal, chronic infection caused by bacteria known as Mycobacterium leprae. Symptoms of leprosy include bumpy rashes, skin indentations, and loss of feeling in the hands and feet. If left untreated, leprosy can cause disfigurement and disability including muscle wasting, loss of toes or limbs, foot dragging, blindness, infertility in men, and a contraction of the fingers referred to as "claw hand". How leprosy is transmitted is not exactly known, but bacteria are thought to be passed through the respiratory (nasal) droplets of an infected person. Contact with infected soil, certain insects, or some infected animals like armadillos may also be a cause of transmission. Contrary to popular opinion, skin-to-skin contact is generally not considered an important means of transmission of leprosy from one person to another. Once it is diagnosed, there are several drugs available to treat leprosy. These drugs include dapsone, Lamprene (clofazimine), and rifampin. All of these drugs work by killing or slowing the growth of the bacteria that causes leprosy. Some antibiotics such as minocycline (Minocin), ofloxacin (Floxin), sparfloxacin (Zagam), or clarithromycin (Biaxin) may also be useful in some patients. The drug treatment for leprosy may involve combinations of these drugs and may need to be continued for several years. Thalidomide has also been used to treat some of the skin problems associated with leprosy.

THALIDOMIDE

QUESTION: I heard that thalidomide is being used for multiple myeloma and other conditions. What can you tell me about this?

ANSWER: 40 years after being removed from the market, thalidomide is now available for use, but its use is very restricted. As you may recall, thalidomide was first marketed in the 1950's as a sedative and to prevent nausea and vomiting. In many countries, pregnant women with morning sickness were treated with thalidomide, resulting in over 12,000 babies being born with fetal malformations including stunted limb growth. After these side effects were discovered, the drug was pulled from the worldwide market in 1961. Surprisingly, thalidomide was never approved for use in the U.S. during this time, because the FDA was concerned about possible nerve damage as a side effect. Today, however, thalidomide (Thalomid) has received approval for the treatment of a skin reaction that can develop in people with leprosy or Hansen's disease. In order to prevent birth defects, a special program known as S.T.E.P.S. (System for Thalidomide Education and Safety) has been established that restricts who can prescribe and dispense the drug. In addition, thalidomide in combination with the corticosteroid, dexamethasone, is now accepted as a treatment of choice for patients with multiple myeloma. Multiple myeloma is a cancer that originates in the bone marrow and is associated with anemia, bleeding, infections, and weakness. It usually occurs in people at least 60 years of age and occurs more frequently in men than in women. Exactly how thalidomide works is not known, but it does have beneficial effects on the immune system, has anti-inflammatory properties, and appears to prevent the development of blood vessels needed by cancer cells. Although not approved for use in other cancers, thalidomide has also shown promising results for the treatment of prostate, liver, ovarian, and cancers involving excessive hormone production, but more study is needed.

QUESTION: I've heard that thalidomide is being used again. Is this true?

ANSWER: Yes. 40 years after being removed from the market, thalidomide is now available for use, but its use is very restricted. Thalidomide (Thalomid) has received approval for the treatment of a skin reaction that can develop in people with leprosy or Hansen's disease. In order to prevent birth defects, a special program known as S.T.E.P.S. (System for Thalidomide Education and Safety) has been established that restricts who can prescribe and dispense the drug. In addition to its approved use for this skin condition, thalidomide is also being studied for other disorders including Crohns disease, HIV-associated weight loss, lupus, and various cancers. It is not known exactly how thalidomide works, but it does affect the immune system and is known as an immunomodulatory agent. It also appears to block the formation of new blood vessels (angiogenesis), which inhibits tumor growth and spread. In addition to causing birth defects, common side effects of thalidomide include constipation, weakness, fatigue, nerve problems, and sedation. Thalidomide capsules (Thalomid) are marketed by Celgene Corporation.

CHAPPED LIPS

QUESTION: What can I use for chapped lips?

ANSWER: Chapped lips can occur anytime during the year, but they are especially common during the winter months. Symptoms of chapped lips include dryness, redness, tenderness, cracking or peeling, and pain. Being in overly windy, sunny, or dry conditions commonly causes chapped lips. They can also be caused by smoking, dehydration, skin disorders like eczema, allergic reactions to skin care products or cosmetics, or the use of certain medications. The outer layer of the lips is thin, and is more sensitive to chapping because the lips do not produce oils like the skin does to protect it from drying out. Some measures that you can take to prevent chapped lips include avoiding licking or biting the lips, wearing a scarf to cover your lips in cold or windy weather, avoiding excessive sun exposure, having properly fitting dentures, drinking enough water to stay hydrated, and using a humidifier in your home. In addition, a number of topical nonprescription products are available to treat or prevent chapped lips. These products usually contain ingredients that assist in healing such as skin protectants, moisturizers, pain relievers, and sunscreens. Some examples of these products are Carmex, Blistex Lip Balm, Chapstick Lip Balm, and Vaseline Lip Therapy. In addition to treating chapped lips, these lip balm products can be used to protect your lips before going out in dry, cold, or windy weather. They can also be applied prior to using lipstick for added protection, especially during the winter months. While chapped lips are seldom associated with serious complications, it should also be noted that if your lips show signs of swelling or bleeding that a physician should be consulted for treatment.

EPILEPSY MEDICATIONS

QUESTION: Can drugs that are used to treat epilepsy increase the risk of suicide?

ANSWER: The FDA recently informed healthcare professionals that the Agency has analyzed reports of suicidality (suicidal behavior or thoughts) from almost 200 clinical studies of eleven drugs used to treat epilepsy as well as psychiatric disorders and other conditions. While the overall incidence was small in the studies, they found that patients taking these drugs had approximately twice the risk of suicidal behavior or thoughts (0.43%) compared to patients taking a placebo "dummy" pill (0.22%). This means that for every 1,000 patients, about 2 more drug-treated patients experienced suicidal thoughts than patients taking a "dummy" pill. The increased risk of suicidal behavior or thoughts was observed as early as one week after starting to take the antiepileptic drug and it continued through 6 months. The risk was higher in patients with epilepsy compared to patients who were given the drug for psychiatric or other conditions. Although only eleven drugs were involved in the FDA's analysis, it expects that the increased risk of suicidality is shared by all antiepileptic drugs. In view of these findings, the FDA encourages all healthcare professionals and family members to closely monitor all patients taking any antiepileptic drug for notable changes in behavior that could indicate the emergence or worsening of suicidal thoughts or behavior or depression. Skipping epilepsy medications can result in seizures and patients taking them should discuss these potential risks with their physician before stopping any drug treatment. The drugs included in the FDA analysis were:

- Carbamazepine (Carbatrol, Equetro, Tegretol, Tegretol XR)
- Felbamate (Felbatol)
- Gabapentin (Neurontin)
- Lamotrigine (Lamictal)
- Levetiracetam (Keppra)
- Oxcarbazpine (Trileptal)
- Pregabalin (Lyrica)
- Tiagabine (Gabitril)
- Topiramate (Topamax)
- Valproate (Depakote, Depakote ER, Depakene, Depacon)
- Zonisamide (Zonegran)

QUESTION: I heard about a new drug for epilepsy. What can you tell me about it?

ANSWER: The FDA recently approved Potiga (ezogabine) tablets for add-on therapy to treat partial-onset seizures in adults. Epilepsy is a brain disorder in which there is abnormal or excessive activity of nerve cells in the brain. Partial seizures affect only a limited or localized area of the brain, but can spread to other parts of the brain. Seizures cause a wide range of symptoms, including repetitive limb movements (spasms), unusual behavior, and generalized convulsions with loss of consciousness. Potiga is the first available drug known as a potassium channel opener to treat epilepsy. It is not known exactly how Potiga works in epilepsy, but it is thought to reduce brain excitability and may help people with partial-onset seizures who are uncontrolled on their current anticonvulsant medications. During clinical studies in over 1,200 adult patients with partial-onset seizures, Potiga was shown to significantly reduce the frequency of seizures when given orally 3 times a day. The most common side effects of Potiga include dizziness, sleepiness, fatigue, confusion, tremor, spinning sensation (vertigo), problems with coordination, double vision, nausea, problems paying attention, and memory impairment. However, Potiga can also cause urinary retention and like other antiepileptic medications may cause neuro-psychiatric problems and suicidal thoughts in a very small number of people. Potiga will be dispensed with a Medication Guide that informs patients of the most important information about the medication.

ASTHMA

QUESTION: Are there any medications that can trigger an asthma attack or worsen the symptoms?

ANSWER: Asthma is a condition in which the airways of the lung (bronchi) narrow in response to certain stimuli. It affects about 17 to 18 million people in the United States and is becoming more common. There are many medications, both prescription and nonprescription, that can cause problems in people with asthma. For example, several over-the-counter pain relievers like aspirin, ibuprofen (Motrin, Advil), and naproxen (Aleve) can trigger severe and even fatal asthma attacks in some people with asthma. The use of nonprescription antihistamines like diphenhydramine (Benadryl) can be a problem in people with asthma due to their drying effects, which can thicken secretions in the respiratory tract. In addition, prescription medications known as beta-blockers used to treat high blood pressure and heart disease such as atenolol (Tenormin), timolol (Blocaden), propranolol (Inderal) and many others can interfere with drugs used to treat asthma, causing a worsening of asthma symptoms. Beta-blockers are also used to treat glaucoma and are found in numerous prescription eye drops such as timolol (Timoptic), betaxalol (Betoptic) and several others. ACE inhibitors used to treat high blood pressure and heart disease such as lisinopril (Zestril), enalapril (Vasotec), quinapril (Accupril) and many others can be a problem in people with asthma. A side effect of these prescription drugs is a very troublesome cough, which can trigger breathing problems. Furthermore, tranquilizers, sedatives, and sleep medications can make a person breathe more slowly and less deeply, which could be dangerous in someone who has lung problems such as asthma. These are only a few examples of some of the problems that can occur with the use of nonprescription and prescription medications in people with asthma. Numerous other medications can cause additional medical problems and drug interactions in people with asthma, so be sure to let your doctor(s) know all the medications that you take to minimize these unwanted effects

QUESTION: What side effects can I get from using oral prednisone for asthma over a long period of time?

ANSWER: A Johns Hopkins Health Alert (**www.johnshopkinshealth alerts.com**, 2007) has warned about the risks of long-term use of oral steroids like prednisone. This Alert points out that since a growing number of people with lung disease are living longer, and more people are taking long-term oral steroids for asthma, chronic obstructive pulmonary disease (COPD), and other chronic lung conditions. Long-term use of oral steroids can cause serious side effects, ranging from osteoporosis to cataracts to high blood pressure and diabetes. If you're taking an oral steroid, it's critical to talk with your doctor about how to minimize these steroid side effects.

Corticosteroids can prevent or reverse inflammation in the airways, making them less sensitive to triggers. If you have severe asthma and you have tried high doses of inhaled steroids without success, your doctor may recommend oral steroids. Some people take oral steroids because they have COPD that other medications can't relieve.

If you take daily oral steroids for months or years, particularly in moderate to high doses, you are at increased risk for developing any of a variety of side effects: cataracts, osteoporosis, diabetes, high blood pressure, muscle weakness, easily bruised skin, hair loss, facial hair growth in women, weight gain, and puffy cheeks. Other possible side effects include hyperexcitability, insomnia, and (in a small number of patients) aggressive behavior or even psychosis.

Steps you can take to avoid osteoporosis and other side effects:

- Ask your doctor about getting regular bone scans to detect osteoporosis.
- Get about 1,500 mg of calcium daily through nutrition or supplements. Because vitamin D helps the body absorb calcium, it may help to take 800 international units (IU) daily of vitamin D.
- If you are diagnosed with osteoporosis, your doctor will recommend medication.
- If you take moderate to high doses of corticosteroids, have regular eye exams to check for glaucoma.
- Ask your doctor whether you can reduce your oral steroid dose by adding other medications.
- Have your blood pressure checked regularly.
- Also have your blood sugar checked frequently. Use of high dose steroids has been associated with the development diabetes.

QUESTION: I heard that the FDA issued a warning about some asthma drugs. What drugs are they?

ANSWER: The FDA recently asked the manufacturers of Singulair (montelukast), Accolate (zarfirlukast), Zyflo and Zyflo CR (zileuton) to include a precaution on the drugs labeling about behavior and mood changes that have been reported in some people taking these asthma medications. All of these drugs are known as leukotriene modifiers or inhibitors. Leukotrienes are chemicals the body releases in response to an inflammatory stimulus, such as when a person breathes in an allergen. Some of the behavior or mood changes reported with these medications included agitation, aggression, anxiousness, dream abnormalities and hallucinations, depression, insomnia, irritability, restlessness, suicidal thinking and behavior, and tremor. In view of these reports, the FDA is asking patients and healthcare professionals to be aware of behavior and mood changes with these drugs and that patients should talk with their healthcare provider if these events occur.

Asthma is a respiratory disease in which the bronchioles, the tubes that carry air from the windpipe to the tiny air sacs in the lungs, tighten, resulting in wheezing and a sensation of being starved for oxygen. It is one of the most common of all chronic respiratory diseases, affecting about 7% of the population. For reasons that are not clearly understood, the incidence and severity of asthma is increasing in the United States, especially among the urban poor.

QUESTION: Why is Primatene Mist being removed from the market?

ANSWER: Primatene Mist (or epinephrine mist) is the only over-the-counter asthma inhaler currently available. It helps to open the airways in the lungs and is approved for temporary relief of shortness of breath, tightness of the chest, and wheezing due to bronchial asthma. However, the FDA is reminding doctors and patients that this product can no longer be made or sold after December 31, 2011 because it contains chlorofluorocarbons (CFCs), which deplete the ozone layer. Chlorofluorocarbons are chemicals that contain fluorine, chlorine, and carbon. With inhalers, they are used as a propellant to move the medication, helping the user to breathe it in. According to The National Library of Science at the National Institutes of Health, once released, the odorless, colorless and nontoxic compounds get into the Earth's atmosphere where they break apart and release chemicals that destroy the Earth's ozone layer. CFCs can last more than 100 years in the atmosphere. The FDA says a number of manufacturers have already replaced their CFC inhalers with a propellant called hydrofluoroalkane, or HFA, which is more environment-friendly, but there's currently no HFA version of an epinephrine inhaler available. This transition to HFA inhalers has been somewhat controversial because they are much more expensive than the CFC inhalers. The FDA is urging asthma patients who use Primatene Mist inhalers to get prescriptions for alternative medications before the end of 2011.

Asthma is a respiratory disease in which the bronchioles, the tubes that carry air from the windpipe to the tiny air sacs in the lungs, tighten, resulting in wheezing and a sensation of being starved for oxygen. It is one of the most common of all chronic respiratory diseases, affecting about 7% of the population. For reasons that are not clearly understood, the incidence and severity of asthma is increasing in the United States, especially among the urban poor.

PROBIOTICS

QUESTION: What are probiotics?

ANSWER: By definition probiotics are live microorganisms given in adequate amounts to produce a beneficial health effect. Most probiotics are various types (strains) of bacteria normally found in the human body. The normal digestive tract contains about 400 types of probiotic bacteria that help to diminish the growth of other harmful bacteria. Various probiotics are available in certain foods (e.g., yogurt, buttermilk, some juices, and soy beverages) and in the form of dietary supplements (capsules, tablets, or powders). The names of commonly available bacteria in commercially available products include Lactobacillus, Bifidobacterium, and Saccharomyces, of which there are many specific types. Probiotics have been used to improve digestion, restore normal bowel function, prevent or reduce the incidence of recurring vaginal infections, and to treat antibiotic-associated diarrhea, traveler's diarrhea, and inflammatory bowel conditions. Many other medical uses for probiotics are also being studied. The use of probiotic supplements has nearly tripled between 1994 and 2003 in the United States and numerous probiotic dietary supplements are available. Examples include Floragen capsules, Align capsules, Culturelle capsules, Flora Q capsules, PhytoPharmica Probiotic Pearls, and many others. The active ingredient(s) in these products are usually shown on the label along with its indicated use(s). For example, Floragen contains the probiotic Lactobacillus acidophilus and is promoted to be used for antibiotic-associated vaginitis, and antibiotic—associated diarrhea. Please read all product labeling and directions carefully prior to use. However, before using any probiotic supplement, patients should seek advice from their healthcare provider. In addition, patients who have a compromised immune system should not use probiotics because of the potential for systemic infection. Much more information about probiotics can be found on the Internet at **www.usprobiotics.org**.

MINOR WOUNDS

QUESTION: What can I do for a minor wound?

ANSWER: Minor wounds caused by falls, cuts, bumps, scratches, etc. are a normal part of everyday living and may be self-treated. The first aid for a minor wound begins with cleansing the wound thoroughly with tap water or sterile normal saline if it is available. This is especially important for abrasion injuries such as a scrape, which is likely to be contaminated with gravel, dirt, grass, and other substances, which can lead to infection. Following this cleaning process the application of an antiseptic or antibiotic can help prevent infection in a minor wound. Safe and effective local antiseptics include denatured ethyl alcohol, isopropyl alcohol, 3% hydrogen peroxide, tincture of iodine, and povidone-iodine. Antibiotic creams and ointments containing polymyxin and/or bacitracin are also useful to help prevent infection. Numerous other first-aid antiseptic/antibiotic products are available. Although not accepted by everyone, current medical wisdom suggests that a moist wound will heal more rapidly than one that is dry. This has led to the development of many occlusive wound dressings that can keep the wound moist. If an abrasion has drainage from it, use of a non-adherent dressing can be helpful. The use of dressings that stick to the wound may cause any drainage to become encrusted in the bandage and its removal can damage the healing process. Like antiseptic/antibiotic products, numerous types of wound dressing products are marketed. Dressings that do not have a self-contained adhesive require tape to secure them. Many newer tapes are hypoallergenic and have only light adhesives that are gentler on the skin when they are removed. Your pharmacist can help you select appropriate products to meet your needs. You should carefully read and follow all directions for use of any of these products. In addition, you should always see a physician if you have a puncture wound, animal or human bite, infected wound, severe burn, gaping wound, long-lasting wound, or a wound that causes you to feel pain or numbness.

MOTION SICKNESS

QUESTION: I'm going on a cruise and I want to prevent motion sickness. What can I use?

ANSWER: Motion sickness (also known as air sickness, sea sickness, car sickness or space sickness) is more common in women and usually occurs when a person is experiencing movement in an aircraft, watercraft, train or other rapid mass transit vehicle, fairground ride, or a car. In these situations, the eyes may not detect motion, but the body feels it, creating a conflict in a person's senses. Nausea and vomiting are the most common symptoms of motion sickness. Usually there is a feeling of discomfort and nausea that gradually increases until the person feels that vomiting is going to occur shortly. A person may also look pale and develop a cold sweat. Others may experience yawning, excessive saliva in the mouth, headaches, drowsiness and rapid breathing.

When taking a boat ride or cruise, motion sickness is more common when the person is below deck without a view of the water. It is best to remain on deck when possible and focus on the horizon. When a person's body moves with the ship, but the head is jerked about, movements of the middle ear may cause motion sickness. It may be helpful to try and keep the head and body still as when lying down with the head and neck in a pillow.

Several different remedies have been used to treat motion sickness, including ginger, acupressure bands and other herbal or homeopathic products. However, these products have not been adequately studied to prove their effectiveness. Medications proven to be effective in the treatment of motion sickness include prescription scopolamine patches, non-prescription oral antihistamines, and a few other prescription drugs. Scopolamine patches (Transderm-Scop) were removed from the market in 1994, but were approved for remarketing by the FDA in November of 1997. They prevent motion sickness very well, but are not effective if nausea and vomiting are already occurring. The patch is placed behind the ear at least four hours before the cruise and it will effectively prevent motion sickness for up to three days. The patch may produce minor side effects such as dry mouth, drowsiness, and blurred vision. Unlike scopolamine patches, antihistamines can both prevent and treat motion sickness. Three effective non-prescription antihistamines are cyclizine (Marezine), meclizine (Bonine), and dimenhydrinate (Dramamine). However, people with breathing problems (emphysema, chronic bronchitis), glaucoma, or having difficulty in urination should not use these products. These antihistamine products can also cause drowsiness, which may be less with Marezine or Bonine.

QUESTION: What can I do to decrease motion sickness without using drugs?

ANSWER: Some non-drug measures to try and decrease motion sickness include:

• Avoid reading during travel.
• Avoid too much food or alcohol before and during extended travel.
• Stay where motion is least experienced, such as the front seat of a car, near the wings of an airplane, or the middle of the ship, preferably on deck.
• Keep your field of vision straight ahead.
• Avoid strong odors, especially from food or tobacco smoke.

Acupressure wristbands are another non-drug method that may be useful in decreasing motion sickness. Acupressure bands use either pressure (Sea Bands) or mild electrical pulses (ReliefBands) to stimulate an acupuncture point over a nerve on the underside of the wrist. It's thought that this stimulation interferes with nausea and vomiting signals. Both of these products are available without a prescription and appear to be safe. Acupressure bands may be used before the onset of anticipated motion sickness or when symptoms first occur. However, people with cardiac pacemakers should not use the ReliefBand.

SOCIAL ANXIETY AND OBSESSIVE-COMPULSIVE DISORDERS

QUESTION: I heard that a once-a-day drug was approved for social anxiety and obsessive-compulsive disorders. What can you tell me about it?

ANSWER: The FDA recently approved Luvox CR (fluvoxamine extended-release capsules for the treatment of social anxiety disorder (SAD) and for the treatment of obsessions and compulsions in patients with obsessive-compulsive disorder (OCD). SAD or social phobia is characterized by the fear and avoidance of social or performance situations that might cause embarrassment. People who experience this fear can suffer a great deal, feeling physical symptoms such as gastrointestinal discomfort, sweating, tremors, or heart palpitations. SAD affects approximately 15 million American adults each year, making it one of the most common psychiatric disorders in the U.S. OCD is also a common psychiatric disorder affecting approximately 2.2 million American adults each year. It causes people to experience unwanted thoughts (obsessions) that can prompt them to carry out repeated actions (compulsions) to reduce the anxiety produced by these thoughts. Common obsessions include excessive fear of contamination, repeated doubts (such as thinking you've harmed someone while driving), or a need for symmetry. Common compulsions include repeated cleaning (such as hand washing), repeated checking (such as checking to see if doors are locked), and counting.

It is not known exactly how Luvox CR works in the treatment of SAD or OCD, but it is presumed to be linked to its ability to increase levels of a chemical known as serotonin in the brain. Luvox CR is taken once daily at bedtime. In clinical studies common side effects of Luvox CR included nausea, sleepiness, weakness, diarrhea, loss of appetite, tremor, and sweating. Antidepressants like Luvox CR can also increase suicidal thoughts and patients should call their doctor right away if they experience any thoughts of suicide. In addition, Luvox CR interacts with numerous other drugs and alcohol so be sure that your doctor(s) and pharmacist(s) know about all the medications that you are taking if this medication is prescribed for you.

EATING DISORDERS

QUESTION: What prescription drugs are used to treat eating disorders?

ANSWER: Eating disorders are usually grouped into the following 3 groups:

Anorexia nervosa is a condition in which individuals starve themselves as a result of misperceptions about the way their bodies look. Symptoms include a refusal to eat, an abnormal fear of weight gain, and an altered body image. Health consequences can include fatigue, depression, an irregular heart rate, growth of baby-fine hair all over the body (known as lanugo), anemia (iron-poor blood), constipation, bloating, brittle nails and hair, and low blood pressure. This insidious disease is difficult to treat and can be life threatening if the individual's weight drops too low. It can also lead to heart disease, bone loss, and nerve damage.

Bulimia nervosa is characterized by a pattern of eating copious amounts and then purging the food by vomiting or abuse of laxatives to prevent weight gain. Many people with this eating disorder are of normal weight. Like anorexia, bulimia can cause serious health consequences, including fatigue; depression; dehydration; electrolyte abnormalities; constipation; damage to teeth, gums, and cheeks (from exposure to stomach acid during vomiting); and an irregular heartbeat.

Binge eating, which is not officially categorized as an eating disorder but may be more common than anorexia and bulimia combined, is diagnosed when someone repeatedly and excessively overeats at one sitting. Binge eaters typically feel like they can't stop eating, then they're ashamed or feel guilty afterwards. They may suffer from fatigue and joint pain and can develop high blood pressure and cholesterol levels, heart disease, type 2 diabetes, or gallbladder disease. They are usually overweight or obese and have a history of weight fluctuations.

Eating disorders are far more common among women, especially younger women, than among men. Heredity factors may play a role in the development of some eating disorders, but social factors are also important. The desire to be thin and look and feel young in our society are contributing factors to the large increase in these disorders. Traumatic life events also may be a cause of eating disorders. The death of a spouse, the onset of menopause, a divorce, and children leaving home may lead midlife and older women to feel like they're losing control of their lives, sparking them to focus too much on things they can control, such as their eating habits and weight.

The treatment of eating disorders often involves cognitive-behavior therapy, where distorted thoughts and behaviors that lead to these disorders are identified and examined, and the person is helped to give them up. Prescription drugs that are effective in the treatment of eating disorders fall into a class of drugs known as selective serotonin reuptake inhibitors or SSRIs. These drugs work by affecting the level of the brain chemical known as serotonin. Some examples include Celexa (citalopram), Lexapro (escitalopram), Prozac (fluoxetine), Zoloft (sertraline), and Paxil (paroxetine). These drugs can also treat the depression and anxiety that may often accompany eating disorders. It is very important for someone with an eating disorder to seek help from their physician, an eating disorder specialist, a psychotherapist, or other qualified mental health professional before it threatens their health.

DRUG ABUSE IN THE ELDERLY

QUESTION: I heard that prescription drug abuse is common in the elderly. What can you tell me about this problem?

ANSWER: Yes, prescription drug abuse is not just something that happens in the young, and people over age 65 are at risk for drug abuse because they take more potentially addictive medications than any other age group. This problem is especially a concern in the elderly because with age, the liver loses the ability to metabolize or get rid of drugs in the body, which can lead to increased side effects. A recent Johns Hopkins Health Alert (**www.johnshopkinshealthalerts.com**, 2010) addresses this problem and identifies those drugs that are most prone to abuse in the elderly.

Which Drugs Are the Riskiest? As with any addictive substance, access increases the risk of abuse. Older people are more likely to get prescriptions for two leading types of drugs with potential for addiction: opioid pain relievers and benzodiazepines.

Drug Abuse With Opioids. Among abused prescription drugs, opioids are the most notorious. These drugs, which include oxycodone (Oxy Contin), oxycodone/acetaminophen (Percocet), and hydrocodone (Vicodin), attach to opioid receptors in the brain that block the perception of pain. They also can produce euphoria by indirectly boosting dopamine levels in the parts of the brain that influence our sensing of pleasure—hence their addictive potential. The most common side effects of opioids are nausea, vomiting, dizziness, sleepiness, constipation, and itching. During an overdose, opioids can slow down breathing, which can be fatal. However, a person who takes pain medication for a legitimate ailment or injury has a slim chance of developing an addiction. The risk increases when opioids are given to someone who has a personal or family history of addiction or has a psychological disorder.

Drug Abuse With Benzodiazepines. Other potentially addictive medications are benzodiazepines such as alprazolam (Xanax), clonazepam (Klonopin), diazepam (Valium), and lorazepam (Ativan). Doctors commonly use these drugs to treat anxiety, panic attacks, insomnia, and acute stress reactions to traumatic experiences, such as the death of a spouse. Benzodiazepines work by slowing brain activity. When used properly—in limited quantities for a short time—addiction is usually not a problem. But taking larger doses or even typical dosages on a daily basis for an extended amount of time can easily lead to tolerance, and an individual will soon need larger and larger doses to get the desired effect. In addition, suddenly going off a benzodiazepine can trigger extreme anxiety and discomfort, prompting a desire to keep taking it. The possibility of tolerance is also present with sleeping medications such as zolpidem (Ambien) and eszopiclone (Lunesta) that work at the same place in the brain as benzodiazepines. The health consequences of benzodiazepine abuse for older people include memory impairment, impaired reasoning, confusion, nodding off, car accidents, and falls, which could be fatal.

LEG CRAMPS AND QUININE

QUESTION: Can quinine help leg cramps?

ANSWER: Quinine may provide some relief from leg cramps, but the FDA does not recommend its use for this condition. This topic was recently reviewed in a Johns Hopkins Health Alert (**www. johnshopkinshealthalerts.com,** 2010).

Muscle cramps are a major problem for people with neurological illnesses such as Parkinson's disease or multiple sclerosis, but muscle cramps also frequently strike otherwise healthy older adults. In fact, it's estimated that upwards of 50% of people older than 65 experience recurring idiopathic (without a known cause) muscle cramps. Quinine is often prescribed off-label for the treatment of muscle cramps. However, the U.S. Food and Drug Administration (FDA) strongly recommends that people only take quinine for its indicated use, which is to treat malaria. Qualaquin, the prescription form of quinine, has been associated with a number of potentially deadly side effects. Between 2005 and 2008, the FDA received 38 reports of quinine-related incidents to its Adverse Event Reporting System. This may not seem like a lot, but the majority of cases were serious. Many of the people involved developed a condition called thrombocytopenia, where their blood platelets dropped to alarmingly low levels, causing excessive bleeding. Fourteen people had a blood platelet count below 5,000 microliters (normal is between 150,000 and 450,000) and five died. A number of other adverse events also were reported, including: GI symptoms, hearing loss, rash, electrolyte imbalance, and drug interactions. In addition, quinine is only mildly effective at stopping muscle cramps or reducing their severity, according to a recent assessment by the American Academy of Neurology (AAN). Other treatments that also fared poorly in the AAN's analysis include the antiseizure drug gabapentin (Neurontin), magnesium, and basic muscle stretching.

SCORPION STINGS

QUESTION: I heard that a drug was approved to treat scorpion stings. What can you tell me about it?

ANSWER: The FDA recently approved Anascorp injection, the first specific treatment for a scorpion sting. Venomous scorpions in the U.S. are mostly found in Arizona. Severe stings occur most frequently in infants and children, and can cause shortness of breath, fluid in the lungs, breathing problems, excess saliva, blurred vision, slurred speech, trouble swallowing, abnormal eye movements, muscle twitching, trouble walking, and other uncoordinated muscle movements. Untreated cases can be fatal. Scorpions are attracted to dark, moist spaces. They like to hide under rocks, wood, loose tree bark or anything else lying on the ground during the day, and they become active at night. Landscapers and others who work outside are at risk of being stung, as are people participating in outdoor activities. Because they're small and adept at climbing, scorpions may hitch a ride into homes in a sack of groceries or piece of clothing. Once indoors, they may get trapped in the sink or bathtub, look for a place to hide in an attic or crawl space, or scale the walls or ceiling. Victims often report being stung while sleeping. About 17,000 scorpion stings were reported to U.S. poison centers nationwide in 2009, with about 11,000 documented in Arizona. Anascorp is made from the plasma of horses that have been immunized with scorpion (Centruroides) venom. Its effectiveness was studied in 15 children with neurological signs of scorpion stings. These signs resolved within 4 hours of treatment in all eight of the children who received Anascorp, but in only one of seven children who received a "dummy" (placebo) injection. The most common side effects of Anascorp are vomiting, fever, rash, nausea, itchiness, headache, runny nose, and muscle pain.

LUPUS

QUESTION: What can you tell me about a new drug approved for lupus?

ANSWER: The FDA approved Benlysta (belimumab) in early 2011 for the treatment of adults with active systemic lupus erythematosus (lupus) who are also receiving existing therapies, such as corticosteroids, antimalarials, immunosuppressives, and nonsteroidal anti-inflammatory drugs (NSAIDs). Benlysta is the first lupus drug to be approved since 1955 and provides a new treatment approach. It is given by intravenous infusion and is designed to target a protein in the body known as the B-lymphocyte stimulator, which may reduce the number of abnormal B cells thought to be a problem in people with lupus. Clinical studies have shown that Benlysta, when used together with existing lupus drugs, can lessen the disease activity. However, African American patients and patients of African heritage do not appear to respond to treatment and more studies are being conducted with Benlysta in these patients. The most common side effects of Benlysta include nausea, diarrhea, fever, and infusion reactions, but other serious adverse reactions including death have been reported.

Lupus is a serious, potentially fatal, autoimmune disease that attacks healthy tissues. It occurs more often in women than men, and usually develops between ages 15 and 44. The disease affects many parts of the body including the joints, the skin, kidneys, lungs, heart, and the brain. When common lupus symptoms appear (flare) they can present as swelling in the joints or joint pain, light sensitivity, fever, chest pain, hair loss, and fatigue. Estimates vary on the number of lupus sufferers in the United States ranging from approximately 300,000 to 1.5 million people. People of all races can have the disease, however, African American women have a 3 times higher incidence (number of new cases) than Caucasian women.

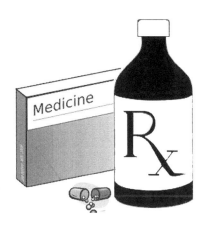

CHAPTER 15
TIPS AND TIDBITS

GENERIC DRUGS

QUESTION: Would you please give your opinion about generic drugs?

ANSWER: Generic drugs are medications that contain the same active ingredients as brand name products and are available both by prescription and over-the-counter (OTC). Common OTC generic products include such items as ibuprofen (trade name Motrin or Advil), diphenhydramine (trade name Benadryl), or acetaminophen (trade name Tylenol) and of course many, many more. Likewise, there are hundreds of generic prescription medications available such as amoxicillin (trade name Amoxil), captopril (trade name Capoten) or metoprolol (trade name Lopressor).

 The Food and Drug Administration (FDA) must approve all new drug products and in order to give manufacturers a chance to recoup their research and development costs, they are granted a patent that prevents other companies from marketing identical products (generics) for approximately 17 years. After this period of time, other manufacturers can then seek to get FDA approval for their generic products and compete with the brand name products. The FDA approves all generic drugs using strict guidelines, including checking for the generic drug's chemistry by evaluating its formulation, potency, stability, and purity. The generic drug must also pass bioequivalency testing that compares the delivery of the generic drug's active ingredient to that of the brand name drug. In addition, after a drug is approved by the FDA (brand or generic), it must maintain its approval within strict manufacturing guidelines, which require the manufacturer to provide samples to the FDA from each batch made for testing. However, since generic manufacturers do not have to re-do all of the original research showing that its product is safe and effective like the original manufacturer, and spends much less on advertising, its costs to produce the product are much less. This is why generic drugs usually cost about 30% to 50% less than brand name products.

It may be of interest to note that many brand or trade name companies may also produce generic products that actually can compete in the marketplace with their own higher priced brand products. It should also be noted that while both brand and generic drugs have the same active ingredients, they may look quite different from each other. The reason for this is that U.S. trademark laws do not allow a generic drug to look exactly the same as a brand name drug. This may be confusing to the patient and since mistakes can occur, always make sure you ask the pharmacist about any drug that looks different from what you're used to getting. Finally, you should also know that many insurance companies require a generic medication to be dispensed for cost savings. If you don't have prescription insurance and you would like to save some money on your medications, ask your doctor to prescribe generics if they are available and ask your pharmacist to dispense them. With the costs of new drugs skyrocketing, generic drugs can provide for cost saving alternatives.

PATENT EXPIRATIONS
OF TRADE NAME DRUGS

<u>QUESTION</u>: What trade name drugs might be available as generics in the near future?

<u>ANSWER</u>: Generic drugs have played an increasing role in our health-care system as a means to address rising drug costs. While prescription drugs account for about 11% of the nation's overall healthcare bill, they continue to gain greater attention by employers, governments, and other payers because of their double-digit growth rates. Retail prices for frequently used brand-name drugs have increased about three times faster than those of commonly used generic drugs. Today, consumers are accepting more than ever before that generic drugs are equivalent to their brand-name counterparts. As I've noted many times before, the FDA approves all generic drugs using strict guidelines, including checking for the generic drug's chemistry by evaluating its formulation, potency, stability, and purity. The generic drug must also pass bio-equivalency testing which compares the delivery into the bloodstream of the generic drug's active ingredient to that of the brand name drug. Generic drugs account for about 40% of prescriptions dispensed.

Numerous brand-name drugs are due to come off patent in the next few years. Although legal battles sometimes occur which can delay the availability of a generic product, new generic drugs are usually ready for FDA approval as the patent expiration date gets closer. I have listed on the next page some of the more popular brand name drugs that will be off patent in the near future. Please note, however, that these dates are subject to change based upon legal challenges or other unforeseen events.

Brand Name Drug (Generic Name) &
Estimated Year Patent Expires
Aciphex (tablets approved but not launched 2/07) (rabeprazole) 2013
Cymbalta (duloxetine) 2013
Eloxatin (oxaliplatin injection) 2013
Evista (raloxifene) 2013

Fosamax Plus D (alendronate/cholecalciferol) 2013
Fuzeon (enfuvirtide injection) 2013
Niaspan (niacin extended-release) 2013
Zomig (zolmitriptan) 2013
Actonel (risedronate) 2014
Advicor (lovastatin/niacin) 2014
Asacol (mesalamine delayed-release tablet) 2014
Avelox (moxifloxacin) 2014
Avodart (dutasteride) 2014
Celebrex (celecoxib) 2014
Copaxone (glatiramer injection) 2014
Exelon (rivastigmine) 2014
Maxalt (rizatriptan) 2014
Micardis (telmisartan) 2014
Micardis HCT (telmisartan/hydrochlorothiazide) 2014
Namenda (memantine) 2014
Nexium (esomeprazole) 2014
Temodar (temozolomide) 2014
Viracept (nelfinavir) 2014
Cipro HC (ciprofloxacin/hydrocortisone otic suspension) 2015
Gleevac (imatinib) 2015
Lovaza (omega-3 acid esters) 2015
Lumigan (bimatoprost ophthalmic solution) 2015
Patanol (olopatadine solution) 2015
Renagel (sevelamer) 2015
Sustiva (efavirenz) 2015
Travatan (travoprost ophthalmic solution) 2015
Welchol (colesevelam) 2015
AndroGel 1% (testosterone) 2016
Benicar (olmesartan) 2016
Crestor (rosuvastatin calcium) 2016
Reyataz (atazanavir) 2016
Sensipar (cinacalcet) 2016
Byetta (exenatide injection) 2017
Relpax (eletriptan) 2017
Strattera (atomoxetine) 2017
Vytorin (ezetimibe/simvastatin) 2017
Zetia (ezetimibe) 2017

Nasonex (mometasone nasal spray) 2018
Spiriva (tiotropium powder for inhalation) 2018
Lyrica (pregabalin) 2019
Detrol LA (tolterodine) 2020
Viagra (sildenafil) 2020
Crixivan (indinavir) 2021

HYDROGEN PEROXIDE

QUESTION: Is high-strength hydrogen peroxide dangerous?

ANSWER: Yes, and the FDA is warning consumers not to purchase or use high-strength hydrogen peroxide products, including a product marketed as 35% Food Grade Hydrogen Peroxide, for medicinal purposes because they can cause serious harm or death when ingested. Commonly available hydrogen peroxide is a 3% topical antiseptic solution that is used for a variety of conditions including the cleansing and disinfection of wounds or diluted half-strength with water and used as an oral rinse. Hydrogen peroxide is an oxidizing agent with antiseptic activity that releases oxygen when applied to tissue. However, the FDA has never approved high-strength hydrogen peroxide, which is more than 10 times stronger than regular-strength hydrogen peroxide and is highly corrosive. Ingesting hydrogen peroxide can cause gastrointestinal irritation or ulceration. Intravenous administration of hydrogen peroxide can cause inflammation of the blood vessel at the injection site, gas embolisms or bubbles in the blood vessels, and potentially life-threatening allergic reactions. Thirty-five percent hydrogen peroxide to be diluted and used in "Hyper-oxygenation Therapy" for AIDS, cancer, and numerous other conditions is fraudulent, dangerous and illegal, and distributors of this product have been actively restrained by the FDA since 1985. Many mail order and Internet distributors promote these products, sometimes called "Biowater" and "H2O2", as an alternative medicine. The FDA is not aware of any medical benefits from consuming hydrogen peroxide in any form and recommends that consumers who are currently using high-strength hydrogen peroxide to stop immediately and consult their health-care provider.

WALKING DEVICES

QUESTION: How do I choose the best walking device?

ANSWER: When walking becomes difficult due to an injury or disability, various types of walking devices are available to help you continue your normal activities. Both canes and walkers can help to reduce the amount of weight on one or both legs, which can ease joint pain and compensate for weakness in the legs. They can also help to prevent falls, which is the leading cause of injuries and injury-related deaths in people over age 65. Canes are usually recommended for people who have moderately impaired walking ability and require only one arm to maintain balance and bear weight. Many people with knee or hip arthritis or mild balance disorders, as well as those who are visually impaired, have a physical injury, or are weak on one side after a stroke may benefit from a cane. There are three basic kinds of canes: standard, offset, and quad (4-legged). Standard canes are made of wood or aluminum and are used by people who need only a minimum amount of support. The length of aluminum canes can be adjusted, while wooden canes need to be custom fitted for the right length. Offset canes have a swan neck, which places the hand directly over the shaft and allows for partial weight bearing. These canes are useful for people with moderate knee or hip arthritis. Small or large based quad canes, which rest on four-rubber tipped points, provide more support for people who need greater weight bearing. An advantage of this type of cane is that it can stand alone and free hands for other tasks if needed. Quad canes with a smaller base may be useful for people with a fast gait. All canes need to be the proper length for good balance and comfort. The length of the cane is measured from the floor to the hip joint, so that your elbow will be flexed at about a 30° angle when you are holding the top of the cane. When being measured for a cane, you should wear your normal walking shoes. Walkers are usually recommended when both upper arms are required to maintain balance or bear wait. A standard walker has four legs that contact the floor at the same time. It is very stable, but people using it must have a slow, controlled gait because they need to lift the walker completely off the ground and place it forward before they take a step. People who walk faster may be better off with a front-wheeled walker. This type of walker allows a more normal walking speed, but is not as stable as a standard walker. Four-wheeled walkers should not be used by people who put too much weight on the walker, because this could cause it to roll away and cause a fall. People needing canes or walkers should contact their physician, a physical therapist, or a pharmacist who specializes in these products for proper selection of the most appropriate assistive device. Here are some suggestions for using walking devices correctly:

Using Canes And Walkers Correctly

- Hold a cane on the same side as your stronger leg. When walking, place your weight on your stronger leg, then step forward with your weaker leg and the cane. Avoid placing the cane too far ahead, as it might slip and cause you to fall.
- To climb stairs with your cane, step off with your stronger leg, then move the cane and your weaker leg to the same step. When descending stairs, step down with the cane and your weaker leg, then move the stronger leg to the same step. An easy way to remember this process is: "Up with the good and down with the bad." If you use a quad cane, a smaller base is best for climbing stairs.
- When using a walker, place it firmly (or roll it) a step's length ahead. Lean slightly forward, holding the walker arms for support, and then take a step.
- Rubber tips on canes or walkers keep them from slipping. Check the tips often. Replace them if they appear worn.
- Invest in sturdy, low-heeled shoes with nonskid soles to help prevent falls and increase stability.
- Avoid wet floors and sidewalks, do not use escalators or revolving doors, and remove loose throw rugs and electrical or telephone cords from your path.
- Consider adding ice tips to the bottom of your device. Ice tips can be flipped down for traction on snow or ice. Also, consider using two canes on winter walks.

PRESCRIPTION PACKAGE INSERTS

QUESTION: Sometimes I ask my pharmacist or doctor for the "package insert" for a medication that I take, but they are hard to read and understand. I heard that they are changing. Can you tell me more?

ANSWER: Package inserts that are included with prescription drugs are very confusing and difficult to understand for doctors, pharmacists, and patients. They are lengthy and detailed with many small-print warnings and even contain chemical structures that are meaningless to most people. Confusing medical information like this is behind many of the estimated 300,000 preventable cases of death or injury that occur each year in our nation's hospitals. This will soon be changing. For the first time in 25 years, the FDA is altering its rules to make these package inserts much easier to read and understand. Under new FDA guidelines, many of the legal warnings will be removed and the drug's chemical structure will be moved to the back of the insert. In their place will be a "Highlights" section that spells out the most important information about a drug's risks and benefits. The insert will also for the first time include a table of contents to help the reader locate specific information about the medication. Some additional features that new prescription drug labels will begin including are the date the drug received approval in the U.S., recent major changes in information about the drug, a toll-free phone number for patients or doctors to report suspected side effects, concise drug interaction information, and a section that prompts doctors on what key facts they should pass on to their patients. These new guidelines will apply to all new drugs within several months and will be phased in over the next seven years for drugs already on the market or currently under FDA review.

MEDICAL LEECHES

QUESTION: I read about the FDA approving the use of leeches for skin grafts. How do they help?

ANSWER: Yes, the FDA recently approved the use of medical leeches as a medical device—not a drug. The use of leeches for medical purposes goes back over 2,000 years when they were used as an alternative treatment to bloodletting for a wide variety of ailments. I can also remember when local pharmacies sold leeches for the treatment of bruising and black eyes many years ago. Today, leeches can be very useful to plastic surgeons in helping heal skin grafts by removing blood that has pooled under the skin and restoring blood circulation in blocked veins by removing pooled blood. They are also useful in some cases of body part reattachment surgery. Leeches are segmented worms closely related to the earthworm, but are more specialized. There are several different types of leeches, but the medicinal leeches known as "hirudo medicinalis" normally make their home in freshwater. They have a segmented body with a powerful clinging sucker at each end and produce a secretion called "hirudin" which prevents blood from clotting. These blood-sucking parasites can ingest several times their own weight at one meal. The company that was approved by the FDA to market medicinal leeches is Ricarimpex, a French company. Leeches have been used for many years in American hospitals, which obtained them from companies that raised and sold leeches in the U.S. prior to 1976. However, the medical device laws passed in 1976 require new companies like Ricarimpex to seek FDA approval. Leeches are to be used only once, then killed and disposed of.

DRUG INTERACTIONS

QUESTION: How can I avoid drug interactions with nonprescription medications?

ANSWER: Many nonprescription medications, herbal products, and vitamins can interact with other over-the-counter medications or prescription drugs. These drug-to-drug interactions may increase the action of a particular drug, may make a particular drug less effective, or can cause unexpected side effects. For example, the decongestant pseudoephedrine, which is found in many nonprescription cold and allergy products, can interact with some prescription antidepressants.

Likewise, the herbal product ginkgo can interact with aspirin or blood-thinning medications to increase the risk of bleeding problems. While I cannot list all of the possible drug interactions with nonprescription medications in this column, there are some steps that can be taken to reduce the risk. First of all, you should always read the "Drug Facts" label on any nonprescription medications that you use. The "Warnings" section of the "Drug Facts" label provides information about important drug interactions. If you are taking any of the medications listed in the "Warnings" section, do not use the product until you talk to your pharmacist or doctor. Also, be sure to tell your doctor(s) and pharmacist(s) about all the nonprescription medicines that you take, including herbal products, vitamins, and other supplements. Don't be afraid to ask your pharmacist for help in choosing the nonprescription products that are right for you. You might also consider using one pharmacy for all of your medication needs to make it easier for the pharmacist to spot potential drug-drug interactions. If you utilize a mail-order pharmacy for some or all of your prescription needs, also let them know what nonprescription medications you use so that they can help to prevent drug-related problems. It should be noted that the risk of drug to drug interactions increases with the number of medications taken, which can be of particular importance in the elderly population who account for about one-third of all prescriptions dispensed, as well as more than one-third of all nonprescription medications sold.

DRUG INTERACTIONS IN THE ELDERLY

QUESTION: You recently wrote that drug interactions are very important in the elderly population. Can you expand on this?

ANSWER: As people get older they are faced with more health problems that require regular drug therapy. In addition, the risk of drug-to-drug interactions in older adults is increased due to body changes that take place as you age. For instance, changes in the gastrointestinal system can affect how fast medications can get into the blood. Changes in body weight can also influence the dose of medications needed. Furthermore, as you age the circulation system may slow down and organ function can diminish, which can affect how fast drugs are removed from the body by the liver and kidneys. Because of all these changes in the body and because the number of medications taken usually increases in the elderly, the risk of drug interactions and side effects is greater in this group of people. As I've noted before, adults over the age of 65 account for more than one-third of all prescription medications dispensed, as well as more than one-third of all nonprescription medications sold. In addition to drugs interacting with other drugs, drug interactions with foods or alcohol can also be a concern for the elderly. In order to try and prevent drug interactions and drug side effects make sure that your doctor(s) and pharmacist(s) are made aware of all the medications that you take—prescription and nonprescription. Don't forget to include eye drops, dietary supplements, vitamins, herbals and topical medications like ointments and creams. Most pharmacies can keep track of the medications that you take on their computer and your pharmacist can help to prevent potentially harmful drug interactions. If you utilize more than one pharmacy or a mail-order pharmacy, let them all know about the medications that you take in order to reduce the risk of drug interactions.

QUESTION: What drugs can cause emergency hospitalizations in older people?

ANSWER: Adverse drug events cause an estimated 100,000 emergency hospitalizations for senior Americans every year, but over two-thirds of these hospitalizations involve only a handful of drugs and drug types. According to a study recently published in the New England Journal of Medicine (2011), only four drugs or drug classes were responsible for the majority of these emergency hospitalizations. The study researchers collected information from 58 hospitals around the country between 2007 and 2009 and estimated that nearly 100,000 emergency hospitalizations each year were due to adverse drug events in adults 65 years of age or older. Nearly one-half of these hospitalizations were among adults 80 years of age or older. Study results showed that over two-thirds of the hospitalizations were due to unintentional overdoses of the following four medications or medication classes:

- Warfarin (Coumadin)—33% of hospitalizations
- Insulins—14% of hospitalizations
- Oral anti-platelet drugs (Aspirin, Plavix, and others)—13% of hospitalizations
- Oral diabetes drugs—11% of hospitalizations

With antiplatelet or blood thinning drugs, bleeding was the main problem. For insulin and other diabetes medications, about two-thirds of cases involved changes in mental status such as confusion, loss of consciousness or seizures.

All of these medications are commonly prescribed to older adults, but their dosage needs to be carefully adjusted to prevent adverse effects. Blood thinners like warfarin and diabetes medications like insulin or oral hypoglycemic agents require blood testing to adjust the doses. Interactions between these medications and other drugs or foods can also cause problems leading to serious side effects, so it is important that your physician and pharmacist know about all the medications (prescription and non-prescription) that you take. Hospitalizations due to adverse drug events are likely to increase as Americans live longer, have more chronic conditions, and take more medications.

MEDICINE CABINET

QUESTION: What should I keep in my medicine cabinet?

ANSWER: Since medicine cabinets are usually in a bathroom, which can get hot and humid, they are not necessarily the best place to store medicines. A better place to store medicine is in a cool, dark, and dry location like a closet (a lockable closet if children are in the household or can visit). That being said, every household should have certain, nonprescription medicinal products available to treat common ailments and minor injuries. You might want to have the following items on hand in your medicine storage area:

- Products for pain and fever such as ibuprofen, acetaminophen, and aspirin.

- Antibiotic ointment and hydrogen peroxide for cuts and scrapes.
- Hydrocortisone cream for itching and inflammation.
- Antacids for upset stomach.
- Antihistamines for allergy symptoms or insect bites.
- Decongestants for colds and flu.
- An anti-diarrhea medication.
- Other products for common ailments that people in your household may have.
- A thermometer.
- Alcohol wipes, disinfectant sprays, and antiseptic sprays to clean scrapes and cuts and to prevent infections.
- Band aids, gauze pads, and adhesive tape for scrapes and cuts.
- A list of emergency phone numbers including the National Poison Hotline (800-222-1222).

In addition, you should periodically check the expiration dates of all products that you store and discard those that are outdated. Also remove any products that have been taken off the market and discard them. Read all product labeling carefully to determine proper storage conditions and expiration dates.

TOOTHBRUSHES

QUESTION: How do I select a good toothbrush?

ANSWER: The practice of using a device to clean teeth can be traced back to the Middle Ages, when wealthy Europeans used twigs made of sweet-smelling wood for this purpose. In 1498, the Emperor of China improved on this idea by embedding hog bristles in bone handles, thus inventing the first toothbrush. This device later became very popular throughout Europe, but because of the high cost of hog bristles, poor people could not always afford their own brush and family members often shared one toothbrush. This all changed in 1938, when the modern toothbrush was invented by Dupont and hog bristles were replaced with nylon ones. Today there are so many types of toothbrushes, from manual to powered ones, that it is mind-boggling for many consumers to make a selection. Probably the most important characteristic of a good toothbrush is that it has soft bristles. Hard bristles can damage enamel on the teeth and cause gum tissue to pull back from the teeth, leading to greater sensitivity to hot or cold beverages. Over time, receding gum tissue can also lead to a need for periodontal correction or tooth loss. Softer bristles are more effective at working themselves into crevices and spaces between the teeth. Furthermore, the size and shape of a toothbrush is very important. A toothbrush should be small enough to allow easy access to all areas of the mouth, teeth, and gums. In addition, the handle size should allow the user to maneuver the brush easily while maintaining a firm grasp. Many types of handles have been developed such as those with angle bends or flexible areas in the handle to help improve contact between the bristles and less-accessible tooth surfaces. Smaller toothbrushes are available for children. Power toothbrushes come in two basic types. Electric toothbrushes generate between 3,000 and 7,000 brush strokes per minute while sonic toothbrushes generate between 30, 000 and 40,000 brush strokes per minute. This compares to about 300 brush strokes per minute generated +with a properly used manual toothbrush. Power toothbrushes may also benefit certain people such as the disabled, the elderly, those wearing braces or orthotic devices, or those who may have difficulty using a manual toothbrush. However, power toothbrushes are more expensive and less portable than manual toothbrushes. The American Dental Association (ADA) recommends that toothbrushes should be rinsed with tap water after each use and should not be shared. Also, that toothbrushes be replaced about every three to four months, or sooner if the bristles become frayed with use. Toothbrushes should be stored in the open air rather than closed containers because microorganisms are less likely to survive in an oxygen rich environment. Your dentist or dental hygienist can help you select the best toothbrush for your specific needs.

QUESTION: You recently wrote about selecting a good toothbrush. I like to use a power toothbrush. Can you discuss the differences between them?

ANSWER: Although manual toothbrushes are still widely used to maintain oral hygiene, most people do not brush well or for an adequate amount of time. Power brushes have been commercially available since the 1960's, but today they are very popular due to many new and improved designs and features. While various factors need to be taken into consideration, there is some evidence that power toothbrushes may be better than manual brushes for plaque removal, and reduction in gingivitis, calculus, and staining. The number of available power toothbrush products is bewildering but there are five basic types:

Types of Power Brushes*
Motion: Side to Side
Mode of Action: Brush heads or bristles move side to side laterally
Product Names: Sonicare, Phillips 550, GEC, LPA/Broxo

Motion: Circular
Mode of Action: Brush head rotates in one direction
Product Names: Rowenta, Teledyne, Aqua Tech

Motion: Counter Oscillation
Mode of Action: Tufts rotate in one direction then another, with other tufts rotating in the opposite direction
Product Names: Interplak, Epident, Plaq and White

Motion: Rotation Oscillation
Mode of Action: Brush head rotates in one direction then in the other
Product Names: Braun Oral B, Phillips Jordan HP 735

Motion: Ultrasonic
Mode of Action: Brush head vibrates at ultrasonic frequencies
Product Names: Ultrasonex

* (From Mann, GB: Power Toothbrushes, **www.dentalcare.com**)

In addition, various brush head shapes are available for adults, children, orthodontic patients as well as for interdental spaces. Some power brushes have replaceable batteries, but as the battery life is reduced, the brush speed also reduces. Other brushes utilize a direct power source or have rechargeable batteries. Additional power brush features include pressure sensors, which interrupts the brush movement to make people aware when too much pressure is being applied, or timers, which enables the user to assess the time spent on brushing. Your dentist can help you decide what type of toothbrush is best for you. Additional useful information about toothbrushes and dental care can be found on the Internet at **www.dentalcare.com**.

BANNED DRUGS IN SPORTS

QUESTION: What nonprescription substances are banned for use in sports?

ANSWER: In addition to many prescription drugs, numerous dietary supplements and other substances have been banned by major sports-governing bodies. These products are marketed to athletes with claims that they will enhance their performance. Some popular supplements have proven performance-enhancing effects, while others do not. Because many of these substances can have serious side effects, they are banned and drug testing programs (doping control) are used to detect if an athlete has used them. Two banned dietary supplements include androstenedione (andro) and dehydroepiandrosterone (DHEA). Both of these agents are promoted to increase levels of the hormone testosterone in he body. Testosterone is claimed to have performance-enhancing ability and DHEA has been touted as a "super hormone". Both of these substances can cause adverse effects and are banned by the National Collegiate Athletic Association (NCAA), the World Anti-Doping Agency (WADA), and other sports-governing agencies. Products containing ephedra or ma huang are also banned by numerous sports-governing bodies. Athletes using herbal ephedra products are at risk of stimulating the heart or nervous system and several deaths have been associated with their use. Because of this, ephedra-containing products were removed from the U.S. market in 2004, but they continue to be available from other countries and through the Internet. Caffeine has also been used in sports as a stimulant to counter drowsiness, to improve endurance, and to enhance body-building workouts. Its side effects include inability to sleep, tremors, nervousness, restlessness, increased heart rate, and irregular heart beats. In addition, caffeine is a diuretic, which can cause electrolyte imbalances and dehydration. Caffeine is restricted by the NCAA, which only allows a urine concentration of 15 mg/liter or less. About 5 cups of regular coffee within a few hours of the urine drug test would put an average size man over the limit. Athletes should be aware that many nonprescription herbal products contain caffeine along with some soft drinks and sport or energy drinks. The use of alcohol can also have a negative effect on athletic performance, particularly for events that require endurance, speed, quick reaction time, balance, and coordination. Short-term side effects of alcohol include drowsiness, sedation, impaired balance, impaired judgment, and impaired physical activity skills. The NCAA and WADA ban the use of alcohol for certain events, such as rifle and archery. Much more information on this topic can be found at the following Internet web sites: **www.idtm.com; www.drugfreesports.com/home.htm; www.usantidoping.org**.

COLOCARE

QUESTION: I heard about a new test to screen for colon cancer that doesn't make you handle fecal material. What can you tell me about it?

ANSWER: Colon cancer is the third leading cancer and the second leading cause of cancer deaths in the U.S. It has been estimated that over 145,000 new cases of colon cancer will be diagnosed in the U.S. this year, and ninety percent of people who get this disease are over the age of 50. In the early stages of colorectal cancer, most patients do not have any symptoms and screening tests can be very useful for cancer detection. The American Cancer Society recommends that beginning at age 50, men and women should have an annual fecal occult blood test (FOBT). The FOBT is a screening test that detects hidden (occult) blood in the stool, which is a warning sign for colorectal cancer and other gastrointestinal diseases. Many people, however, have avoided using the at-home FOBT because of the unpleasantness of handling fecal material. Recently, a new nonprescription FOBT for at-home use has been developed that does not require collection of a stool sample. ColoCare is a throw-in-the-bowl FOBT that is disposable, accurate, easy to use, and does not require the handling of fecal material. ColoCare utilizes a test pad that floats on the water surface in the toilet bowl and detects hidden blood in the toilet water within 30 seconds following a bowel movement. The test pad is made of specially treated biodegradable paper that produces a blue or green color when blood is detected. Following the test reading, the ColoCare pad is flushed down the toilet with the bowel movement. It is recommended that you test 3 consecutive bowel movements and if any test is positive, that you consult your physician for further evaluation and testing. Patients using ColoCare are advised to maintain a normal, well balanced, fully cooked, and unaltered diet for 2 days prior to testing. Red or raw meats, vitamin C (over 250 mg/day), and certain medications may interfere with test results, so patients should read the test instructions very carefully and consult with their doctor and pharmacist if necessary. Other factors that can alter the test results include bleeding from hemorrhoids or menstruation, use of rectal preparations, toilet bowl cleaners or deodorizers, and mineral oil laxatives.

TEETH WHITENERS

QUESTION: How do nonprescription teeth-whitening products work?

ANSWER: Just about everyone would like their teeth to be "movie-star" white and the popularity of nonprescription teeth-whitening products has escalated in recent years. Tooth discoloration can occur due to aging (increased yellowing), certain diseases, injury, or the use of tetracycline antibiotics. Staining of the teeth is commonly caused by smoking, chewing tobacco, or the consumption of certain foods or drinks such as coffee, tea, or wine. Basically, there are two methods of teeth whitening available: bleaching and non-bleaching. The active ingredients in bleaching products are either hydrogen peroxide or carbamide peroxide. Both of these chemicals are oxidizing agents that release oxygen when applied to teeth and mouth tissues providing cleansing and antiseptic effects. However, hydrogen peroxide is a stronger oxidizing agent than carbamide peroxide. Nonprescription bleaching products are available as strips (e.g., Crest Whitestrips), brush-on gels (e.g., Colgate Simply White), applicator pens (e.g., Oral-B Rembrandt Whitening Pen), and mouth trays with gels (e.g., Oral-B Rembrandt Plus Kit). Depending on the product, they are used from 30 minutes to 2 hours a day for approximately 5 to 14 days. The most common side effects of these products is tooth sensitivity (increased response to cold) and gingival irritation. Non-bleaching products usually contain abrasive ingredients such as sodium bicarbonate (baking soda) and hydrated silica. These products are marketed as whitening toothpastes and can also be combined with peroxides. When used daily as part of a good oral hygiene practice, these non-bleaching products can help to polish away surface stains. It should be noted that nonprescription teeth-whitening agents are considered to be cosmetic products and therefore are not regulated by the FDA. In addition, it is advisable to see a dentist before and while using a bleaching product. People also need to know that these products are only to be used on healthy natural teeth and not on fillings, crowns, veneers, or other dental work. Furthermore, these products should not be used for longer periods than recommended on package labels unless they are used under the supervision of a dentist.

ACETAMINOPHEN AND LIVER FAILURE

QUESTION: I take Tylenol for my arthritis and Tylenol-PM to help me sleep. Can too much Tylenol be harmful?

ANSWER: Both Tylenol and Tylenol-PM contain acetaminophen, which is an effective drug to relieve pain and reduce fever. Acetaminophen (abbreviated APAP) is also an ingredient in numerous other nonprescription and prescription generic and tradename products. When acetaminophen is taken in recommended doses it is safe and effective. However, when it is taken in large doses it can cause liver problems. In fact, accidental poisonings from acetaminophen is the leading cause of acute liver failure in the U.S. In 1998, acetaminophen was to blame in 28% of liver poisonings, but it was responsible for 51% of liver poisoning cases in 2003. While most of these patients survived after intensive care in the hospital, 74 died and 23 others required a liver transplant. Approximately 44% of the poisoning cases were suicide attempts, but 48% were unintentional overdoses, which could have been avoided. Since so many prescription and nonprescription medications contain acetaminophen, consumers need to make sure that they are not taking more than the maximum recommended total daily dose of 4,000 mg (4 grams) for adults. This maximum dose is the combined total daily dose from all acetaminophen-containing products that are being used in a given day. In order to prevent unintentional overdoses of acetaminophen, consumers need to read all product labels carefully to determine if they contain acetaminophen and in what amount. They also need to know if their prescription medications contain acetaminophen and in what amount, so that if they are taken together not more than a total of 4,000 mg of acetaminophen is taken per day for adults. If someone is a regular user of alcohol, it is recommended that the total daily dose of acetaminophen be limited to 2,000 mg (2 grams) per day or less or not used at all. In addition, many prescription drugs can interact with acetaminophen, making it more likely to cause liver problems. In view of this, be sure to ask your physician and pharmacist about any potential drug interaction problems if you are taking acetaminophen. While it is beyond the scope of this column to identify all products that contain acetaminophen, many nonprescription and prescription pain relievers, cold and flu preparations, and fever reducing products contain acetaminophen in various amounts. Please read all product labels carefully and if you have any concerns or questions, ask the pharmacist or your physician for advice.

QUESTION: Why is the FDA limiting the amount of acetaminophen in prescription pain relievers like Vicodin and Percocet?

ANSWER: In January of 2011 the FDA announced that it will be asking manufacturers of combination prescription pain relievers to limit the amount of acetaminophen to no more than 325 milligrams (mg) in each tablet or capsule. The reason for this limit is to reduce the risk of liver injury, which can occur when patients combine these products with other acetaminophen-containing medications like Tylenol and other over-the-counter (OTC) medications. The FDA also is requiring manufacturers to update labels of all prescription combination acetaminophen products to warn of the potential risk for severe liver injury. Acetaminophen, also called APAP, is a drug that relieves pain and fever. It is combined in many prescription products with other ingredients, usually opioids such as codeine (Tylenol with Codeine), oxycodone (Percocet), and hydrocodone (Vicodin). OTC acetaminophen products are not affected by the new dosage limit. The elimination of higher-dose prescription combination acetaminophen products will be phased in over three years and should not create a shortage of pain medication. Patients and health care professionals are being notified of the new limitation on acetaminophen content, and of the labeling change, in a drug safety communication. The FDA believes that prescription combination products containing no more than 325 mg of acetaminophen per tablet are effective for treating pain. Acetaminophen is the leading cause of liver failure in the U.S. and sends 56,000 people to the emergency room annually. Many of these patients will die or require a liver transplant. Since so many prescription and nonprescription medications contain acetaminophen, consumers need to make sure that they are not taking more than the maximum recommended total daily dose of 4,000 mg (4 grams) for adults. This maximum dose is the combined total daily dose from all acetaminophen-containing products that are being used in a given day. In order to prevent unintentional overdoses of acetaminophen, consumers need to read all product labels carefully to determine if they contain acetaminophen and in what amount. They also need to know if their prescription medications contain acetaminophen and in what amount, so that if they are taken together not more than a total of 4,000 mg of acetaminophen is taken per day. If someone is a regular user of alcohol, it is recommended that the total daily dose of acetaminophen be limited to 2,000 mg (2 grams) per day or less or not used at all. Please be sure to ask your physician and pharmacist about any potential drug interaction problems if you are taking acetaminophen. While it is beyond the scope of this column to identify all products that contain acetaminophen, many nonprescription and prescription pain relievers, cold and flu preparations, and fever reducing products contain acetaminophen in various amounts.

MEDICAL MAGGOTS

<u>QUESTION</u>: You recently wrote about the use of medical leeches. What about maggots?

<u>ANSWER</u>: Yes, the FDA also recently approved the use of medical maggots as a medical device—not a drug. The lifecycle of a maggot starts with the parent housefly (or similar species) laying eggs. After the eggs hatch, the caterpillar-like larval stage begins and after about 15 days the housefly emerges. Maggots are most useful for medical therapy during the feeding stage and the use of medical maggots is also known as larval therapy. Maggots have been used for helping to heal wounds since the 16th century. Their use became more widespread after an American doctor during World War I noticed that soldiers whose wounds became infected with maggots were less likely to die from infection than those who did not. However, when antibiotics became available in the 1940's, the use of maggot therapy for wound healing became less popular. More recently maggot therapy has been revived for the treatment of wounds, burns, and necrotic tumors. It is used in numerous hospitals in the United Kingdom. Maggot therapy appears to work in three ways. First of all, maggots liquefy dead (necrotic) tissue by secreting enzymes; secondly, they produce a substance that kills bacteria; and thirdly, they speed wound healing. Normal tissue is not affected by medical maggots. Medical maggot therapy is particularly beneficial when used for moist wounds in areas that have a poor blood supply and where antibiotic penetration is poor. The maggots used for medical purposes do not burrow under the patient's skin and they do not multiply. The maggots are usually covered by a dressing and are flushed out of a wound after several days. The only U.S. supplier of disinfected maggots is the non-profit Biotherapeutics Education and Research Foundation in California.

NANOTECHNOLOGY

<u>QUESTION</u>: I heard about a new cancer drug that uses nanotechnology. What is nanotechnology?

ANSWER: The FDA recently approved a new drug for treating patients with certain types of metastatic breast cancer that was developed using "nanotechnology". In the future, you will be hearing more and more about this technology being used to develop new drugs. Scientists are learning more about how the human body functions on a smaller and smaller scale. The term "nano" means one billionth and a "nanometer" is 1/1,000,000,000 of a meter (nine zeros). To get an idea about how small a nanometer is, the smallest object visible with an unaided eye is about 10,000 nanometers in size. Human hair measures 50,000 nanometers across and a single cell of bacteria is a few hundred nanometers. The most complicated organisms are made up of tiny cells that are made from nanoscale building blocks. Pharmaceutical nanotechnology and nanoscience studies and utilizes nano particles to develop improved drug therapy on a molecular level. The National Cancer Institute (NCI) is so excited about this new development that it has committed to a $144 million, five-year project to develop and apply nanotechnology for the prevention, diagnosis, and treatment of cancer. The new nanotechnology drug that you heard about is Abraxane, which was approved for use in patients with metastatic breast cancer who have not responded to other drug therapies. Abraxane contains the anticancer drug, paclitaxel, obtained from the Pacific Yew tree. However, the paclitaxel particles in the new product are only 130 nanometers in size and they are attached to protein (albumin). This nanoparticle protein engineered product reduces the incidence of certain side effects from the drug and allows for a higher dosage to be given with better treatment results. In clinical studies, patients receiving Abraxane had almost a double response rate compared to patients receiving the regular paclitaxel product. Many other drugs are being developed using nanotechnology and you will be seeing many of these new products in the future.

SEROTONIN SYNDROME

QUESTION: I heard that certain migraine medications can interact with some antidepressants. What can happen if they are taken together?

ANSWER: The FDA recently issued a Public Health Advisory about taking triptan drugs, which are used to treat migraine headaches, together with certain antidepressant medications. The antidepressants of concern are known chemically as selective serotonin reuptake inhibitors (SSRI's) and selective serotonin/norepinephrine reuptake inhibitors (SNRI's). Antidepressants in these two categories include Celexa (citalopram), fluvoxamine, Lexapro (escitalopram), Paxil (paroxetine), Prozac (fluoxetine), Symbyax (olanzapine/fluoxetine), Zoloft (sertraline), Cymbalta (duloxetine), and Effexor (venlafaxine). They are primarily used to treat depression and other mood disorders and are very effective. However, when taken together with triptan drugs used to treat migraine headaches, a life-threatening condition called "serotonin syndrome" may occur. This syndrome occurs when the body has too much serotonin, which is a chemical found in the nervous system. Symptoms of this condition may include restlessness, hallucinations, loss of coordination, fast heart beat, rapid changes in blood pressure, increased temperature, overactive reflexes, nausea, vomiting, and diarrhea. The antidepressants listed above and triptan drugs both increase serotonin levels and when taken together can cause levels of this chemical to increase too much. Triptan drugs used to treat migraine headaches include Amerge (naratriptan), Axert (almotriptan), Frova (frovatriptan), Imitrex (sumatriptan), Maxalt and Maxalt-MLT (rizatriptan), Relpax (eletriptan) and Zomig or Zomig ZMT (zolmitriptan). The FDA recommends that patients taking these triptans along with the antidepressants noted above should talk to their doctor before stopping their medications and to seek medical attention immediately if they experience symptoms of "serotonin syndrome" described earlier. This health advisory points out the importance of making sure that all of your healthcare providers (physicians, pharmacists, nurses) know about every medication (prescription and nonprescription) that you are taking so that serious drug interactions can be avoided.

TABLET SPLITTING

QUESTION: Is it okay to split drug tablets to save money?

ANSWER: In order to try and save money, many people are asking their physicians to prescribe medications in a higher dosage than required so that they can split their tablets to get more doses. The American Medical Association and the American Pharmacists Association are both against this practice, but they don't pay for the increasingly expensive medications needed by patients without prescription insurance. Your pharmacist can help you to decide if tablet splitting is a good idea for your medications, but let me offer a few considerations. First of all, many tablets are not "scored" (have an indentation line across the tablet), which helps to split the tablet evenly. This makes it more difficult to split the tablet into two or more correct doses even using a tablet splitting device. A recent study has shown that tablet fragments may contain anywhere from 50% to 150% of the desired amount of active drug ingredient when split using a tablet splitter or a kitchen knife to divide the tablet. In addition, drug products that are long-acting or sustained release formulations should not be split. Tablets that contain a combination of ingredients should also not be split because you may not get the right combination of drugs in each split dose. Tablet splitting may not be appropriate if the drug dose is critical for therapy, if the tablet is film coated, or if the tablet crumbles when split. Furthermore, some patients may be physically incapable of splitting tablets because they lack manual dexterity, strength, or good vision. Others may take several medications and tablet splitting could make their drug therapy regimen even more confusing. The bottom line is that in some cases tablet splitting may be appropriate to save money on medications, but in other situations it could make matters worse or even endanger a patient's health. You should seek the advice and assistance of your pharmacist to determine if tablet splitting is a reasonable thing for you to do.

WEIGHT GAIN

QUESTION: Can some drugs cause you to gain weight?

ANSWER: Yes, certain prescription drugs can cause weight gain in some people. The amount of weight gain can range from a few pounds to more than 100 pounds, depending upon the type of drug or drugs being taken. This extra weight can be a problem for people with high blood pressure, cardiovascular problems, diabetes, high cholesterol, or osteoarthritis. Why some prescription drugs can cause weight gain is not always clear, but they increase a person's appetite or make people crave certain foods. In addition, some drugs can alter one's metabolism, causing them to burn calories more slowly or to store fat. Other drugs, like corticosteroids (e.g., prednisone, methylprednisolone) can make the body less able to absorb sugar from the blood, leading to fat deposits. Furthermore, some medications can cause fatigue or shortness of breath, making the person less active, or can cause retention of water. However just because a drug can cause weight gain doesn't mean that everyone taking it will gain weight. In many cases it is impossible to identify if a medication is the cause of weight gain. If you think that you're putting on weight because of a medication that you are taking, talk to your doctor about it. Your doctor may want you to switch to another drug, take a lower dose, change your eating habits, or increase your physical activity. Don't stop taking a prescribed medication without first talking to your doctor. Below are some drugs that have been associated with weight gain:

Drug Type
Examples (Generic/Tradename)
- **Antihypertensives**
    Propranolol (Inderal)
    Nisoldipine (Sular)
    Hydralazine (Apresoline)
    Minoxidil (Loniten)
- **Diabetes drugs**
    Insulin
    Glipizide (Glucotrol)
    Glyburide (DiaBeta, Glynase, Micronase)
    Glimepiride (Amaryl)
    Pioglitazone (Actos)
    Rosiglitazone (Avandia)
- **Antidepressants/Mood stabilizers**
    Clozapine (Clozaril)
    Risperidone (Risperdal)

Olanzapine (Zyprexa)
Lithium
Paroxetine (Paxil)
Mirtazapine (Remeron)
Amitriptyline (Elavil, Vanatrip)
Imipramine (Tofranil)
Trimipramine (Surmontil)
Doxepin (Sinequan)
- **Anticonvulsants**
  Carbamazepine (Carbatrol, Epitrol, Tegretol)
  Valproate (Depakene, Depakote)
- **Cortocosteroids**
  Prednisone (Deltasone)
  Methylprednisolone (Medrol)

CAFFEINE

QUESTION: My doctor told me to avoid caffeine. What are some common sources of caffeine including non-prescription medications?

ANSWER: Caffeine is one of the oldest and most commonly used stimulants in the world. It has a well-known effect on the central nervous system to increase alertness and prevent drowsiness. However, in higher doses it also can produce side effects such as tremors, anxiety, nervousness, insomnia, heart palpitations, increased stomach acid, and increased urination. Because of these side effects, doctors will often recommend that people with certain stomach disorders, heart disorders and other conditions to try and avoid too much caffeine. Because of its stimulant effects, caffeine is often used in combination with pain relievers to increase their effects and in OTC (over-the-counter) preparations as an aid in staying awake or restoring mental alertness. Below and on the next pageI have listed several common sources of dietary caffeine and caffeine containing non-prescription medications.

Dietary Source
Amount of Caffeine (Milligrams)

- Coffee (1 cup regular)
  100 mg
- Coffee (1 cup decaffeinated)
  2-3 mg
- Tea (instant, 5 oz)
  28 mg
- Tea (brewed, 5 oz)
  20-110 mg
- Tea (iced, 12 oz)
  70 mg
- Coke (12 oz)
  46 mg
- Dr. Pepper (12 oz)
  40 mg
- Pepsi (12 oz)
  36 mg
- Mountain Dew (12 oz)
  55 mg
- Milk chocolate (1 oz)
  6 mg
- Baking chocolate (1 oz)
  26 mg
- Bittersweet chocolate (1 oz)
  20 mg

OTC Medications
Amount of Caffeine per Tablet, Capsule or Powder (mg)

- No Doz maximum strength
  200 mg
- Vivarin
  200 mg
- Anacin
  32 mg
- Excedrin
  65 mg

- Midol maximum strength
  60 mg
- Tirend
  100 mg
- Quick Pep
  150 mg
- Caffedrine (time release)
  200 mg
- BC Powder
  32 mg
- BC Powder (arthritis strength)
  36 mg
- Goody's Powder
  33 mg
- Goody's extra strength tablet
  16 mg
- Vanquish
  33 mg

In addition, several medications can increase the level of caffeine in the blood when taken with caffeine by preventing the body from getting rid of caffeine. These include Tagamet (cimetidine), birth control pills, Antabuse, Cipro, and Penetrex. When these drugs are taken together with caffeine, increased stimulant effects can occur.

DRUGS THAT
DISCOLOR URINE OR FECES

QUESTION: I've noticed that my urine or stool sometimes changes color when I'm taking medications. Can you tell me what drugs will do this?

ANSWER: Numerous medications (and vitamins) can discolor the urine or stool. I've provided a listing of many (but not all) of these medications on the next page.

Drugs That Can Discolor The Urine
Color
Generic Name (Example Trade Names)

Blue
   Triamterene (Dyrenium)
Blue-green
   Amitriptyline (Elavil, Endep)
Orange-yellow
   Heparin (Hep-Lock)
   Phenazopyridine (Azp-Standard, Baridium, Urogesic)
   Rifampin (Rifadin, Rimactane)
   Sulfasalazine (Azulfadine, Azulfadine EN-tabs)
   Warfarin (Coumadin)
Red-pink
   Heparin (Hep-Lock)
   Ibuprofen (Motrin, Advil, Nuprin, Rufen)
   Phenytoin (Dilantin)
   Rifampin (Rifadin, Rimactane)
   Senna (Ex-Lax Gentle Nature)
Black, brown or dark
   Cascara (Cascara Segrada)
   Chloroquine (Aralen)
   Ferrous salts (iron) (Feosol, Mol-Iron, Feratab)
   Metronidazole (Flagyl, MetroGel)
   Nitrofurantion (Furadantin, Macrobid, Macrodantin)
   Quinine (Formula Q)
   Senna (Ex-Lax Gentle Nature)

Drugs That Can Discolor The Feces
Color
Generic Name (Example Trade Names)

Blue
   Chloramphenicol (Chloromycetin, AK-chlor)
Green
   Indomethacin (Indocin)
   Medroxyprogesterone (Cycrin, Provera)
Yellow/yellow-green
   Senna (Ex-Lax Gentle Nature)

Orange-red
Phenazopyridine (Azo-Standard, Baridium, Urogesic)
Rifampin (Rifadin, Rimactane)
Pink-red
Anticoagulants (Warfarin, Dicumarol)
Aspirin (Many products)
Heparin (Hep-Lock)
Tetracycline syrup (Achromycin, Sumycin)
White-speckling
Antibiotics (oral) (Many products)
Black
Acetazolamide (Diamox, Diamox Sequels)
Aluminum hydroxide (Alu-Cap, Amphojel, many antacid products)
Aminophylline (Phylocontin, Truphylline)
Bismuth salts (PeptoBismol, Bismatrol)
Chlorpropamide (Diabenese)
Clindamycin (Cleocin)
Corticosteroids(Many products (cortisone, hydrocortisone, prednisone, etc.))
Cyclophosphamide (Cytoxan, Neosar)
Ethacrynic acid (Edecrin)
Ferrous salts (iron) (Feosol, Mol-Iron, Feratab)
Hydralazine (Apresoline)
Hydrocortisone (Many products)
Mephalen (Alkeran)
Methotrexate (Rheumatrex, Folex)
Methylprednisolone (Medrol, A-Methapred)
Phenylephrine (Numerous decongestant products)
Potassium salts (Slow-K, K-dur, Micro-K, many more)
Prednisolone (AK-Pred, Econopred, Prelone, many more)
Procarbazine (Matulane)
Sulfonamides (Azulfadine, Gantanol, Thiosulfil Forte)
Tetracycline (Achromycin, Sumycin, Tretracyn)
Theophylline (Aerolate, Elixophyllin, Theobid, many more)
Triamcinolone (Aristocort, Kenacort)
Warfarin (Coumadin)

TRAVEL CONCERNS

<u>QUESTION</u>: I am planning to take a two-week vacation outside of the U.S. What advice can you give me regarding medication use?

<u>ANSWER</u>: Many people plan vacations to foreign countries without giving much thought to medications they may need to take prior to or during their trip. However, in one-third to one-half of travelers, health problems may spoil a trip. In fact, travelers "lose" about three out of fourteen vacation days because of illness and almost one out of five remain ill after their return home. On a personal note I recall having had diarrhea and weight loss due to a parasite infection over a nine-week period following a trip to the South Pacific several years ago. With advance planning, many health related problems can be prevented or minimized. Far enough in advance of your trip you should do the following:

- Create a brief summary of your major illnesses.
- Make a list of the medications that you take (prescription, nonprescription, herbal, etc.), why you take them, and their dosage.
- Get a sufficient supply of your medicines with some to spare and keep all medications in their original containers. These should be and carried with you.
- Make a list of your drug allergies, if any.
- Make a list including your doctor's name, pharmacy, person to contact in case of an emergency, including telephone and fax numbers, street and E-mail addresses.
- If you have diabetes, or must give yourself injections for any reason, carry a personal supply of disposable syringes and needles. If you give yourself insulin, you should work with your doctor to adjust your dosage according to the number of time zones crossed during your trip.
- Prescriptions to treat or prevent travel related illnesses (e.g., malaria, motion sickness, jet-lag, traveler's diarrhea) may be obtained from your doctor.
- Check into the need for routine vaccinations and country-specific immunizations. The Center for Disease Control and Prevention is a good resource for current recommendations (1-888-232-3228) or (web site **www.cdc.gov**).

Some nonprescription medicines that may be helpful during your trip may include dimenhydrinate (Dramamine) or meclizine (Bonine) to prevent motion sickness; diphenhydramine (Benadryl), doxylamine (Unisom), or melatonin for jet-lag; Pepto-Bismol or Imodium for traveler's diarrhea; nasal decongestants or nasal saline drops; sunscreen; and insect repellants. It is also a good idea to avoid nonprescription medications in foreign countries, since many lack warning labels and may contain potentially toxic ingredients. Multivitamins may also be useful for long trips to areas where food or water may be contaminated. Finally, report any symptoms of fever, diarrhea, or weight loss to your doctor upon your return—even if they occur six months after returning home.

CHECKING BLOOD PRESSURE

QUESTION: I always check my blood pressure using a machine at the pharmacy. What level is normal and if it's too high what can I do to lower it?

ANSWER: Although blood pressure machines are handy and can be useful for determining your blood pressure, they also can be inaccurate at times, so always have a healthcare professional take your blood pressure to verify machine results. For an accurate reading you should avoid heavy exercise, eating a heavy meal, consuming caffeine, smoking, or drinking alcohol prior to a blood pressure measurement. The "normal" target for blood pressure is usually less than 140/90 but this can vary with age and other medical conditions. In addition, the National Heart, Lung and Blood Institute (NHLBI) recently revised its blood pressure guidelines so that people with a blood pressure between 120/80 and 139/89 are now considered to have "pre-hypertension". The higher number refers to your systolic pressure, which is the pressure in your blood vessels when the heart contracts to force blood out into the circulation. The lower number is the diastolic pressure, which is the pressure in your blood vessels between heartbeats when the heart relaxes. High blood pressure (also called hypertension) occurs when your heart has to exert more pressure to force enough blood through your blood vessels. This causes your heart to work harder and can lead to an enlarged heart, heart attack, or stroke. High blood pressure is called the "silent killer" because there are usually no symptoms unless the pressure is very high.

Lifestyle changes can help to lower a person's blood pressure and if this is not effective, various medicines can be useful. Lifestyle changes for lowering blood pressure include the following:

- Weight reduction
- Regular exercise (30-45 minutes most days of the week)
- Reduce the consumption of salt, cholesterol, and saturated fat
- Reduce alcohol consumption
- Stop smoking
- Maintain adequate intake of potassium, calcium, and magnesium in your diet by eating fruits, vegetables, low fat milk and cheese

If lifestyle changes do not lower your blood pressure to the normal range, then drug therapy prescribed by your doctor is usually needed in addition. For patients with uncomplicated hypertension, thiazide diuretics and/or beta blockers can be very effective in lowering blood pressure. Thiazide diuretics reduce fluid in the body, which reduces pressure in the blood vessels. Beta blockers reduce the heart rate, which also lowers blood pressure. In some patients other medications know as ACE inhibitors, calcium channel blockers, or alpha blockers are also useful to lower high blood pressure. ACE inhibitors, alpha blockers, and calcium channel blockers help the blood vessels to expand (dilate), which reduces blood pressure. A number of other medications can also be used for hypertension depending upon the patient's condition and other illnesses that they may have. Needless to say, all of these drugs can produce side effects and you may need special instructions, so ask your doctor and pharmacist for additional information when they are prescribed.

QUESTION: I want to get a blood pressure monitor to use at home. What can you tell me about them?

ANSWER: High blood pressure or hypertension affects about 50 million people in the U.S. and nearly one-third of them don't know they have it. While high blood pressure produces few symptoms, if it is not corrected it can lead to a stroke, heart attack, or heart disease. Because of this, it is a good idea to periodically check your blood pressure whether you have hypertension or not. Home monitoring of blood pressure may be particularly useful for those people (like myself) who experience high blood pressure when it is taken by a health professional—known as the "white coat" syndrome. Home monitoring also allows patients to keep a record of their measurements that they can share with their physicians, who can use these records to determine how a patient's medicine is working.

Blood pressure is determined by the amount of blood the heart pumps and the resistance to its flow in the arteries. The more blood the heart pumps and the narrower the arteries, the higher the blood pressure. Blood pressure varies throughout the day and rises with increased activity and decreases with rest. The top number or systolic pressure is the peak pressure when the heart contracts and pumps blood out through the arteries. The bottom number is the diastolic pressure when the heart relaxes to allow blood flow into the heart. Normal blood pressure readings are approximately 120/80. However, recently the National Heart, Lung and Blood Institute revised its blood pressure guidelines so that people with a blood pressure between 120/80 and 139/89 are categorized as having "pre-hypertensive".

There are several types of blood pressure monitors available. The least expensive are called "aneroid" monitor. With these monitors, blood pressure readings are taken from a dial gauge after the cuff has been inflated using a rubber bulb. They usually come with a built-in stethoscope. They are very accurate and reliable, but good eyesight and hearing are needed for good results. Another type of monitor is the "digital" monitor which either manually or automatically inflates the arm cuff, then flashes the blood pressure reading on a small screen. They are accurate, easy to use, and require batteries. Make sure that when you purchase a monitor that the arm cuff size is appropriate or readings will be inaccurate. A third type of monitor is a "finger" monitor. With this monitor a small cuff is placed over the finger, but they may be less accurate because the finger is a longer distance from the heart. They also require that you hold the finger at the exact level of the heart.

After you select a blood pressure monitor, take it to your physician to have it checked for accuracy. Also, when measuring your blood pressure:

- Rest for 3 to 5 minutes before testing. Try not to talk during this time.
- Sit in a comfortable position, with your back supported and legs and arms uncrossed.
- Place your arm, raised to the level of your heart, on a desk or table.
- Wrap the cuff smoothly and snugly against the upper part of your bare arm. There should be room for one fingertip under the cuff.
- The bottom of the cuff should be 1 inch above the elbow.
- Keep records of your measurements and provide them to your physician. Also, be sure to read and follow the directions that come with your blood pressure monitoring product.

FEVER AND THERMOMETER USE

QUESTION: When my forehead is hot because of a fever, what over-the-counter medication should I take?

ANSWER: Just feeling your forehead is usually not a good way to tell if you have a fever because many things like physical activity or excess clothing can increase your skin temperature. On the other hand, your forehead may feel normal even when you do have a fever. The best way to tell if you have a fever is to take your temperature with a thermometer. Many types are available at the pharmacy, but the least expensive are either oral or rectal mercury thermometers. The best way to use an oral thermometer is as follows:

- Do not eat or drink anything warm or cold within 10 minutes before taking your temperature.
- Wipe the thermometer with a cotton ball or piece of gauze that has been soaked in rubbing alcohol. Rinse the thermometer with cool water.

- Shake the thermometer so that the mercury goes below 94 degrees F.
- Place the thermometer under your tongue and slightly to one side of your mouth. Hold the thermometer in your mouth for at least 3 minutes. Then remove and read it right away.
- Wipe the thermometer off with rubbing alcohol like you did before using it and rinse it. Store thermometers out of the reach of children.

Most fevers are due to an infection and are non-threatening in healthy people, lasting only a couple of days. However, in some cases fever may indicate a serious medical problem. Because of this a physician should be consulted if: the fever is higher than 102 degrees F in children or 104 degrees F in adults; the fever lasts for more than 2 or 3 days; or seizures (convulsions) occur.

Over-the-counter (OTC) medications for fever include acetaminophen (Tylenol), aspirin, ibuprofen (Advil, Motrin, etc.), ketoprofen (Orudis KT, Actron), naproxen (Aleve) and salicylates (Arthropan, Doan's). These products will help to reduce fever and relieve minor aches and pains. The best OTC medication for you depends on your age, symptoms, medical history, allergies, and other medications that you take. Your pharmacist can help you select the best product for your. Do not take the fever medication for more than 3 days unless you talk to your physician and follow the directions on the package label. Keeping your room cool and taking a lukewarm shower, bath, or sponge bath may also help to make yourself more comfortable while you have a fever.

DRUGS THAT SHOULD NOT BE CRUSHED

QUESTION: I take care of my father and he has difficulty swallowing his medications. Can I crush them up to make them easier to swallow?

ANSWER: There are many types of oral medications that should not be crushed prior to taking them for a variety of reasons. Extended-release tablets or capsules are designed to release the drug over an extended period of time and should not be crushed because they will lose their long acting effects. Some of these drugs have the letters SR (sustained release) or LA (long acting) in their trade names. Many times multiple tablet layers and drug beads within capsules are used for this purpose or a wax is used that melts in the gastrointestinal tract. Enteric-coated tablets are another example of medications that should not be crushed. The coating on these tablets (e.g. enteric coated aspirin) allows the tablet to pass through the stomach with the drug then released in the intestines. Enteric coating is useful for drugs that are destroyed by stomach acid, to prevent stomach irritation by the drug, and to delay the time for some drugs to start working. Furthermore, sublingual medication and effervescent tablets should not be crushed prior to use. Sublingual medication is placed under the tongue and is designed to dissolve quickly in the mouth for rapid action. Likewise, effervescent tablets are made to quickly dissolve when dropped into a liquid, and when crushed lose their ability to do so. Finally, there are some medications that contain a special coating because they can irritate the mouth, are extremely bitter or are foul tasting, or contain dyes that could stain the teeth or mouth. If you have any question about crushing a medication before use, be sure to "Ask The Pharmacist".

ASPARTAME

QUESTION: My wife drinks Diet Pepsi and Diet Coke on a very regular basis. Can the artificial sweetener Aspartame be harmful?

ANSWER: Probably not. Aspartame is an alternative sweetener that is about 200 times sweeter than sugar (sucrose). In the past century, the increased intake of simple carbohydrates like sugar has contributed to a number of medical problems such as obesity, dental caries, and diabetes. In view of this, a number of alternative sweeteners have been developed including fructose, sorbitol, xylitol, sacchrin, and aspartame. Of these, aspartame appears to be the safest alternative sweetener available. It was approved by the FDA for dry foods in 1980 and in carbonated beverages in 1983. A number of adverse effects have been reported following the use of aspartame, such as headache, psychiatric or behavioral symptoms, seizures, gastrointestinal problems, and hypersensitivity or skin reactions. It has also been suggested that aspartame use may be linked with systemic lupus, multiple sclerosis, Gulf-War Syndrome, myalgia, and Alzheimer's disease. However, the available research does not provide evidence that the use of aspartame is a serious healthcare risk. The safety of aspartame has been demonstrated in healthy adults, lactating and pregnant women, children, adolescents, and people with diabetes. But people with a condition known as phenylketonuria or PKU should avoid excessive use of aspartame. The acceptable daily intake of aspartame recommended by the FDA is 50 mg per kilogram of body weight per day (one kilogram equals 2.2 pounds). This is equivalent to approximately 17 twelve-ounce cans of soda drink (100% aspartame sweetened) per day for someone weighing about 150 pounds. The American Dietetic Association has also concluded that the long-term consumption of aspartame is safe and not associated with adverse health effects.

DRUGS THAT INCREASE POTASSIUM

QUESTION: The level of potassium in my blood is slightly high. Can any drugs cause this?

ANSWER: High potassium levels in the blood is known as "hyperkalemia" and low potassium levels is known as "hypokalemia". Normally the level of potassium in the blood is 3.5 to 5 milliequivalents (mEQ) per liter of blood, but this range may vary a little from one laboratory to another. Potassium is a mineral that plays an important role in maintaining normal muscle activity and helps to keep body fluids in balance. Too much potassium in the blood can lead to changes in heartbeat and muscle weakness. Mild hyperkalemia causes few if any symptoms and is usually first diagnosed by routine blood tests. Hyperkalemia can be caused by kidney problems, diabetes, and by injuries to muscle tissue. It can also result from the use of a variety of drugs. Some of the oral drugs that can lead to an increase in blood levels of potassium include potassium chloride supplements (SlowK,

Klotrix, K-Lyte, Micro-K and many other products); potassium sparing diuretics such as spironolactone (Aldactone), triamterene (Dyrenium), or amiloride (Midamor); cyclosporine (Sandimmune, Neoral, Gengraf); ACE inhibitors such as captopril (Capoten), fosinopril (Monopril), benazepril (Lotensin), lisinopril (Prinivil, Zestril), enalapril (Vasotec), quinapril (Accupril), and others; lithium; digoxin (Lanoxin); NSAIDs such as ibuprofen (Motrin, Advil, etc.), indomethacin (Indocin), Ketoprofen (Orudis, Oruvail), Naproxen (Naprosyn), celecoxib (Celebrex), and many others; in addition to some anti-cancer medications. Numerous salt substitutes such as Adolphs, No Salt, Morton Season Salt Free, Nu Salt, Papa Dash, Morton Lite Salt, and Lawry's Season Salt Substitute also contain high amounts of potassium and can lead to hyperkalemia.

DRUGS THAT LOWER MAGNESIUM LEVELS

QUESTION: In a previous column you mentioned that some heartburn drugs might lower the amount of iron absorbed. What about magnesium?

ANSWER: The FDA has recently warned that heartburn drugs known as proton pump inhibitors or PPIs may cause low levels of magnesium in the blood if taken for prolonged periods of time (in most cases, longer than a year). Low levels of magnesium can result in serious adverse events including muscle spasm, irregular heartbeats (arrhythmias), and convulsions (seizures); however, patients do not always have these symptoms. The treatment of low magnesium levels or hypomagnesemia usually requires the use of magnesium supplements, but in about one-fourth of the cases reviewed by the FDA, magnesium supplementation did not improve the low levels and the PPI had to be discontinued. Low magnesium levels are especially important for people who take PPIs with other medications that can cause hypomagnesemia such as diuretics (water pills) or the heart medication digoxin (Lanoxin). Healthcare professionals should consider obtaining magnesium levels periodically in these patients as well as patients taking PPIs for long periods of time.

Ppis work by reducing the amount of acid in the stomach and are used to treat gastroesophageal reflux disease (GERD), stomach and small intestine ulcers, and inflammation of the esophagus. Prescription PPIs include Nexium (esomeprazole magnesium), Dexilant (dexlansoprazole), Prilosec (omeprazole), Zegerid (omeprazole and sodium bicarbonate), Prevacid (lansoprazole), Protonix (pantoprazole sodium), AcipHex (rabeprazole sodium), and Vimovo (a prescription combination drug product that contains a PPI (esomeprazole magnesium and naproxen). Over-the-counter (OTC) PPIs include Prilosec OTC (omeprazole), Zegerid OTC (omeprazole and sodium bicarbonate), and Prevacid 24HR (lansoprazole).

SYNTHROID

QUESTION: I take a daily Synthroid tablet for my thyroid, a calcium supplement 3 times a day for osteoporosis, and Neurontin (a drug for seizures). I was told not to take my Synthroid within 4 hours of my calcium supplement. How should I schedule to take them?

ANSWER: Synthroid is the tradename for the thyroid hormone levothyroxine also known as T4. Levothyroxine is used to treat people with an underactive thyroid gland that does not produce enough thyroid hormone. This condition is known as hypothyroidism or myxedema. Thyroid hormones control the speed at which the body's chemical reactions proceed (metabolism) and a lack of these hormones can produce a number of symptoms such as a slow pulse, hoarse voice, slowed speech, puffy face, loss of eyebrows, dropping eyelids, intolerance to cold, constipation, weight gain, sparse hair, dry skin, carpal tunnel syndrome, confusion, depression, dementia, and many others. Hypothyroidism can result from an inability of the thyroid gland to make hormones due to a variety of reasons or from the effects of surgery, radiation, or drugs. The treatment of choice is usually daily replacement therapy with levothyroxine tablets. The appropriate dosage of levothyroxine is determined by monitoring the results of laboratory tests for thyroid hormone levels in the blood. It is usually taken as a single daily dose, preferably one-half to one-hour before breakfast. Synthroid is better absorbed on an empty stomach. It is also recommended that Synthroid be taken at least 4 hours apart from other medications that are known to interfere with its absorption. As you noted, the calcium that you take for osteoporosis can interfere with the absorption of the Synthroid leading to less drug getting into the bloodstream and poor thyroid control. It appears that the calcium binds to the Synthroid and forms a complex compound that cannot be easily absorbed in the gastrointestinal tract. I am not aware of a drug interaction between Neurontin and Synthroid, but some other anti-seizure medications can be a problem. In order to prevent any interference with your sleep schedule, I would suggest that you take your Synthroid dose upon arising in the morning, 30-60 minutes prior to breakfast. The calcium supplement could then be taken 4 hours later, mid-afternoon, and at bedtime. However, you should check with your doctor before making any dosing schedule change. Your pharmacist and physician can help you schedule your specific medications appropriately and should be consulted whenever you are unsure about the proper dosage timing and potential for drug interactions.

MEDICATION/PRESCRIPTION ASSISTANCE PROGRAMS

QUESTION: Are there any programs available to help people get prescription medications that can't afford them?

ANSWER: Yes, there are medication assistance programs available sponsored by drug manufacturers that help some indigent and uninsured patients in getting prescription medications for free or at reduced prices. Usually, people that qualify for government assistance are not eligible for these programs. Approximately 70 patient-assistance programs are offered from 55 different drug companies, but not all medications are available. The definition of "indigent" varies widely from program to program. A few programs offer payment limits for patients who need expensive and long-term medications. The application process for these programs also varies from program to program but before the patient's application is approved, most programs screen patient's assets, including bank accounts, stock and real estate holdings, and retirement funds before approval. Also, in many programs the patient's physician or patient advocate must initiate the application process. Information about pharmaceutical company-sponsored medication assistance programs can be obtained directly from the companies and from Web sites on the Internet.

- **www.needymeds.com**
- **www.themedicineprogram.com**
- **www.rxassist.org**
- **www.rxhope.com**
- **www.eohayes.com/indigent.html**
- **www.volunteersinhealthcare.org**
- **www.phrma.org/patients)**

The Partnership for Prescription Assistance may also be a useful program to contact (1-888-477-2669). Your pharmacist, social workers, and other healthcare providers should be able to help. Another good resource is the Directory of Prescription Drug Patient Assistance Programs, which can be obtained by writing the Pharmaceutical Research and Manufacturers of America at 1100 15th Street, N.W., Washington, D.C. 20005.

DIRECT-TO-CONSUMER ADVERTISING

QUESTION: What do you think about all the ads on TV for prescription drugs?

ANSWER: You can hardly watch the evening news or other TV programs these days without seeing advertisements about prescription drugs. Years ago the FDA had rules that kept these advertisements off of TV, but now pharmaceutical companies are permitted to advertise directly to consumers. This direct-to-consumer (DTC) advertising reaches the majority of Americans and often motivates them to visit their doctors and request prescriptions for a wide variety of medical problems. Initially, these commercials were for minor problems such as hair loss or indigestion. Today, however, you can see TV ads for just about every medical problem including depression, inability to sleep, high cholesterol, overactive bladder, erectile dysfunction, heart problems, and even cancer. Drug companies now spend over $3 billion dollars each year on these ads to lure the public to their products. A recent survey by the National Consumers League shows that more than three-quarters of American adults said that they had seen or heard advertising for prescription medications in the past year. In addition, more than half of these people were moved by these ads to talk with their doctors about the medication. Another report by the General Accounting Office says that each year, over 8 million Americans ask for and receive prescriptions from their doctors for medications they've seen advertised on TV or in printed form. On one hand, these ads may provide consumers with useful information. On the other hand, these ads may entice people to use expensive brand name drugs for which they may or may not have a real medical need. Another point to consider is that all medications can cause side effects, many of which can be serious. Remember that an estimated 100,000 people die each year because of prescription errors, drug side effects, and interactions between drugs or foods. It may be difficult to think of side effects when you are seeing smiling and happy people celebrating about the pain reliever Celebrex or with Bob Dole promoting Viagra for erectile dysfunction. A final point to be made is that these ads are almost always for expensive brand name drugs without any comparative information about less expensive medications that may work just as good. Your doctor and pharmacist can help with these product comparisons so that the best and most economical medication is prescribed for all your medical needs.

PRESCRIPTION DRUG ABUSE

QUESTION: What is the government doing to prevent the abuse of prescription drugs?

ANSWER: The U.S. Government recently announced a plan called Epidemic: Responding to America's Prescription Drug Abuse Crisis, which is aimed at reducing the "epidemic" of prescription drug abuse in the U.S. This plan includes a Food and Drug Administration (FDA) backed education program that concentrates on reducing the misuse and misprescribing of opioids. It is a collaborative effort involving agencies from the departments of Justice, Health and Human Services, Veterans Affairs, Defense, and others, which provides a national framework for reducing prescription drug abuse and the diversion of prescription drugs for recreational use. Key elements of this plan include:

• Expansion of state-based prescription drug monitoring programs
• Recommending convenient and environmentally responsible ways to dispose of unused medications from homes
• Supporting education for patients and health care providers
• Reducing the number of "pill mills" and doctor-shopping through law enforcement

In conjunction with the plan, the FDA announced a new risk reduction program called a Risk Evaluation and Mitigation Strategy (REMS) for all extended-release and long-acting opioid medications. Opioids, such as morphine and oxycodone, are synthetic versions of opium and are used to treat moderate and severe pain. Over the past few decades, drug makers have developed extended-release opioid formulas to treat people in pain over a long period. FDA experts say extended-release and long-acting opioids—including OxyContin, Avinza, Dolophine, Duragesic, and eight other brand names—are extensively misprescribed, misused, and abused, leading to overdoses, addiction, and even deaths across the United States. The new REMS plan focuses primarily on educating doctors about proper pain management, patient selection, and other requirements and improving patient awareness about how to use these drugs safely. As part of the plan, the FDA wants drug companies to give patients education materials, including a medication guide that uses consumer friendly language to explain safe use and disposal. Doctor training, patient counseling, and other risk reduction measures developed by opioid makers as part of the REMS are expected to become effective by early 2012. They will be required for various brand name products known under the generic names:

- hydromorphone
- oxycodone
- morphine
- oxymorphone
- methadone
- transdermal fentanyl
- transdermal buprenorphine

The FDA estimates that more than 33 million Americans age 12 and older misused extended-release and long-acting opioids during 2007—up from 29 million just five years earlier. A 2007 survey reported by the FDA revealed that more than half of opioid abusers obtained the drug from a friend or relative. In 2006, nearly 50,000 emergency room visits were related to opioids.

METHAMPHETAMINE ABUSE

QUESTION: I heard that the sale of some popular nasal decongestants is being restricted in Oklahoma—why?

ANSWER: The popular nonprescription nasal decongestant pseudoephedrine (contained in Sudafed, Drixoral non-drowsy formula, Dimetapp non-drowsy formula, Claritin-D, Trinalin, Chlor-Trimeton Allergy-D, Actifed Cold & Allergy, and many other products) has recently been classified as a Schedule V controlled substance by the state of Oklahoma. Products in Schedule V can be purchased without a prescription, but the purchaser must be at least 18 years of age and must show identification and sign a log book when the purchase is made. The reason for this restriction is that pseudoephedrine can be made into methamphetamine by illegal laboratories. Police in Oklahoma broke up nearly 1,300 illegal meth labs during 2003 and the abuse of methamphetamine has become a big problem in our country. On the street, methamphetamine is called "speed", "meth", "chalk", "glass", Ice", and "crystal". It is a popular drug, especially with young adults and teens that go to dance clubs and parties. Methamphetamines are swallowed, inhaled, smoked, or injected into a vein to produce an intense "high", called a "rush" or "flash". Users may become addicted quickly, and use it with increasing frequency and in increased doses. However, methamphetamine can cause serious medical problems including damage to the brain with permanent memory and body movement problems. Methamphetamine is a stimulant that increases a person's heart rate, breathing, and blood pressure. It also causes sweating, headaches, blurred vision, dry mouth, hot flashes, convulsions, dizziness, tremors, anxiety, paranoia, depression, and aggressiveness. High body temperature and convulsions can result in death. The increase in blood pressure and heart rate can also lead to strokes, and fatal cardiovascular collapse. In view of the abuse potential for methamphetamine and its damaging effects, we may see tighter controls on the sale of products containing pseudoephedrine throughout the country in the future.

PLEASE NOTE: The Combat Methamphetamine Epidemic Act became effective in September 2006. This new federal law allows the sale of pseudoephedrine only from locked cabinets or behind the counter. It also limits the monthly amount any individual can purchase, requires photo ID to purchase these medications, and requires retailers to keep personal information about these customers for at least 2 years after the purchase.

THERMOMETER DISPOSAL

QUESTION: What is the best way to dispose of mercury thermometers?

ANSWER: Glass thermometers containing mercury have been in use for over a century. Advantages of mercury-in-glass thermometers include their low cost, light weight, compact size, and patient familiarity with using them. However, these thermometers can break and release their mercury. Contamination of the environment from improper disposal of mercury-containing products is an environmental and health concern. The mercury content of one small fever thermometer is about 700 milligrams (just under 1 gram). When this mercury is released into the environment it can enter lakes and streams where microorganisms transform it into methylmercury, which is highly toxic. The accumulation of methylmercury can lead to toxic mercury levels in fish. If not properly disposed of, as little as 1 gram of mercury per year (just a little more than that found in one thermometer) has the potential to contaminate all the fish in a 20-acre lake. Unlike the elemental mercury found in thermometers, which is not absorbed from the gastrointestinal tract, methylmercury is almost 100% absorbed when ingested. Once methylmercury is absorbed, it accumulates in the liver, kidney, brain, and blood and can adversely affect the central nervous system. In view of this, the following procedures are recommended for the proper disposal of mercury containing thermometers.

- Collect all mercury beads in a double plastic bag by using tape, stiff cardboard, or a suction device such as an eyedropper.
- Label the plastic bag as "Mercury Hazardous Waste".
- Deposit all mercury and mercury-contaminated items at county household hazardous waste sites.
- Keep the area of contamination quarantined from pets and children during cleanup to prevent further contamination.
- Keep the contaminated area well ventilated for 48 hours. If possible, it is advised that the temperature in the contaminated area be kept below 70 degrees F to prevent mercury vaporization.
- Remove the mercury-soiled carpeting from the premises, wrapping it in plastic and disposing of it at the county hazardous waste site.
- Mercury spills should never be vacuumed, thrown into the household trash, or deposited down the sink.

DISPOSAL OF MEDICATION NEEDLES

QUESTION: How should I dispose of used medication needles and other "sharps"?

ANSWER: It is very important that patients and caregivers safely dispose of needles and other so-called "sharps" that could end up in places potentially causing harm to people. In view of this, the FDA has recently provided guidelines for their proper disposal.

Sharps is a term for medical devices with sharp points or edges that can puncture or cut the skin. Such medical devices include hypodermic needles and syringes used to administer medication; lancets or fingerstick devices to collect blood for testing; needle and tubing systems for infusing intravenous and subcutaneous medicines; and connection needles used for home hemodialysis.

After being used, many sharps end up in home and public trash cans or flushed down toilets. This kind of improper disposal puts people, such as sanitation workers, sewage treatment workers, janitors, housekeepers, family members and children at risk for needle stick injuries or infection with viruses such as Hepatitis B and C and Human Immunodeficiency Virus (HIV). With more diseases and conditions such as diabetes, cancer, allergies, arthritis and HIV being managed outside of hospitals and doctors' offices, the number of sharps used in homes and work offices is increasing. In addition, pets are being treated in homes and livestock are being treated on farms, which are also contributing to the increased number of sharps outside of veterinary hospitals. The U.S. Environmental Protection Agency estimates that more than 3 billion needles and other sharps are used in homes in the United States each year. Sharps disposal guidelines and programs vary by jurisdiction. For example, in 2008, California passed legislation banning throwing needles in household trash. Florida, New Jersey and New York have established community drop off programs at hospitals and other health care facilities. People using sharps at home or work or while traveling should check with their local trash removal services or health department to find out about disposal methods available in their area.

For the safe disposal of needles and other sharps used outside of the health care setting, the FDA recommends the following:

DO:
• Immediately place used sharps in an FDA-cleared sharps disposal container to reduce the risk of needle-sticks, cuts or punctures from loose sharps. (A list of products and companies with FDA-cleared sharps disposal containers is available on the FDA web site. Although the products on the list have received FDA clearance, all products may not be currently available on the market.)

- If an FDA-cleared container is not available, some associations and community guidelines recommend using a heavy-duty plastic household container as an alternative. The container should be leak-resistant, remain upright during use and have a tight fitting, puncture-resistant lid, such as a plastic laundry detergent container.
- Keep sharps and sharps disposal containers out of reach of children and pets.
- Call your local trash or public health department in your phone book to find out about sharps disposal programs in your area.
- Follow your community guidelines for getting rid of your sharps disposal container.

DO NOT:
- Throw loose sharps into the trash.
- Flush sharps down the toilet.
- Put sharps in a recycling bin; they are not recyclable.
- Try to remove, bend, break or recap sharps used by another person.
- Attempt to remove a needle without a needle clipper device.
- If you are accidently stuck by another person's used needle or other sharp:
- Wash the exposed area right away with water and soap or use a skin disinfectant (antiseptic) such as rubbing alcohol or hand sanitizer.
- Seek immediate medical attention by calling your physician or local hospital.

RADIATION EMERGENCY

QUESTION: I heard about some pills to protect against radiation escape from a nuclear power plant. What can you tell me about them?

ANSWER: Potassium iodide tablets (Thyro-Block), available to State and Federal agencies, are used in situations where there is a radiation emergency involving the release of radioactive iodine into the environment. This is a concern for people who live near nuclear power plants, especially in view of the recent terrorist attacks. Prescription products containing potassium iodide have been available for a long time and are used to treat a variety of medical conditions including some lung diseases, various skin problems, and hyperthyroidism (overactive thyroid). Potassium iodide is known as a thyroid-blocking agent that is useful in preventing radiation injury to the thyroid gland from radioactive iodine. The thyroid gland needs iodine to function normally and make thyroid hormones. The administration of potassium iodide saturates the thyroid gland with non-radioactive iodine. This then blocks the thyroid from taking up radioactive iodine entering the body from the air, contaminated water, milk, or other foods. Potassium iodide can block about 90% of radioactive iodine absorption if the first dose is given a few hours before or immediately after intake of radioactive iodine, but even if the first dose is given 3 to 4 hours after exposure it can still block about 50% of absorption. However, the use of potassium iodide is not a panacea in a radiation emergency. It does not reduce the effects of radioactive materials other than radioactive iodine or provide protection against external radiation. Possible side effects of potassium iodide include allergic reactions, gastrointestinal irritation, rash, thyroid problems, swelling of the neck and throat, confusion, irregular heartbeat, extremity numbness, tingling pain, weakness, and fever. Iodism can also occur, which produces a metallic taste, burning mouth and throat, sore teeth and gums, symptoms of a head cold, stomach upset, and diarrhea. Potassium iodide should only be used as directed by state and local public health authorities for radiation emergencies. It is my understanding that the Nuclear Regulatory Commission will be distributing potassium iodide tablets to states with nuclear plants for use in an emergency.

QUESTION: I've read that people in Japan are taking a medication to protect their thyroid from radiation exposure. I live near the nuclear power plant in Crystal River, Florida and would like more information about this medication.

ANSWER: A breach-of-containment nuclear reactor accident at a functioning nuclear power plant can release radioactive iodine and other radionuclides. Human exposure can result from inhalation of iodine particles or aerosols, or from ingestion of contaminated water, vegetation, dairy products or meat; grazing cows that feed on radioactive iodine-contaminated vegetation secrete radioactive iodine in their milk. Children, adolescents and young adults who as children were exposed to even small amounts of radioactive iodine from the Chernobyl reactor accident have had a marked increase, beginning 4 years after exposure, in the incidence of thyroid nodules and cancer. The risk is greatest for children, adolescents and pregnant women. Adults more than 40 ears old have a much lower risk.

Potassium iodide tablets, available to State and Federal agencies, are used in situations where there is a radiation emergency involving the release of radioactive iodine into the environment. This is a concern for people who live near nuclear power plants, especially in view of terrorist attacks and the recent tragedy in Japan. Potassium iodide is known as a thyroid-blocking agent that is useful in preventing radiation injury to the thyroid gland from radioactive iodine. The thyroid gland needs iodine to function normally and make thyroid hormones. The administration of potassium iodide saturates the thyroid gland with non-radioactive iodine. This then blocks the thyroid from taking up radioactive iodine entering the body from the air, contaminated water, milk, or other foods. Potassium iodide can block about 90% of radioactive iodine absorption if the first dose is given a few hours before or immediately after intake of radioactive iodine, but even if the first dose is given 3 to 4 hours after exposure it can still block about 50% of absorption. However, the use of potassium iodide is not a panacea in a radiation emergency. It does not reduce the effects of radioactive materials other than radioactive iodine or provide protection against external radiation. Possible side effects of potassium iodide include allergic reactions, gastrointestinal irritation, rash, thyroid problems, swelling of the neck and throat, confusion, irregular heartbeat, extremity numbness, tingling pain, weakness, and fever. Iodism can also occur, which produces a metallic taste, burning mouth and throat, sore teeth and gums, symptoms of a head cold, stomach upset, and diarrhea. Potassium iodide should only be used as directed by state and local public health authorities for radiation emergencies. It is my understanding that in some states, people who live within 10 miles of a nuclear reactor are eligible to receive free potassium iodide supplied by the U.S. Nuclear Regulatory Commission (**www.nrc.com**) and that people who live 10-20 miles from a nuclear reactor can receive free potassium iodide supplied by the Federal Emergency Management Agency (**www.fema.gov**).

OXYCODONE ABUSE

QUESTION: I heard about someone dying from an overdose of a drug called oxycodone. What can you tell me about this drug?

ANSWER: Oxycodone is known as an opiate or opioid drug. Other drugs in this class include morphine, codeine, hydrocodone (Dilaudid), methadone, meperidine (Demerol), hydrocodone (Hycodan), propoxyphene (Darvon), pentazocine (Talwin), and others. They are all narcotic-like drugs that depress the central nervous system and are used as analgesics to treat pain. Heroin also falls into this class of drugs. Some tradename products that contain oxycodone are Percodan, Percocet, Roxicet, Tylox, Percolone, Oxycontin, and Roxicodone.

Many of these opiod drugs are also drugs of abuse on the street, where oxycodone tablets are known as "percs". They are abused because of the temporary "euphoria" or sense of well being that they produce. Opiate abusers can also include people with chronic pain and health care professionals like physicians, nurses, and pharmacists that have easy access to the drugs. Street abusers usually begin by using opiates occasionally after experimenting with alcohol or marijuana, and perhaps other depressants or stimulants. Cocaine can also be administered with an opiate in a mixture known as a "Speedball". Once persistent opiate use is established, at least 25% are likely to die within 10-20 years of active abuse, with death from suicide, homicide, accidents, or infections like TB, hepatitis, or AIDs. Below are many of the analgesics abused in the street.

Analgesic
Example Trade Name
Street Name
- **Codeine**
  Empirin #3
  Schoolboy
- **Morphine**
  Roxanol
  "M", Morph, Horse, Smack
- **Diacetylmorphine**
  Heroin (common name)

"H", Speedball (with cocaine)
- **Hydrocodone**
  Hycodan
  None
- **Hydromorphone**
  Dilaudid
  Juice, Dillies
- **Oxycodone**
  Percodan
  Percs
- **Merperidine**
  Demerol
  Demmies, pain killer
- **Methadone**
  Dolophine
  Dollies, Meth
- **Pentazocine**
  Talwin
  T's
- **Propoxyphene**
  Darvon
  Pain killer

QUESTION: What can you tell me about the drug OxyContin?

ANSWER: OxyContin contains the pain reliever oxycodone in a controlled-release dosage form. Oxycodone is known as an opiate or opioid narcotic-like drug that depresses the central nervous system and relieves moderate to severe pain. Drugs that contain oxycodone are one of the most widely abused prescription medications that addicts snort, chew, or inject to get high. On the street, they are nicknamed "oxy" or "percs". OxyContin has also been referred to as the "heroin" of rural America. These drugs are abused because they produce a temporary intense "euphoria" or sense of well-being. Opiate abusers can include people with chronic pain as well as health care professionals like physicians, nurses, and pharmacists who have easy access to the drugs. Once addicted, abusers may require increasing doses of these drugs to get the same effect. In fact, approximately two years ago the FDA strengthened warnings about OxyContin after reports of widespread abuse and misuse of the medication. Normally OxyContin tablets are to be swallowed whole and are not to be broken, chewed, or crushed because they are a controlled-release formulation. Abusers, however, will sometimes crush the tablets to get an immediate "high", but this may lead to a potentially fatal dose of oxycodone.

QUESTION: What is the difference between oxycodone and OxyContin?

ANSWER: Oxycodone and OxyContin are known as opioid analgesics and are used to treat pain. Oxycodone is an "immediate-release" dosage form that is used for the management of moderate to severe pain. It is usually given in a dose of 5 to 15 mg every 4 to 6 hours as needed for pain. For control of chronic pain, it may be given on a regularly scheduled basis to prevent the reoccurrence of pain rather than treating the pain after it has occurred. If the pain increases in severity, the dosage may be increased. Oxycodone is available as a generic drug made by numerous manufacturers and as a tradename product (M-oxy, Roxicodone). It is also available in combination with acetaminophen in generic drug products and tradename products (Magnacet, Percocet, Primlev, Endocet, Roxicet, Roxilox, Tylox, Xolox), in combination with ibuprofen (Combunox), and in combination with aspirin (Percodan). OxyContin, on the other hand, is a tradename controlled-release formulation of oxycodone that is prescribed for patients needing continuous around-the-clock therapy for pain and is given every 12 hours. It is not appropriate for occasional or "as needed" use, or for the short-term treatment of pain. OxyContin also contains oxycodone as the active ingredient, but it is formulated to gradually release the drug into the bloodstream over a 12-hour period of time. Controlled-release oxycodone tablets are also available as generic products, but not in combination products. Because oxycodone (OxyContin) controlled release products contain larger amounts of the active ingredient, oxycodone (10-80 mg), the dangers of an overdose are more pronounced. This is especially true for first time users and in the case of addicts, who may crush the tablets, which are then ingested, injected, snorted, or inhaled. In summary, oxycodone is a short acting pain reliever that works for about 4 to 6 hours. OxyContin on the other hand, is a higher dose controlled-release formulation of oxycodone that works for about 12 hours and is more likely to be abused, leading to an overdose.

SPORTS CREAM

QUESTION: I heard that a high school track star died from using a sports cream. What can you tell me about this?

ANSWER: According to published reports, a 17-year-old high school track and cross country star died from a toxic level of methyl salicylate in her body. The medical examiner in this tragic case reported that the high school student had more than 6 times the safe amount of this substance in her system. It was the first time that the New York City medical examiner had seen a death from methyl salicylate. Methyl salicylate is the active ingredient in numerous sports creams including Bengay Cream, Icy Hot Cream, Exocaine Plus Rub, ArthriCare Triple-Medicated Gel, Musterole Deep Strength Rub, and others. Methyl salicylate is a "counterirritant" that is used topically on the skin to help relieve muscle aches and pains. Counterirritants produce a temporary irritation or inflammation of the skin causing itching, burning, warmth, or cooling which is thought to mask the pain occurring more deeply in the body. While toxic exposure to topical methyl salicylate is rare, high levels in the body can result in salicylate toxicity, which may cause rapid deep breathing, rapid heart rate, nausea, vomiting, ringing in the ears, blood changes, fluid in the lungs, coma, and seizures. The patient in this case was reportedly using 3 topical products containing methyl salicylate—Ultra Strength Bengay, adhesive pads, and a third unspecified product to relieve muscle aches and pains after exercise. Besides using multiple products, one possible explanation for how toxic levels of methyl salicylate were found in this student is that heat and exercise may have increased the rate of drug absorption through the skin into the bloodstream. Manufacturers of products containing methyl salicylate recommend that they should not be used more than 3-4 times per day and for no more than 7 days. These products are also not recommended to be taken orally, used by children under 12, used on any open cuts, wounds, damaged skin, or used in combination with heating pads. The use of other salicylate products may also contribute to toxicity and should be avoided. Please read all product labeling carefully and consult with your pharmacist and physician if you have any questions regarding the use of nonprescription medication.

PET DRUGS ONLINE

QUESTION: Can I purchase drugs for my pet online?

ANSWER: Yes, but be careful. The FDA has found companies that sell unapproved pet drugs and counterfeit products, make fraudulent claims, dispense prescription drugs without requiring a prescription, and sell expired drugs. The FDA's Center for Veterinary Medicine (CVM) regulates the manufacture and distribution of animal drugs, while individual state pharmacy boards regulate the dispensing of prescription veterinary products. Some foreign Internet pharmacies advertise that veterinary prescription drugs are available to United States citizens without a prescription, but there is a risk of the drugs not being FDA-approved. While a foreign or domestic pharmacy may claim that one of its veterinarians on staff will "evaluate" the pet after looking over a form filled out by the pet's owner, the FDA recommends that a veterinarian should physically examine an animal prior to making a diagnosis to determine the appropriate drug therapy. The CVM is especially concerned about pet owners going online to buy nonsteroidal anti-inflammatory drugs (NSAIDs) and heartworm preventatives. Some tips for buying pet drugs online include the following:

• Order from a web site that belongs to a Verified Internet Pharmacy Practice Site (VIPPS) that has been certified by the National Association of Boards of Pharmacy (NABP). NABP gives the VIPPS seal to online pharmacies that comply with stringent licensing and inspection requirements. Only pharmacies that sell human drugs are certified at this time, but sometimes veterinarians will prescribe human drugs to pets when there is no animal drug approved for the pet's illness.

- Mail the prescription provided by your veterinarian to the pharmacy after your pet receives a physical examination.
- Order from an outsourced prescription management service that your veterinarian uses. Also, ask your veterinary hospital if it uses an Internet pharmacy service.

For more information on this subject go to **www.fda.gov/cvm/nsaids. htm** and **www.fda.gov/buyonline**.

SINGLE-DOSE ANTIBIOTIC FOR DOGS & CATS

QUESTION: I heard that a single-dose antibiotic for dogs and cats was approved. What can you tell me about it?

ANSWER: The FDA recently approved Convenia (cefovecin), the first and only single-dose antibiotic for skin infections in dogs and cats. Convenia is a cephalosporin antibiotic that stays in the body for a much longer period of time than other antibiotics. Because of this, Convenia can be given to cats and dogs in a single veterinarian-administered injection, which provides up to 14 days of antibiotic treatment for common skin infections. By relieving pet owners of the responsibility of giving medications to their pets several times a day for weeks at a time, Convenia ensures that the antibiotic course of treatment is completed on time, giving the pet the best chance for treatment success. When antibiotic doses are not given on time or when they are missed or stopped prematurely, pets do not receive optimal treatment and risk treatment failure, deterioration of health, and additional veterinary visits. Convenia appears to be well tolerated in adult dogs and cats as well as in puppies and kittens. The most common side effects seen with Convenia are similar to other antibiotics and include vomiting, diarrhea, decreased appetite, and tiredness. In clinical studies, Convenia given as a single injection was found to be as effective as a 14-day course of oral cephalosporin antibiotics against naturally occurring skin infections in dogs and cats. Skin infections, which are caused by a variety of bacteria, are the main reason dogs and cats receive antibiotic treatment. In dogs, skin infections are typically a response to an allergy or parasite infestations that result in scratching, licking, and biting that can weaken skin and make it susceptible to bacterial infections. In cats, skin infections are typically in response to wounds or bites that become infected.

FLU VACCINE FOR DOGS

QUESTION: I heard that a new flu vaccine was approved for dogs. What can you tell me about it?

ANSWER: As we await the availability of a human swine flu vaccine caused by the H1N1 virus, the U.S. Department of Agriculture's Animal and Plant Health Inspection Service (APHIS) recently announced conditional approval to Intervet/Schering-Plough Animal Health for a canine influenza virus (H2H8) vaccine. It is the first flu vaccine to be approved for dogs. The vaccine, which is made from killed virus, is intended to reduce the incidence and severity of lung lesions, as well as the duration of coughing and viral shedding. Dog flu was first identified as a disease in U.S. dogs in 2004, after an outbreak of respiratory disease in racing greyhounds in Florida. Since then, it has continued to spread and has now been detected in dogs in 30 states and the District of Columbia. Dogs have no natural immunity to the H3N8 virus, which can produce cough, high fever and nasal discharge. While most cases are mild, severe illness can lead to pneumonia and become fatal. This dog flu virus does not affect people but can be passed among dogs, especially at animal shelters, adoption groups, pet stores, boarding kennels, veterinary clinics and any locations where dogs congregate. It also appears to be particularly dangerous to dogs with a pushed-in nose, such as a Pekinese, a Pug, or Shi-Tzu because they have a short, bent respiratory tract. The dog flu vaccine is administered by subcutaneous injection in two doses, two to four weeks apart. During its conditional approval, the vaccine may be distributed and used by, or under the supervision of veterinarians while the product's performance is further monitored. If you have a dog you might want to talk to your veterinarian about getting him or her vaccinated for the flu.

ADVERSE DRUG REACTIONS

QUESTION: How many adverse drug reactions are reported to the FDA?

ANSWER: According to the Institute for Safe Medication Practices, which monitors adverse drug events (ADEs), the FDA received 179,855 reports of serious or fatal adverse drug reactions in 2011. However, there is a general consensus in the drug world that only about 1% of serious events ever get reported to the FDA, so this number is probably very conservative. The top 10 drugs with the largest number of reports sent directly to the FDA by healthcare practitioners and consumers in 2011, in order of frequency, were Pradaxa (dabigatran), Coumadin (warfarin), Levaquin (levofloxacin), carboplatin, Zestril (lisinopril), cisplatin, Zocor (simvastatin), Cymbalta (duloxetine), Cipro (ciprofloxacin), and Bactrim (trimethoprim/sulfamethoxazole or TMP-SMZ). It is interesting to note that Pradaxa surpassed all other monitored drugs in several categories, including overall number of reports (3,781), deaths (542), hemorrhage (2,367), acute renal failure (291), and stroke (644). It was also suspect in 15 cases of liver failure. Coumadin (warfarin) has been prominent in the rankings for many years. It accounted for 1,106 reported ADEs overall, including 731 reports of hemorrhage and 72 deaths.

REPORTING SIDE EFFECTS

QUESTION: How do I report side effects of my medication to the FDA?

ANSWER: The U.S. Food and Drug Administration (FDA) relies on adverse event (side effects) reports to help identify potential risks of medical products following their introduction to the marketplace. This information may provide a better understanding of risk previously identified during clinical development or identification of new risks. Although the FDA requires rigorous safety analysis of any new product prior to approval, not all adverse events are evident prior to marketing.

Once a product is marketed, it is often used by a much larger and broader population that may have different clinical characteristics than those studied, and the greater population may use the product in a manner that differs from that used in clinical trials. Postmarketing surveillance through programs such as MedWatch captures data about adverse events in these broader conditions, and is helpful in improving understanding of a product's overall benefits and risks. Based on knowledge generated by postmarket surveillance:

- Manufacturers can update product labeling, modify availability of the product, and/or revise educational efforts.
- Pharmacists and other health care professionals can make better clinical judgments about the appropriateness of a medication for their patients.
- Patients can identify risks associated with medical products and prompt discussion about these risks between patients and their health care team.

There are three options for submitting a voluntary adverse event report:
1. Complete Form 3500 online at **https://www.accessdata.fda.gov/ scripts/medwatch**.
2. Call 1-800-FDA-1088 to report by telephone.
3. Download a copy of Form 3500 at **http://www.fda.gov/medwatch/ SAFETY/3500.pdf** and either fax it to 1-800-FDA-0178 or mail it back using the postage-paid addressed form.

It is very important for consumers to report side effects from their medication to the FDA.

BAD REACTIONS TO COSMETICS

<u>QUESTION</u>: You have written columns about reporting a drug's side effects to the FDA. What about bad reactions to cosmetics?

<u>ANSWER</u>: Yes, if you've had a bad reaction to a beauty, personal hygiene, or makeup product the Food and Drug Administration (FDA) wants to hear from you. The federal Food, Drug, and Cosmetic Act defines "cosmetics" as products that are intended to be applied to the body "for cleansing, beautifying, promoting attractiveness, or altering the appearance." But the legal definition includes items that most people might not ordinarily think of as cosmetics, including:

- face and body cleansers
- deodorants
- moisturizers and other skin lotions and creams
- baby lotions and oils
- hair care products, dyes, conditioners, straighteners, perms
- makeup
- hair removal creams
- nail polishes
- shaving products
- perfumes and colognes
- face paints and temporary tattoos
- permanent tattoos and permanent makeup

Consumers should contact the FDA if they experience a rash, hair loss, infection, or any other problem—even if they didn't follow product directions. The FDA also wants to know if a product has a bad smell or unusual color—which could signal contamination—or if the item's label is incomplete or inaccurate. If you have any concerns about a cosmetic contact MedWatch, the FDA's problem-reporting program, on the Web (**www.fda.gov**, click on MedWatch and Begin) or by calling 1-800-332-1088. When you contact the FDA, include the following information in your report:

- the name and contact information for the person who had the reaction;

- the age, gender, and ethnicity of the product's user;
- the name of the product and manufacturer;
- a description of the reaction—and treatment, if any;
- the healthcare provider's name and contact information, if medical attention was provided; and
- when and where the product was purchased.

When a consumer report is received, the FDA enters the information into a database of negative reactions. Experts then look for reports related to the same product or similar ones. FDA scientists will use the information to determine if the product has a history of problems and represents a public health concern that needs to be addressed. If you file a consumer report, your identity will remain confidential.

BLACK BOX WARNING

QUESTION: You often write about "black box" warnings for drugs. What exactly is a "black box" warning?

ANSWER: The FDA often requires drug manufacturers to include a "black box" warning in the labeling (package insert) of their drug products. These warnings have been required for many drugs including certain antidepressants which may increase the risk of suicidal thinking and behavior and for the prescription drug Regranex, which is used to treat dangerous foot and leg ulcers in diabetic patients but has also been linked to an increase in cancer deaths. The "black box" warning is the FDA's highest warning level for prescription drug products. A "black box" warning, commonly referred to as a boxed warning, is a notification to medical practitioners from the FDA that 1 of 3 situations has occurred: (1) There is an adverse reaction so serious in proportion to the potential benefit from the drug that it is essential that it be considered in assessing the risks and benefits of using a drug, (2) There is a serious adverse event reaction that can be prevented or reduced in frequency or severity by appropriate use of the drug, or (3) The FDA approved the drug with restrictions to assure its safe use because the

FDA concluded that the drug can be safely used only if its distribution or use is restricted.

Does this mean that a drug with a "black box" warning should not be used? No, it does not. The FDA requires the warning to be placed in the package insert so that medical practitioners can heed the warnings. Medications with a "black box" warning have either shown or are expected to have a serious adverse event or possibly cause death. Therefore, patients who are on these medications should be carefully monitored on a regular basis.

SOFT DRINKS & THE FDA

QUESTION: Does the Food and Drug Administration (FDA) monitor the safety of soft drinks?

ANSWER: Yes, The Food and Drug Administration (FDA) ensures that carbonated soft drinks are safe, sanitary, and honestly labeled. In fact, the FDA has established "Current Good Manufacturing Practices" (CGMPs) for carbonated soft drinks, which describe the basic steps manufacturers and distributors must follow to make sure carbonated soft drinks are safe.

Only food and color additives that are determined to be safe, based on scientific information available to the FDA, may be used in carbonated soft drinks. For example, this might include additives such as citric acid as a flavoring or a preservative, or caramel coloring. In addition, the materials the carbonated soft drink comes in contact with, such as the bottles and cans in which it is sold, also are strictly regulated for safety.

The Nutrition Facts Panel on carbonated soft drinks typically includes the serving size and the nutrients provided in a serving: calories, total fat, sodium, total carbohydrate, sugars (if present), and protein. If a nutrient content claim, such as "Very Low Sodium," appears on the label, the manufacturer must also add the statement "Not a significant source of _____," with the blank filled in by the names of nutrients that are present only at insignificant levels. Soft drink containers must also list:

- Name and address of the manufacturer, packer or distributor.
- The amount of carbonated soft drink in the container.
- All the ingredients, listed in order of predominance by weight. In other words, the ingredient that weighs the most is listed first, and the ingredient that weighs the least is last. For carbonated soft drinks, the first ingredient usually will be carbonated water.
- Any chemical preservatives used, with an explanation of their function. Examples include "preservative," "to retard spoilage," "a mold inhibitor," "to help protect flavor," "to preserve freshness," or "to promote color retention."
- Diet carbonated soft drinks containing phenylalanine must also include the statement, "PHENYLKETONURICS: CONTAINS PHENYLALANINE," for individuals who suffer from phenylketonuria, a genetic disorder in which the body can't process that amino acid. If the phenylalanine level gets too high in these individuals, it can damage the brain.

OSMOPREP

QUESTION: I recently saw an ad in the AARP magazine about OsmoPrep for a colonoscopy. What can you tell me about it?

ANSWER: OsmoPrep is a prescription drug product in tablet form that is used to clean the colon prior to a colonoscopy examination. It is a virtually tasteless product and may be a useful alternative for people unable to tolerate liquid bowel cleansing products. OsmoPrep tablets contain salts of sodium phosphate, which act to cleanse the colon by drawing large amounts of water into the colon, promoting diarrhea. OsmoPrep tablets are taken the evening before the colonoscopy procedure (4 tablets with 8 ounces of clear liquids every 15 minutes until 20 tablets have been taken) and on the day of the colonoscopy starting 3-5 hours before the procedure (4 tablets with 8 ounces of clear liquids every 15 minutes until 12 tablets are taken). The most common side effects of OsmoPrep include abdominal pain, nausea, and vomiting. However, other adverse effects can occur and before considering OsmoPrep and you should tell your doctor about all your medical conditions, including heart or kidney problems, abdominal problems such as bowel obstruction or motility issues, and any history of seizures. In addition, you should tell your doctor about any medications that you are taking or if you may be pregnant.

The majority of colonoscopies performed in the U.S. are for colorectal cancer screening. Colon cancer is the second leading cause of death in the U.S. Nearly 1 in 18 Americans will develop colon cancer, with 90% of cases occurring in those over the age of 50. While it is recommended that anyone over the age of 50 have a colonoscopy performed every 10 years, it has been estimated that 66% of patients avoid colonoscopy because of reservations about the bowel prep.

QUESTION: Are products for bowel cleansing before a colonoscopy safe?

ANSWER: The FDA recently announced that it will add a Boxed Warning to the prescription labeling for Visicol and OsmoPrep to warn consumers about the potential risk of acute injury to the kidneys when using these products. People routinely take these products to cleanse the bowel before a colonoscopy and other procedures. The FDA is also concerned about the risks associated with the use of similar products that are available over-the-counter, such as Fleet Phospho-soda, which may be used in high doses for bowel cleansing. Current information, however, does not show a risk of acute kidney injury when these non-prescription products are used in lower doses for laxative use. The FDA is recommending that consumers do not use over-the-counter products like Fleet Phospho-soda for bowel cleansing. These oral prescription and non-prescription products contain sodium phosphate, which can form deposits in the kidney and cause permanent damage. While this side effect is rare, it is recommended that these products be used with caution for bowel cleansing in the following risk groups:

- People over 55 years of age.
- People who suffer from dehydration, kidney disease, acute colitis, or delayed bowel emptying.
- People taking certain medications that affect kidney function, such as diuretics (water pills), certain blood pressure medications (ACE

inhibitors or ARBs), and possibly nonsteroidal anti-inflammatory drugs like ibuprofen or other arthritis medications.

In addition, these oral phosphate products should not be used by children under 18 years of age or in combination with other laxative products containing sodium phosphate. Please check with your physician and pharmacist if you have any questions in using bowel cleansing/laxative products.

FILLING PRESCRIPTIONS ABROAD

QUESTION: Can it be a problem getting a prescription filled in another country?

ANSWER: Yes, getting a prescription filled in another country can be a problem. The FDA has issued a Public Health Advisory warning that consumers filling United States prescriptions abroad may get the wrong active ingredient because of confusing drug names. In fact, some FDA-approved prescription products have the same brand names as drug products that are marketed outside the United States but contain completely different ingredients. Over 100 U.S. brand names are so similar to foreign brand names used for products with different active ingredients that patients who fill prescriptions abroad may inadvertently get the wrong drugs. Consumers who fill U.S. prescriptions abroad, either while traveling or when shopping at foreign internet pharmacies, need to take caution because foreign drugs may use identical or potentially confusing brand names for products with different active ingredients. To minimize confusion within the U.S., the FDA has procedures in place to review brand names, but no international regulatory system exists to ensure that new brand names are sufficiently different from existing ones elsewhere in the world to prevent undue confusion outside the country. The Institute for Save Medication Practices has received a number of reports involving brand name medications that may contain different active ingredients in another country. In one report, a patient was prescribed Dilacor XR for high blood pressure. While traveling to Serbia, he ran out of medication.

A Serbian pharmacist filled the prescription, but actually dispensed digoxin (a heart failure medication) since Dilacor is a brand name for digoxin in Serbia. The patient developed digoxin toxicity and had to be admitted to a hospital for treatment. Another example of brand name confusion includes Cartia XT, a drug used to treat high blood pressure and angina in the U.S., but in New Zealand and Australia, Cartia is an enteric-coated aspirin product. Please be cautious of drug information obtained on the Internet, which knows no national boundaries, and when you travel always carry an adequate supply of medications and a list of them by generic and brand names. For a list of drug names in which identical or nearly identical names used in other countries but containing different ingredients, please visit the FDA web site at: **www. fda.gov/oc/opacom/reports/confusingnames.html**.

TUMOR NECROSIS FACTOR (TNF) BLOCKERS

QUESTION: I heard that the FDA is warning people about using some drugs used to treat rheumatoid arthritis and other conditions. What can you tell me about these drugs?

ANSWER: The FDA recently announced that the manufacturers of Cimzia, Enbrel, Humira, and Remicade must strengthen their product warnings about the risk of developing potentially fatal invasive fungal infections. These drugs are known as tumor necrosis factor (TNF) blockers, which suppress the immune system and are approved to treat a variety of conditions including rheumatoid arthritis, juvenile idiopathic arthritis, psoriatic arthritis, plaque psoriasis, ankylosing spondylitis, and Crohns disease. Patients taking these drugs should be aware that they are more susceptible to serious fungal infections and those that develop a persistent fever, cough, shortness of breath, and fatigue should promptly seek medical attention. The FDA has reviewed over 240 reports of invasive fungal infections due to the fungus Histoplasma in patients treated with these medications, including several deaths. The majority of these reports involved people in the Ohio River and Mississippi River valleys, where this fungus is commonly found. In addition, several other fungal infections have been reported in patients treated with these drugs, which weaken a patient's immune system.

CONFUSION WITH MAALOX PRODUCTS

QUESTION: Why is the FDA warning people about using Maalox Total Relief?

ANSWER: The FDA recently warned consumers about the potential for serious side effects from mistakenly using Maalox Total Relief instead of other Maalox products. Maalox Total Relief is an anti-diarrheal and upset stomach reliever, while traditional Maalox products (Maalox Advanced Regular Strength and Maalox Advanced Maximum Strength) are antacids and anti-gas medications. Even though these products both have the name Maalox in their labeling, they contain different ingredients. The active ingredient in Maalox Total Relief is bismuth subsalicylate, which is chemically related to aspirin and may cause similar harmful side effects such as bleeding. Because of this, Maalox Total Relief is not appropriate for people with a history of gastrointestinal ulcer disease or a bleeding disorder. It should also not be taken by children and teens if they are recovering from a viral infection, nor by individuals who are taking certain medications including: oral anti-diabetic drugs, blood thinners such as warfarin (Coumadin) or clopidogrel (Plavix), non-steroidal anti-inflammatory drugs (NSAIDs) such as ibuprofen (Motrin) or naproxen (Aleve), and other anti-inflammatory drugs. At least 5 reports of serious side effects have been received by the FDA in people who took Maalox Total Relief thinking it was Maalox antacid. Because of this confusion in product labeling, the maker of Maalox products has agreed to drop the name Maalox from the label of Maalox Total Relief and will also change the product label design. The renamed product is expected to be available in September, 2010. Until then, consumers should carefully check the labels of all Maalox products to ensure that the appropriate product is being selected for the patient's symptoms. If you have any doubts, please Ask The Pharmacist for advice.

ANTITHROMBIN MADE BY GOATS

QUESTION: Is it true that the FDA approved a new drug made by goats?

ANSWER: Yes, the FDA recently approved the first drug made by genetically altered goats. In order to make the drug ATryn or antithrombin, scientists combined human genetic material (DNA) coded to make antithrombin with goat DNA in such a way that the goat's milk (mammary) glands would produce human antithrombin in its milk. The human antithrombin drug is then extracted from the goat's milk, purified, and made into a usable product. By utilizing goats as "factories" to produce the human antithrombin, it can be manufactured faster and more cheaply than by other processes. Goats were selected for making antithrombin because it takes only 18 months to raise a goat genetically altered to produce milk with this drug. As part of the approval process, the manufacturer of ATryn had to assure the FDA that the goats used in this process were not harmed and that the goats cannot be used for food or feed.

The drug produced by these goats, ATryn or antithrombin, is used to treat a rare blood disorder known as hereditary antithrombin deficiency, which occurs in about 1 in 5,000 people in the United States. People with this disease are at high risk of blood clots during surgery, and before, during and after childbirth. The drug, antithrombin, is a protein that naturally occurs in healthy individuals and helps to keep blood from clotting in the veins and arteries. The purified antithrombin in ATryn has the same chemical structure as human antithrombin and must be administered by intravenous injection in a hospital setting. The manufacturer of ATryn is also looking to develop additional products using this unique process known as transgenic animal technology.

SKIN NUMBING PRODUCTS

QUESTION: Can nonprescription skin numbing products be dangerous to use?

ANSWER: The FDA recently issued a Public Health Advisory to alert consumers, patients, health care professionals, and caregivers about potentially serious and life-threatening side effects from the improper use of skin numbing products. The products, also known as topical anesthetics, are available in over-the-counter (OTC) and prescription forms. Skin numbing products are used to desensitize nerve endings that lie near the surface of the skin, causing a numbness of the skin. Commonly used nonprescription topical anesthetic products contain anesthetic drugs such as dibucaine, lidocaine, benzocaine, or pramoxine and can be found in creams, ointments, liquids, gels, and sprays. These products are used for topical numbing of the skin in local skin disorders such as itching and pain due to minor burns, insect bites, eczema, and hemorrhoids. By relieving the itch, these anesthetic agents help to protect the tissues from further scratching injury and may reduce the risk of a secondary infection. They may also be found in products in combination with other ingredients. However, when applied to the skin, they may also be absorbed into the blood stream and, if used improperly, may cause life-threatening side effects such as irregular heartbeat, seizures, breathing difficulties, coma, or even death. In view of this, the FDA suggests that patients for whom an over-the-counter (OTC) or prescription topical anesthetic is recommended should consider using a topical anesthetic that contains the lowest amount possible of medication that will relieve your pain. The FDA strongly advises consumers NOT to:

- make heavy application of topical anesthetic products over large areas of skin;
- use formulations that are stronger or more concentrated than necessary;
- apply these products to irritated or broken skin;
- wrap the treated skin with plastic wrap or other dressings; and
- apply heat from a heating pad to skin treated with these products.

In addition, the FDA advises patients that if they use a topical anesthetic to:
- use a topical anesthetic that contains the lowest strength, and amount, of medication that will relieve the pain;

- apply the topical anesthetic sparingly and only to the area where pain exists or is expected to occur;
- do not apply the topical anesthetic to broken or irritated skin;
- ask their healthcare professional what side effects are possible and how to lower their chance of having life-threatening side effects from anesthetic drugs; and
- be aware that wrapping or covering the skin treated with topical anesthetics with any type of material or dressing can increase the chance of serious side effects, as can applying heat to the treated area while the medication is still present.

HOW THE BODY DISRIBUTES MEDICATION

QUESTION: What happens to a medication after I swallow it?

ANSWER: A lot of things happen to a drug after a person swallows it. Once it reaches the stomach some of the drug may be lost as it moves through the gastrointestinal tract. Many digestive enzymes and bacteria in the stomach and intestines can break down drugs. In addition, medications can interact with foods and beverages in the gastrointestinal tract, which may reduce or increase the amount of drug that gets absorbed into the bloodstream. Once the drug is absorbed, it travels to the liver via the portal vein. In the liver most of the drug changes (metabolism) take place. Drugs are primarily metabolized in the liver by a number of enzymes that can make the drug more active, less active, or even toxic. Whatever remains of the medication after metabolism in the liver then enters the vein in the liver that carries blood from the liver to the heart (hepatic vein). The heart then pumps the drug molecules out into the general circulation, which carries the drug throughout the body to its eventual target site(s) in the body and to other locations as well. Any medication that remains after traveling through the blood circulatory, system eventually goes back to the liver via the hepatic artery, where additional metabolism can occur. The body ultimately gets rid of (excretes) the metabolized medication, which is made more water-soluble in the liver, via the kidneys into the urine. Some of the metabolized drug may also pass back from the liver into the digestive tract through bile and end up in the stool. Some medications may also leave the body in saliva, sweat, exhaled air, or a mother's breast milk.

NONPRESCRIPTION PRODUCTS FOR SEXUALLY TRANSMITTED DISEASES

QUESTION: I understand that the FDA is warning about non-prescription products for sexually transmitted diseases (STDs). What can you tell me about this?

ANSWER: On May 3, 2011, the U.S. Food and Drug Administration (FDA) and the Federal Trade Commission (FTC) jointly announced the Fraudulent STD Products Initiative. Fraudulent STD products are products that make unproven claims to prevent, cure, and/or treat sexually transmitted diseases (STDs). Some of the products included in this action are marketed as dietary supplements and others are marketed as drugs. These products have not been evaluated by the FDA for safety and effectiveness and may pose health risks to consumers who are misled to believe they are receiving safe, effective treatment. Consumers who use fraudulent STD products may not seek the medical attention they need, delaying appropriate and effective treatment, and potentially spreading infections to sexual partners because they falsely believe they are being treated for their disease. Currently there are no FDA approved drugs or dietary supplements available over-the-counter (OTC) that can prevent, cure, and/or treat STDs. Condoms are the only products cleared by FDA to help prevent sexually transmitted infections. FDA approved drugs and vaccines for the treatment and prevention of STDs can only be obtained by prescription through a licensed healthcare professional. Fraudulent STD products are sold primarily over the Internet, but some are also available in local retail stores.

The following list provides several manufacturers of these products, but this list is not all inclusive.

Manufacturer Name
Product Name

- Immuneglory (Arenvy Laboratories, Inc)
  ImmuneGlory
- Viruxo
  Viruxo
- Masterpeace, Inc.
  Disintegrate Formula, Echinacea/Golden Seal, Detox Formula,
  Burdock Extract
- Int'l Inst of Holistic Health (doctorAJAdams)
  Oil of Oregano P73 Physician's Strength, Essaic Tonic Liquid
  Drops, Colloidal Silver 500ppm (Liquid)
- Gene-Eden, PolyDNA
  Gene-Eden
- Pacific Naturals
  Herpeset, Wartrol
- Derma Remedies
  H-Stop Dx, H-Guard Dx, Molluscum Dx, Wart Dx
- Flor Nutraceuticals
  Herpaflör Outbreak Response Topical Liquid, Herpaflör
  Outbreak Response Tablets, Herpaflör Outbreak Response
  Combo Pack, Herpaflör Daily Formula Tablets, Herpaflör
  Complete Package
- Medavir
  Medavir, ViraBalm, Vyristic Immune Support, Medavir
  H-Elimination Kit
- Never An Outbreak
  O2xygen Force (Oxygen Force/OxyForce), DMSO Cream,
  DMSO Roll-on, DMSO Cream w/Aloe, AlkaLife
- EverCLR3
  EverCLR3
- Chlamydia-Clinic.com
  C-Cure

The FDA advises consumers who believe they might have used or
are currently using a fraudulent STD product to stop using and discard
the product, and see a licensed health care professional, as they might
be at risk for having an STD. Correct diagnosis and treatment of an

STD requires the supervision of a trained healthcare professional. The FDA recommends consumers contact a healthcare professional if they have symptoms of an STD, believe they may have been exposed to an STD, and/or are using OTC products to treat symptoms of an STD. Symptoms of common STDs include: pain or burning sensation during urination, pain during sexual intercourse, abdominal pain, abnormal discharge from the vagina or penis, abnormal vaginal bleeding, genital itching, genital warts, and/or blisters or sores in the genital area. However, the majority of people with sexually transmitted infections have no symptoms, so consumers should talk to a healthcare professional about STD testing if they are sexually active, have unprotected sex, or have been exposed to a STD.

There are several FDA approved drugs and vaccines available to treat and prevent many STDs, and these products have met federal standards for safety, effectiveness, and quality but are only available by prescription through a licensed healthcare professional and pharmacy.

REGENERATIVE MEDICINES

QUESTION: What types of regenerative medicines are being tested?

ANSWER: Regenerative medicine is defined as the clinical application of biologic approaches to repair, replace, and restore functional living tissue. In the world of biotechnology, several types of regenerative therapies are in early-stage testing, for use in patients with spinal cord injuries, age-related macular degeneration (AMD), Type 1 diabetes, cancer, Parkinson's disease, chronic wounds, AIDS, and even hair loss. Approximately 1.3 million Americans live with chronic spinal cord injuries that result in paralysis. Studies are now underway in animals and humans to see if special types of human stem cells injected into injured spinal cord tissues can grow into new nerve fibers. AMD, the leading cause of vision loss in the developed world, is caused by the death of cells within the retina of the eye. Researchers are now looking at the possibility of injecting retinal cells into the eye to rescue these dying cells and restore vision. A California company is testing a system which can be implanted in people with Type 1 diabetes to help them grow new beta cells, which produce insulin in the pancreas. Another California biotech firm is testing the use of specialized proteins that can be used to stimulate hair growth as well as to cause cancer cells to die. Yet another California-based biotech company is studying how a virus can be used to deliver a human protein into the brain, which would help keep brain cells (neurons) alive and functioning in people with Parkinson's disease. In addition, a possible cure for HIV/AIDS is being studied, which uses specialized proteins that can make cells that are resistant to the HIV virus. One type of regenerative medicine that is already approved for treating chronic leg ulcers and diabetic foot ulcers is a biotechnology product named Apligraf. This product contains living cells, proteins, and other substances that help to promote healing. Many companies around the world are actively pursuing regenerative medicine research programs and the future in this area of study holds great promise.

MEDICATION ERROR PREVENTION

QUESTION: What is the FDA doing to help protect consumers from medication errors?

ANSWER: The FDA's Center for Drug Evaluation and Research (CDER) has formalized a long standing relationship with the Institute for Safe Medication Practices (ISMP), a non-profit organization based in Horsham, Pa. ISMP's mission is to educate the health care community and consumers. Medication errors are preventable mistakes that can happen in labeling, packaging, prescribing, dispensing, and communications when the medication is ordered. Causes include:

• Incomplete patient information, with the health care professional not knowing about allergies and other medications the patient is using
• Miscommunication between physicians, pharmacists and other health care professionals. For example, drug orders can be communicated incorrectly because of poor handwriting
• Name confusion from drug names that look or sound alike

- Confusing drug labeling
- Identical or similar packaging for different doses
- Drug abbreviations that can be misinterpreted

As a part of its ongoing effort to fight these and other risks, CDER has entered into an agreement with ISMP to develop collaborative efforts to reduce preventable harm from medicines, and to more effectively reach consumers with information on how to use medicines safely.

The FDA and ISMP each have well-established online pathways for the reporting of medication errors. ISMP hears from "front line practitioners"—like pharmacists, nurses and physicians—via its national Medication Errors Reporting Program. ISMP also has a medication error reporting program for consumers. ISMP shares these reports with MedWatch, the FDA's safety information and adverse event reporting system, which covers bad experiences with medical procedures and products that include drugs, devices, supplements and cosmetics.

The collaboration is also designed to provide more informational and educational materials for both consumers and health care professionals. And the relationship will broaden FDA's ability to reach out to these groups when there are issues with product safety and effectiveness. ISMP also has two useful, medication error web sites:

- **www.ConsumerMedSafety.org** : This site is designed to help consumers get involved in preventing medication errors. The extensive information here includes interactive features. For example, typing in the name of a medication will bring up information about side-effects, duplicative treatments and drug interactions. A free safety alert service, about medications patients or their family members are taking, also is available.
- **www.ismp.org** : This site is designed more for health care professionals, with information that includes medication safety tools and resources, as well as educational and professional webinars and training programs.

Both ISMP web sites have lists of potential medication safety issues, such as the drugs most likely to be involved in harmful errors, medications with look-alike or sound-alike names, and error-prone abbreviations.

EXPIRATION DATES

QUESTION: Are medications that have passed their expiration dates good to use, or should they be discarded?

ANSWER: This is a very good question and one that has recently been addressed by a Johns Hopkins Health Alert (**www. johnshopkinshealthalerts.com**, 2011). Think of expiration dates—which the U.S. Food and Drug Administration (FDA) requires be placed on most prescription and over-the-counter medications—as a very conservative guide to longevity. The expiration date is a guarantee from the manufacturer that a medication will remain chemically stable—and thus maintain its full potency and safety—prior to that date. In a study conducted by the FDA on a large stockpile of medications purchased by the military, 90% of more than 100 medications were safe and effective to use years after the expiration date. The drugs in the FDA study, however, were stored under ideal conditions—not in a bathroom medicine cabinet, where heat and humidity can cause drugs to degrade. You should discard any pills that have become discolored, turned powdery, or smell strong; any liquids that appear cloudy or filmy; or any tubes of cream that are hardened or cracked. To help maintain potency, store your medications in a closet or cabinet located in a cool, dry room. Also, don't mix medications in one container: chemicals from different medications can interact to interfere with potency or cause harmful side effects. If two or more medications have been mingled for any period of time, discard them. A few medications, like insulin and some liquid antibiotics, do degrade quickly and should definitely not be used beyond the expiration date. You should also replace any outdated medications that you're taking for a serious health problem, since its potency is more critical than that of an over-the-counter drug you take for a headache or hay fever. In 2012, the FDA also issued a consumer ommunication regarding this topic which includes the following information.

- Using expired medical products is risky and possibly harmful to your health. In the late 1970s, the FDA began requiring an expiration date on prescription and over-the counter medicines. Expiration dates on medical products are a critical part of determining if the product is safe to use and will work as intended.
- Expired medical products can be less effective or risky due to a change in chemical composition or decrease in potency. Improper storage (such as a humid bathroom cabinet) can also contribute to decreased effectiveness in medicines that have not reached their posted expiration date. To help ensure the proper shelf life of your medicine, it is better to store medicine in a controlled climate.
- If you have expired medicine, it should be disposed of properly. Read the label for disposal instructions that may be included.
- If no instructions are provided, a drug take-back program, if available, is a good way to dispose of expired, unwanted or unused medicine. Check with your local government to see if there is a drug take-back program available in your area. If no take-back program is available, federal guidelines recommend throwing medicine away in the household trash by placing it in a bag or container and mixing with coffee grounds or kitty litter.

DARVON NO LONGER AVAILABLE

QUESTION: Why is Darvon being taken off the market?

ANSWER: On November 19, 2010 the FDA asked that the popular prescription pain reliever propoxyphene be removed from the market because of the potential for serious heart problems. This withdrawal includes all propoxyphene-containing products, both brand name and generic. The FDA sought market withdrawal of propoxyphene after receiving new clinical data showing that the drug puts patients at risk of potentially serious or even fatal heart rhythm abnormalities. As a result of these data, combined with other information, including new epidemiological data, the agency concluded that the risks of the medication outweigh the benefits. The FDA is advising health care professionals to stop prescribing propoxyphene to their patients, and patients who are currently taking the drug should contact their health care professional as soon as possible to discuss switching to another pain management therapy. Propoxyphene is an opioid used to treat mild to moderate pain. First approved by the FDA in 1957, propoxyphene is sold by prescription under various names both alone (e.g., Darvon) or in combination with acetaminophen (e.g., Darvocet). It has been estimated that 10 million people used a propoxyphene-containing product in 2009, however, numerous other effective prescription pain relievers are available. Long-term users of propoxyphene also need to know that the heart rhythm abnormalities associated with propoxyphene are not cumulative, and once patients stop taking the drug, the risk will go away.

BOTTLED WATER

QUESTION: Does the Food and Drug Administration (FDA) monitor the safety of bottled water?

ANSWER: Yes, the Food and Drug Administration (FDA) and the Environmental Protection Agency (EPA) are both responsible for the safety of drinking water. The EPA regulates public drinking water (tap water), while the FDA regulates bottled drinking water. Under FDA labeling rules, bottled water includes products labeled:

- Bottled water
- Drinking water
- Artesian water
- Mineral water
- Sparkling bottled water
- Spring water
- Purified water (distilled, demineralized, deionized, reverse osmosis water)

Waters with added carbonation, soda water (or club soda), tonic water and seltzer historically are regulated by FDA as soft drinks.

The FDA has set Current Good Manufacturing Practices (CGMPs) specifically for bottled water. They require bottled water producers to:
- Process, bottle, hold, and transport bottled water under sanitary conditions
- Protect water sources from bacteria, chemicals, and other contaminants
- Use quality control processes to ensure the bacteriological and chemical safety of the water
- Sample and test both source water and the final product for contaminants

The FDA monitors and inspects bottled water products and processing plants under its food safety program. When the FDA inspects plants, the agency verifies:
- That the plant's product water and operational water supply are obtained from an approved source
- Inspects washing and sanitizing procedures
- Inspects bottling operations
- Determines whether the companies analyze their source water and product water for contaminants

New types of flavored and/or nutrient-added water beverages have begun to appear in stores and on food service menus. Some are simply bottled water with flavoring, others may also contain added nutrients such as vitamins, electrolytes like sodium and potassium, and amino acids. The bottled water ingredients of these flavored and nutrient-added water beverages must meet the bottled water requirements if the term "water" is highlighted on the label, as in, for example, a product named Berry Flavored Spring Water Beverage. In addition, the flavorings and nutrients added to these beverages must comply with all applicable FDA safety requirements and they must be identified in the ingredient list on the label.

According to the International Bottled Water Association, bottled water was the second most popular beverage in the U.S. in 2005, with Americans consuming more than 7.5 million gallons of bottled water—an average of 26 gallons per person. Today, only carbonated soft drinks out sell bottled water.

DRUG APPROVAL PROCESS

QUESTION: How are new drugs approved?

ANSWER: The drug approval process in the U.S. involves a lengthy research and approval process that can take as long as 15 years to develop a potential new treatment. The process begins with laboratory and animal studies, which assess the safety and biological activity of a potential new drug compound. This "Preclinical Testing" can take several years. If the drug being studied looks like a promising candidate, an Investigational New Drug (IND) application is filed with the Food and Drug Administration (FDA). Once an IND is filed and approved, "Clinical Testing" can begin in humans and consists of 3 phases. Phase 1 testing typically involves about 20-100 healthy volunteers to determine if the potential new drug is safe for humans and at what dosage. This phase may take a year or more. If the new drug candidate makes it through Phase 1, it goes into Phase 2 testing. This phase usually involves 100-300 patient volunteers and evaluates a potential new drug treatment's safety and effectiveness for a particular disease. Phase 2 testing may take two or more years and if completed successfully, the next phase can begin. Approximately 33% of potential new drugs make it to the third phase. Phase 3 testing involves approximately 1,000 to 3,000 patient volunteers and is required to confirm the safety and effectiveness of a potential new drug and to determine if its treatment benefits outweigh its risks. Phase 3 testing takes longer than Phase 1 or 2 testing and is usually conducted at numerous testing sites. Following successful Phase 3 testing, the potential new drug's sponsor (manufacturer) will file a New Drug Application with the FDA. If the FDA approves this potential new drug to be marketed, Phase 4 studies may also be conducted to help determine its long-term safety and potential new uses for other conditions. Approximately 27% of initial IND applications will make it into Phase 3 testing and ultimately be approved by the FDA.

INSECT REPELLENTS

QUESTION: We have been getting bitten by a lot of mosquitoes lately. What can you tell me about using insect repellents.

ANSWER: Mosquitoes have been a big problem lately in our area due to all the rain and storms. Recently (2012) the FDA provided some useful information for consumers about using insect repellents.

Applying insect repellent is not complicated, but before you do, be sure to read the label for any warnings and to see the active ingredients. All insect repellents, including products combined with sunscreen, should be used according to instructions on the label. Insect repellents can be used in all ages unless the label specifically states an age limitation or precaution. As long as you read and follow label directions and take proper precautions, insect repellents with active ingredients registered by the U.S. Environmental Protection Agency (EPA) do not present health or safety concerns. The FDA recommends using products that contain active ingredients registered by the EPA for use on skin and clothing. EPA registration of insect repellent active ingredients indicates that the materials have been reviewed and approved for human safety and effectiveness when applied according to instructions on the label. The active ingredients DEET and picaridin are conventional man-made, chemical repellents according to the EPA. Oil of lemon eucalyptus, oil of citronella and IR3535 are repellents made from natural materials such as plants, bacteria, and certain minerals.

Insect repellents containing DEET should not be used on children under 2 months of age. Oil of lemon eucalyptus products should not be used on children under 3 years of age. When applying insect repellents to children, avoid their hands, around the eyes, and cut or irritated skin. Do not allow children to handle insect repellents. When using on children, apply to your own hands and then put it on the child. After returning indoors, wash your child's treated skin or bathe the child. Clothes exposed to insect repellants should be washed with soap and water.

If a sunscreen containing DEET is used, then a sunscreen-only product should be used if additional sunscreen is needed. The sunscreen that contains DEET should not be reapplied because repeated applications may increase potential toxic effects. For sunscreen products made with natural insect repellent ingredients follow package directions. Re-application of the combination product may be all right depending upon the particular formulation. After returning indoors, wash treated skin with soap and water, especially if using repellents repeatedly in a day or on consecutive days.

Although higher concentrations of any of the active ingredients provides longer protection, concentrations above 50% generally do not increase protection time. Products with less than 10% of the active ingredient offer only limited protection, about one or two hours. Protection and duration vary considerably among products and insect species. Temperature, perspiration, exposure to water, and other factors affect the product's duration and effectiveness.

SAFE USE OF DRUGS
DURING NATURAL DISASTERS

QUESTION: What medication concerns should I have in case of a flood or other natural disaster?

ANSWER: This is a good question, especially during hurricane season. The FDA recently (2012) issued a consumer bulletin for the safe use of drugs that have been potentially affected by fire, flooding or unsafe water, and lack of refrigeration after a natural disaster.

Drugs Exposed to Excessive Heat, Such As Fire

The effectiveness of drugs can be destroyed by high temperatures. You should consider replacing your medications if there's a possibility that your medication was exposed to excessive heat, such as in a fire. It is especially important to assure the effectiveness of lifesaving drugs and these should be replaced as soon as possible. However, if the lifesaving medication in its container looks normal to you, the medication can be used until a replacement is available.

Drugs Exposed to Unsafe Water

Drugs (pills, oral liquids, drugs for injection, inhalers, skin medications) that are exposed to flood or unsafe municipal water may become contaminated and lead to diseases that can cause serious health effects. The FDA recommends that drug products–even those in their original containers–should be discarded if they have come into contact with flood or contaminated water. In the ideal setting, capsules, tablets, and liquids in drug containers with screw-top caps, snap lids, or droppers, should be discarded if they are contaminated. In addition, medications that have been placed in any alternative storage containers should be discarded if they have come in contact with flood or contaminated water. In many situations, these drugs may be lifesaving and replacements may not be readily available. For these lifesaving drugs, if the container is contaminated but the contents appear unaffected (i.e., if the pills are dry) they may be used until replacements can be obtained. However, if a pill is wet, it is contaminated and should be discarded.

Reconstituted Drugs

For children's drugs that have to be made into a liquid using water (reconstituted), the drug should only be reconstituted with purified or bottled water. Liquids other than water should not be used to reconstitute these products.

Drugs That Need Refrigeration

Some drugs require refrigeration (for example, insulin, somatropin, and drugs that have been reconstituted). If electrical power has been off for a long time, the drug should be discarded. However, if the drug is absolutely necessary to sustain life (insulin, for example), it may be used until a new supply is available. Because temperature sensitive drugs lose potency if not refrigerated, they should be replaced with a new supply as soon as possible. For example, insulin that is not refrigerated has a shorter shelf life than the labeled expiration date. If a contaminated product is considered medically necessary and would be difficult to replace quickly, you should contact a healthcare provider (for example, Red Cross, poison control, health departments, etc.) for guidance.

If you are concerned about the efficacy or safety of a particular product, contact your pharmacist, healthcare provider or the manufacturer's customer service department.

TATTOOS

QUESTION: Can tattoos be risky to get?

ANSWER: Many people young and old get tattoos these days, but they are not without risk. The Food and Drug Administration (FDA) recently (2012) provided a consumer update about them. The FDA is particularly concerned about a family of bacteria called nontuberculous Mycobacteria (NTM) that has been found in a recent outbreak of illnesses linked to contaminated tattoo inks. M. chelonae, one of several disease-causing NTM species, can cause lung disease, joint infection, eye problems and other organ infections. These infections can be difficult to diagnose and can require treatment lasting six months or more. Some of these contaminated inks have caused serious infections in at least four states in late 2011 and early 2012. The FDA is reaching out to tattoo artists, ink and pigment manufacturers, public health officials, health care professionals, and consumers to warn them of the potential for infection. The FDA also warns that tattoo inks, and the pigments used to color them, can become contaminated by other bacteria, mold and fungi. Tattoo artists can minimize the risk of infection by using inks that have been formulated or processed to ensure they are free from disease-causing bacteria, and avoid using non-sterile water to dilute the inks or wash the skin. Non-sterile water includes tap, bottled, filtered or distilled water.

Consumers should also know that the ointments often provided by tattoo parlors are not effective against these infections. NTM infections may look similar to allergic reactions, which means they might be easily misdiagnosed and treated ineffectively. Once an infection is diagnosed, health care providers will prescribe appropriate antibiotic treatment. Such treatment might have uncomfortable side effects, such as nausea or gastrointestinal problems. However, without prompt and proper treatment an infection could spread beyond the tattoo or become complicated by a secondary infection. If you suspect you may have a tattoo-related infection, the FDA recommends the following:

- Contact your health care professional if you see a red rash with swelling, possibly accompanied by itching or pain in the tattooed area, usually appearing 2-3 weeks after tattooing.
- Report the problem to the tattoo artist.
- Report the problem to MedWatch by calling 1-800-332-1088 or by going to their Internet site **(www.fda.gov/safety/medwatch)**.

About the Author

Richard P. Hoffmann received his Bachelor of Science and Doctor of Pharmacy degrees from Wayne State University (Detroit, Michigan) in 1970 and 1972 respectively. Since that time he has practiced pharmacy in a variety of settings including community pharmacies, nursing home pharmacies, compounding pharmacies, and numerous hospitals. Dr. Hoffmann has over 40 years of drug information and medical writing experience. His publications include several hundred professional and scientific papers, in addition to a book on adverse drug reactions and medication errors. He is the recipient of numerous professional awards including the prestigious national Award for Achievement in the Professional Practice of Hospital Pharmacy from the American Society of Health-System Pharmacists and was named Michigan Hospital Pharmacist of the Year in 1988. In addition, he has been an adjunct faculty member for three different colleges. Dr. Hoffmann is now retired and lives in Florida with his wife, Meg. He currently participates in volunteer endeavors and freelance professional activities including his weekly "Ask The Pharmacist" column and serves as the Consumer Representative for the FDA's Peripheral and Central Nervous System Advisory Committee. Dr. Hoffmann has two sons, Rick and Bill, who live in Michigan.

Other Books By Dr. Hoffmann

Drug Death – A Danger of Hospitalization
Time Is Life – A Practical Guide To Early Retirement
Ask The Pharmacist – First, Second, Third, Fourth, 10th Anniversary,
2009, 7th, and Last Edition.

Index

Polypill 72
Potassium 44, 83, 157, 499, 653, 661, 672, 674
Potassium iodide 672, 674
Potiga 607
Pradaxa 111, 682
Pramipexole 473, 474, 512
Prandimet 359
Pravachol 21, 57, 59, 79, 80, 81, 86, 88, 91, 94, 95, 96, 97, 104, 129, 175, 413, 561, 563
Pravastatin 21, 91
Precose 360
Pregnancy 4, 110, 248, 395, 529
Premarin 268
Premenstrual syndrome 273
Prempro 266, 268, 270, 271
Prescription abbreviations 1
Prescription assistance 665
Prescription programs 664
Prevacid 54, 215, 216, 217, 219, 220, 221, 513, 663
Prevar 301
PRICE therapy 522
Prilosec 21, 53, 54, 55, 56, 136, 215, 216, 217, 218, 219, 220, 221, 512, 663
Prinivil 23, 48, 61, 62, 67, 662
Privine 427, 501
Probiotics 612
Propecia 126, 130, 131, 135, 149, 150, 151
Propoxyphene 9, 10, 14, 120, 676, 702
Propranolol 67, 147, 525, 648
Propulsid 17, 214, 215
Proquin 421
Proscar 115, 116, 117, 122, 126, 131, 135, 149

Prostate 79, 114, 115, 116, 117, 118, 119, 122, 123, 125, 126, 127, 128, 129, 130, 131, 132, 135, 136, 141, 142, 143, 144, 151, 152, 169, 170, 181, 210, 211, 337, 410, 426, 427, 429, 431, 433, 563, 600, 605
Prostate cancer 79, 125, 126, 127, 128, 129, 130, 131, 135, 136, 143, 152, 169, 170, 181, 600
Proton pump inhibitors (PPIs) 53, 219, 220, 221, 512, 662, 663
Provenge 125, 153
Prozac 13, 55, 148, 163, 270, 500, 527, 543, 572, 618, 646
PSA 127, 130, 136, 170
Pseudoephedrine 122, 206, 427
Psoriasis 313, 331

Q
Qsymia 452
Quinine 21, 620, 652
Qutenza 382

R
Radiation emergency 672, 674
Rapaflo 122
Raptiva 332
Rasagiline 473, 476, 477, 484
Razadyne 557
Reclast 127, 577, 580, 581, 582, 583
Regranex 375, 376, 685
Relenza 305, 386, 387, 406, 408
Relpax 493, 626, 646
Remeron 14, 38, 543, 570, 649
Remicade 227, 228, 230, 313, 456, 690
RepHresh 277, 278
Reporting side effects 682